# The Founders of Operative Surgery

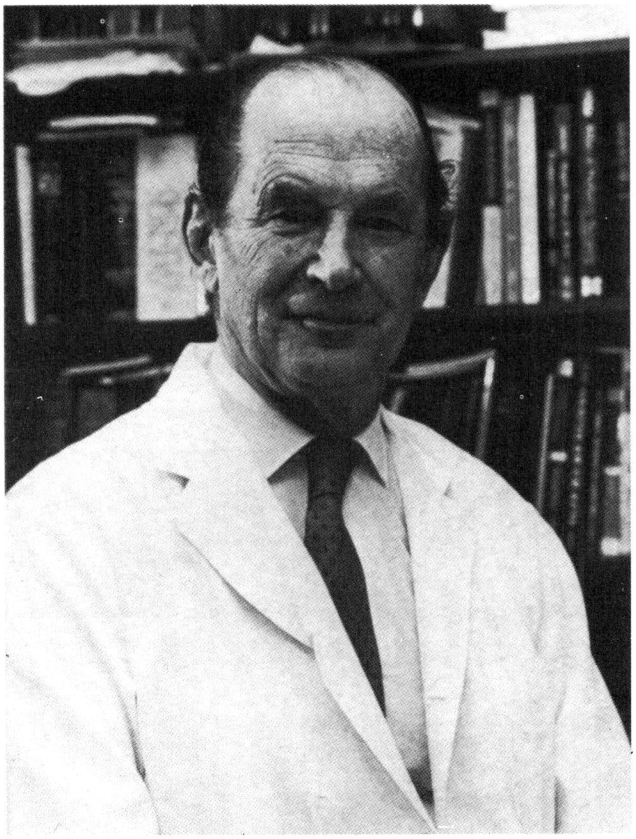

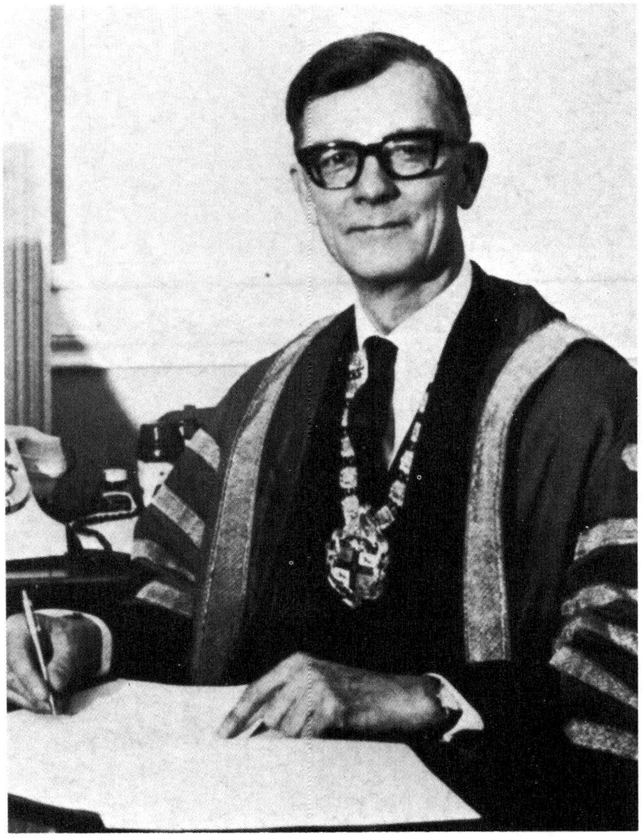

**Charles Granville Rob** MC, MChir, FRCS, FACS
Professor of Surgery, Uniformed Services University of the Health Sciences, E Edward Hébert School of Medicine, Bethesda, Maryland
Quondam: Professor of Surgery, St Mary's Hospital Medical School, London 1950–1960
Professor and Chairman, Department of Surgery, University of Rochester, New York, 1960–1978
Professor of Surgery, East Carolina University, 1978–1983

**Lord Smith of Marlow** KBE, MS, FRCS, Hon DSc (Exeter and Leeds), Hon MD (Zurich), Hon FRACS, Hon FRCS(Ed), Hon FACS, Hon FRCS(Can), Hon FRCSI, Hon FRCS(SA), Hon FDS
Honorary Consulting Surgeon, St George's Hospital, London
Quondam: Surgeon, St George's Hospital, London, 1946–1978
President of the Royal College of Surgeons of England, 1973–1977

Rob & Smith's

# Operative Surgery

## Neurosurgery

**Fourth Edition**

Rob & Smith's

# Operative Surgery

General Editors

**Hugh Dudley** ChM, FRCS(Ed), FRACS, FRCS
Emeritus Professor, St Mary's Hospital, London, UK

**David C. Carter** MD, FRCS(Ed), FRCS(Glas)
Regius Professor of Clinical Surgery, Royal Infirmary, Edinburgh, UK

**R. C. G. Russell** MS, FRCS
Consultant Surgeon, Middlesex Hospital, St John's Hospital for Diseases of the Skin; Royal National Nose, Throat and Ear Hospital, London, UK

Rob & Smith's

# Operative Surgery

## Neurosurgery

### Fourth Edition


Edited by

**Lindsay Symon** TD, FRCS
Professor of Neurosurgery, Gough-Cooper Department of Neurological Surgery, Institute of Neurology, National Hospitals for Nervous Diseases, London, UK

**David G. T. Thomas** MRCP, FRCSE
Senior Lecturer and Consultant Neurosurgeon, Institute of Neurology, National Hospitals for Nervous Diseases, London, UK

**Kemp Clark** MD, FACS
Professor of Neurosurgery, Division of Neurological Surgery, Southwestern Medical School, Dallas, Texas, USA



**Butterworths**
London Boston Sydney Wellington Singapore

PART OF REED INTERNATIONAL P.L.C.



First published 1989



First edition published in eight volumes 1956–1958
Second edition published in fourteen volumes 1968–1971
Third edition published in nineteen volumes 1976–1981
Fourth edition published 1983–

**British Library Cataloguing in Publication Data**

Rob, Charles, *1913–*
Rob & Smith's operative surgery. – 4th ed.
Neurosurgery/edited by Lindsay Symon, David G T Thomas, Kemp Clark
1. Medicine. Surgery
I. Title II. Smith, Rodney Smith, Baron, *1914–*
III. Symon, Lindsay IV. Thomas, David G T (David Glynder Treharne) V. Clark, Kemp
VI. Rob, Charles, *1913–*. Operative surgery
617

ISBN 0-407-00668-0

**Library of Congress Cataloging in Publication Data**
(Revised for Vol. 12)

Rob & Smith's operative surgery.

Rev. ed. of: Operative surgery. 3rd ed. 1976–
Includes bibliographies and index.
Contents: [1] Alimentary tract and abdominal wall.
1. General principles, oesophagus, stomach, duodenum, small intestine, abdominal wall, hernia/edited by Hugh Dudley – [2] Urology; – [etc.] – [11] Trauma surgery; [12] Neurosurgery.
1. Surgery, Operative 2. Surgery, Operative
I. Rob, Charles II. Smith of Marlow, Rodney Smith, Baron, 1914– III. Dudley, Hugh A. F. (Hugh Arnold Freeman) IV. Pories, Walter J. V. Carter, David C. (David Craig) [DNLM: 1. Operative Surgery. [W0 500 061 1982]
[RD32.06 1983] 617'.91 83-14465

Photoset by Butterworths Litho Preparation Department
Printed and bound by Robert Hartnoll, Bodmin, Cornwall

# Volumes and Editors

## Alimentary Tract and Abdominal Wall

**1 General Principles · Oesophagus · Stomach · Duodenum · Small Intestine · Abdominal Wall · Hernia**

**Hugh Dudley ChM, FRCS(Ed), FRACS, FRCS**
Emeritus Professor, St Mary's Hospital, London, UK

**2 Liver · Portal Hypertension · Spleen · Biliary Tract · Pancreas**

**Hugh Dudley ChM, FRCS(Ed), FRACS, FRCS**
Emeritus Professor, St Mary's Hospital, London, UK

**3 Colon, Rectum and Anus**

**Ian P. Todd MS, MD(Tor), FRCS, DCH**
Consulting Surgeon, St Bartholomew's Hospital, London;
Consultant Surgeon, St Mark's Hospital and
King Edward VII Hospital for Officers, London, UK

**L. P. Fielding MB, FRCS**
Chief of Surgery, St Mary's Hospital, Waterbury, Connecticut, USA;
Associate Professor of Surgery, Yale University, Connecticut, USA

## Cardiac Surgery

**Stuart W. Jamieson MB, FRCS, FACS**
Professor and Head, Cardiothoracic Surgery,
University of Minnesota, Minneapolis, Minnesota, USA

**Norman E. Schumway MD, PhD, FRCS**
Professor and Chairman, Department of Cardiovascular Surgery,
Stanford University School of Medicine, California, USA

## The Ear

**John C. Ballantyne FRCS, HonFRCSI, DLO**
Consultant Ear, Nose and Throat Surgeon,
Royal Free and King Edward VII Hospital for Officers, London, UK;
Honorary Consultant in Otolaryngology to the Army

**Andrew Morrison FRCS, DLO**
Senior Consultant Otolaryngologist, The London Hospital, UK

## General Principles, Breast and Extracranial Endocrines

**Hugh Dudley ChM, FRCS(Ed), FRACS, FRCS**
Emeritus Professor, St Mary's Hospital, London, UK

**Walter J. Pories MD, FACS**
Professor and Chairman, Department of Surgery, School of Medicine,
East Carolina University, Greenville, North Carolina, USA

## Gynaecology and Obstetrics

**J. M. Monaghan MBChB, FRCS(Ed), FRCOG**
Consultant Gynaecological Surgeon, Head of the Regional
Department of Gynaecological Oncology, Queen Elizabeth Hospital,
Gateshead, Tyne and Wear, UK

## The Hand

**Rolfe Birch FRCS**
Consultant Orthopaedic Surgeon, PNI Unit and Hand Clinic, Royal National Orthopaedic Hospital, London and St Mary's Hospital, London, UK

**Donal Brooks MA, MB, FRCS, FRSCI**
Consulting Orthopaedic Surgeon, University College Hospital and Royal National Orthopaedic Hospital, London, UK; Civilian Consultant in Hand Surgery to the Royal Navy and Royal Air Force, UK

## Neurosurgery

**Lindsay Symon TD, FRCS**
Professor of Neurosurgery, Gough-Cooper Department of Neurological Surgery, Institute of Neurology, The National Hospitals for Nervous Diseases, London, UK

**David G. T. Thomas MRCP, FRCSE**
Senior Lecturer and Consultant Neurosurgeon, Institute of Neurology, National Hospitals for Nervous Diseases, London, UK

**Kemp Clark MD, FACS**
Professor of Neurosurgery, Division of Neurological Surgery, Southwestern Medical School, Dallas, Texas, USA

## Nose and Throat

**John C. Ballantyne FRCS, HonFRCSI, DLO**
Consultant Ear, Nose and Throat Surgeon, Royal Free and King Edward VII Hospital for Officers, London, UK; Honorary Consultant in Otolaryngology to the Army

**D. F. N. Harrison MD, MS, FRCS, FRACS**
Professor of Laryngology and Otology, Royal National Throat, Nose and Ear Hospital, London, UK

## Ophthalmic Surgery

**Thomas A. Rice MD**
Assistant Clinical Professor of Ophthalmology, Case Western Reserve University School of Medicine, Cleveland, Ohio, USA; formerly of the Wilmer Ophthalmological Institute

**Ronald G. Michels MD**
Professor of Ophthalmology, The Wilmer Ophthalmological Institute, The Johns Hopkins University School of Medicine, Maryland, USA

**Walter W. J. Stark MD**
Professor of Ophthalmology, The Wilmer Ophthalmological Institute, The Johns Hopkins University School of Medicine, Maryland, USA

## Orthopaedics

**George Bentley ChM, FRCS**
Professor of Orthopaedic Surgery, Institute of Orthopaedics, Royal National Orthopaedic Hospital, London, UK

**Robert B. Greer III MD, FACS**
Professor of Orthopedic Surgery, The Milton S. Hershey Medical Center and College of Medicine of the Pennsylvania State University, Hershey, Pennsylvania, USA

## Paediatric Surgery

**L. Spitz MB ChB, PhD, FRCS(Ed), FRCS(Eng), FAAP(Hon)**
Nuffield Professor of Paediatric Surgery, Institute of Child Health, University of London; Consultant Paediatric Surgeon, London, UK

**H. Homewood Nixon MA, MB BChir, FRCS(Eng), FRCSI(Hon), FACS(Hon), FAAP(Hon)**
Consultant Paediatric Surgeon, The Hospital for Sick Children, Great Ormond Street, London and St Mary's Hospital, Paddington, London, UK

## Plastic Surgery

**T. L. Barclay ChM, FRCS**
Consultant Plastic Surgeon, St Luke's Hospital, Bradford, West Yorkshire, UK

**Desmond A. Kernahan MD**
Chief, Division of Plastic Surgery, The Children's Memorial Hospital, Chicago, Illinois, USA

## Thoracic Surgery

**J. W. Jackson MCh, FRCS**
(Late) Consultant Thoracic Surgeon, Harefield Hospital, Middlesex, UK

**D. K. C. Cooper MD, PhD, FRCS**
Department of Cardiac Surgery, University of Cape Town Medical School, Cape Town, South Africa

## Trauma Surgery

**Howard R. Champion FRCS(Ed), FACS**
Chief, Trauma Service;
Director, Surgery Critical Care Services,
The Washington Hospital Center, Washington DC;
Professor of Surgery, Chief of Division of Surgery for Trauma, Department of Surgery, Uniformed Services University of the Health Sciences, Bethesda, Maryland, USA

**John V. Robbs ChM, FRCS(Ed)**
Professor of Surgery; Head, Metropolitan Vascular Services;
Head, Division of Surgery, University of Natal, Durban, Natal, South Africa

**Donald D. Trunkey MD, FACS**
Chairman, Department of Surgery, University of Portland, Portland, Oregon, USA

## Urology

**W. Scott McDougal MD**
Professor and Chairman, Department of Urology, Vanderbilt University Medical Center, Nashville, Tennessee, USA

## Vascular Surgery

**James A. DeWeese MD**
Professor and Chairman, Division of Cardiothoracic Surgery, University of Rochester Medical Center, Rochester, New York, USA

## Head and Neck

**Ian McGregor ChM, FRCS**
Formerly Director, Plastic and Oral Surgery Unit, Canniesburn Hospital, Glasgow, UK

**David J. Howard FRCS, FRCS(Ed)**
Deputy Director, Professorial Unit, Institute of Laryngology and Otology, London and the Royal National Throat, Nose and Ear Hospital, London, UK

# Contributors

**C. B. T. Adams** MChir, FRCS
Consultant Neurosurgeon, The Radcliffe Infirmary, Oxford, UK

**H. Hunt Batjer** MD
Assistant Professor, Division of Neurological Surgery, University of Texas Southwestern Medical Center, Dallas, Texas, USA

**George A. S. Blair** MDS, FFD
Consultant in Restorative Dentistry, Royal Victoria Hospital, Belfast, UK

**Peter R. Bronec** MD
Division of Neurosurgery, Department of Surgery, Duke University Medical Center, Durham, North Carolina, USA

**A. D. Cheesman** FRCS
Consultant Otolaryngologist, Charing Cross Hospital, London; Royal National Throat, Nose and Ear Hospital, London, UK

**Kemp Clark** MD, FACS
Professor of Neurosurgery, Division of Neurological Surgery, Southwestern Medical School, Dallas, Texas, USA

**Charles G. Drake** OC, MD, FRCS(C)
Professor and Chairman, Department of Surgery; Professor, Division of Neurosurgery, Department of Clinical Neurosurgical Sciences, Faculty of Medicine, The University of Western Ontario, Canada

**Charles A. Fager** MD
Chairman Emeritus, Department of Neurosurgery, Lahey Clinic Medical Center, Burlington, Massachusetts, USA

**J. L. Firth** FRCP(Ed)
Consultant Neurosurgeon, Regional Department of Neurosurgery and Neurology, University Hospital, Nottingham; Leicester Royal Infirmary; Harlow Wood Orthopaedic Hospital, Mansfield, UK

**S. Galbraith** MD, FRCS
Formerly Consultant Neurosurgeon, University of Glasgow, Institute of Neurological Sciences, The Southern General Hospital, Glasgow, UK

**John Garfield** MA, MChir, FRCP, FRCS
Consultant Neurosurgeon, Wessex Neurological Centre, Southampton General Hospital; Clinical Teacher in Neurosurgery, University of Southampton, Southampton, Hampshire, UK

**Sidney Goldring** MD
Head of Neurological Surgery; Washington University School of Medicine, St Louis, Missouri, USA

**Derek S. Gordon** MCh, FRCS
Consultant Neurosurgeon, Royal Victoria Hospital, Belfast, UK

**Erik M. Gregorie** MD
Chief, Neurosurgery Service, Brooke Army Medical Center, Fort Sam Houston, Texas, USA

**Phillip Harris** FRCS(Ed), FRCS(Glas), FRCP(Ed), FRS(Ed)
Senior Lecturer in Neurological Surgery, University of Edinburgh; Consultant Neurosurgeon, Western General Hospital, Edinburgh; The Royal Infirmary, Edinburgh; The Spinal Unit, Edenhall Hospital, Musselburgh, UK

**Richard Hayward** MB BS, FRCS
Consultant Neurosurgeon, The Hospital for Sick Children, London; National Hospitals for Nervous Diseases, London; St Mary's Hospital, London, UK

**Roberto C. Heros** MD
Associate Professor of Surgery, Neurosurgery, Harvard Medical School; Director of Cerebrovascular Surgery, Massachusetts General Hospital, Boston, Massachusetts, USA

**Edward Hitchcock** ChM, FRCS
Professor and Head of Department of Neurosurgery, University of Birmingham, Birmingham, UK

**R. D. Illingworth** FRCS
Consultant Neurosurgeon, Regional Neurosciences Centre, Charing Cross Hospital, London; Honorary Consultant Neurosurgeon, Westminster and Central Middlesex Hospitals, London, UK

**H. R. Ingham** FRCPath, DipBact
Consultant Microbiologist, General Hospital, Newcastle-upon-Tyne, UK

**Patrick J. Kelly** MD
Department of Neurosurgery, Mayo Clinic and Mayo Medical School, Rochester, Minnesota, USA

**Brian E. Kendall** FRCP, FRCR
Lysholm Radiological Department, The National Hospital, London, UK

**T. T. King** FRCS
Consultant Neurosurgeon, The London Hospital, London, UK

**Valentine Logue** FRCS, FRCP
Emeritus Professor of Neurosurgery, Institute of Neurology, London, UK

**J. J. Maccabe** FRCS(Ed)
Consultant Neurosurgeon, King's College Hospital and Maudsley Hospital, London, UK

**Thomas Herrick Milhorat** MD
Professor and Chairman, Department of Neurosurgery, State University of New York Health Sciences Center at Brooklyn, Brooklyn, New York, USA

**A. W. Morrison** FRCS, DLO
Consultant Ear, Nose and Throat Surgeon, The London Hospital, London, UK

**Blaine S. Nashold Jr** MD
Division of Neurosurgery, Department of Surgery, Duke University Medical Center, Durham, North Carolina, USA

**Phanor L. Perot Jr** MD, PhD
Professor and Chairman, Department of Neurological Surgery, Medical University of South Carolina, Charleston, South Carolina, USA

**Albert L. Rhoton Jr** MD
R. D. Keene Family Professor and Chairman, Department of Neurological Surgery, University of Florida College of Medicine, Gainseville, Florida, USA

**M. Rice-Edwards** MA, FRCS
Consultant Neurosurgeon, Department of Neurosurgery, Regional Neurosciences Centre, Charing Cross Hospital, London, UK

**Duke S. Samson** MD
Professor and Chairman, Division of Neurological Surgery, University of Texas Southwestern Medical Center, Dallas, Texas, USA

**Stephen C. Saris** MD
Surgical Neurology Branch, National Institute of Health, Bethesda, Maryland, USA

**R. D. Smith** MD
Department of Neurosurgery, Louisiana State University Medical Center, New Orleans, Louisiana, USA

**A. J. Strong** MA, FRCSE
Consultant Neurosurgeon, The Neurosurgical Unit of Guy's, Maudsley and King's College Hospitals, London, UK

**Thoralf M. Sundt Jr** MD
Professor and Chairman of Neurosurgery, Department of Neurosurgery, Mayo Clinic, Rochester, Minnesota, USA

**Lindsay Symon** TD, FRCS
Professor of Neurosurgery, Gough-Cooper Department of Neurological Surgery, Institute of Neurology, National Hospitals for Nervous Diseases, London, UK

**G. M. Teasdale** FRCP, FRCS(Ed), FRCS(Glas)
Professor and Head of Department of Neurosurgery, University of Glasgow, Institute of Neurological Sciences, The Southern General Hospital, Glasgow, UK

**Rene Tempelhoff** MD
Chief of Neuroanesthesia, Washington University School of Medicine, St Louis, Missouri, USA

**D. G. T. Thomas** FRCP, FRCS
Senior Lecturer and Consultant Neurosurgeon, Institute of Neurology, The National Hospitals for Nervous Diseases, London, UK

**M. G. Yaşargil** MD
Professor and Director, Neurosurgical University Clinic, Kantonsspital Zürich, Switzerland

# Contributing Medical Artists

**Margaret E. Barry** MA
Medical Illustrator, Department of Neurosurgery, The University of Florida School of Medicine, Box J-265 JHMHC, Gainesville, Florida 32610, USA

**A. Besterman**

**J. M. P. Booth**

**Angela Christie**
14 West End Avenue, Pinner, Middlesex HA5 1BJ, UK

**John W. Desley**
Mayo Clinic, Rochester, Minnesota, USA

**Robert Gordon**
Medical Artistry, Duke University Medical Center, Durham, North Carolina, USA

**Anne S. Greene** MA
Medical Illustrator, Lahey Clinical Medical Center, Burlington, Massachusetts, USA

**D. Hutchinson**

**Barbara Hyams** MA, AMI
Medical Illustrator, Poynings, Northchurch Common, Northchurch, Berkhamsted, Hertfordshire, UK

**Ludwig G. Kempe** MD, FACS
Diplomate of Board of Neurological Surgery, 19 Logan Street, Charleston, South Carolina 29401, USA

**Robert N. Lane** MMAA
Medical Illustrator, Studio 19A, Edith Grove, London SW10, UK

**David Peace** MS
Medical Illustrator, Department of Neurosurgery, The University of Florida School of Medicine, Box J-265 JHMHC, Gainesville, Florida 32610, USA

# Contents

# Preface

Ten years have passed since the third edition of this book appeared. The time lapse is a testimony both to the sound opinions expressed in the second edition and perhaps less happily to the delays inevitably consequent upon such a wide-ranging multiauthor book. It has seemed important, however, to update those chapters which have served as a basis for neurosurgical thinking for many years. Readers will notice the disappearance of ventriculography and the inevitably greater emphasis on neuroimaging which the present book contains. A number of new authors, particularly from the United States, have been added and in each case the techniques have been explained by surgeons internationally known for their expertise.

We are much indebted to the authors who have updated and revised their contributions. Once again, no praise is too high for the work of the medical illustrators nor to the long suffering efforts of the publishing staff at Butterworths.

Lindsay Symon
David G. T. Thomas
Kemp Clark

Illustrations by Robert N. Lane and Angela Christie

# Control of intracranial tension

**Lindsay Symon** TD, FRCS
Professor of Neurosurgery, Gough-Cooper Department of Neurological Surgery, Institute of Neurology, National Hospitals for Nervous Diseases, London, UK

## Introduction

Significant advances in anaesthesia and pharmacology, allied with wider appreciation of the physiological background, have in recent years appreciably lessened the problems of management of raised intracranial tension. Success in management of neurosurgical patients, however, and the successful completion of any operation on the brain, still depend upon the control of intracranial tension.

In preoperative and postoperative periods, the inelastic skull dictates that swelling around the diseased area or at the site of operation is unable to expand into either a surface or an elastic-walled cavity, and the result is a considerable rise in intracranial pressure. This in turn compresses low-pressure areas of the vascular system or of the cerebrospinal fluid pathways, and may result in further secondary pressure increases.

Considerable changes in intracranial blood volume take place under the influence of alteration in blood gas tensions (particularly arterial $P\mathrm{CO_2}$); such changes may be accompanied by large alterations in intracranial pressure[1]; indeed, active changes in the vascular system are more common in practice than obstruction of the effluent veins, although such obstruction may give rise to raised pressure.

Cerebral oedema, partly a process of cellular imbibition and partly a process of egress of fluid into the interstitial spaces, particularly in white matter, may occur in the open skull with great rapidity, and occasion the prolapse of important functional areas through the wound. Subsequent rupture of pia mater and distortion of white matter may adversely affect the functional results of operation.

The nature of the circulation of the cerebrospinal fluid means that small lesions in the posterior fossa or periaqueductal zone soon result in the damming back of fluid from both lateral ventricles and, with the persistent filtration power of the choroid plexuses, this results in a rise of pressure, the magnitude of which depends upon the rapidity of the process. In rapidly growing lesions, or particularly postoperatively, such obstruction to cerebrospinal fluid allows little scope for secondary adaptive mechanisms, and the resulting acute rise in intracranial pressure constitutes one of the most serious neurosurgical emergencies.

In this brief review, these three main factors – changes in the cerebral circulation, development of cerebral oedema and obstruction of the cerebrospinal fluid pathways – will be seen to emerge as dominant in the production of rapid changes in intracranial pressure.

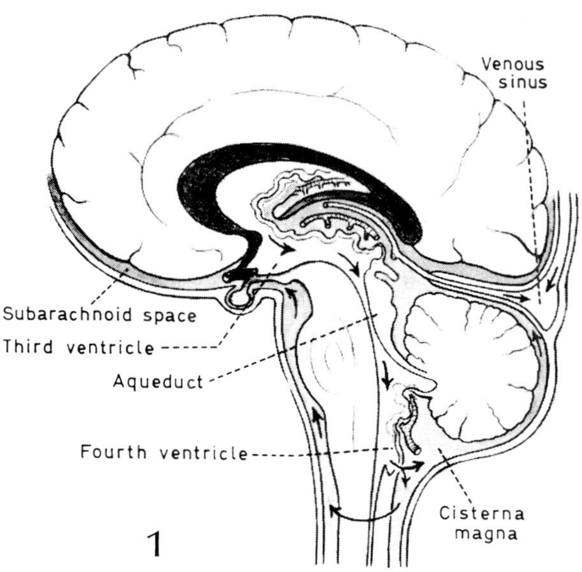


1

1

### Circulation of cerebrospinal fluid

Cerebrospinal fluid from the lateral and third ventricles passes down the aqueduct, emerges into the cisterna magna from the fourth ventricle and circulates over the top of the hemispheres in the subarachnoid space. From there it is absorbed into the venous sinuses.

# Control of vascular factors

## VENOUS PRESSURE AND PERFUSION

### Position of patient

The venous system of the brain, neck and thorax has no functioning valves; a major factor in the level of intracranial venous pressure is, therefore, the height of the head above the right atrium. The influence of posture depends on two factors: the height of the head above the right atrium (greater if the patient is in the sitting position than if he is prone), and the original level of cerebral venous pressure. If the original cerebral venous pressure is normal, the assumption of the sitting position may produce a negative pressure if a vein is opened, with the consequent danger of air embolism.

The majority of intracranial operations are conducted with a modest amount (approximately 20–30°) of foot-down tilt. By abolishing this modest tilt, the surgeon has the capacity to provide swift autotransfusion in the case of sudden or unexpected hypotension.

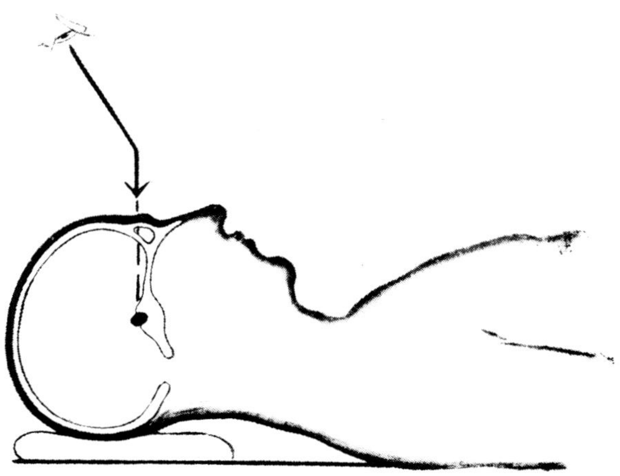

2a

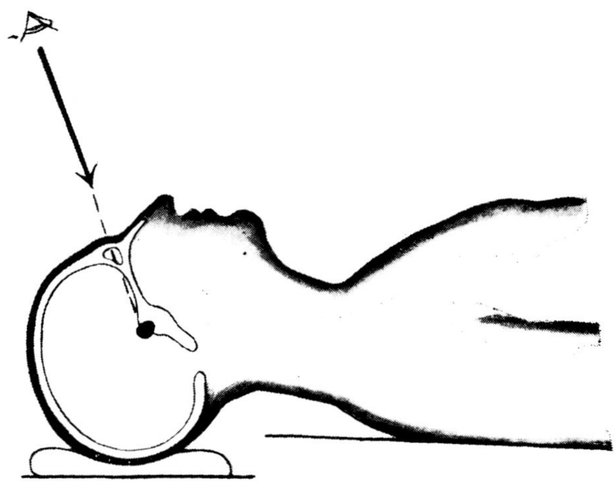

2b

# 2a & b

The position of the lesion to be reached must be remembered, and head position planned for optimal access. The position of the operator in relation for example to the pituitary fossa can affect access. Slight extension of the head allows a more direct subfrontal approach. The supine position with adequate rotation of the head allows access to frontal, parietal and temporal lesions, and variation in neck flexion permits comfortable access to the hemisphere and parasagittal zone as far back as the postparietal region.

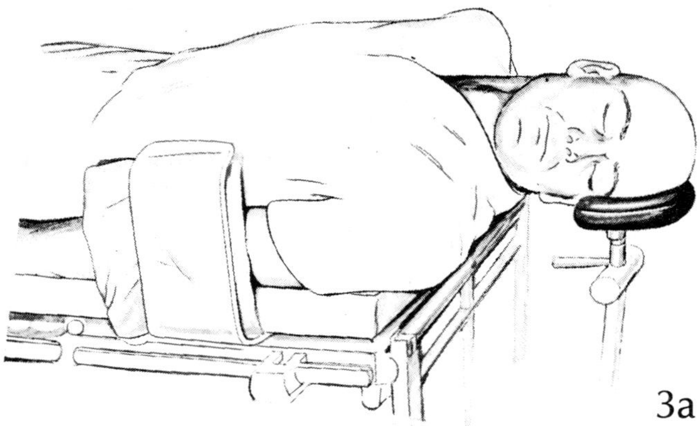

3a

# 3a & b

It is important to remember that brachial plexus traction is easily produced in an unconscious patient, and therefore lateral rotation of the head should be accompanied by elevation of the occipital shoulder on sandbags, with prevention of undue lateral flexion of the neck.

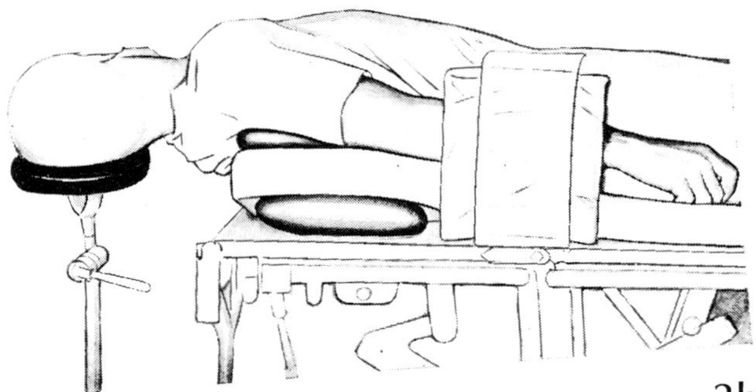

3b

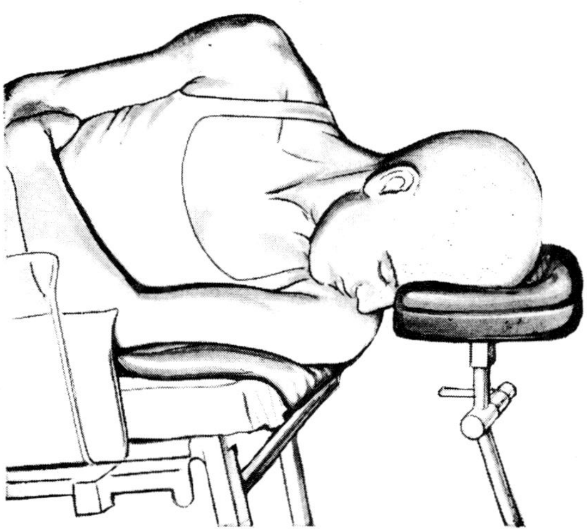

4a

# 4a & b

For occipital lesions and certain lesions in the posterior fossa, particularly in the cerebellopontine angle, a lateral position of the body may be preferred with varying degrees of rotation and lateral flexion of the head to produce a greater or lesser degree of brow-down posture, and to open up and elongate the upward facing lateral aspect of the posterior fossa and neck. The advantage of this position is that, unlike the prone position, it permits free and unimpeded respiration. It demands careful protection of the downward prominences – shoulder, greater trochanter and the circumflex, radial and lateral popliteal nerves. The weight of the thorax is taken upon an axillary pillow, with careful padding of points of contact on the downward arm which is relieved of weightbearing capacity; other pressure areas should be protected by soft Sorbo rubber sponges. Slight traction upon the upward shoulder prevents it riding upwards and obscuring the posterior fossa; again, care is necessary in this manoeuvre to avoid traction injury of the brachial plexus.

The fully prone position is little used in intracranial surgery since access to the posterior fossa is limited. However, with careful support of the pelvis and thorax to leave the abdomen free, it is possible to prevent a rise in central venous pressure resulting from thoracic or abdominal compression; the position is therefore a popular one for operations upon the spine from the cervical level downwards.

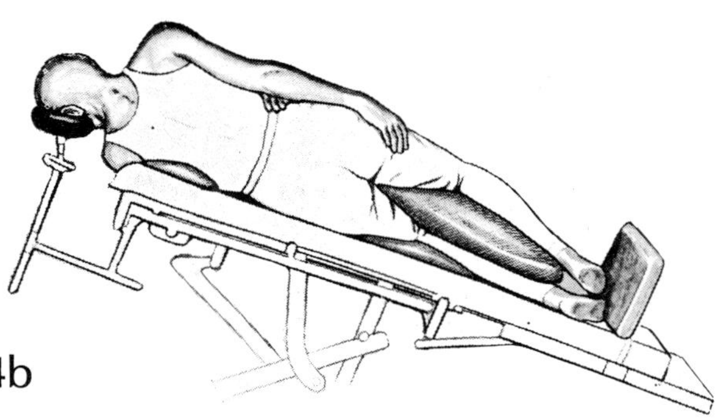

4b

# 5

The seated position is of value in the approach to lesions in the posterior fossa, particularly in the presence of raised intracranial pressure where the larger height differential between the posterior fossa veins and the right atrium is useful. The seated position as used for posterior fossa craniotomy is illustrated. The anti-gravity suit, used to elevate venous pressure, and a spirometer, used to record the respiratory excursions, are indicated. Most of these procedures, however, are now performed with intermittent positive-pressure ventilation.

In addition to affording access to the fourth ventricle, the upper and lower surfaces of the cerebellum, and the region of the foramen magnum, the seated position enables free egress of blood and cerebrospinal fluid from the site of operation. The chief potential hazard is air embolus, but the cases in which this position is most advantageous are those in which the likelihood of air embolus is least, because of the very high resting intracranial venous pressures. Nevertheless, because of the danger of air embolism, the full seated position with the legs dependent has been abandoned by many surgeons in favour of a semi-seated position with the legs elevated as illustrated. With the additional availability of such measures as an anti-gravity suit to apply pressure to the venous beds of the legs and abdomen, and with the capacity to load the expiratory resistance in the airway circuit[2] or by the use of intermittent positive-pressure ventilation, the central venous pressure may be rapidly increased if cranial venous pressure becomes so low as to render air embolism likely.

A helpful routine is to elevate the central venous pressure intermittently as dissection through the layers of the wound proceeds, so that the veins are temporarily distended in each layer. Open veins are readily detected and occluded by diathermy, silver clips, or plugging with bone wax or Surgicel (Ethicon, UK). Elevation of central venous pressure for 3–4 minutes proves quite adequate for such safety precaution, but maintenance of appreciably raised central venous pressure for longer periods is to be avoided.

The more usual use of the seated position combines the anti-gravity suit with the use of positive end-expiratory pressure of up to 10 cm$H_2O$ on artificial ventilation when the central venous pressure, measured in the superior vena cava, is observed to be low. Where raised intracranial pressure is no problem, the central venous pressure may be raised by the addition of a fluid load of about 0.5–1.0 litre of Hartmann's solution; this is of particular value in dehydrated patients, for example in elderly patients with cerebellar tumour who may have been vomiting for some time.

The sitting position may also be used in the approach to occipital lesions, where special care is necessary in the area of the mastoid emissary veins and large dural sinuses to prevent air embolism.

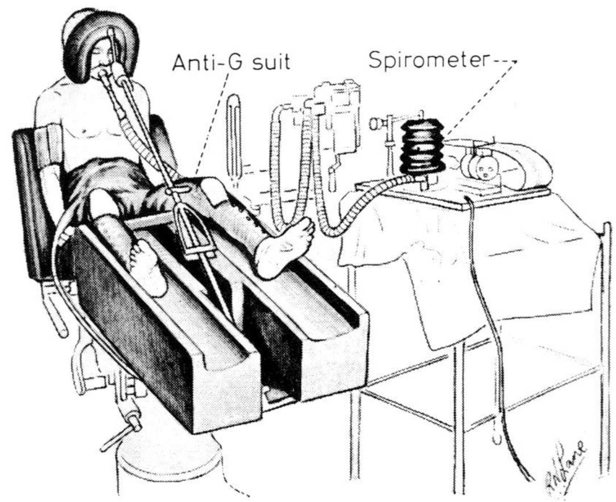


5

# 6

A further position which has been much used in our clinic in recent years is referred to as the 'praying mantis' position, described elsewhere as the 'concorde' position. It is particularly useful for midline vermian, cerebellar, or upper cervical arteriovenous malformations where induced hypotension may be thought necessary. In the seated position, which might be thought to be an alternative, the induction of hypotension is fraught with hazard. The 'praying mantis' position, in which ready adjustment is made simply by changing the tilt of the table, is very much safer. Points to be noted are that the patient should be held to the table by a strap across the buttocks, that there should be the usual adequate padding under the thorax to leave the abdomen free, and that there should be padding beneath the knees which are taking weight on the modified foot-rest of the table.

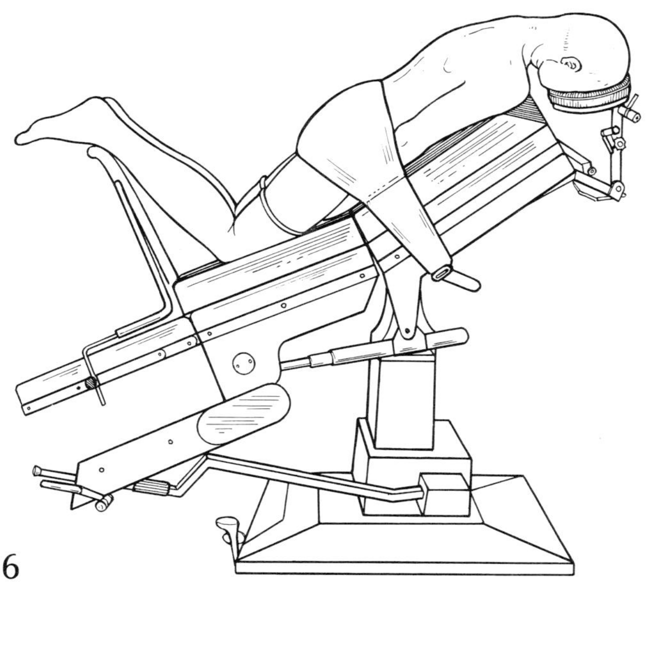

6

## Control of respiration

# 7 & 8

Alteration of the arterial $P_{CO_2}$ is now recognized as the chief extraneous factor available to modify cerebral blood flow. Increase in arterial $P_{CO_2}$, besides raising cerebral blood flow, also raises intracranial pressure owing to the increased blood content within the brain. The accompanying illustrations show that elevation of the arterial $P_{CO_2}$ increases both the pressure within the closed skull and also the directly measured cortical venous pressure. *Illustration 7* shows the effect of 3 per cent carbon dioxide in inspired air on central venous pressure (CVP), systemic arterial pressure (BP), cerebrospinal fluid pressure in the cisterna magna (CSFP), extradural intracranial pressure recorded by transducer in the closed skull (ICP) and end-tidal carbon dioxide concentration in a baboon.

*Illustration 8* shows the effect of increase in arterial $P_{CO_2}$ from 37.5 to 48 mmHg (SBP, systemic arterial pressure; MCAP, arterial pressure in a parietal branch of the middle cerebral artery; MCVP, venous pressure in a parietal branch of the middle cerebral vein emerging from the cortex; $ETCO_2$, end-tidal carbon dioxide record). The increase in brain bulk which can be produced by retention of carbon dioxide is so great that many neurosurgical operations are now conducted with the arterial $P_{CO_2}$ artificially lowered by mechanical ventilation. Indeed, this is now the most generally applicable method of control of intracranial pressure during the neurosurgical operation itself.

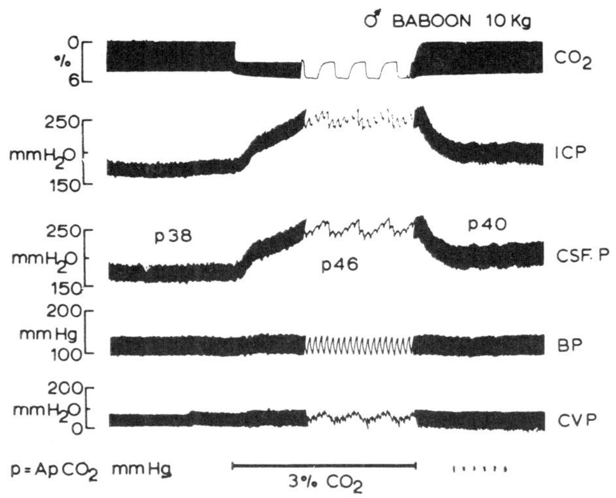


7

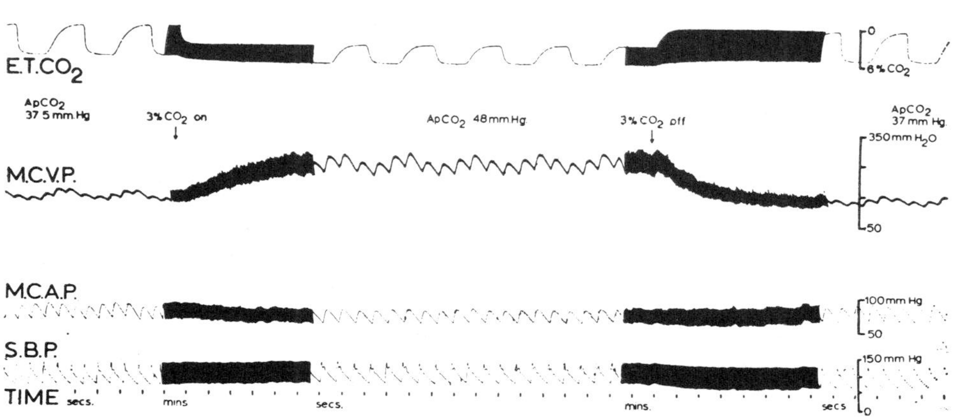


8

### Advantages of controlled ventilation

As a method of control of arterial $P_{CO_2}$, ventilation shares the advantages of gaseous anaesthetics: it is readily induced and readily reversed. It requires cuffed endotracheal anaesthesia with a suitable mechanical ventilator such as the Cape–Wayne, Manley, East–Radcliffe or Barnet ventilators. The first two are the most commonly employed. There is no great advantage in lowering the arterial $P_{CO_2}$ below 20 mmHg, and, indeed, excessive reduction may be dangerous. An adult exchange volume of between 8 and 15 litres per minute is usually adequate. This may be achieved by intermittent positive pressure, and the attendant mild hypotension may prove advantageous. If it is desirable to avoid hypotension completely, a negative phase may be added to achieve ventilation with less interference to the venous return to the heart. The patient's respiratory activity is usually suppressed by the intermittent administration of a respiratory paralysant such as tubocurarine, although it is possible by variations of anaesthetic gas concentration to maintain adequate hyperventilation without relaxants.

It is the author's practice to return to spontaneous ventilation before dural closure, so that some idea of the immediate postoperative intracranial tension may be obtained and, for example, the adequacy of palliative resection for a glioma assured, while the profound arteriolar vasoconstriction induced by hyperventilation relaxes and the adequacy of haemostasis is confirmed.

### Disadvantages of hyperventilation

The chief disadvantage of respiratory control is the loss of the patient's own respiration as a monitor of diencephalic or brain-stem function. Manipulations in the region of the hypothalamus, third ventricle, brain stem or the vessels of the posterior fossa commonly produce slight respiratory irregularities[3] which are of value as a guide to avoiding prolonged distortion of vital structures. This is lost when hyperventilation is induced. For this reason some surgeons are reluctant to use assisted respiration in the surgery of posterior fossa tumours. The various advantages and dangers must be weighed by the surgeon and anaesthetist concerned, and a dialogue between the two should be established so that operating ease and anaesthetic safety are judiciously combined.

An inevitable accompaniment of lowered arterial $P_{CO_2}$ is diminished tissue perfusion, which may at very low $P_{CO_2}$ levels induce anaerobic glucose utilization[4] in the neural tissue with an increased arteriovenous $P_{CO_2}$ gradient[5]. Cohen *et al.*[6] indicate that there may be accompanying tissue hypoxia. The extent of this hazard is far from clear at this stage but it would seem wise to include the highest concentration of oxygen possible in the ventilating mixture.

### CONTROL OF SYSTEMIC BLOOD PRESSURE

### Hypotensive anaesthesia

Hypotensive anaesthesia has been much employed in recent years as an adjunct to neurosurgery. The agents commonly employed have been ganglion-blocking agents such as hexamethonium or trimetaphan (Arfonad, Roche, Welwyn Garden, UK). Sodium nitroprusside in a solution of 20 µg/ml in saline may also be used. A suitable solution of the hypotensive agent is administered by continuous intravenous drip, the rate being titrated against blood pressure. Trimetaphan in a dilution of 100 µg/ml is commonly employed.

The advantage of hypotensive anaesthesia is the reduction of arterial bleeding. Because of the autoregulatory capacity of the cerebral circulation, however, the reduction in cerebral blood flow by no means parallels the reduction in the arterial blood pressure, and venous bleeding is much less reduced than, for example, by hyperventilation. For the same reason, reduction in intracranial pressure is slight and the use of active hypotension is probably best restricted to cases where considerable arterial haemorrhage is envisaged, such as in the surgery of intracranial aneurysms, certain vascular meningiomas, and arteriovenous malformations.

Evidence suggests that traumatized areas of brain such as those around pathological processes, or those subject to retraction at operation, do not display the normal autoregulatory control of tissue perfusion, but are instead 'pressure passive', with blood flow falling with decline in blood pressure[7]. Such areas also show a decline in flow with raised carbon dioxide tension[8]. For these reasons a judicious combination of hyperventilation and hypotension is preferable to hypotension alone.

Dangers also lie in the extensive reduction of tissue perfusion in areas other than the brain, which if prolonged may result in necrosis of the edge of a turned-back scalp flap or, more important, in renal damage, perhaps progressing to renal failure.

## Control of cerebral oedema

### Dehydrating agents

If a hyperosmolar and relatively non-diffusable solution is introduced into the vascular compartment, it attracts fluid from the extravascular space and diminishes any pathological collection of interstitial fluid as in cerebral oedema. The first solutions used, 50 per cent sucrose or glucose, were given in small volumes; their effect was slight and transient, and repeated use carried a danger of damage to the tubular cells of the kidney. Lyophilized urea, however, was shown to produce a sustained fall in intracranial pressure[9] and although as with the earlier solutions there was a later rise or 'rebound', this was delayed and not great. By judicious repeated use, control of raised intracranial pressure, particularly in supratentorial pathology, could be achieved with much greater certainty than had hitherto been possible.

Solutions of mannitol have been found to possess certain advantages over urea solutions[10], and in most neurosurgical practices mannitol has replaced urea as the dehydrating agent of choice.

#### *Mode of action of intravenous dehydrating agents*

Dehydrating agents act by inducing hyperosmolarity in the serum, creating a gradient of osmolarity between serum and cerebrospinal fluid. The diffusional characteristics of urea and mannitol differ slightly in that mannitol does not diffuse into intracellular spaces. Throughout its action, therefore, it continues to abstract fluid from the intracellular compartment. It equilibrates slowly with the extracellular spaces only, and there is a considerable gradient between intravascular and extracellular spaces. Urea, on the other hand, slowly diffuses over the cell membranes and is ultimately distributed in all tissues. During its therapeutically active stage, however, the relative slowness of this diffusion enables the creation of osmolar gradients upon which its action depends. It has been suggested that the smaller rebound phenomena after mannitol may perhaps depend upon the different diffusion characteristics of the two drugs.

Certain diuretic agents show a surprisingly similar degree of effectiveness, notably frusemide (Lasix, Hoechst, Middlesex, UK) which has to some extent replaced urea and mannitol in routine practice. Its action depends upon the rapid excretion of water and electrolytes from the intravascular compartment and the creation of an osmolar gradient between this compartment and the tissues of the body generally.

### *Indications for use of dehydrating agents*

Dehydrating agents are primarily indicated where surgery is not contemplated, or where surgery must be deferred for some reason.

In the treatment of severe head injuries where intracranial haematoma has been excluded, repeated administration of dehydrating agents, such as urea or mannitol in doses of 1–2 g/kg body weight or of frusemide 40 mg 6–12-hourly, has constituted the chief method of control of intracranial pressure, although Gordon and Rossanda[11] suggest that prolonged hyperventilation may have a place in management. When a patient with intracranial tumour suddenly deteriorates, perhaps with the development of a tentorial or foraminal cone, the administration of similar doses of dehydrating agents may prove life-saving while steps are taken to transfer him to the care of a surgeon. In the 48 hours following operation, when cerebral oedema may prejudice function and particularly when the condition is known to be a self-limiting one, the intermittent use of dehydrating agents may preserve function and obtain the optimum result of operation.

### *Disadvantages of dehydrating agents*

The chief disadvantage of dehydrating agents lies in their very effectiveness. If a patient is ill owing to a space-occupying lesion, the logical procedure is to remove the space-occupying lesion and not to shrink the brain to accommodate the disease still more, especially since these drugs act most upon normal brain and least on areas imperfectly perfused and oedematous. If the space-occupying lesion is a haematoma, perhaps after an operation, then the shrinking of normal brain or of oedematous reactive brain simply ensures the further expansion of the haematoma, so that as the action wears off the patient's condition is rather worse than before. One should have a clear idea of the nature of the circumstance which one wishes to treat before these agents are employed. The CT scan is most helpful in this regard.

A further serious disadvantage is that urea in particular is extremely irritating to tissues, and produces a disastrous slough if it escapes from the vein during infusion. Mannitol may produce the same effect to a lesser extent. For this reason forearm veins are best avoided, and the solution is given by catheter percutaneously introduced into the lumen of a continuously flowing vein in the leg despite the fact that these drugs may induce thrombosis of veins.

Administration of urea is contraindicated in cases of renal failure. It is important that the blood urea at least be estimated before a hypertonic solution of urea is administered. Mannitol possesses a clear advantage in this respect – indeed the drug may be used in the treatment of renal failure.

Frusemide shares the dangers of urea and mannitol in relation to intracerebral expanding lesions, but is free from the disadvantages of tissue damage at the site of administration. It may be given intravenously or intramuscularly in doses of 40–80 mg as a single injection. All of the dehydrating agents mentioned increase the excretion of electrolytes from the kidney. This loss of electrolytes and water is of little consequence if the use is episodic over 1 or 2 days only, but if continued, a serious state of depletion may result. Serum electrolytes and haematocrit must be estimated if recurrent dehydration is contemplated; this is of particular importance in vascular cases where haemoconcentration may constitute an additional hazard in an already imperfectly perfused vascular bed.

## Control of intracranial pressure during induction of anaesthesia

There is clear evidence that substantial rises in intracranial pressure occur during the induction of anaesthesia[12]. Because of this, for a time many surgeons employed urea or mannitol 30 minutes or so before the commencement of surgery. However, with the increasing use of artificial ventilation and with wider recognition of the dangers of a rise in intracranial pressure during induction, this is now less frequently employed. Disadvantages were the marked increase in blood flow[13] and usually also in systemic blood pressure accompanying reduction in intracranial pressure and general hypervolaemia; the unfortunate surgeon, therefore, opened the cranium in the face of extremely high intracranial and extracranial blood flows. Hyperventilation controls intracranial pressure with *reduction* of intracranial blood flow, so that the ease and comfort of operation is considerably increased.

## Use of steroids

Steroids alleviate symptoms in patients with brain tumour or with postoperative cerebral oedema, an effect usually explained by their action in reducing cerebral oedema, shown experimentally[14] and confirmed clinically by the observation of reduced intracranial pressure in patients with brain tumour[15]. Dexamethasone or betamethasone may be used in the preoperative and postoperative phase, the dose schedule varying considerably from one clinic to another. The effect, however, is not instantaneous, and it is usual to place the patient on a moderate dose of steroids (say 4–6 mg four times a day) for some days before operation, to maintain the treatment at this level for 3 or 4 days postoperatively, and then to tail off with progressively reduced dosage over the succeeding 7–10 days.

It is now general practice in the majority of neurosurgical units to place all patients with brain tumour on this moderate steroid dosage, and to accept the theoretical disadvantages of steroid administration, these being slight slowing of wound healing and a demonstrable reduction of the patient's resistance to infection. Where direct dissection of tumours from the substance of the spinal cord is to be attempted, as has become increasingly the practice in recent years, a similar steroid dosage may be employed.

There is less general agreement on the place of steroids in the management of intracranial aneurysm both before and after surgery, but it is the author's practice to place all subarachnoid cases on standard steroid dosage before arteriography and to maintain this throughout any surgical procedure and for a few days thereafter. Possible compromise of the circulation during surgery will then occur, with whatever potential protective effect steroids may have on membrane permeability. Experimental evidence suggests that steroid preloading will reduce such ischaemically induced swelling, though there is less convincing evidence that it will influence ischaemic oedema once this is established.

The possibility that an extremely high steroid dosage (up to 100 mg dexamethasone per day) may be of value, for example in the control of intracranial tension after head injury, has been suggested by the use of such steroid dosages in inoperable brain tumours, although evidence of more than transitory benefit has yet to be presented.

Steroid therapy has proved particularly useful in the treatment of inoperable intracranial metastases, or in the management of the later phases of infiltrative brain tumours, where terminal rises in intracranial pressure produce a distressing reduction in visual acuity secondary to papilloedema. Steroids have also been shown to influence the course of benign intracranial hypertension, and their use is clearly justified in severe examples of this condition. They may also be employed in association with radiotherapy in the treatment of gliomas.

# Cerebrospinal fluid drainage

## 9

Raised intracranial pressure may be produced by obstruction of the cerebrospinal fluid pathways, and since this commonly occurs quite gradually, considerable dilatation of the ventricular spaces above the level of the block may occur. For example, with an aqueductal obstruction the third ventricle and both lateral ventricles are commonly very dilated. At first this dilatation seems to occur with only episodic rises in intracranial pressure[16], but gradually intracranial pressure becomes constantly raised, despite the attempted accommodation produced by white matter compression and ventricular dilatation. The greater part of the patient's symptoms may be produced by the cerebrospinal fluid obstruction rather than by the original disorder. Where this is irremovable, for example with aqueduct stenosis, diversion of the fluid may cure the symptoms. Where the original cause of symptoms is removable, however, for example with a posterior fossa tumour, cerebrospinal fluid drainage may temporarily control intracranial pressure before surgery and perhaps for a period of time afterwards.

The method usually employed is to pass a No. 3 or 4 English gauge rubber catheter from a postparietal burr hole (the normal ventricular burr hole), leaving 4–5 cm of catheter within the ventricle. The ventricle is located with a standard Dandy brain cannula, its depth from the dural surface assessed, and the appropriate calculations of length made. The catheter must be passed into the body of the ventricle and not into the temporal horn where it will not drain satisfactorily. The ventricular burr hole wound is closed around the catheter; alternatively the catheter may be brought obliquely through a separate stab incision, but there is little advantage in this latter procedure. The catheter may then be drained intermittently or, as shown, connected to a drainage apparatus. The height of the ventricular drainage can be adjusted as desired. Adjustment of the height of the system sets the intracranial pressure at any desired level. If the intracranial pressure has been much raised for any length of time, it is wise to decompress the ventricular system very slowly, lowering the drainage flask over a period of about 24 hours until a level of 40–50 mm above the patient's forehead is reached.

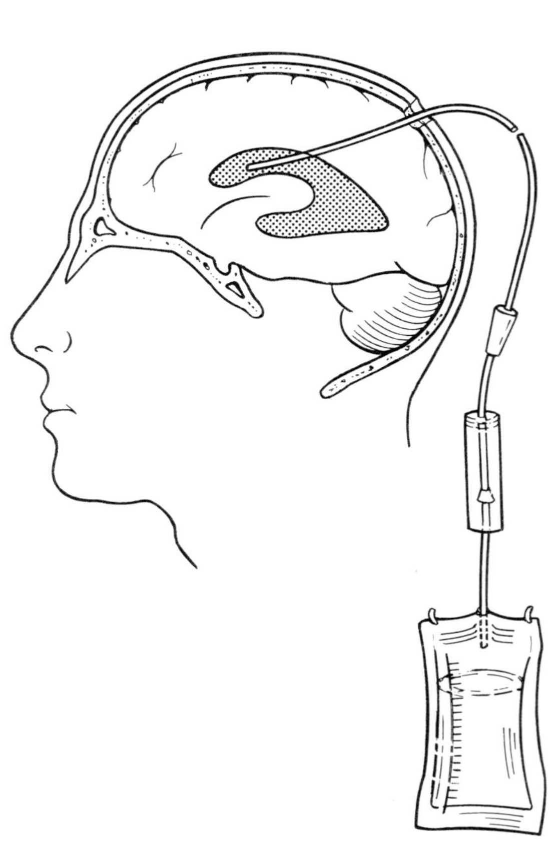

9

More permanent cerebrospinal fluid diversion by drainage of the ventricular fluid through a valve system into the vena cava has been used in certain North American clinics as a preliminary to the management of posterior fossa lesions[17], but this has not found great favour in the UK.

External ventricular drainage in the presence of a dilated ventricular system is simple and effective in the temporary management of raised pressure, but should not be used without careful consideration. With care, effective drainage can usually be established, but the catheter may produce a reaction within the ventricular system; there is also the everpresent danger of infection, and good reason to believe that subsequent performance of a more permanent ventriculovenous or ventriculoatrial shunt is more prone to infection than normally. It is the author's practice, therefore, to drain the ventricles for short periods of 7–10 days only. During this time treatment of the original condition may have abolished the need for ventricular drainage, or it may have become clear that more permanent diversion of cerebrospinal fluid is necessary, in which case the patient can be prepared for a shunt procedure.

### *Infection*

Routine administration of antibiotics to patients with indwelling ventricular drains has little merit; infection is best avoided by scrupulous attention to occlusive dressings protecting the point of exit of the ventricular catheter from the scalp, and by the employment of modern fully closed drainage systems. These should be changed when necessary as a full sterile ward procedure.

### *Long-term catheterization*

In certain special circumstances[16], fine ventricular catheters may be employed for very much longer periods of time, and successful use has been made of them in monitoring intracranial pressure during the management of intracranial tumours or obstructions to the cerebrospinal fluid pathways. It is likely, however, that this procedure will remain in the province of research rather than of routine practice.

## Lumbar spinal drainage

As a short-term method for the evacuation of cerebrospinal fluid, lumbar spinal drainage still has a place – for example in the approach to posterior fossa tumours with the patient in the lateral position, where drainage of the fluid when the dura has been opened prevents troublesome collections in the depths of the wound. A flexible lumbar puncture needle is introduced at the L4–L5 level, bent over, and strapped to the skin with drainage into any convenient closed system of plastic tubing and reservoir. It is the author's practice to discontinue this immediately on the completion of the operation and, if further fluid drainage should be necessary, to rely either on intermittent ventricular tapping or on continuous ventricular drainage for a few days.

The development of disposable lumbar drainage sets, in which a needle of Tuohy design is supplied together with a suitable narrow polyethylene tube, has revived the use of spinal drainage for a few days postoperatively in the control of cerebrospinal fluid leaks from posterior fossa or spinal wounds. Drainage may be encouraged by the establishment of a modest negative pressure through the system by the use of a suction pump with 5–6 mmHg pressure through a reservoir bottle. The technique, however, is unsatisfactory for even temporary control of intracranial pressure, and in raised pressure cases applied negative pressure should never be employed.

## CURRENT MONITORING IN NEUROSURGERY

Recent monitoring techniques make it possible for the neurosurgeon and anaesthetist to follow the condition of a patient very closely. The full complexity of modern monitoring may not be applicable to every neurosurgical case, but there are certain essential principles which may be stated briefly.

## Recording arterial blood pressure

For many years neurosurgeons have relied upon intermittent monitoring of the arterial blood pressure by auscultative or tonometric methods. These methods have proved satisfactory for routine use, but the rapid changes in blood pressure produced by transient neurological disturbances are not recorded. In prolonged operations in the region of the brain stem, continuous blood pressure recording from a catheter in the radial or brachial artery via a suitable transducer may be employed. Brachial catheterization for periods of up to 2 days is safe in skilled hands, although catheterization of the radial artery is generally employed and is more satisfactory. For short-term recording the strain gauge and catheters may be filled with normal saline containing 2 IU/ml heparin, and intermittent flushing of the catheter system arranged either through the strain gauge or by suitable three-way connections. For longer-term recording, continuous slow perfusion of the catheter system is used, so that while the catheter and flushing system are perfused with physiological solutions containing small quantities of anticoagulants, the gauges themselves may be filled with antiseptic solution which does not pass into the patient.

## Respiratory monitoring

Respiratory monitoring presents fewer technical problems than continuous monitoring of intra-arterial pressure, and the apparatus necessary is both less complicated and less expensive[2]. Since respiratory disturbances may be evoked from a wide area of the neuraxis, extending from the subfrontal grey matter through the diencephalon to the main respiratory centres of the brain stem itself, transient disturbances of respiration may provide valuable warning of disturbance in a variety of neurosurgical procedures. Recording of respiratory patterns may be achieved by a spirometer bleeding out from the respiratory pathway and connected to an ink-writing system.

# 10

More commonly now, however, tracheal air is sampled for analysis by an infrared gas analyser, and additional quantitative information on end-tidal carbon dioxide concentration thereby obtained. Characteristic respiratory patterns resulting from disturbance of the respiratory centres in the brain stem have been described, and several are shown. In Trace 1, a non-specific response from traction on the fifth nerve is shown at A. At B dissection of the medial part of an acoustic neuroma capsule from the upper brain stem occasioned development of periodic respiration.

Trace 2 shows a transient respiratory disturbance associated with a similar dissection (also a case of acoustic neuroma). The respiratory spikes which have here followed the incident are often seen separately and are by themselves of no significance.

Respiratory monitoring is not applicable where continuous moderate hyperventilation is employed. In the management of most supratentorial lesions, the advantages gained from moderate hyperventilation are so great that abandonment of the respiratory monitor is justified; however, it may be desirable where complicated dissection in the region of the brain stem or upper cervical spine is contemplated, to return the patient to spontaneous respiration at this stage, to obtain the added guidance of the respiratory monitor.

## Monitoring central venous pressure

Continuous monitoring of the central venous pressure by a strain gauge from a catheter passed through a peripheral arm vein into the superior vena cava presents few technical difficulties beyond the sterilization of the system and the assurance of adequate perfusion of the catheter.

The information obtained is of value when the patient is in the sitting position where air embolus is a possible hazard. In these circumstances the central venous pressure record may be used to check the effectiveness of an anti-gravity suit and increased expiratory resistance in the airway, and also, if need be, to aspirate air from the right atrium. It is doubtful, however, whether central venous pressure recording has much to offer in routine neurosurgical practice apart from this.

## Electrocardiogram monitoring

The absolute indications for electrocardiogram monitoring relate to circumstances in which the heart is at particular risk, such as in established heart disease, or when the general body temperature is being lowered in operations for aneurysm or certain vascular anomalies. The limiting factor in the induction of hypothermia is the development of cardiac irregularities, and continuous electrocardiogram monitoring is then essential. The detection of the earliest ventricular extrasystoles may enable the cooling process to be slowed before ventricular fibrillation supervenes. Electrocardiographic monitoring is now routine in most neurosurgical units, whatever procedure is being undertaken.

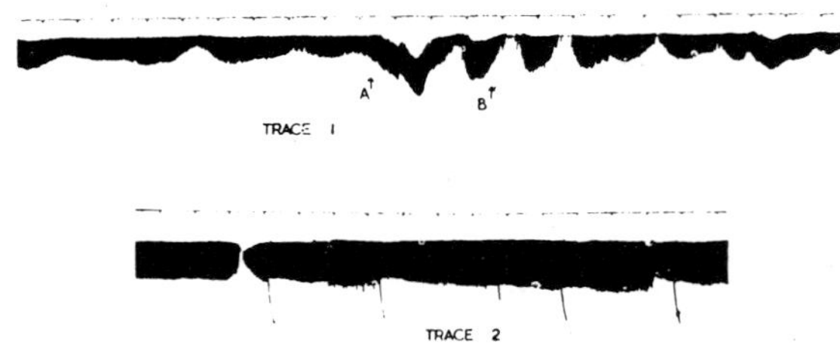


10

## Electrophysiological monitoring

Over the past 10 years much interest has arisen in monitoring of other electrophysiological parameters during surgery. Thus the observed relationship between the amplitude and latency of a primary somatosensory evoked response and the perfusion of the cortex, described as a threshold relationship by Branston *et al.*[18], gives insight into the adequacy of cerebral perfusion during carotid surgery, during hypotensive anaesthesia, or during transient occlusion of major cerebral arteries in aneurysm surgery[19].

Visual evoked responses may likewise be employed, light-emitting diode containing goggles being applied to the eyes during surgery on the visual pathways, the monitored parameter being the delay to the P100 wave induced either by anaesthesia or by manipulation of the pathways.

In the auditory system, continuous monitoring of brain-stem auditory evoked responses has been employed during decompression of cranial nerves in acoustic neuroma surgery or during surgery in the posterior fossa generally. Electrocochleography monitoring potentials in the cochlear and distal part of the acoustic nerve has also been used in an attempt to preserve hearing in the surgery of acoustic neuromas. The next decade is likely to see a considerable expansion in the use of electrophysiological monitoring, although at the present stage it remains confined to specialist units with particular interests.

## Auditory monitoring for air embolism

In the sitting position, the occurrence of a small air embolus need not necessarily be fatal, provided that prompt measures are taken to prevent the embolization of large volumes of air. One of the earliest signs is the presence of a slight irregularity on the respiratory trace. If air is detected at this stage, it may be possible by quickly lowering the patient's head to prevent a massive air embolus. Even with a small amount of air, auscultation over the precordium reveals a typical rhythmic crunching, as of footsteps in the snow. It has been suggested that auscultation from the oesophagus is more sensitive but, like all auscultatory procedures, it demands either intermittent attention on the part of the anaesthetist or a more complicated auditory amplification which will not be justified for routine use.

Many units now employ a precordial Doppler apparatus which will rapidly detect the presence of air in afferent veins to the heart. Experience is necessary in the use of this machinery, however, as minor incursions of air with no clinical significance are liable to evoke over-reaction in inexperienced hands.

## References


1. Risberg, J., Sundbarg, G. (1968) Regional cerebral blood volume during plateau waves. Acta Neurologica Scandinavica, 44, 252–255

2. Hewer, A. J. H., Logue, V. (1962) Methods of increasing the safety of neuroanaesthesia in the sitting position. Anaesthesia, 17, 476–481

3. Hewer, A. J. H., Logue, V., Symon, L. (1966) Respiratory recording in posterior fossa surgery. Proceedings of the Third International Congress on Neurological Surgery, pp. 828–832. Excerpta Medica Foundation

4. Alexander, S. C., Cohen, P. J., Woolman, H., Smith, J. C., Reivich, M., van der Molen, R. A. (1965) Cerebral carbohydrate metabolism during hypocarbia in man studies during nitrous oxide anaesthesia. Anesthesiology, 26, 624–632

5. Schettini, A. (1967) Hyperventilation in craniotomy in brain tumour. Anesthesiology, 28, 363–371

6. Cohen, P. J., Alexander, S. C., Woolman, H. (1968) Proceedings of the International Symposium on CSF and CBF. Scandinavian Journal of Clinical and Laboratory Investigation, Supplement 102, IV A

7. Brock, M. (1968) Regional cerebral blood flow (rCBF) changes following local brain compression in the cat. Proceedings of the International Symposium on CSF and CBF. Scandinavian Journal of Clinical and Laboratory Investigation, Supplement, 104, XIV A

8. Symon, L. (1969) The concept of intracerebral steal. In International Anesthesiology Clinics, vol. 7. Boston: Little, Brown

9. Javid, M. (1958) A valuable new method for the reduction of benign intracranial and intraocular pressure by the use of urea. Transactions of the American Neurological Association, 113

10. Wise, B. L. (1963) Effects of infusion of hypertonic mannitol on electrolyte balance and on osmolarity of serum and cerebrospinal fluid. Journal of Neurosurgery, 20, 961–967

11. Gordon, E., Rossanda, M. (1968) The importance of cerebrospinal fluid acid base status in the treatment of unconscious patients with brain lesions. Proceedings of the International Symposium on CSF and CBF. Scandinavian Journal of Clinical and Laboratory Investigation, Supplement 102, IX C

12. McDowall, D. S. G., Barker, J., Jennett, W. B. (1966) Cerebrospinal fluid pressure measurements during anaesthesia. Anaesthesia, 21, 189

13. Taylor, A. R., Bell, T. K. (1968) In: Blood Flow Through Organs and Tissues, p. 314. Edinburgh: Churchill Livingstone

14. Rose, A. L., Millac, P. (1965) The treatment of benign intracranial hypertension with frusemide. Journal of the Neurological Sciences, 3, 606–608

15. Kullberg, G. (1965) Influence of corticosteroids on the ventricular fluid pressure. Acta Neurologica Scandinavica, 14, Supplement 13, 445–452

16. Lundberg, N. (1960) Acta Psychiatrica at Neurologica Scandinavica, Supplement 149, 193 pp

17. Hekmatpanah, J., Mullan, S. (1967) Ventriculo-caval shunt in the management of posterior fossa. Journal of Neurosurgery, 26, 609–613

18. Branston, N. M., Symon, L., Crockard, H. A., Pasztor, E. (1974) Relationship between the cortical evoked potential and local cortical blood flow following acute middle cerebral artery occlusion in the baboon. Experimental Neurology, 45, 195–208

19. Wang, A. D., Cone, J., Symon, L., Costa e Silva, I. E. (1984) Somatosensory evoked potential monitoring during the management of aneurysmal subarachnoid hemorrhage. Journal of Neurosurgery, 60, 264–268

Illustrations by Barbara Hyams

# Burr holes, trephine and craniotomy

**R. D. Illingworth** FRCS
Consultant Neurosurgeon, Regional Neurosciences Centre, Charing Cross Hospital, London; Honorary Consultant Neurosurgeon, Westminster and Central Middlesex Hospitals, London, UK

## BURR HOLES

### Indications

Since CT scanning has become widely available there has rarely been a need to make exploratory burr holes in patients with head injury. The procedure is now used mainly for the drainage of chronic subdural haematomas, and for the biopsy of malignant cerebral tumours. Burr holes are also used to provide access for ventricular drainage, for intracranial pressure monitoring, and for drainage of deep cerebral abscesses and haematomas.

Burr hole and needle biopsy of a cerebral tumour is not a completely reliable way of obtaining a histological diagnosis and it may be preferable to explore through a craniotomy or trephine. However, this technique is generally indicated where the tumour lies deep, particularly if it is in the dominant hemisphere and there is no prospect of attempting to remove it. Intracerebral haematomas are often clotted and may be easier to remove through a trephine under direct vision.

### Anaesthesia

Burr holes may be made under local anaesthetic in conscious, cooperative adult patients and in unconscious patients who are not restless. A little premedication may be given to conscious patients to allay anxiety but heavy sedation should be avoided since the cooperation of the patient is essential.

In all other circumstances general anaesthesia with endotracheal intubation is necessary to prevent movement of the patient and to ensure a good airway. General anaesthesia is also essential if there is any possibility of proceeding from burr holes to craniotomy. In patients under general anaesthetic, spontaneous respiration may be maintained, unless the intracranial pressure is raised, when hyperventilation anaesthesia may be preferable. When local anaesthetic is used, only the skin need be anaesthetized since the bone is insensitive to pain and the dura nearly so. The skin is infiltrated along the line of the incision with 1 per cent lignocaine with or without adrenaline 1:200 000.

### Position of patient

Burr holes are generally made with the patient supine. In this position there is easy access to the front of the head on both sides. If access to the back of the head is required the operating table must be tilted head-up and the patient's head raised by flexing the neck to bring the back of the head as high as necessary. In the occasional head injury where burr holes without CT are indicated, the patient should be positioned in this way so that there is access to the whole of the skull vault except the occipital region and the posterior fossa. To explore the posterior fossa, the patient will need to be repositioned on the side, in the sitting position, or prone.

### Skin preparation and towelling

Where a single burr hole is to be made, the scalp should be shaved for at least 5 cm around the incision. Where exploratory burr holes are being made in patients with head injury, the whole scalp should be shaved to allow as many burr holes as are necessary to be made, and to allow burr holes to be converted into a craniotomy. It is advisable to shave and prepare the whole head even if the clinical signs indicate a unilateral lesion, so that both sides may be explored. The skin is cleaned using first an aqueous soapy solution to remove any dirt and skin debris and then with 0.5 per cent chlorhexidine in 70 per cent alcohol. The planned incisions for the burr holes should be marked with ink or by scratching the scalp with a scalpel. The prepared skin can be covered with an adhesive plastic drape or with fabric which may be soaked in antiseptic solution. The rest of the head is covered with sterile sheets.

# The operation

## 1

### The incision

The incision, which need only be about 2 cm long, is made by cutting right down onto the bone. A small self-retaining retractor is inserted and opened widely and this will generally control any skin bleeding. Any persistent bleeding should be controlled with diathermy, but this should be used sparingly near the skin edge. The pericranium is incised and scraped to each side with a small periosteal elevator.

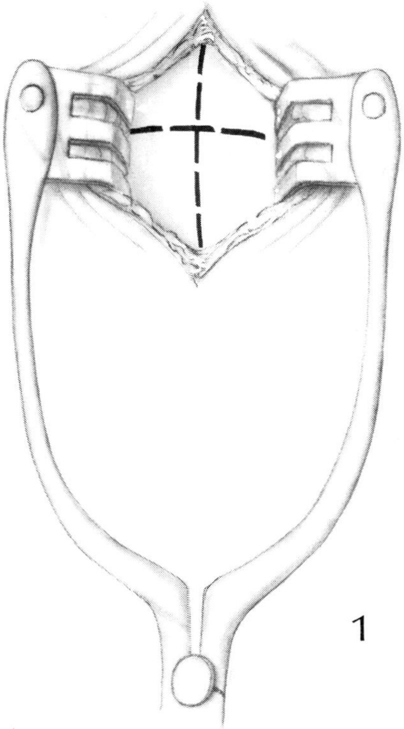

1

## 2a, b & c

### Cutting the burr hole

The burr hole is cut in two stages using a Hudson's brace. This is fitted first with a skull perforator, which is used until there is a small hole through the inner table (*a*). Care should be taken at this stage since the instrument can penetrate deeply into the brain if the bone gives way; pressure on the instrument should be made from the shoulder rather than with the weight of the body. The progress of the drilling can be checked from time to time and when the inner table is penetrated a slight change in the feel of the drill may be detected. Once the inner table has been penetrated the skull perforator is exchanged for a conical burr (*b*) or Soutar's drill (*c*) and the hole enlarged until it is parallel-sided. Care should be taken to avoid separating the dura from the bone around the burr hole since this may result in troublesome extradural venous bleeding. Bleeding from the bone is controlled with bone wax and extradural bleeding from under the bone may be stopped with oxidized cellulose or gelatin sponge. Bleeding from the dura is controlled with light diathermy.

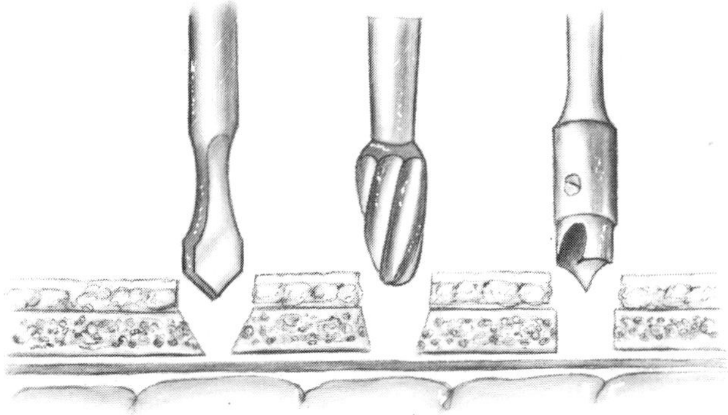

2a 2b 2c

## 3

### Opening the dura

If the dura is to be opened, it is elevated with a sharp hook and lightly incised with a small scalpel blade. Care must be taken to avoid injury to the underlying brain and its blood vessels. Once the initial opening is made it can be extended to a cruciate incision with scissors. Any bleeding from the edge of the dura is stopped with diathermy.

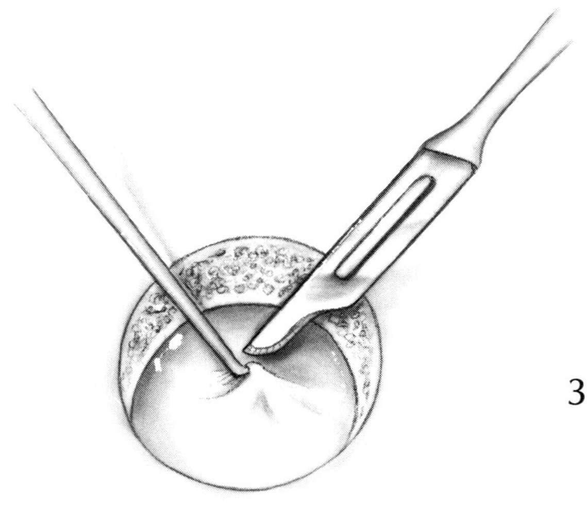

3

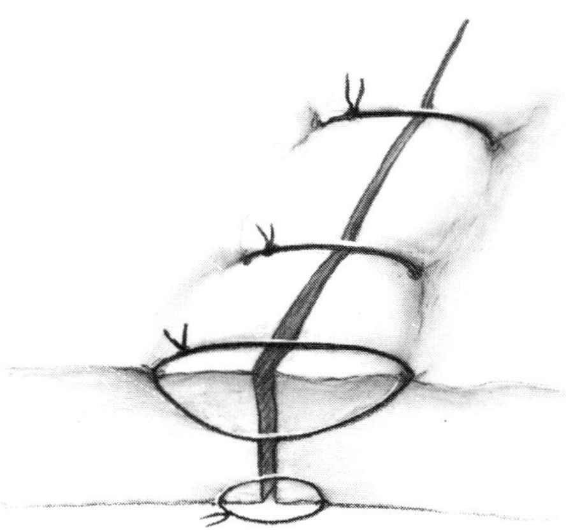

4

## 4

### Closure

When closing the incision, the dura is not sutured but is covered with gelatin sponge. The galea is closed with two or three interrupted sutures, the knots being buried and the ends cut short. The skin is closed with interrupted sutures which will control all but major bleeding. This method is preferable to excessive use of diathermy. The head may be dressed with a thick layer of gauze and wool held with bandages, but a small piece of gauze which just covers the sutures and is held in place with adhesive paper strips serves equally well.

# Postoperative care and complications

The sutures can be removed on the fifth day and normally the dressings need not be disturbed until that time. Complications after burr holes are rare. Intracranial haematoma is unusual unless bleeding from the dura or brain has not been stopped. Infection of the wound may have serious consequences if the dura has been opened since this can allow spread into the subdural space with abscess formation. Necrosis of the skin edge may occur if the skin sutures have been inserted too near together and tied too tightly.

# TREPHINE

### Indications

Generally this technique is used when a burr hole will not provide adequate access and yet the situation does not require the much wider exposure that a craniotomy can afford. Examples are the removal under direct vision of an intracerebral haematoma or the biopsy and removal of a cerebral glioma where the exact location is known and the limited exposure of a trephine can be chosen with confidence that it will be adequate. The procedure can also be used where the approach is necessarily limited to a narrow track in the brain. An example is a tumour in the third ventricle which can be explored through the foramen of Monro by frontal trephine, since a wide exposure of the cerebral cortex is no additional advantage. Trephine should not be used where wide exposure of the cortex may be required, as in the removal of a meningioma.

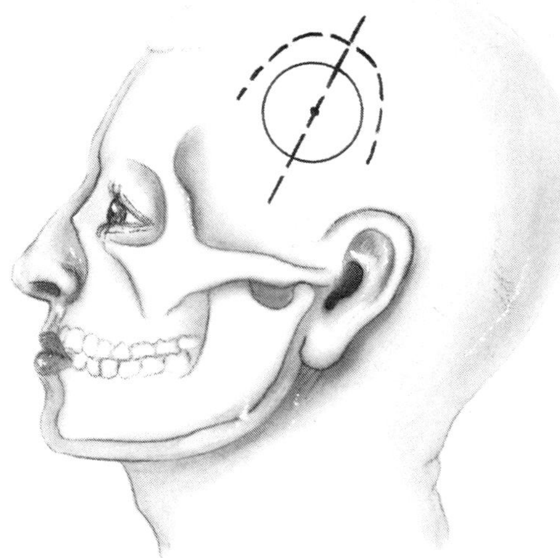

5

## The operation

### Surgical technique

## 5

The incision may be linear or a small flap. A linear incision will need to be longer than the diameter of the trephine and the skin margins will need to be widely retracted with a self-retaining retractor. Firm retraction will stop most skin bleeding and diathermy should be used sparingly near the skin edge.

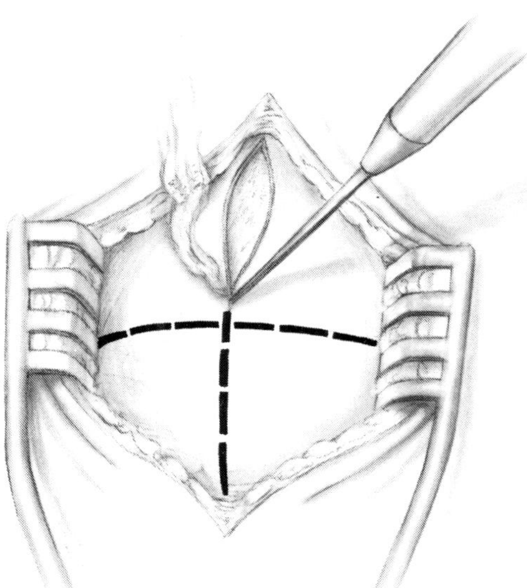

6

## 6

The pericranium is incised with diathermy and reflected from the skull with a periosteal elevator.

# 7a, b & c

Trephines come in graduated sizes of between 0.5 and 2 inches (13–51 mm) in diameter, the size being used depending on the exposure required. The bone disc is cut in three stages. First a small hole is drilled in the centre of the proposed disc using a guarded drill (*a*). Next the trephine, fitted with a centring pin which engages in the hole, is used to cut a circular groove (*b*). Once the cutting edge of the trephine will remain in the groove, the centring pin is removed, and the skull cut until the dura is exposed in at least part of the circumference, with the remainder of the bone being cut to almost full depth. At this point, the bone disc can be levered out without difficulty using a periosteal elevator (*c*). Bleeding from the bone is stopped with bone wax and any ragged bone edges should be trimmed from the bone disc or from the skull to allow the bone disc to fit when replaced. A small shelf of the inner table can be left to prevent the bone disc sinking in when replaced. Bleeding from the dura is stopped with diathermy.

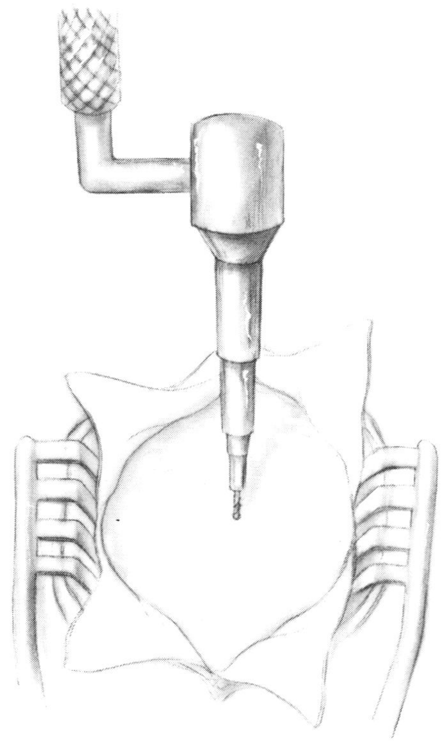

7a

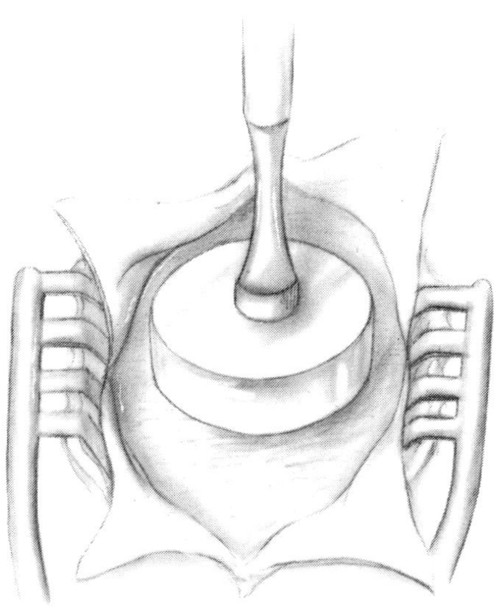

7b

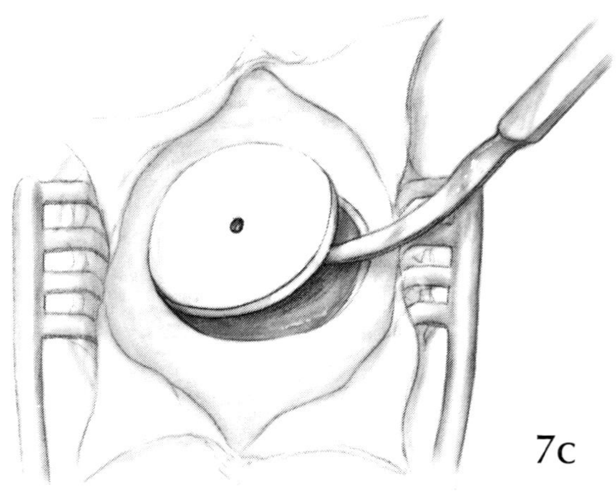

7c

# 8

The dura is opened by elevating the centre with a sharp hook and lightly incising it. The dura can then be opened in a cruciate incision using scissors, taking care not to cut the underlying brain or blood vessels. When closing, the dura should be brought together as far as possible with interrupted sutures and covered with gelatin sponge. The bone disc can be held by a suture from the centre of the dura passed through the drill hole in the bone and tied over a straightened haemostatic clip. The pericranium is drawn back over the bone and the incision closed in layers with interrupted sutures to the galea and to the skin. The dressing and postoperative management are as for a burr hole.

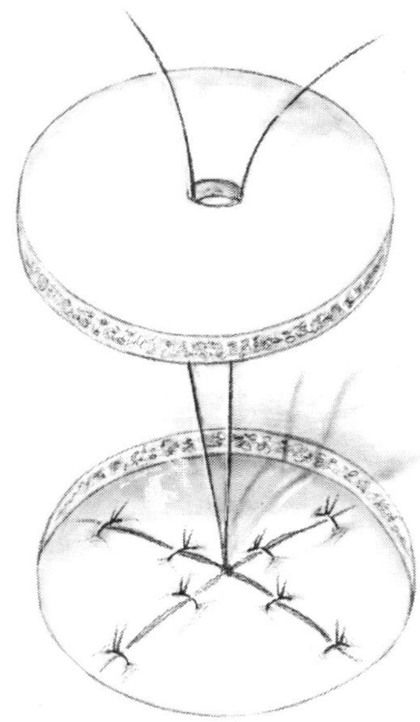

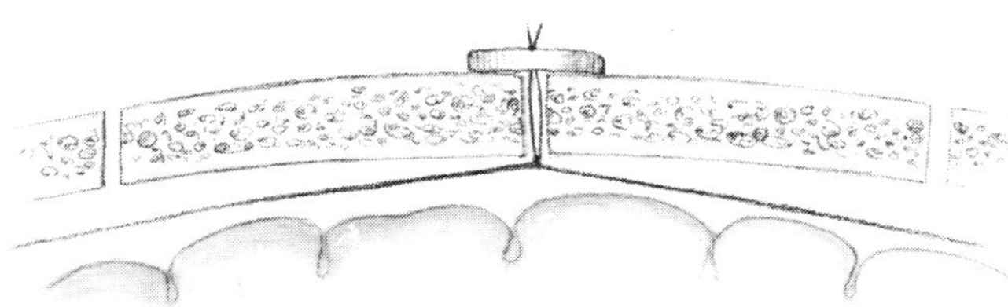

8

# CRANIOTOMY

## Preoperative

### Indications and contraindications

Craniotomy is indicated for the diagnosis or treatment of intracranial lesions demonstrated by neuroradiology where there is adequate clinical indication. With modern diagnostic facilities, truly exploratory procedures will rarely be needed.

Contraindications may be the nature of the lesion, the speed of progression of symptoms and also the patient's age and fitness. The few absolute contraindications include overwhelming infection or abnormalities of blood coagulation. Poor neurological condition of the patient need not be a contraindication, since surgical treatment of an intracranial mass will usually be required before improvement can occur.

When considering treatment of elderly people there may be a need to predict whether the patient is likely to benefit from operation. There may on occasion be a case for performing a lesser procedure such as biopsy, or advising against operation, and individual judgements will often be required.

### Premedication and anaesthesia

It is customary to use light non-sedative premedication for intracranial operations to allow patients to be assessed immediately before operation, and so that recovery of consciousness after operation is not delayed. Dexamethasone 4 mg 6-hourly started 24–48 hours before operation will often improve the neurological state of patients with intracranial tumours and appears to reduce the cerebral oedema which may follow operative manipulation of the brain.

Endotracheal intubation with hyperventilation, and hypotension if required, is standard practice for most craniotomies. This reduces intracranial pressure and brain bulk and allows easy manipulation of the brain, especially if preoperative dexamethasone has been given. Mannitol can be given to reduce brain bulk during the operation, but has the disadvantage of increasing blood volume and hence bleeding, and may mislead the surgeon about the extent of the decompression achieved in partial removal of gliomas.

Occasionally the reduction of brain bulk achieved by mannitol may be so great that cortical veins draining into the venous sinuses become torn and an acute subdural haematoma may result.

### Positioning the patient

Positioning the patient is discussed elsewhere. It is so important in making the planned procedure easier that the surgeon will wish to do this himself. In general the following apply.

1. The plane of the craniotomy should be approximately horizontal
2. The position of the head should allow any dissection at depth to be in the normal line of vision of the surgeon
3. The airway must be protected and venous drainage from the head not obstructed
4. Vulnerable points on the patient should be protected from pressure, either from the patient's weight or from fittings on the operating table

### Placement of skin incision

This, like the positioning of the patient, is crucial and any operation, however straightforward, may be made infinitely more difficult if the wrong skin incision, and consequently the wrong bone flap, is cut. The skin incision should be planned with three factors in mind: *(1)* surgical access to the lesion; *(2)* the skin blood supply; *(3)* the cosmetic effect of the scar.

#### *Craniotomy flaps*

In general craniotomy flaps fall into five main groups.

1. Flaps to expose the surface of the cerebral hemisphere
2. Flaps to expose the base of the brain
3. Flaps to expose the midline and medial surface of the cerebral hemisphere
4. Flaps for frontal or occipital lobectomy
5. Flaps for temporal exploration

# 9

*Flaps to expose the surface of the cerebral hemisphere* These should be centred on the lesion and made sufficiently large to allow adequate access with some margin for error. A semicircular or rectangular skin incision can be used. The width of the base of the flap should not be narrower than the widest point of the flap and the length of the flap should not exceed the width of the base. These flaps will generally be entirely behind the hair line, but if exposure anterior to this is required the skin flap should be based anteriorly with one limb of the incision on the midline.

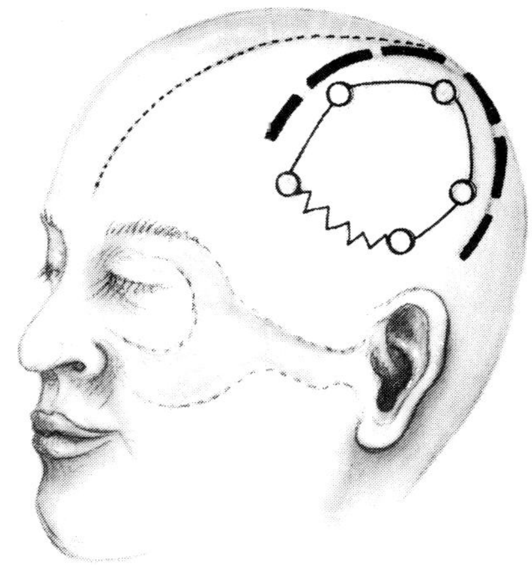

9

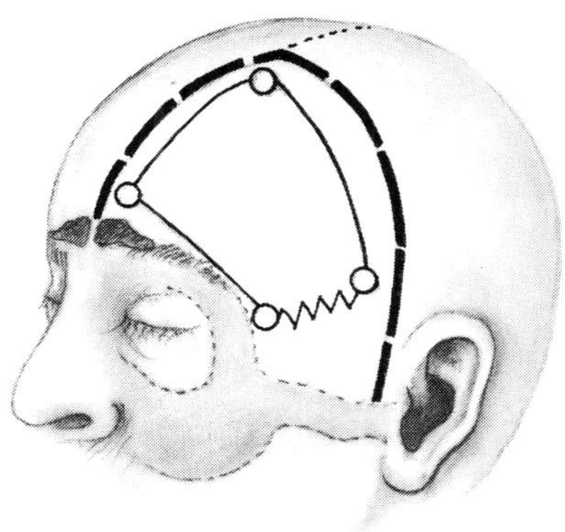

10a

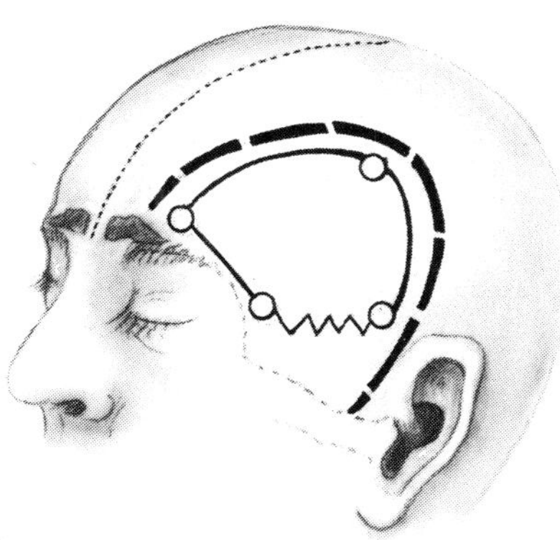

10b

# 10a & b

*Flaps to expose the base of the brain* These are required for the removal of basal tumours such as meningiomas and pituitary adenomas, and for the treatment of intracranial aneurysms. The skin incision used is generally a frontal (*a*) or frontotemporal (*b*) flap. The anterior limb of the flap may pass down the midline onto the forehead or run obliquely forward on the forehead near the midline. If only a small bone flap is required, such as for treating an aneurysm, it may be possible to avoid making a visible scar on the forehead by keeping the anterior part of the skin incision within the hair line and extending the incision medially. The forehead skin is then undermined and retracted towards the eye to allow the anterior burr hole to be placed low enough as in *Illustration 10b*. If bifrontal exposure is required a coronal skin incision is used, and this can also be used if a scar on the forehead is to be avoided. The skin flap need not be large but must be taken down to the level of the frontal sinus in the midline anteriorly and to the level of the zygomatic arch in the temporal region. The skin flap must be dissected down until the superior orbital margin can be seen, to allow the bone cut above the orbit to be made level with the floor of the anterior cranial fossa. This is essential if brain retraction is to be minimized. The anterior burr hole should be made just above the frontal sinus and a further burr hole made either on the outer end of the sphenoidal wing, as will be described for temporal craniotomy, or immediately anterior to this but level with the floor of the anterior cranial fossa. The bone flap need not include the temporal region unless this additional exposure is required.

# 11a & b

If large, the frontal sinus may be divided deliberately to improve access (*a*). If the mucosa is left intact, it need not be disturbed, but if the mucosa of the sinus is opened it must be completely removed from the upper part of the sinus within the bone flap and the hole into the sinus closed with a piece of temporalis fascia held with sutures through dura and pericranium (*b*). It may be advisable in this circumstance not to use high vacuum suction drainage beneath the skin flap to avoid sucking through from the nose.

If a burr hole has been made on or posterior to the lesser sphenoidal wing, this may be rongeured away further to improve access.

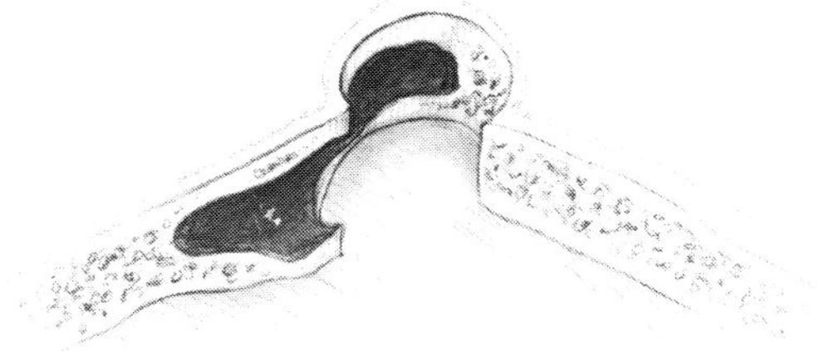

11a

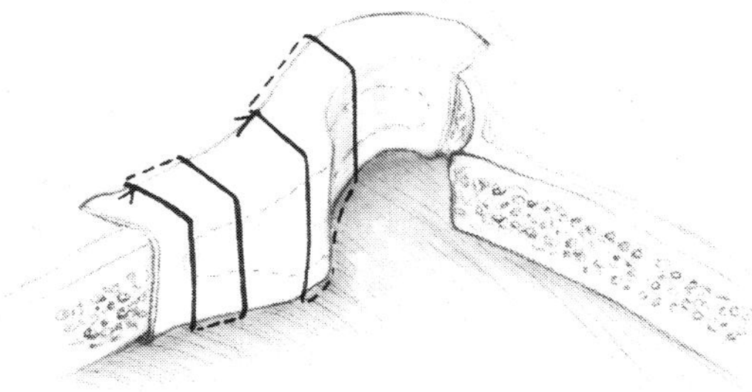

11b

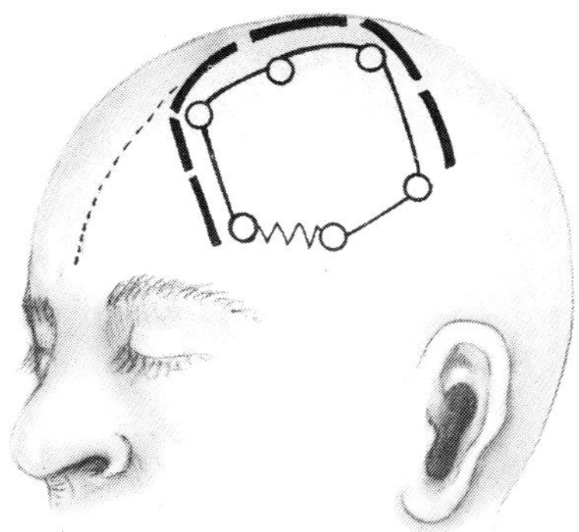

12

# 12

*Midline flaps* These are used for parasagittal and falx meningiomas and for pericallosal aneurysms. For these the midline limb of both the skin and bone flaps should be made precisely on the midline, since even a small overhang of bone may add considerably to the operative difficulties. There is generally some venous bleeding when the dura is separated from the bone at the midline although with modern anaesthesia this is usually not excessive. There may, however, be considerable bleeding if there is a parasagittal or falx meningioma and it is advisable to leave the midline bone cuts until last when turning such a flap. Some difficulty may be experienced anteriorly where there may be a sharp ridge of bone continuing up the midline from the base of the skull. The dura may be torn if power tools are used at this point and the most anterior frontal burr hole is most conveniently cut by hand.

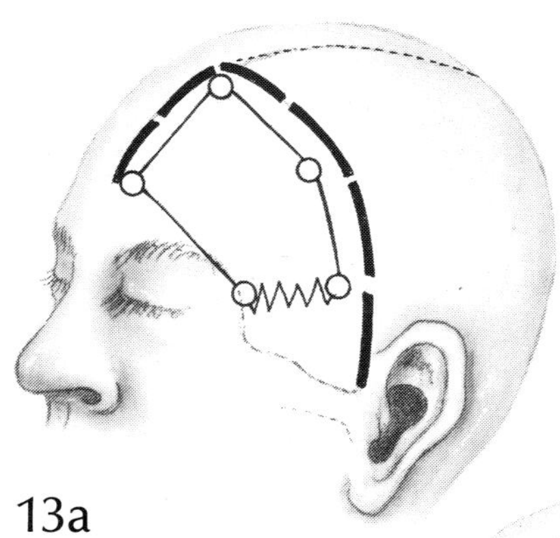

13a

# 13a & b

*Flaps for frontal (a) and occipital (b) lobectomy* These must extend up to the midline and also down to the base of the skull for lobectomy to be easily achieved. Flaps which do not reach the midline cause difficulty with the most medial part of the dissection, and flaps which do not reach the base of the skull similarly cause difficulty with the cut across the orbital surface of the frontal lobe or the tentorial surface of the occipital lobe. The skin incision should therefore pass from anteriorly or, in the case of an occipital flap, from posteriorly, up the midline and then turn down to the anterior or posterior temporal region. These flaps are a combination of basal and midline exposures.

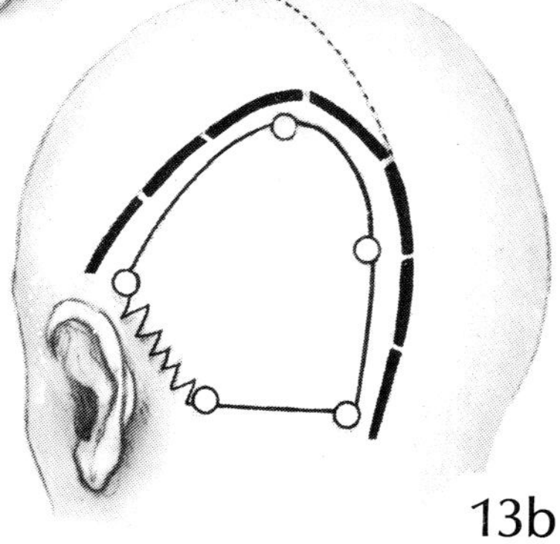

13b

# 14a & b

*Flaps for temporal exploration* These must be planned to expose as much of the temporal lobe as possible or the exposure will prove to be more parietal than temporal. Two types of incision may be used. In type one, the incision is started on the zygomatic arch, immediately in front of the ear so that the superficial temporal artery is preserved. It then curves upwards and forwards and passes obliquely across the forehead near the midline (*a*). The incision must be made low enough at each end to allow the skin flap to be turned down to expose the outer end of the lesser sphenoidal wing. Type two starts on the zygomatic arch 1 cm in front of the tragus of the ear so that it lies anterior to the superficial temporal artery. The incision runs forward in a low curve to a point no less than 2 cm above the outer end of the eyebrow and then curves upwards and backwards to pass back behind the ear. This incision allows a little anterior flap to be dissected downwards and so improves the exposure anteriorly, and it can be taken as far posteriorly as necessary (*b*). If the incision is taken lower than 2 cm above the outer end of the eyebrow the frontal branch of the facial nerve may be cut, with unsightly paralysis of the frontalis muscle. Care must be taken to preserve the superficial temporal artery and not to make the anterior curve of the flap too acute or ischaemic necrosis of the most anterior part of the flap may result. The incision must not go below the zygomatic arch or the facial nerve may be cut.

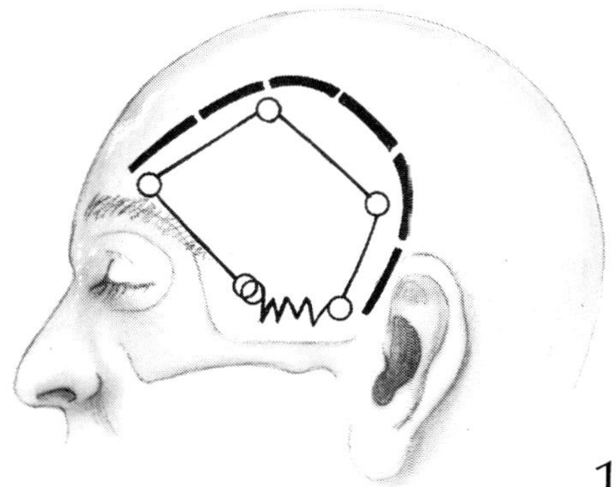

14a

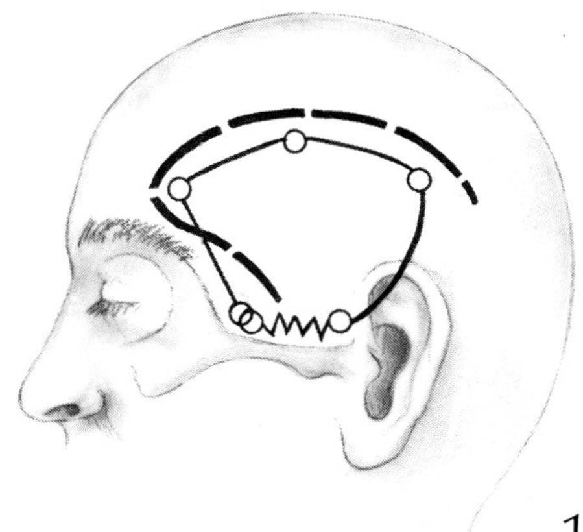

14b

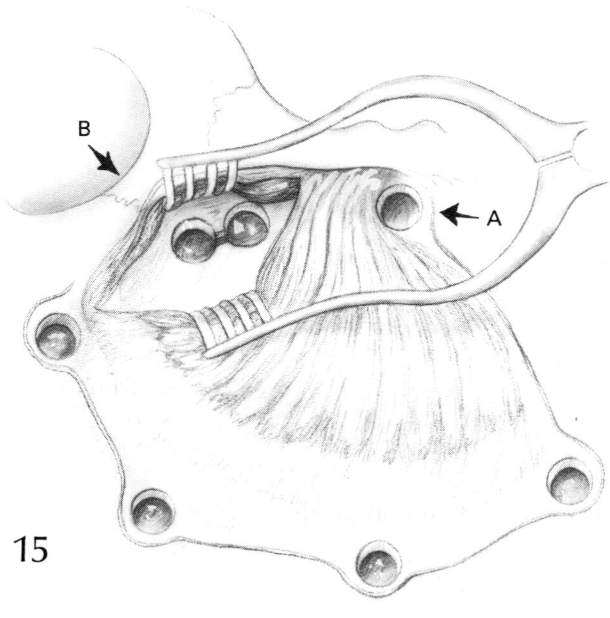


15

# 15

In both these exposures the temporalis muscle is incised, posteriorly down to the level of the zygomatic arch and anteriorly from just above the orbital margin deep into the anterior part of the muscle to expose the external groove on the temporal bone which indicates the position of the lesser sphenoidal wing. The burr holes made at these points are the keys to the exposure. Posteriorly the burr hole must be made as low as possible onto the floor of the middle fossa (A). Anteriorly the exposure can be improved if a double burr hole is made on the lesser sphenoidal wing (B). The drill is directed anteriorly into the anterior cranial fossa, and posteriorly and inferiorly into the middle cranial fossa. This will often leave a ridge of the lesser sphenoidal wing in between and this may be nibbled through with bone forceps. If the anterior burr hole is made lower, the orbit may easily be entered. The sphenoidal wing may be nibbled away and the exposure generally needs to be extended anteriorly by nibbling bone away from the front and the anterior part of the lateral wall of the middle cranial fossa. The bulk of the temporalis muscle may obscure the exposure here and the bone flap and muscle can be retracted with a large self-retaining retractor.

# The operation

## Skin preparation and towelling

The patient, having first been positioned and the flap planned, has the scalp cleaned, first with a dilute aqueous solution of chlorhexidine and cetrimide and then with chlorhexidine 0.5 per cent in 70 per cent methylated spirit. The skin incision is marked with ink or a skin scratch and the line of the incision may be infiltrated with adrenaline 1:200 000. The head is covered with an adhesive plastic drape or with fabric which may be soaked in antiseptic solution. Sheets are placed around and held with towel clips. A table over the patient is useful to place instruments on and to lift the sheets off the patient so that the anaesthetist has access. This overtable and the rest of the patient may be covered with a large sheet which leaves only the operative site exposed.

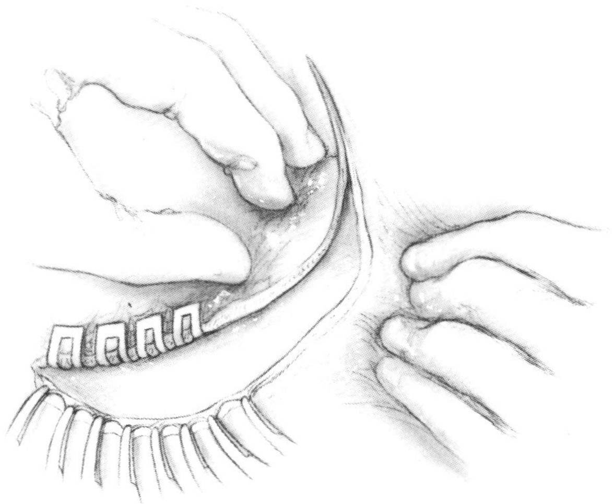

16

# 16

## Skin incision and haemostasis

The incision is made in short lengths through both skin and galea, the bleeding being controlled initially by pressure from the surgeon's and assistant's fingers. Bleeding on the side of the flap is stopped with Raney clips and on the side of the scalp by applying curved artery forceps to the galea. The weight of the forceps, which are gathered into groups with rubber bands, is generally sufficient to stop most bleeding. Artery forceps may be applied to the scalp flap instead of Raney clips but the extra bulk tends to be cumbersome. When the incision has been made all round, the scalp flap is elevated from the underlying pericranium by gentle sharp dissection. Bleeding from the deep surface of the scalp or from the pericranium is stopped with diathermy and the flap is then covered with damp gauze.

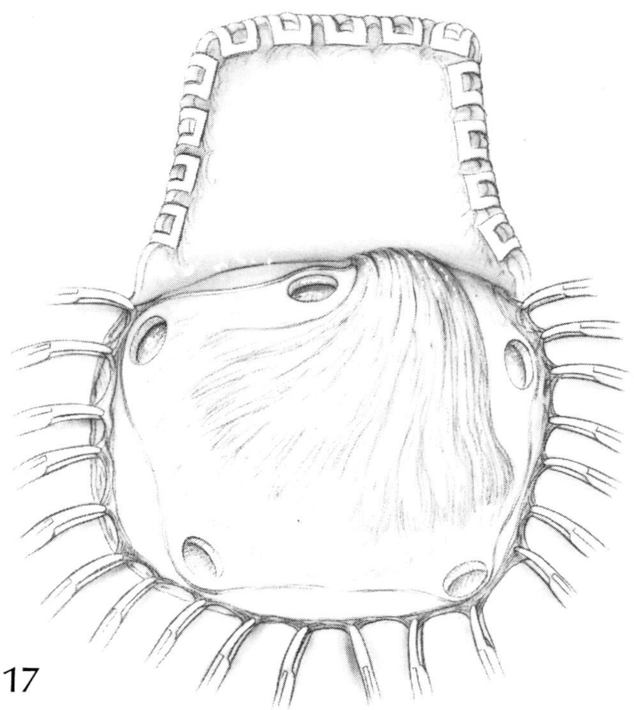

17

## Cutting the bone flap

# 17

The pericranium and muscle are incised with cutting diathermy in the line of the intended bone flap except inferiorly where a pedicle of pericranium or temporalis muscle is left uncut to allow some blood supply to the bone to remain. Alternatively, the pericranium and muscle may be detached completely from the intended bone flap but this generally produces little advantage in the exposure and the completely detached bone flap may be absorbed after replacement. The pericranium is reflected with a broad periosteal elevator and the temporalis muscle held back with self-retaining retractors. The bone flap is cut using either hand instruments or power tools.

By hand, the flap is cut by making a series of burr holes about 6 or 7 cm apart. The burr holes will need to be nearer together if the bone is very thick or the dura very adherent. Using gentle dissection with a blunt curved Adson periosteal elevator, the dura is separated from the bone between the burr holes. Some difficulty may be experienced in this, particularly in older patients, and care should be taken to keep the tip of the instrument against the bone to avoid tearing the dura.

# 18a & b

The cuts between the burr holes are made using a Gigli saw which is passed between the burr holes using the malleable saw guide (*a*). The cuts are made with a steady sawing motion with handles attached to the ends of the saw and the surgeon's hands well separated (*b*). The angle of the cut should be bevelled outwards to allow the bone flap to rest on the surrounding skull when replaced.

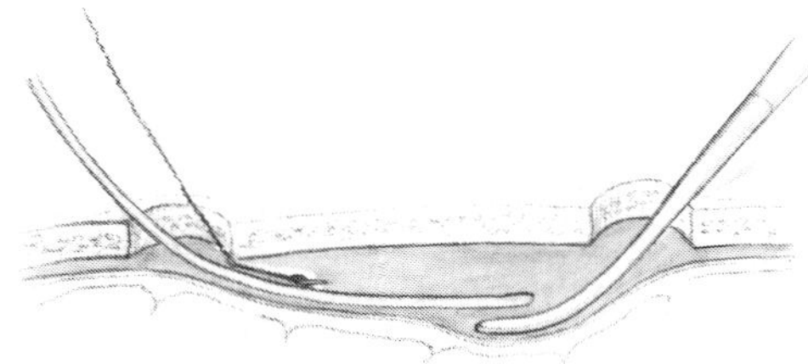

18a

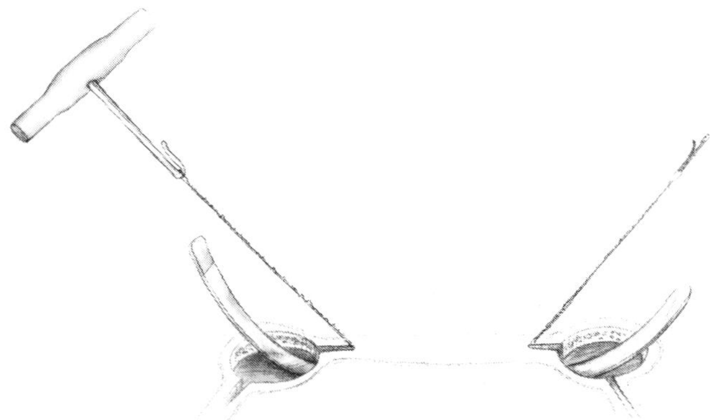

18b

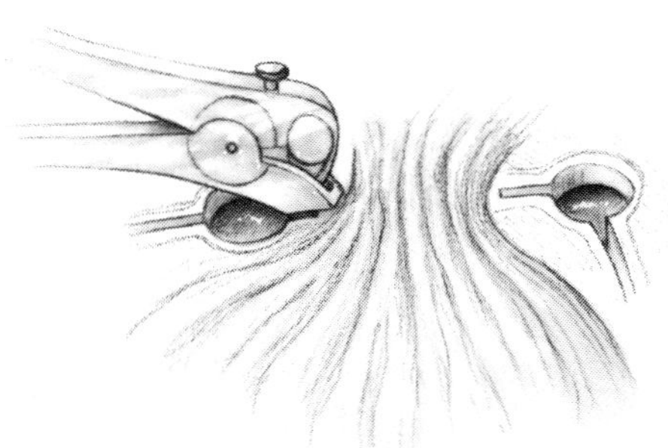

19

# 19

At the base of the flap the cut is not made with a saw but by cutting between the burr holes, using the de Vilbis bone forceps until the remaining bridge of bone is weak enough to break easily when the flap is elevated.

# 20

The flap is elevated by levering it upwards with two Horsley's elevators, carefully separating the dura from the bone as this is done. If the base of the flap has been made narrow enough the bone should break straight between the burr holes.

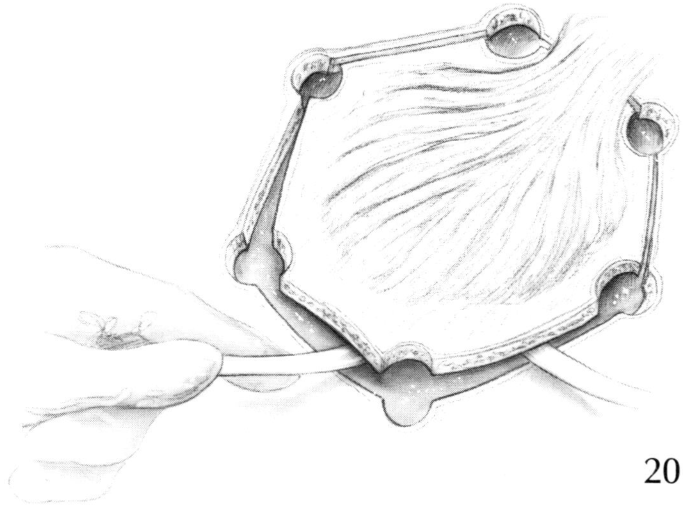

20

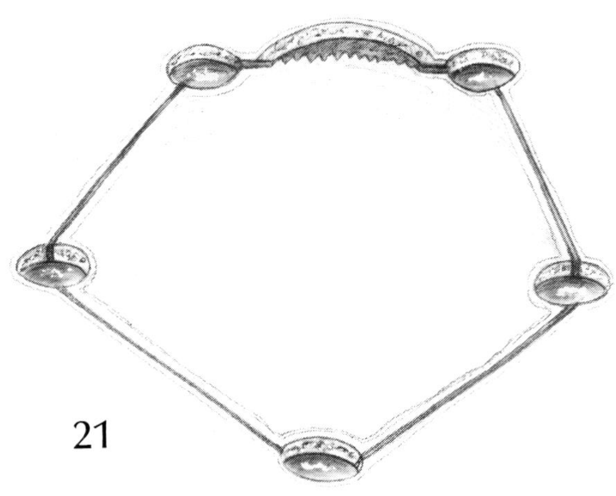

21

# 21

A little bone must be trimmed from the skull side of the fracture to allow the bone flap to fit when replaced, but subtemporal decompression is rarely required.

The disadvantage of this method is that it may be very slow and laborious if the bone is thick and dense.

# 22

Alternatively, the bone flap may be cut using power tools. Only two burr holes may be necessary at the base of the flap and these are cut using the skull perforator attachment of the drill.

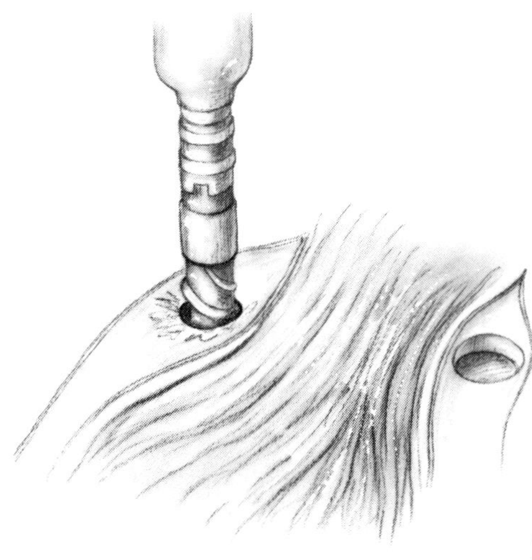

22

# 23

The dura is then separated from the bone at the burr holes and a large bone flap may then be rapidly cut using the dural guard and the cutting blade.

If the burr holes at the base of the flap have not been made close together, the bony bridge can be narrowed using de Vilbis forceps or the power drill. The technique is a very rapid way of cutting a bone flap, but the dura may be extensively lacerated if it does not separate easily from the inner table and this may cause major difficulties if the sagittal sinus or large veins draining into it are damaged. There may also be difficulty if the bone is irregular as it may be near the base of the skull, and the dural guard may catch. The channel cut by the power drill tends to be rather broad and a small bone flap may need to be held by sutures through drill holes if it is not to become depressed. In general the power drill is most suitable for cutting large convexity bone flaps where the dura can be separated easily rather than those near the midline or the base of the skull. As a compromise, since cutting the burr holes is the most laborious part of the procedure, these can be made with the power drill and the cuts between made by hand using Gigli's saws. If the bone flap is to be held in place with sutures at the end of the operation the drill holes necessary to do this should be made at this stage. The bone flap should be held up by hand away from the brain as this is done. Three or four holes should be made at intervals close to the edge of the bone flap. Corresponding drill holes are made in the skull while the underlying brain is protected with a broad brain retractor or similar instrument. The drill holes in the centre of the bone flap should also be made at this stage (*see Illustrations 26a, b and c*).

The bone flap is wrapped in damp gauze and held away from the area with towel clips or a self-retaining retractor.

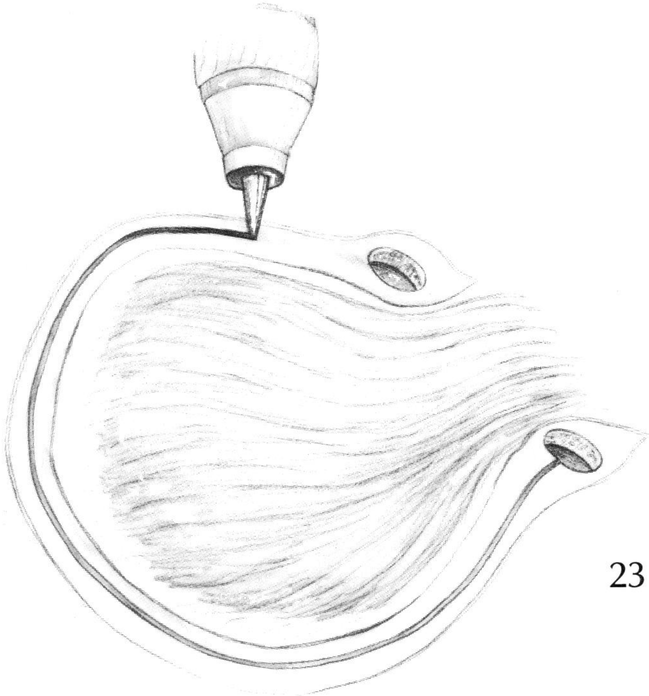

23

## Extradural haemostasis

Bleeding from the cut edge of the bone is stopped with bone wax. Bleeding vessels on the dura are lightly coagulated with diathermy and venous bleeding which may be troublesome near the midline or at the base of the skull is controlled with gelatin sponge which is held in place with gentle pressure. The sutures which will hold the bone flap at the end of the operation are now placed through the drill holes in the skull and the ends held with artery forceps. Wire can be used but heavy polyglactin 910 is now preferred.

# 24

Duropericranial sutures are next inserted all round the edge of the bone to hold the dura up to the inner table of the skull to prevent a postoperative extradural haematoma developing. The sutures, which are placed right against the cut edge of the bone, just pass through the dura so as to avoid piercing the brain, and are tied through the adjacent pericranium or muscle. The sutures are generally not inserted at the midline or over the transverse sinus.

Major meningeal vessels may be underrun and tied by the sutures and this will markedly reduce the bleeding from a convexity or parasagittal meningioma. Care should be taken not to detach the dura beyond the edges of the bone flap since this may result in an extradural haematoma developing postoperatively beyond the limits of the exposure. This is a risk where a self-retaining brain retractor is attached to the edge of the bone. Good extradural haemostasis should be achieved before the dura is opened to avoid the field becoming obscured by blood running in from outside. The skin and bone edges are covered with strips of moistened lintine and wound towels are applied before the dura is opened.

24

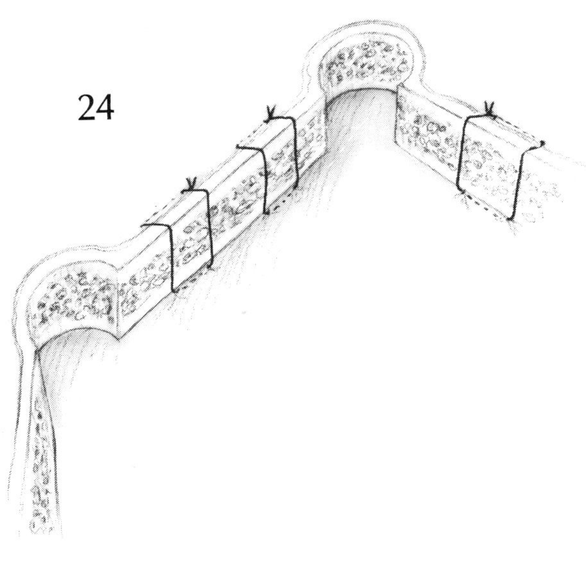

# 25a–d

## Opening the dura

The dura is opened by elevating it with a sharp hook and lightly incising it with a scalpel. Care must be taken, particularly when intracranial pressure is raised, to avoid injuring the underlying brain. Once the initial opening is made, the incision may be extended as required using scissors with rounded ends. The dura may be opened with a flap (*a*) or a straight incision which may be extended with side cuts (*b*). Straight incisions have the advantage of being easier to make and close, and when the intracranial pressure is raised the dura may be opened with a straight incision over the tumour to avoid problems with bulging brain. Once sufficient tumour has been removed to lower the pressure, the dura may be opened more widely. Straight incisions allow inspection of the operative site to check haemostasis until a late stage of the dural closure.

Dural flaps are based towards the midline to avoid injury to large cortical veins which often run from the brain onto the dura at some distance from the sagittal sinus. Dural incisions should not be taken too near the bone edge since this may cause difficulty with closure. Straight incisions are generally more convenient in the temporal region, where the dura may be opened in a Y-shaped incision with side cuts (*c*), and for basal exploration, where a low curved incision which extends down to the bone edge at each end is adequate (*d*). Bleeding from the edge of the dura is stopped by haemostatic clips. Monopolar diathermy should be avoided since it causes the dura to shrink. Once opened, the dura is retracted with sutures weighted with artery forceps to hold it out of the way.

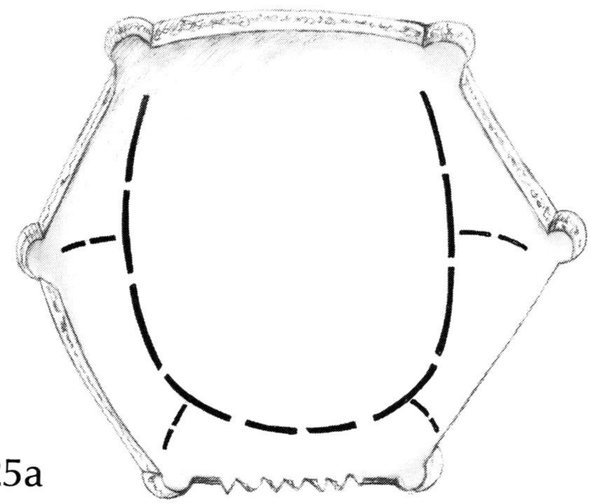

25a

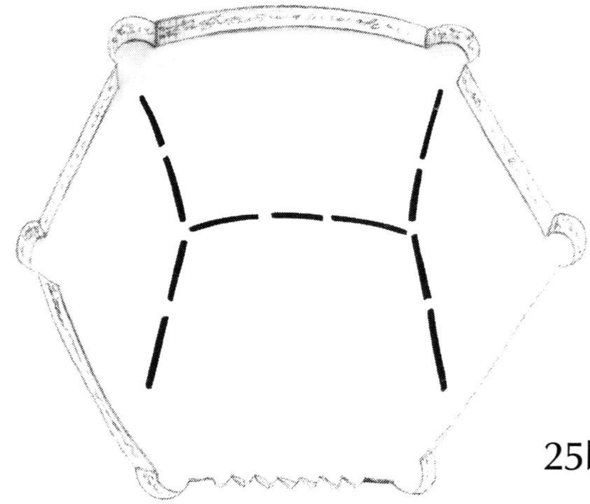

25b

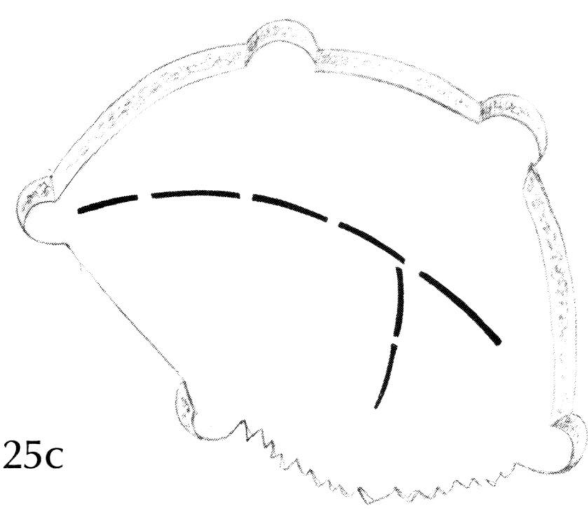

25c

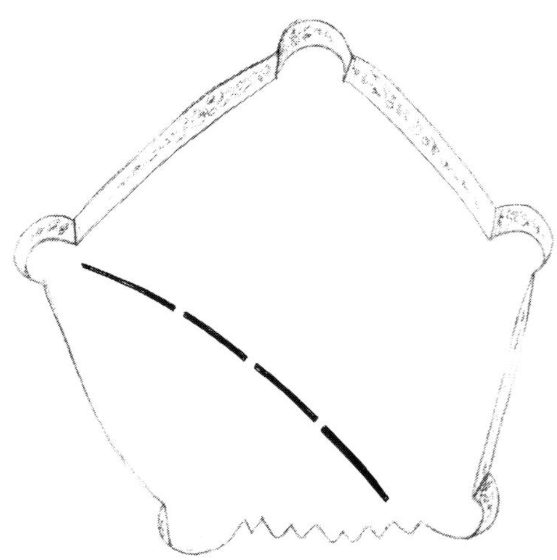

25d

## Closing the dura

Before closing the dura it is advisable to confirm absolute haemostasis at the operative site by elevating the blood pressure to at least normal and by returning the arterial $P\mathrm{CO}_2$ to normal if hyperventilation anaesthesia has been used. The anaesthetist may be asked to compress the jugular veins in the neck to confirm that no veins are open. The dura may be closed with interrupted sutures or by a continuous suture. If the dura cannot be closed because of raised intracranial pressure it is advisable to leave it widely open to prevent herniation and strangulation of the brain through a narrow opening. The unsutured dura can be laid back over the brain and the brain covered with sheets of gelatin sponge. Where the dura has been torn while cutting the bone flap, it may be closed as far as possible and any defects covered with sheets of gelatin sponge.

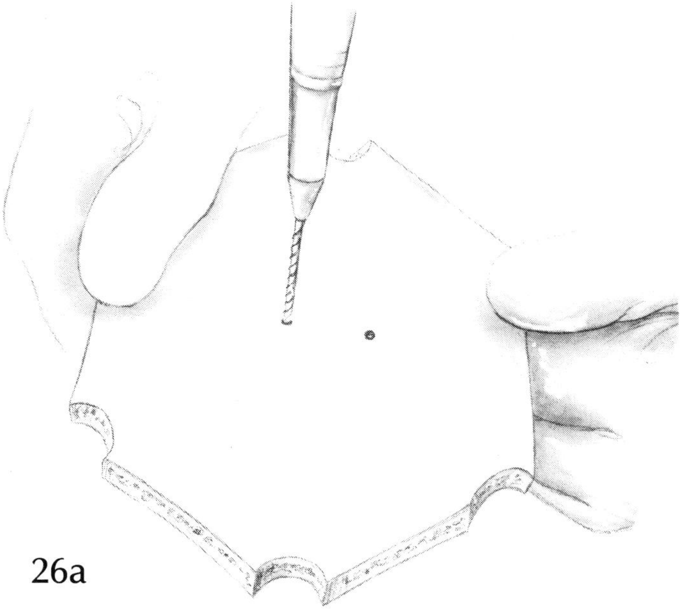

26a

# 26a, b & c

In addition to the sutures already inserted between the dura and the pericranium, one or more sutures can be used to hold up the dura to the bone flap. These are inserted by making a drill hole in the bone flap (*a*). The bone flap is laid back into the opening and a mark made on the dura with light diathermy by passing a brain needle stilette through the hole in the bone (*b*). A suture is placed through the dura at this point and passed through the drill hole and tied over a straightened haemostatic clip when the bone flap is replaced (*c*). Alternatively two drill holes can be made about 0.5 cm apart and the ends of the suture passed through the holes and tied on the surface of the bone. For a small bone flap one such suture is sufficient but if larger, two or more may be required.

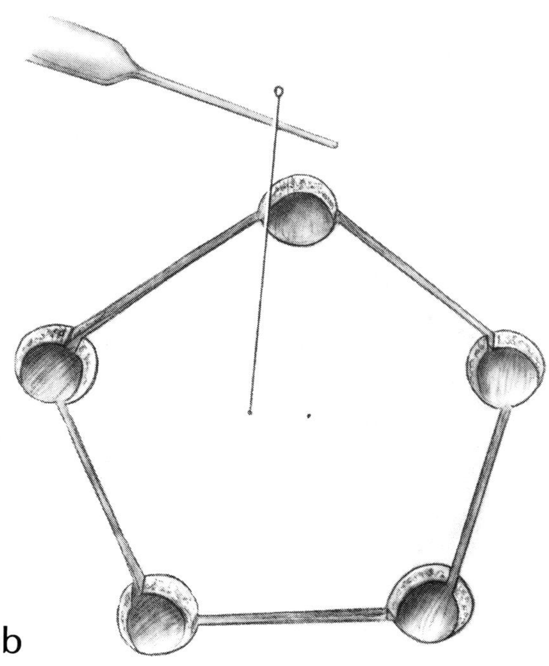

26b

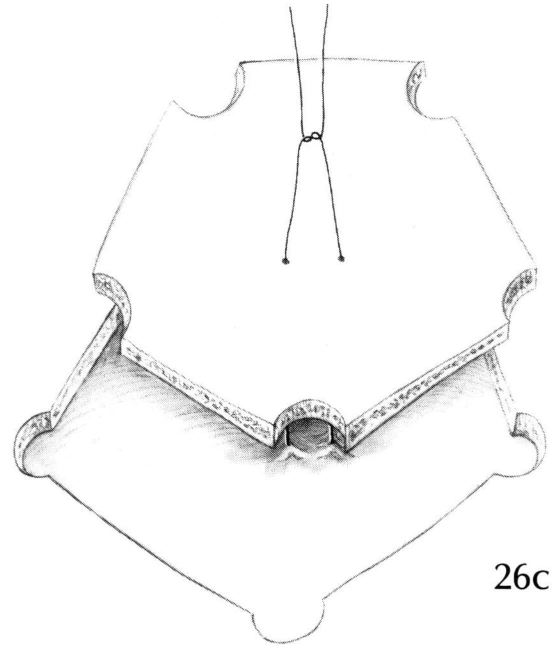

26c

# 27

The bone flap is held in place by interrupted sutures through the pericranium and muscle.

Alternatively, drill holes may be made and sutures used as described earlier (*see Section 23*). If the bone flap is partly in front of the hair line, fixation should start anteriorly so that an accurate fit is obtained in an area where any irregularity may be visible. For the same reason any burr holes that lie anterior to the hair line should be filled with bone dust to prevent unsightly dents developing. If the thick muscle in the anterior part of the temporal region has been incised, the deep part as well as the superficial part should be closed with a few interrupted sutures to avoid subsequent development of an unsightly groove.

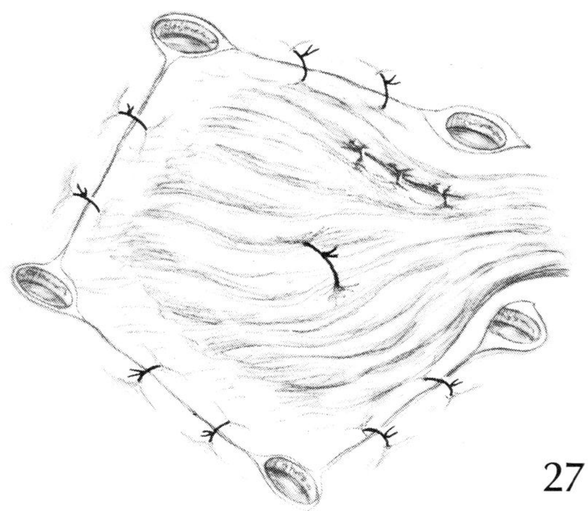

27

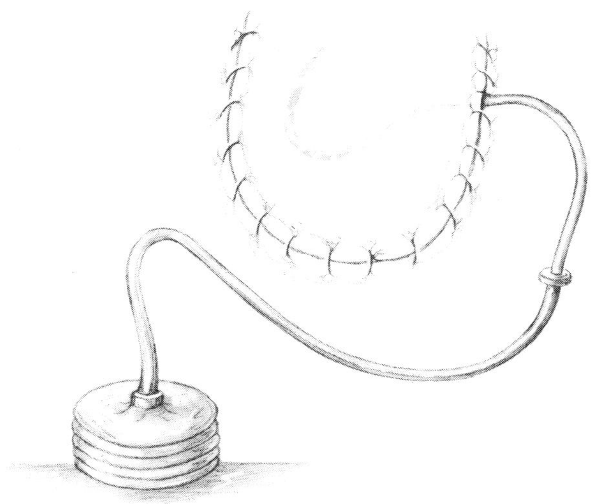

28a

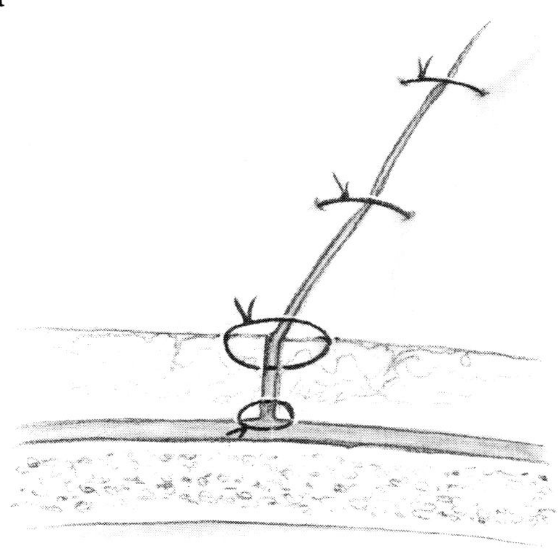

28b

# 28a & b

A suction drainage tube may be introduced through the skin outside the line of the incision and connected to a vacuum bottle to prevent subcutaneous haematoma developing (*a*). The incision is closed in two layers using interrupted sutures with buried knots through the galea, and interrupted sutures, which do not pass through the galea, or metal staples, for the skin (*b*).

### Dressing and wound care

Conventionally the head may be covered with many layers of cotton gauze held in place with crêpe bandages, but alternatively narrow strips of gauze held in place with adhesive paper strips to cover just the skin incisions may be used. The suction drainage tube may be removed after 24 hours and although this will prevent much of the facial bruising and swelling that occurs after frontal craniotomy, some swelling may develop on the day following removal of the drain. If this drainage is not used blood will tend to collect under the flap and may require aspiration using a wide-bore needle. Even this will generally not prevent marked bruising and swelling of the eyes developing after a frontal or temporal craniotomy and infection may be introduced. Where the skin incision has been closed in two layers as described, the skin sutures may be removed at between 2 and 5 days postoperatively, according to preference.

## Postoperative care

Ideally the patient should be extubated without straining or coughing occurring and yet should rapidly regain consciousness to allow early assessment. Considerable anaesthetic skill is required to achieve this ideal since if patients are allowed to become lightly anaesthetized towards the end of the procedure, they may move when the skin sutures are inserted and cough or strain when the endotracheal tube is removed. In general, patients are nursed supine with the same degree of head-up tilt as was used for the operation. The blood pressure tends to rise as the patients regain consciousness and they may then sit up further. Observations of pulse, blood pressure, respiration, consciousness level and neurological signs are made at 15-minute intervals and recorded during the early postoperative phase. If the patient's postoperative course is satisfactory and the condition is stable, the frequency of the observations may be reduced to half-hourly after a few hours, but it is inadvisable to reduce the frequency of the observations further during the first 24 hours. The purpose of the observations is to detect any deterioration which may be due to the development of a postoperative intracranial haematoma, although such an event should nowadays be rare if the steps described under extradural haemostasis have been followed and the blood pressure elevated to normal before closure. If deterioration occurs, suggesting the development of a postoperative haematoma, the patient will need to be returned to the operating room promptly for re-exploration, since a haematoma is a serious complication which may result in the patient's death or survival with severe disability. Postoperative sedation is not used lest the assessment of consciousness level is obscured, and strong analgesics are not generally required. There is no evidence that antibiotics are helpful in preventing wound infection in clean uncomplicated operations. The stage at which the patient gets out of bed depends on the progress and the surgeon's preference. When progress is satisfactory, patients may sit out of bed on the second postoperative day. Dexamethasone, if given to cover the procedure, should be rapidly reduced, starting on the first or second postoperative day, and discontinued within 1 week. If this is not done major gastrointestinal problems, such as perforation or bleeding, may occur.

Illustrations by Barbara Hyams

# Head injuries

**G. M. Teasdale** FRCP, FRCS(Ed), FRCS(Glas)
Professor and Head of Department of Neurosurgery, University of Glasgow, Institute of Neurological Sciences, The Southern General Hospital, Glasgow, UK

**S. Galbraith** MD, FRCS
Formerly Consultant Neurosurgeon, University of Glasgow, Institute of Neurological Sciences, The Southern General Hospital, Glasgow, UK

## Introduction

The aims of early treatment of the head-injured patient are the following.

1. To ensure the best conditions for recovery from any primary brain damage sustained at the time of the injury.
2. To prevent any secondary brain damage resulting from complications of the injury. *Intracranial complications* leading to secondary damage that may need operation are intracranial haematoma and any open injury of the vault or base of the skull. *Extracranial complications* are very common causes of secondary brain damage after high speed injuries, for example, road traffic accidents. Overall, one-third of head injuries admitted to hospital have another injury.

# Preoperative management

## Diagnosis

Diagnosis can be difficult after a head injury. It is necessary to answer three questions. (*1*) Has the patient indeed suffered a head injury, and if so what degree of brain damage has already been sustained? (*2*) Is there evidence of threatened or developing damage from secondary complications? (*3*) Is there *only* a head injury? When there is doubt, the finding of a skull fracture, either clinically or by X-ray, can confirm that the patient has sustained a head injury and will also indicate an increased risk of complications.

## Assessing brain damage

The level of consciousness is the best index of the initial effect of the injury upon the brain. Changes in consciousness are also the best guide to the rate of recovery or to the development of complications.

It is now widespread practice to assess consciousness in neurosurgical patients using the Glasgow coma scale. This is based upon a separate assessment of three aspects of responsiveness: (*1*) the stimulus needed to make the patient open his or her eyes, (*2*) the best verbal response, and (*3*) the best motor response. These can be assessed quickly and reliably and can be recorded regularly to provide a clear picture of the patient's progress (*see Table 1*). Focal neurological signs such as differences in the movement of the limbs or changes in response of the pupils are also important, but usually develop later than changes in consciousness.

## Extracranial injuries

There are great dangers in overlooking serious extracranial complications, and this is a particular risk in patients with impaired consciousness. It is essential that extracranial problems are known before embarking upon an operation on the head. Life-threatening extracranial complications take precedence over performance of intracranial surgery.

It is necessary to establish and secure a clear airway (in the case of injuries to the face and jaws), to ensure adequate oxygenation (where ventilation and gas exchange in the lungs may be impaired by chest injuries), and to maintain adequate cardiac output. Hypotension is rarely due to a head injury and is usually a sign of concealed extracranial bleeding. Failure to replenish the blood volume can lead to a catastrophic fall in blood pressure during operation, particularly after cerebral compression is relieved. Cervical spinal injuries should also be excluded before anaesthesia.

## Prognosis

The likelihood of a poor outcome can be a factor in deciding whether or not to operate on an unconscious patient. The more profound and prolonged the depression of consciousness, and the older the patient, the less good are the prospects for recovery. On the other hand, decisions about operation should not be taken before effective initial resuscitation. General guidelines are not appropriate, but we have not seen recovery from evacuation of a supratentorial haematoma in a patient with established apnoea.

## Anaesthesia for head injuries

An almost invariable rule is that the patient should be intubated, paralysed and ventilated in order to secure the airway and to ensure adequate oxygenation throughout the operation. A large-bore intravenous cannula should be inserted for administration of fluids, and arrangements instituted for cross-matching of blood. The need for transfusion may be sudden if replacement after extracranial bleeding has been inadequate. In a child, shock may result simply from the reflection of a scalp flap and the evacuation of a haematoma.

**Table 1 Institute of Neurological Sciences, Glasgow. Observation chart**

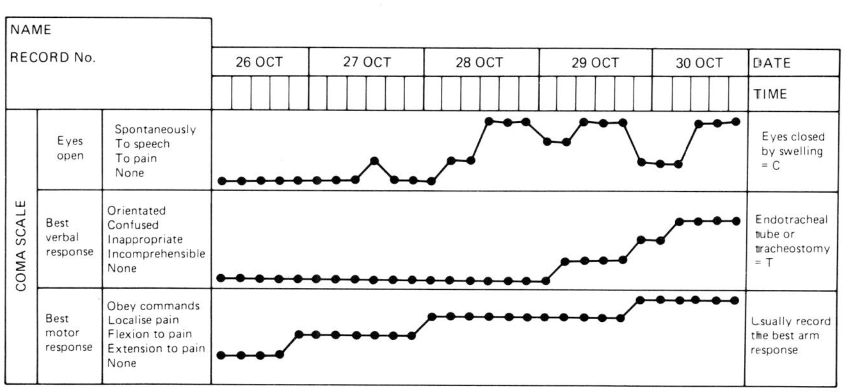

# TRAUMATIC INTRACRANIAL HAEMATOMA

## Principles

There is an important distinction between an extradural haematoma and the range of intradural haematomas. The operative treatment of an intradural lesion is much more complex and requires neurosurgical expertise. Only one in five clots is a pure *extradural haematoma*. Intradural haematomas include *subdural* and *intracerebral clots,* and many patients have a *burst lobe,* a combination of subdural and intracerebral lesions, connected through a laceration of the frontal or temporal lobes.

## Detection and diagnosis

The effects of an acute traumatic haematoma are due to compression of the brain, raised intracranial pressure, and brain shift and herniation. These events are expressed clinically by a deteriorating level of consciousness. Delaying the diagnosis until clinical deterioration is clearly established carries considerable risk of irreversible ischaemic damage to the brain. It is far better to achieve early detection before deterioration; evacuation of the clot will then ensure the optimum outcome. Although computerized tomography (CT) remains the mainstay of investigations, magnetic resonance imaging (MRI) can also detect both acute and chronic haematomas, and it provides more information about the degree of damage.

Early detection has become possible as a result of a number of advances. A guide to the likelihood of a haematoma which needs evacuation can be obtained from information about the patient's level of consciousness, and the result of a skull X-ray performed at the time of the first attendance at hospital (*see Table 2*). When this likelihood is judged to be present, CT scanning should be carried out as soon as feasible, without awaiting deterioration. The pictures produced by CT also give a very clear guide to the site and number of lesions, so that surgery can be planned more accurately. The criteria for use of CT currently applied in the UK are shown in *Table 3*. This tactic has greatly reduced the need for emergency exploratory surgery in head-injured patients and has resulted in improved outcomes.

# EXTRADURAL HAEMATOMA

## Principles

Most patients with an extradural clot have not sustained primary brain damage, and timely evacuation normally results in recovery. When a CT shows an extradural clot, operation is indicated unless the collection is very thin.

## Skull preparation and flap position

The patient should be positioned with the head 15° up and turned with the side of the clot uppermost. Unless there has been recent rapid clinical deterioration, the head should be shaved and prepared as for an ordinary neurosurgical operation.

**Table 2 Risks of an intracranial haematoma in a recently head-injured adult**

| *Skull fracture* | *Consciousness level on arrival at hospital* | *Risk* |
|---|---|---|
| Absent | Normal | 1:6000 |
| Absent | Impaired | 1:100 |
| Present | Normal | 1:30 |
| Present | Impaired | 1:4 |

**Table 3 Indications for CT scan after head injury**

1. Fractured skull
   - with confusion or worse impairment of consciousness
   - with focal neurological signs
   - with fits
   - with any other neurological symptoms or signs
2. Coma continuing after resuscitation – even if skull fracture absent
3. Deterioration in level of consciousness or other neurological signs
4. Confusion or other neurological disturbances persisting for more than 6–8 hours, even if skull fracture is absent

## The operation

### Incisions

# 1a–d

The sites of the skin incision and osteoplastic bone flap vary according to the location of the lesion as demonstrated by CT.

*Figure 1 CT scans of extradural haematoma: (a) temporal, (b) subtemporal, (c) frontal, (d) occipital haematoma. The incision shown in Illustration 2 (lower) would be performed if a CT scan as shown in Illustration 1a were seen; Illustration 2 (upper) relates to Illustration 1b; Illustration 3 relates to Illustration 1c; Illustration 4 relates to Illustration 1d.*

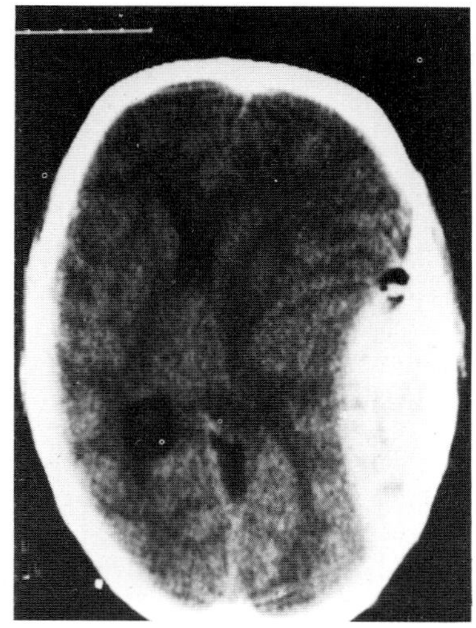

1a

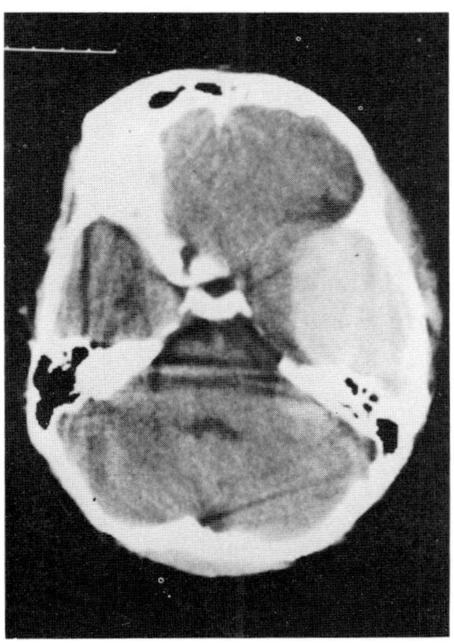

1b

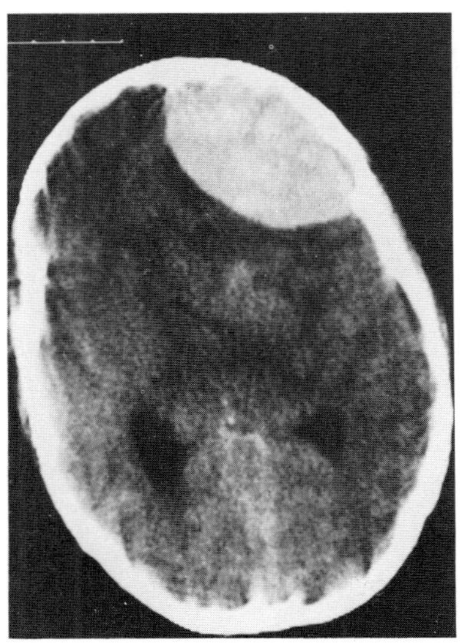

1c

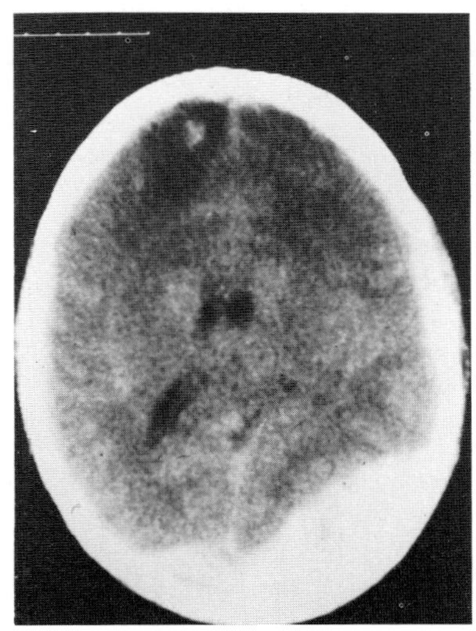

1d

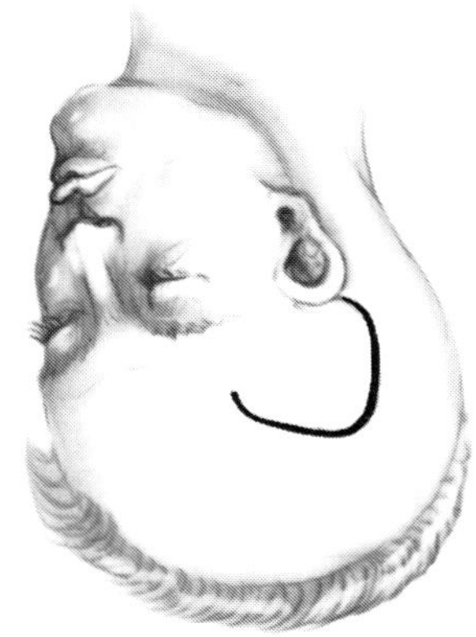

## 2, 3 & 4

The majority of extradural clots are in the temporal region, and normally an anterior temporal 'question mark' flap or a posterior temporal U-shaped flap, centred on the ear, is used (*see Illustration 2*). Clots in the frontal or subfrontal region require a frontal flap (*see Illustration 3*). It is important to remember the possibility of extradural haematoma overlying the vertex or in the posterior fossa (*see Illustration 1c and 4*), each related to a fracture crossing the major venous sinuses.

The skin flap is reflected and retracted and the temporalis muscle and pericranium incised with cutting diathermy.

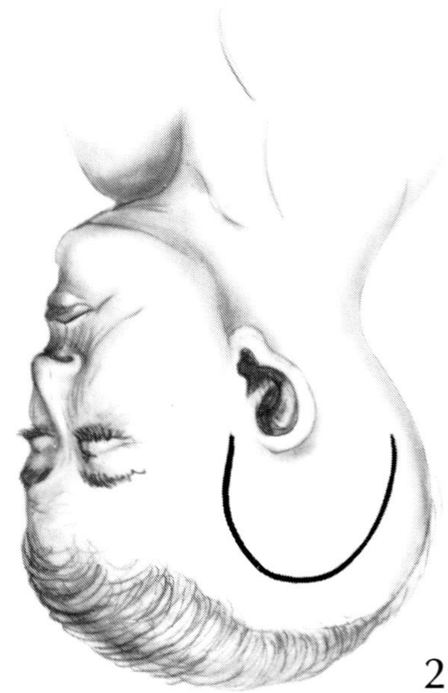

2

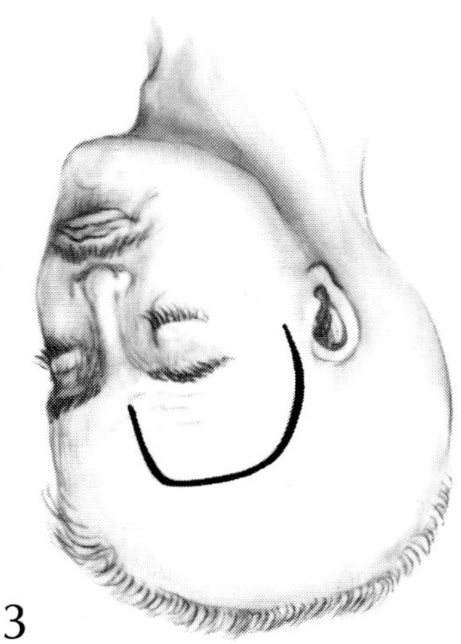

3

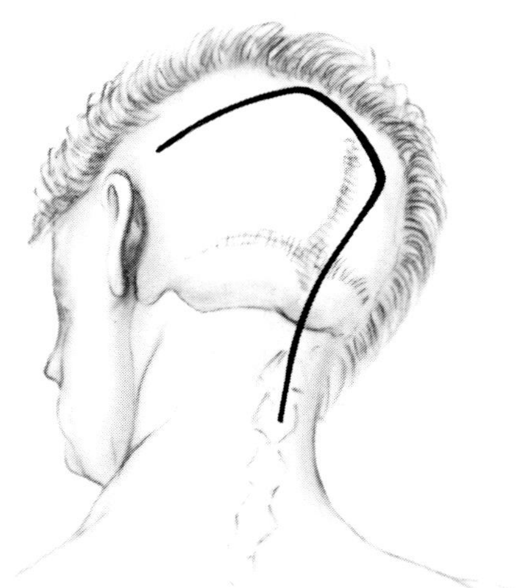

4

# 5

The muscle and pericranium are retracted with a sharp periosteal elevator. This may disclose the site of the fracture.

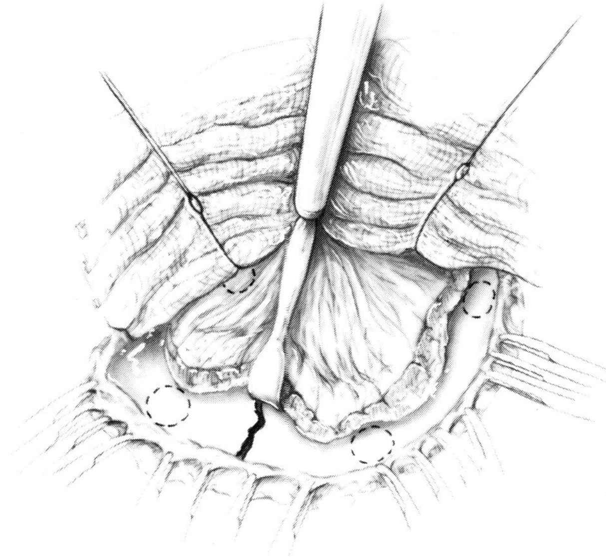

5

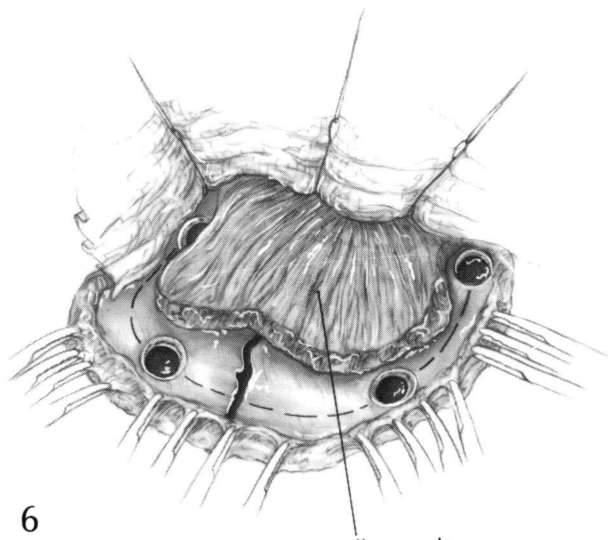


6

# 6

Burr holes are then placed, ideally at the edge of the clot, and are joined with the Gigli saw. The base of the flap is cracked across to allow reflection of the bone flap.

# 7

The clot is usually solid, with little continuing bleeding.

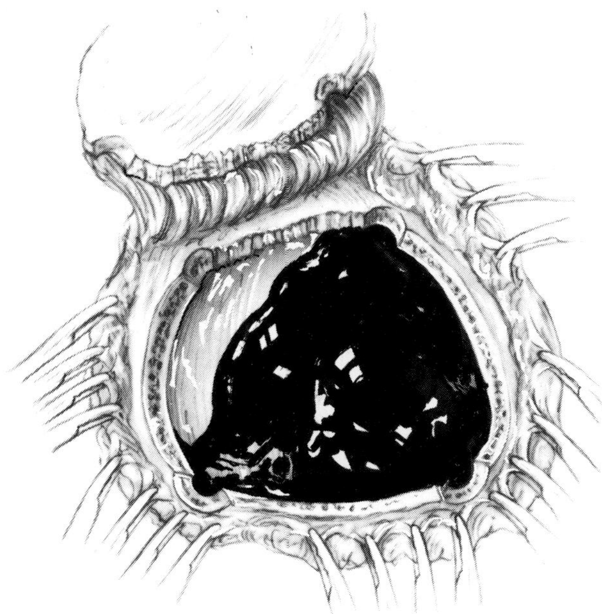

7

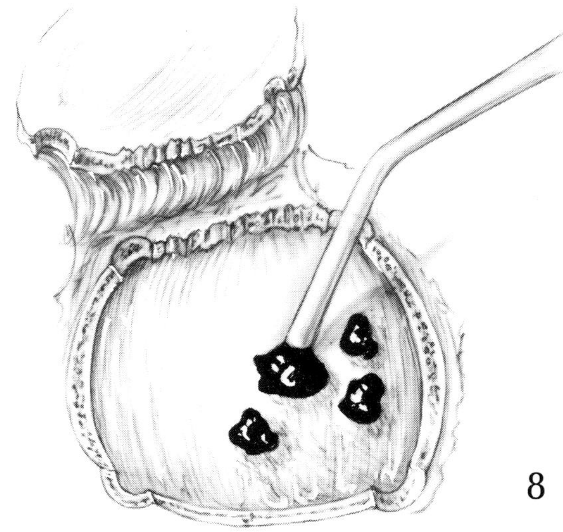

8

## Evacuation

# 8 & 9

The clot is removed by a combination of suction, irrigation and scooping.

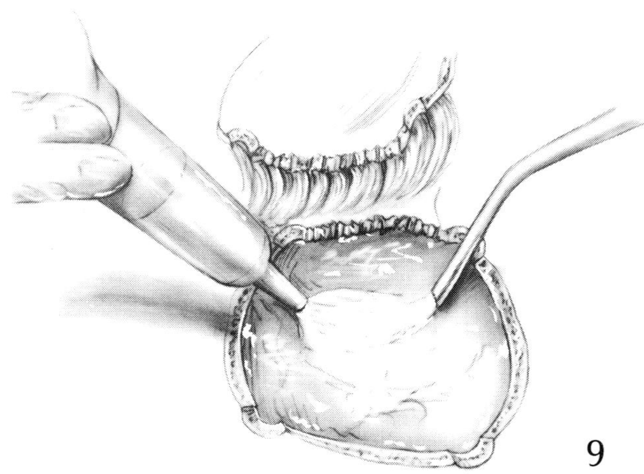

9

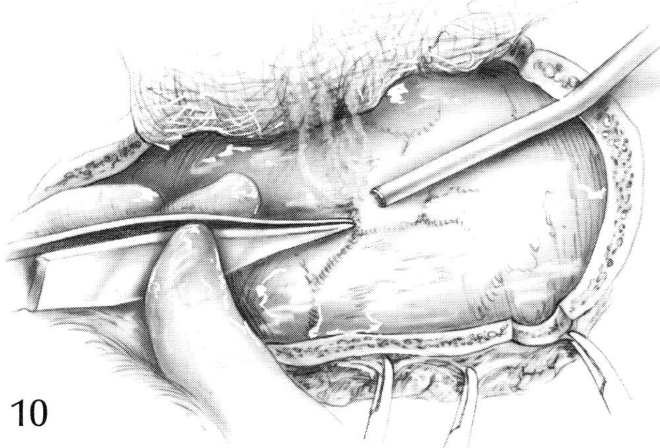

10

# 10

Sources of bleeding from the dura are identified with the aid of irrigation. Sometimes there is a discrete point which can be stopped with diathermy. Often the exposed dura bleeds in many sites and this is best controlled with haemostatic gauze. The dura is not opened routinely unless the preoperative CT scan showed an adjacent intradural lesion. If the dura rapidly becomes tense, a small exploratory opening may disclose an accessible subdural clot, but it is often better to close the wound and carry out a CT scan.

### Closure

**11**

Closure is by standard techniques. The hitch stitches inserted between the dura and the temporalis muscle are particularly important in order to limit any reformation of the haematoma.

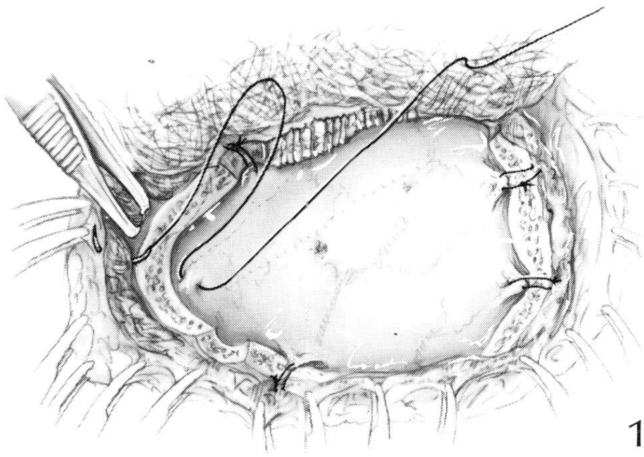

11

## Postoperative care

Suction drainage is continued for 24–48 hours. Clinical neurological and general monitoring are performed until the patient is discharged. Intracranial pressure monitoring is performed if the patient was in coma before operation, or if the CT scan showed another intradural lesion.

## Results

Overall mortality has been reduced from 30 per cent to between 10 and 20 per cent. The results depend upon the presence of an associated intradural lesion, which worsens the outcome, and upon the level of consciousness before operation. For patients who are still talking, recovery is the rule in 90 per cent of cases, and mortality approaches zero. In patients who have deteriorated into coma, mortality may be as high as 50 per cent.

# INTRADURAL HAEMATOMA

### Principles

Many patients with intradural haematomas also have primary brain damage. Nevertheless, prompt and effective operation can be rewarded by good recovery.

### Indications for operation

If CT or other investigations show a large haematoma, or if the patient is deteriorating, operation should be performed urgently. On the other hand, the scan sometimes shows a small, inaccessible lesion, and these patients will not normally benefit from operation. Between these extremes are patients in whom there is initial uncertainty about whether or not to remove the haematoma. If there is midline shift of more than 10 mm, or if there are CT findings indicating raised intracranial pressure (obliteration of the third ventricle or basal cisterns, or dilatation of the contralateral temporal horn), the clot should be removed. If doubt remains, it is useful also to monitor the intracranial pressure. If this is above 20–30 mmHg, deterioration is likely and the haematoma should be removed forthwith.

# The operation

## The incision

# 12a, b & c

The patient is placed supine with the head rotated to bring the clot uppermost. In the majority of patients it will be necessary to expose both the frontal and the temporal lobes, but the precise position and size of the flap can be adjusted depending on the CT scan appearances.

*Figure 12 CT scans of intradural haematoma: (a) subdural, (b) frontal subdural and intracerebral, (c) temporal intracerebral haematoma*

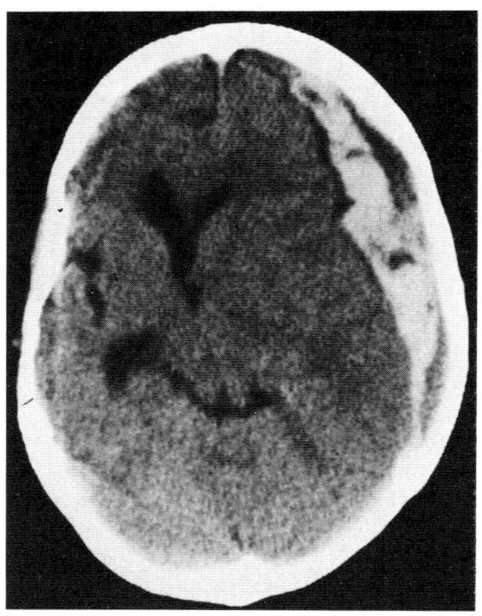

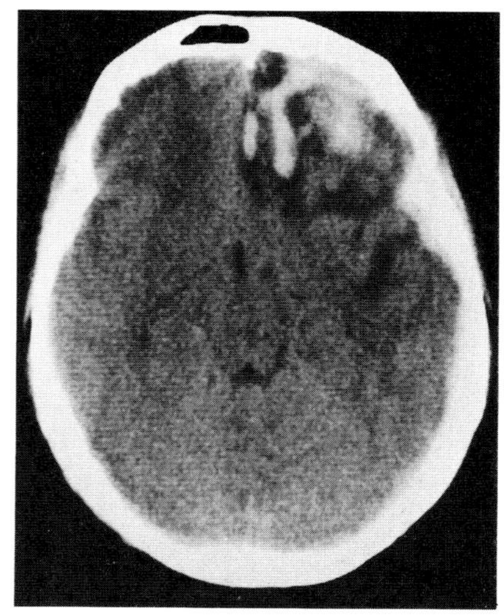

12b

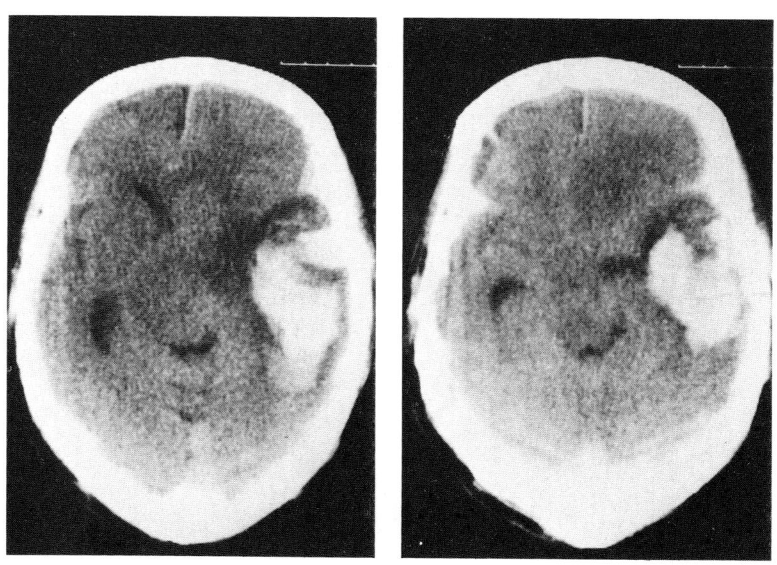

12c

## 13

A large frontotemporoparietal flap is usual. The skin should be cut close to the midline and down close to the front of the ear.

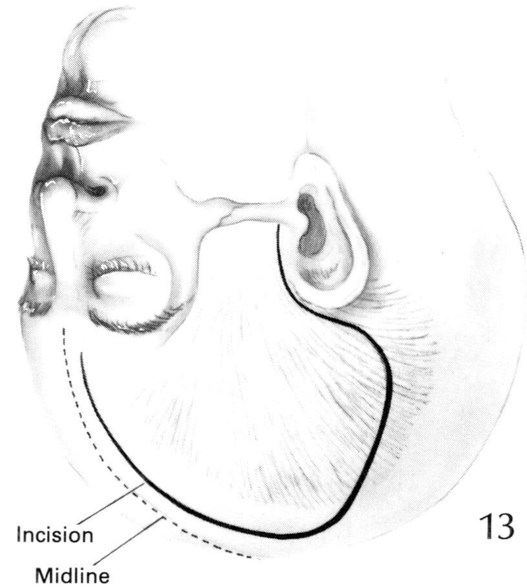


13

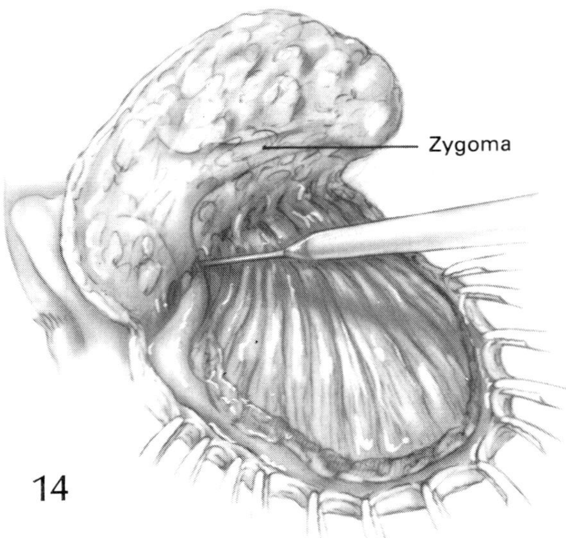


14

### Exposure

## 14

After turning down the skin flap the temporalis muscle is exposed. In order to get low in the temporal fossa and to ensure that the view is not obscured by overlying temporalis, the muscle is incised low and deeply, with the diathermy cut angled anteriorly towards the pterygoid fossa. After the bone flap has been lifted, the muscle can be retracted out of the temporal fossa.

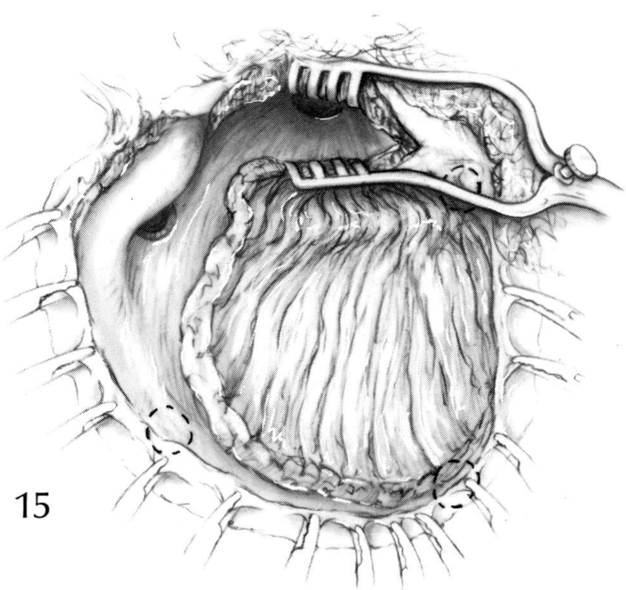

15

## 15

With the temporalis muscle cut and retracted to expose the temporal fossa, burr holes are cut. One is placed anteriorly in the temporal fossa, just above the sphenoid wing and alongside the orbit.

## 16

After the bone flap has been lifted the remainder of the temporal bone is rongeured down to the floor of the fossa. The sphenoid wing is removed as far as the superior orbital fissure.

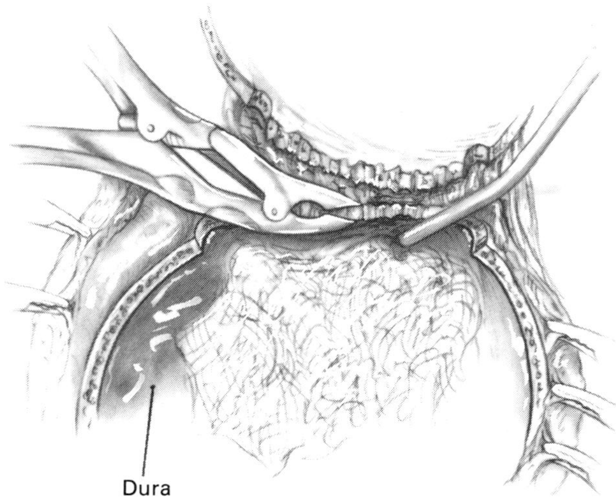


16

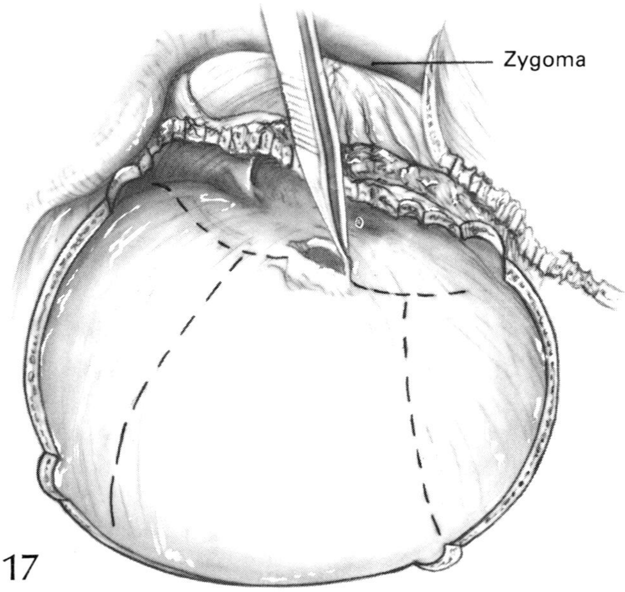


17

## 17

A semicircular dural opening is made, based around the sphenoid wing.

## 18

The flap of dura is stitched back to the muscle. Radiate incisions are then placed as necessary.

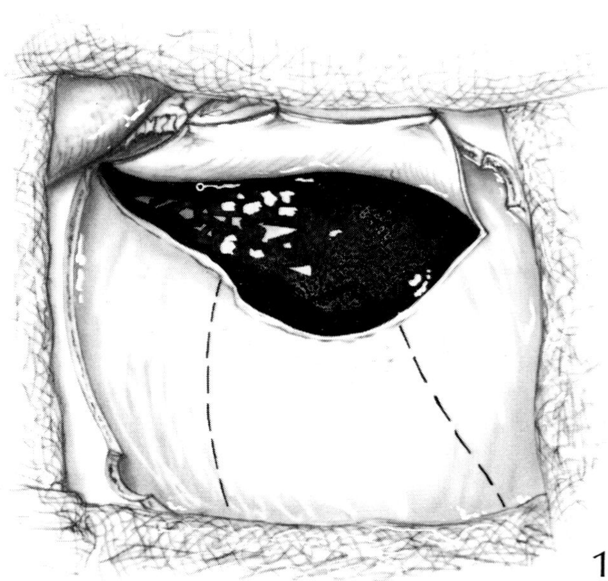

18

# 19

The subdural clot is removed by a combination of washing and gentle suction.

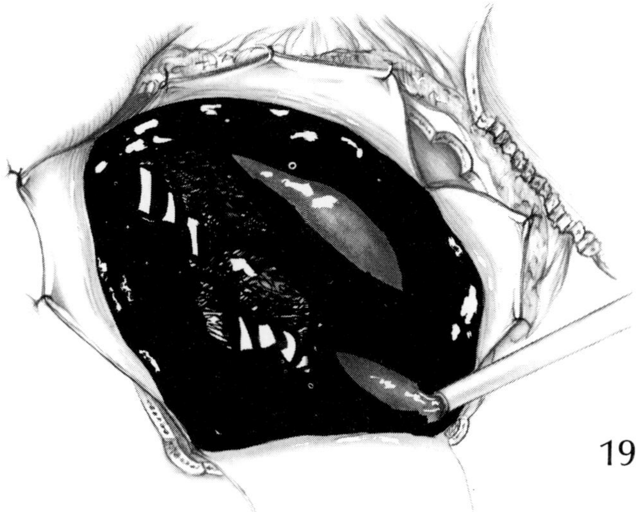

19

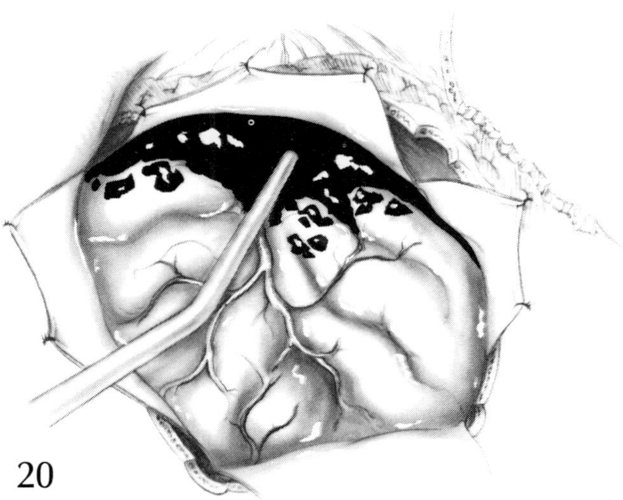

20

# 20

After removal of the subdural clot, the burst lobes are exposed. Each will be a combination of intracerebral blood and surrounding contused brain.

# 21

The temporal lobe is retracted and the bridging veins entering the sphenoparietal sinus are coagulated and cut. These veins are often the source of the subdural clot. If bleeding is not controlled, it may recur after operation.

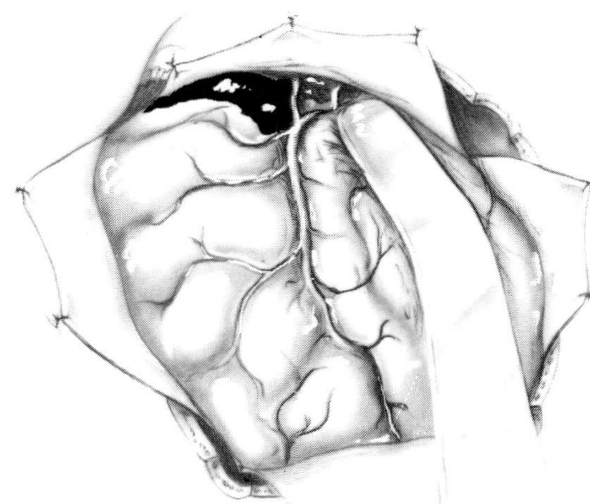

21

## Evacuation

### 22

Intracerebral blood clots are removed along with non-viable brain; this is softer than normal brain and is removed more easily by suction. The line of dissection passes along the edge of the slightly contused but viable brain. The limit is defined by suction. The cortical blood vessels crossing the line of excision are diathermied and cut.

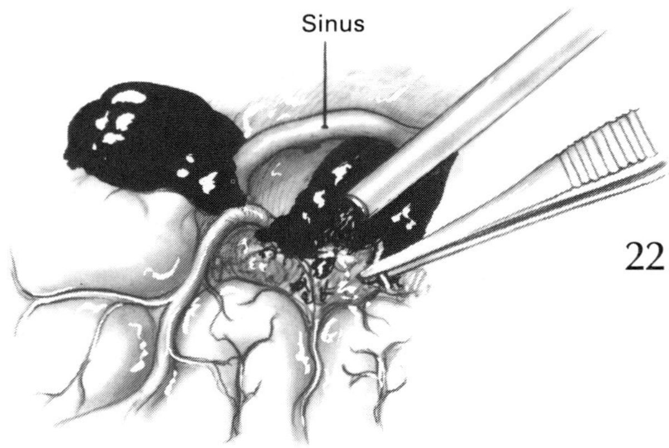


22

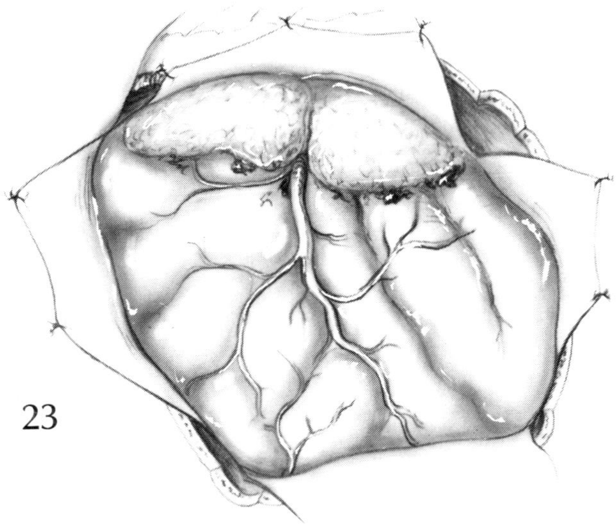

23

### 23

After clot and abnormal brain are removed, haemostasis is achieved. Initially the defect is gently packed with cotton wool balls.

### 24

The cotton wool balls are removed, and final haemostasis is obtained by covering the brain surface with a layer of Surgicel (Ethicon, UK) over which further temporary packing may be applied.

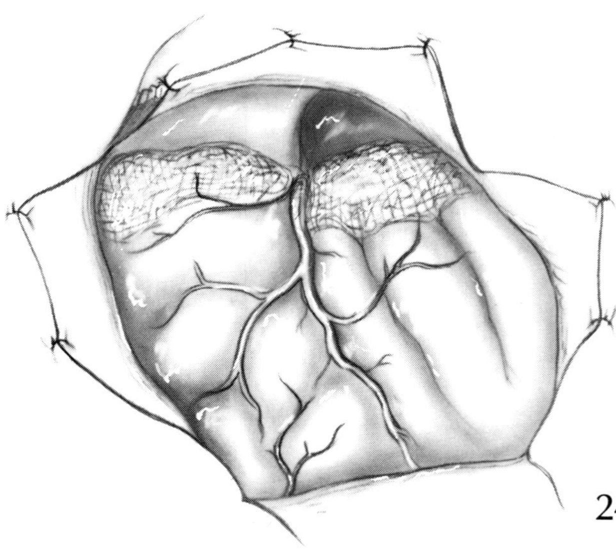

24

### Closure

## 25

The dura should always be closed. This prevents a decrease in the interstitial pressure in the underlying brain which would promote oedema and brain swelling. If the dura is left open the swollen brain will bulge through the defect; it infarcts and then acts as a further space-occupying lesion.

To achieve closure it may be necessary to patch the dura. This is best done by placing fascia or artificial dural substitute inside the original dura and either gluing it in position or inserting interrupted stitches. The bone flap is replaced and the skin closed in the customary way.

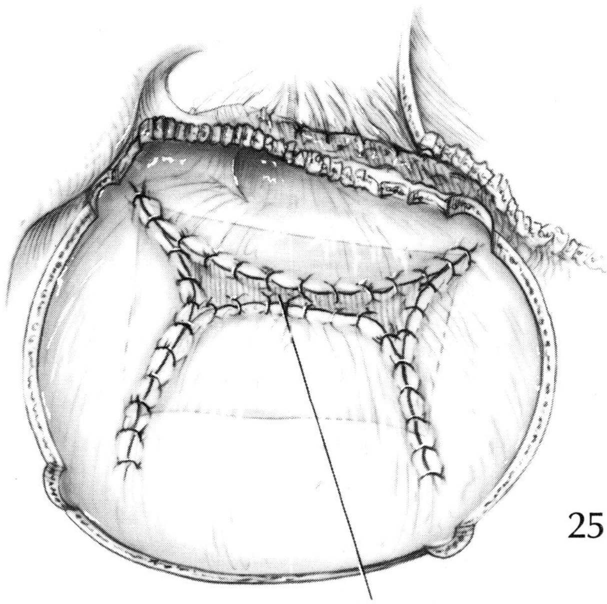


25

## Postoperative care

If the patient was in coma before operation it is customary to continue ventilation overnight. Thereafter, if the patient's respiratory function is satisfactory, prolonged hyperventilation does not have proven benefits.

Raised intracranial pressure is found most commonly after operation for an intradural haematoma. It may be due to the development of a new lesion which will require a further operation, or brain swelling which may respond to osmotic diuretics. We therefore advise the monitoring of intracranial pressure for 2–3 days after operation. If there is a sustained elevation, a further CT scan is indicated.

## Results

Early detection and evacuation have reduced mortality from intradural haematoma from around 50 per cent to 30–40 per cent. There is little difference in recovery rates between the three types of lesion; intracerebral clots have a lower mortality, but more survivors are disabled. The level of consciousness is important prognostically: in patients in coma, mortality is 60 per cent; of those still talking, less than 10 per cent die.

# EXPLORATORY SURGERY

It is not always possible to establish a precise diagnosis before operation. The necessary radiological facilities may not be readily available, or the patient may be deteriorating so rapidly that operation cannot be delayed. The more 'classical' the clinical picture, and the more remote the radiological facilities, the greater may be the justification for exploratory surgery. Nevertheless, any decision not to establish the diagnosis before operation should be influenced by the interval that can be gained by the administration of mannitol, and also by the short time taken to obtain sufficient information from a limited CT scan. Only about one in five patients has a simple extradural haematoma, and even in these the classical clinical picture is exceptional. A negative exploration only delays effective treatment.

# The operation

The patient's head should be fully shaved; this allows a precise assessment of the location of any scalp damage. Furthermore, if a burr hole discloses a clot, the head is prepared for the more extensive operation needed to remove the collection.

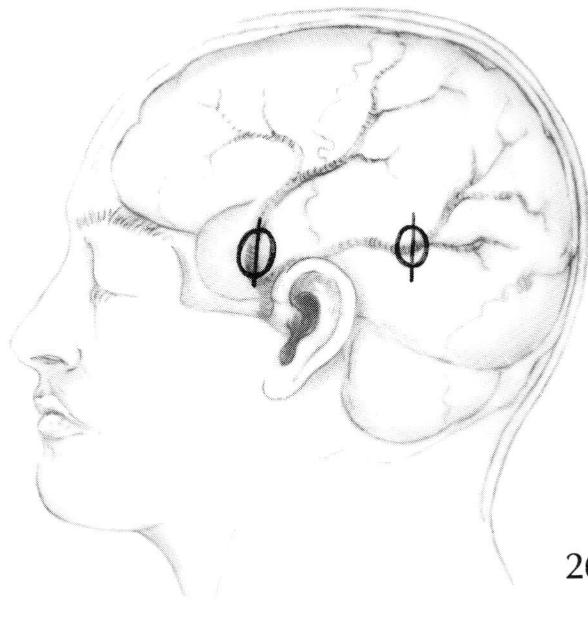

26

## Localization of the lesion

The most appropriate site for the exploration may be indicated by a number of factors. These are as follows.

1. *Signs of local trauma to the scalp.* These will usually overlie an extradural collection at some point.
2. *The site of a fracture shown radiologically.* When associated with an extradural haematoma, the fracture line virtually always crosses the collection at some point. Characteristically this is where it crosses the line of a meningeal vessel but in more than one-third of patients with an intradural haematoma the collection lies on the opposite side of the head from the fracture.
3. *Localizing neurological signs.* When there is a hemiplegia or some other difference between responses of the limbs on the two sides, the intracranial haematoma lies on the side of the head opposite the less responsive limbs in 80 per cent of cases. When it is known that pupillary abnormalities have developed at some time after the initial injury, the haematoma will be ipsilateral to the pupil which first becomes abnormal in 90 per cent of cases. However, it must be remembered that pupillary abnormalities carry such a grave prognosis that all efforts should be directed at preventing their development rather than using them as a guide to intracranial operation.

# 26

4. *Traditional anatomical landmarks.* These can be misleading because the inexperienced operator finds it difficult to translate them to the intact head. A common error is for a burr hole aimed at the middle meningeal artery to be made much too high. If a horizontal skin incision is made, it will greatly complicate a subsequent definitive operation.

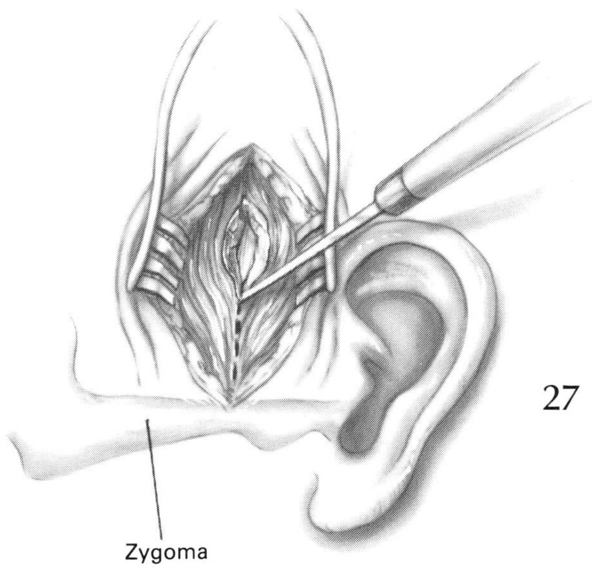


27

# 27

The anterior temporal incision should be made just in front of the ear, with its lower end reaching to the zygoma. After retracting the skin, the temporalis muscle is incised with cutting diathermy and retracted. The burr hole is cut as described in the chapter on 'Burr holes, trephine and craniotomy', pp. 12–29.

## Interpretation of findings

It can be far from simple to decide what has actually been found by a burr hole. The exploration itself can produce substantial bleeding from a number of sites: from the deep temporal vessels lying between the temporalis muscle and the outer surface of the skull; from diploic veins between the inner and outer tables of the skull; and from normal vessels in the epidural space where venous bleeding is particularly common. Moreover, when an opening is made in the dura, it can provoke brisk and unremitting bleeding, either from vessels within the layers of the dura or from underlying cortical arteries and veins.

Bleeding at any of these sites may be difficult for the inexperienced to stem, and can lead to the erroneous conclusion that the operation has found the cause of the patient's deterioration.

# 28

An extradural haematoma is usually seen as a solid, dark clot which protrudes through the burr hole. Sometimes evacuation of the surface clot is followed by fresh arterial bleeding. These findings need to be distinguished from the epidural bleeding which normally accompanies the cutting of a burr hole.

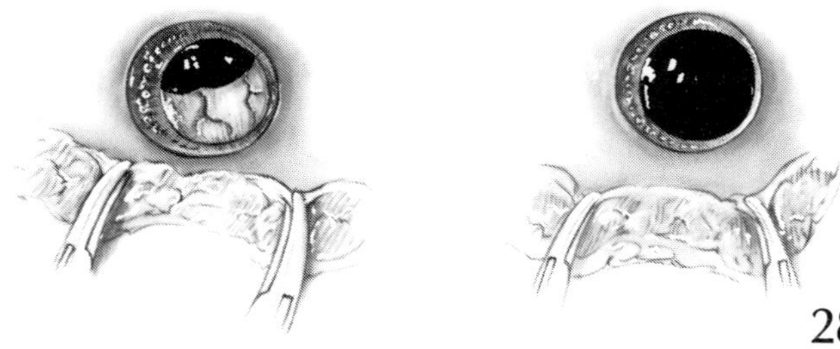

28

## Extension of a burr hole

# 29

The volume of a significant extradural haematoma will be at least 25 ml, and more commonly 50 ml or more. It is usually possible to remove only a fraction through a burr hole, and although this may provide some temporary relief, definitive evacuation requires exposure of the full extent of the clot. This can be done by extending the skin incision and progressively enlarging the bone opening by nibbling its edges.

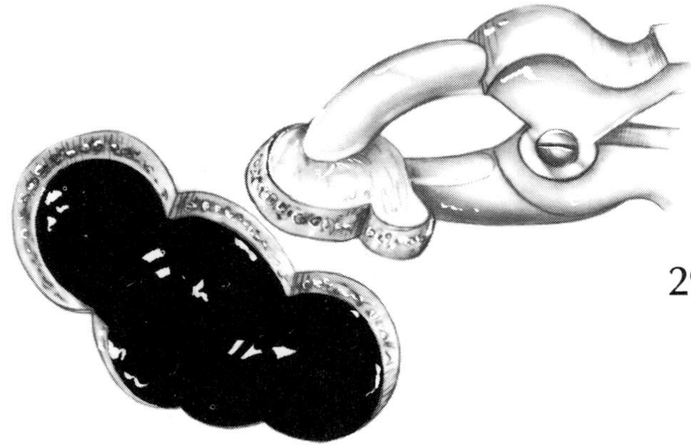

29

# 30

It is usually necessary to 'follow the clot' for several centimetres until normal dura is reached; a large craniectomy thereby results. A more satisfactory method, if the operator has the required expertise, is to turn an appropriately located formal craniotomy flap, as previously described.

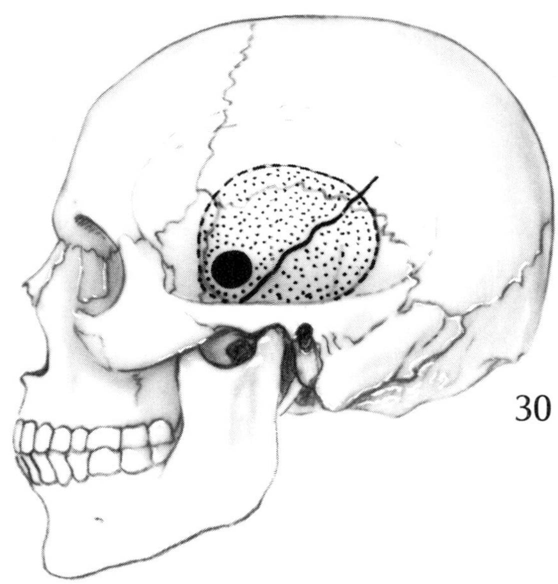

30

## What to do if an extradural haematoma is not discovered

Inexperienced operators may be tempted to ask themselves two questions. (*1*) Can I tell through the burr hole if the intracranial pressure is high? (*2*) Should I open the dura?

In practice, it is impossible to gauge the intracranial pressure from the apparent tension of the dura in the burr hole. Moreover, even when an acute subdural clot does lie under a burr hole, it cannot be evacuated without more extensive surgery. If the dura is incised through a burr hole over a subdural haematoma, only a few fragments of the clot will be extruded before the adjacent brain impacts against the dura and closes the aperture. Attempts to dislodge further clot either by scooping or irrigation are ineffective and can often provoke further damage.

## When to stop looking

If the burr hole site(s) chosen for exploration on the basis of the patient's localizing features does not yield a clot, it is usually preferable to stop and to arrange for definitive radiological studies. More burr holes may simply delay the eventual relief of compression. A burr hole may miss a large extradural clot by only a few millimetres. Even when performed by practised neurosurgeons, exploratory burr holes miss one-third of significant intracranial clots.

# CHRONIC SUBDURAL HAEMATOMA

## Principles

The diagnosis of chronic subdural haematoma is much more often suspected than confirmed. The condition never gives rise to such dramatic deterioration that investigation is precluded. The diagnosis can be suspected from isotope scanning, and made definite by CT or MRI scanning. Even when the collection is not hypodense, the associated shift and compression of the ventricular system will suggest the diagnosis.

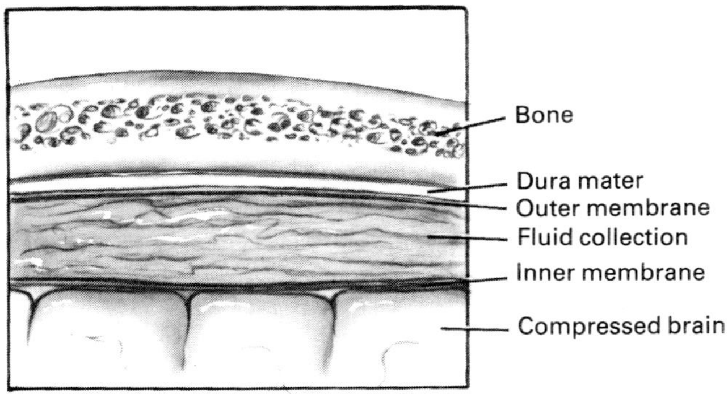


31

## Characteristics

### 31

A chronic subdural haematoma characteristically consists of a thick, dark fluid collection bounded by firm fibrous membranes on its inner and outer surfaces, the latter often fused with the inner surface of the dura. Recurrent bleeding from the membranes plays an important part in the persistence of the collection, and produces the symptoms.

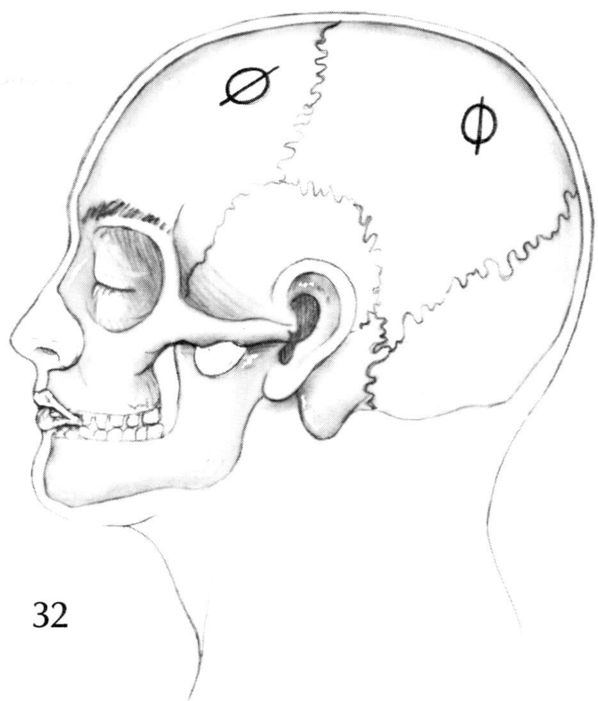

32

## Treatment

### 32

Simple drainage is almost always effective in relieving the symptoms. This can be achieved through a burr hole, or by the use of a twist-drill.

Drainage is usually achieved by making a burr hole, incising the dura and outer membrane, and releasing the fluid collection. Customarily, burr holes are placed at the frontal and parietal eminence. After drainage of the collection the cavity is irrigated with saline. Some surgeons make only one burr hole and rely upon irrigation to achieve the desired effect.

## Postoperative care and results

Many surgeons drain the cavity of a chronic subdural haematoma through a catheter into a drainage bottle at the level of the patient's head. The drain is retained for 24–48 hours, depending upon the volume of fluid obtained.

The patient's clinical condition is the most important monitor of progress. Routine repeated CT scanning is not helpful; there is little correspondence between its findings and a successful clinical result. On the other hand, if the patient fails to improve as quickly as anticipated, CT scanning should be performed in order to detect persistence of the original collection, or of a component loculus, or the development of another complication such as cerebral infarction or hydrocephalus. A small proportion of patients require repeated drainage; this carries the risk of introducing infection into the cavity and thus should be done with scrupulous attention to sterile technique.

Recovery is the rule in more than 90 per cent of patients.

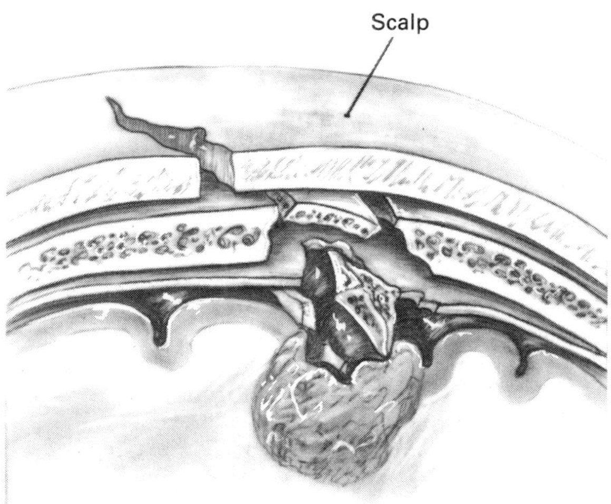


33

# OPEN INJURIES

## Depressed fracture of the skull vault

The indications for operation on a depressed fracture of the skull depend upon whether it is *closed* or *compound*.

### CLOSED DEPRESSED FRACTURE

These are uncommon in adults; any local violence that fractures and forces the bones inward directly under the impact usually also lacerates the overlying scalp. The degree of depression with a closed fracture is usually slight, and only rarely is operation needed on cosmetic grounds. The risk of epilepsy from a depressed fracture is not an indication for operation because this risk is not affected by elevation of the depression. The technique of operation is essentially the same as for a compound fracture.

### COMPOUND DEPRESSED FRACTURE

#### Principles

The main aim of treatment of a compound fracture is to minimize the risk of intracranial infection. A much less frequent complication is serious intracranial bleeding, either from the cerebral cortex underlying the fracture or from major vessels in the dura. There is a high risk of epilepsy with a compound fracture, but operation does not ameliorate this risk.

Diagnosis depends upon a high index of clinical suspicion, thorough inspection of scalp wounds, and satisfactory skull radiography.

When the wound is relatively clean and the fracture overlies a major venous sinus, it may be prudent simply to clean and to close the scalp, and then to treat the patient with an antibiotic.

## 33

The anatomy of a depressed fracture and its underlying complications are illustrated.

# The operation

## Exposure

### 34

The first step is to clean and shave the surrounding area for at least one inch. The skin edges are excised if they are very devitalized and contaminated. The wound is then extended into an S shape with suitable incisions. When the fracture is in the forehead it is usually preferable to turn a formal frontal skin flap rather than extend the primary wound.

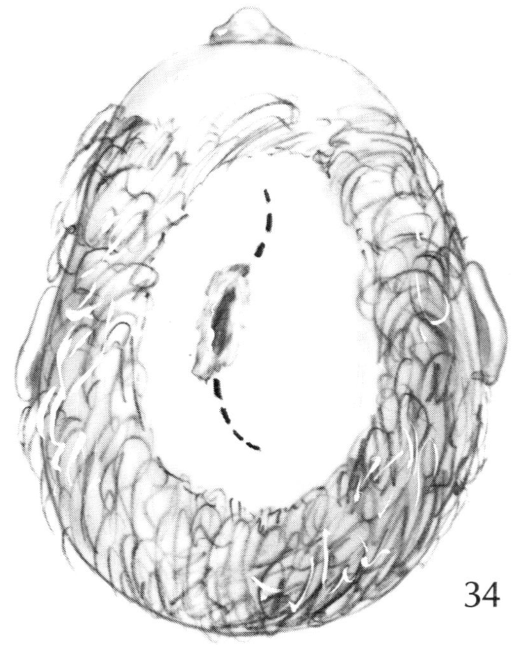

34

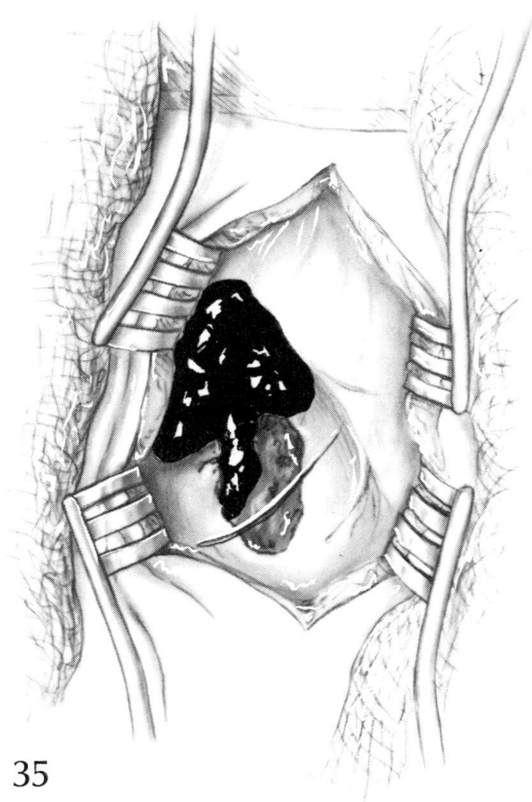

35

### 35

Self-retaining retractors are inserted to retract the skin edges and to expose the region of the fracture. This is usually covered by blood clot, contaminated by fragments of hair.

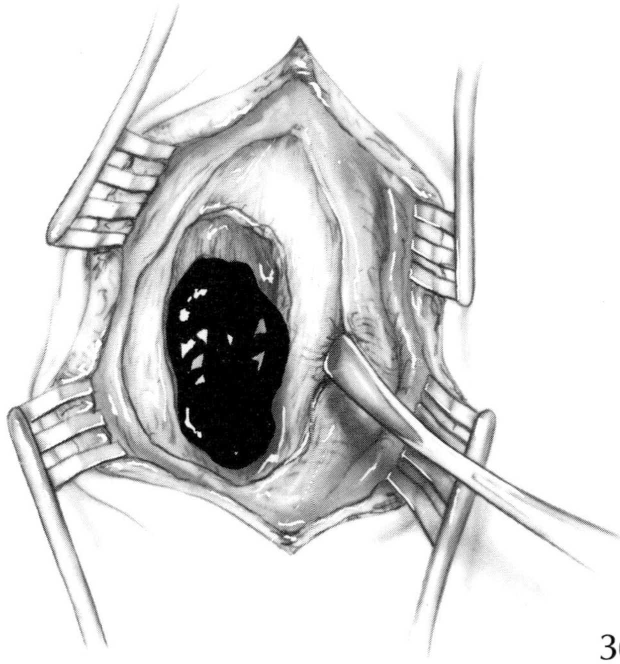

36

# 36 & 37

The pericranium around the fracture is incised and stripped back using a sharp periosteal elevator. Blood clot and any fragments of hair or other indriven substances are removed with suction. This exposes the bone fragments.

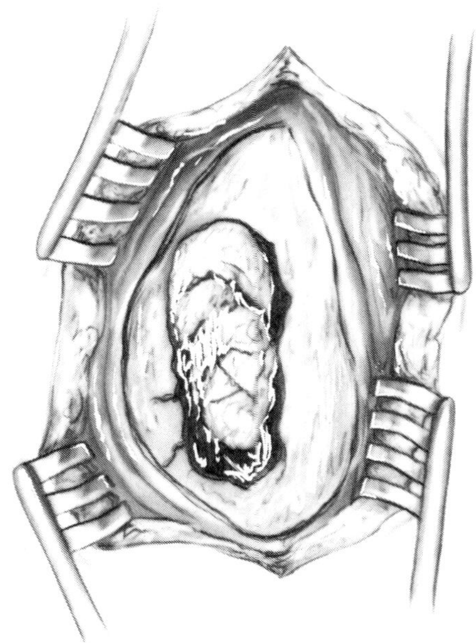

37

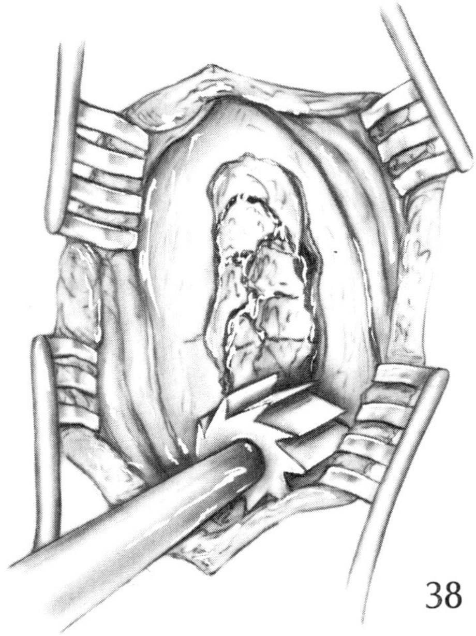

38

# 38 & 39

A burr hole is placed alongside the outer edge of the fracture where the fragments are stable.

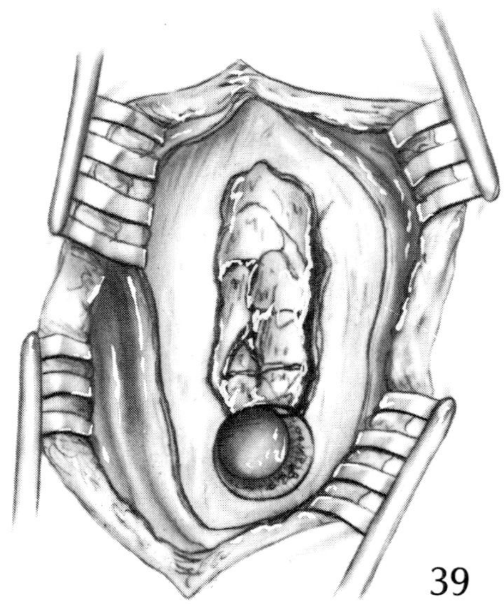

39

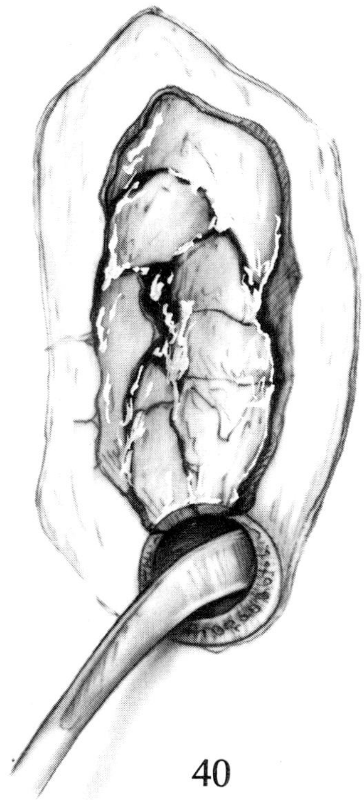

40

# 40 & 41

A periosteal elevator is used to separate the dura from the inner surfaces of the skull, first at the edge of the burr hole, then under the fracture. Bone nibbling is started at the edge of the burr hole alongside the fracture and then extended into and along the margins of the fracture.

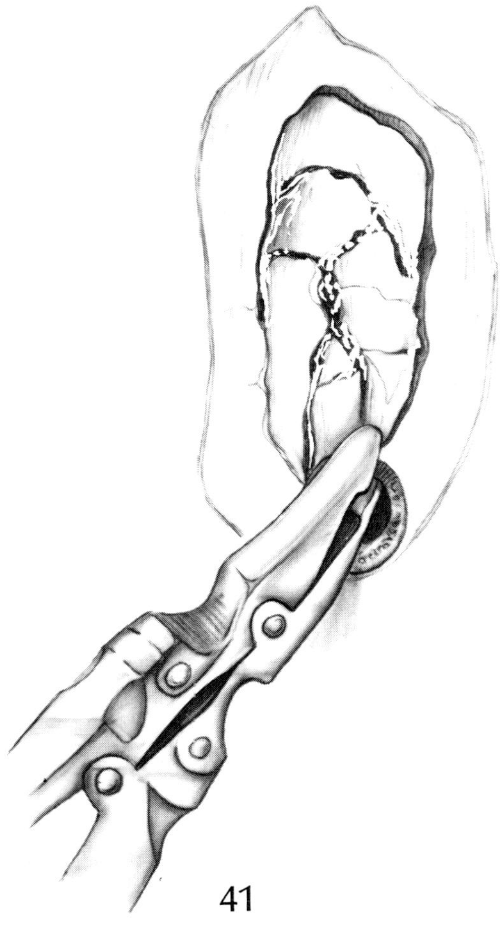

41

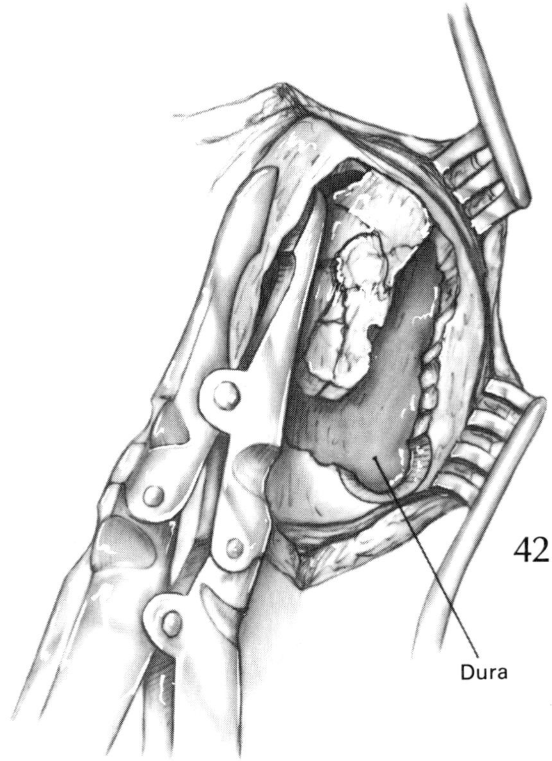


42

# 42 & 43

Bone nibbling is continued around the margin of the fracture, exposing the dura, until the depressed fragment is isolated and mobile. It is necessary to avoid further impaction of the depressed fragments; this may provoke haemorrhage from the cortical vessels which at this stage are inaccessible, and hence any bleeding will be difficult to control.

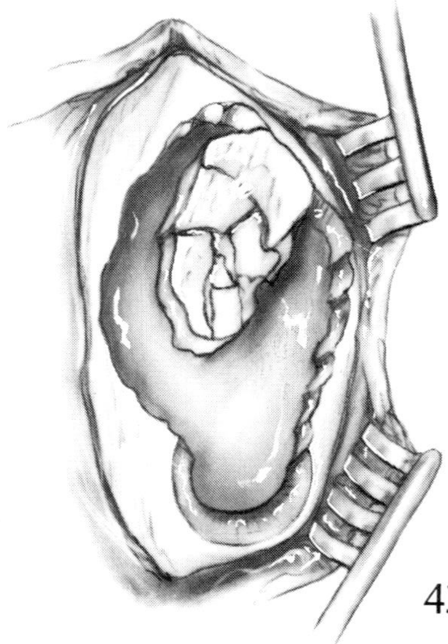

43

# 44 & 45

When there is adequate access and the indriven fragment is mobile, it is grasped firmly and drawn out from any remaining overhanging lip of skull.

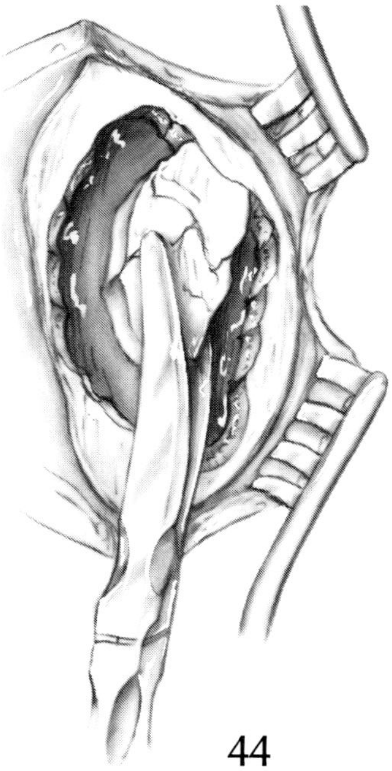

44

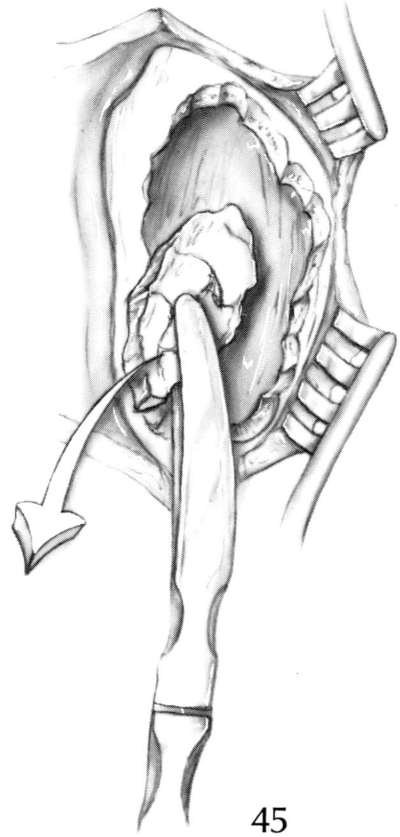

45

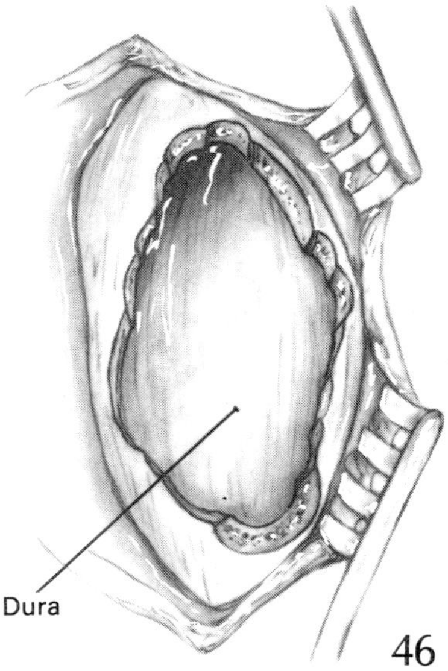


46

### Inspection of the dura

## 46 & 47

The dura mater is inspected; blood clot and any foreign substances are removed, and large bleeding points coagulated. If the dura is not torn it is covered with Surgicel (Ethicon, UK).

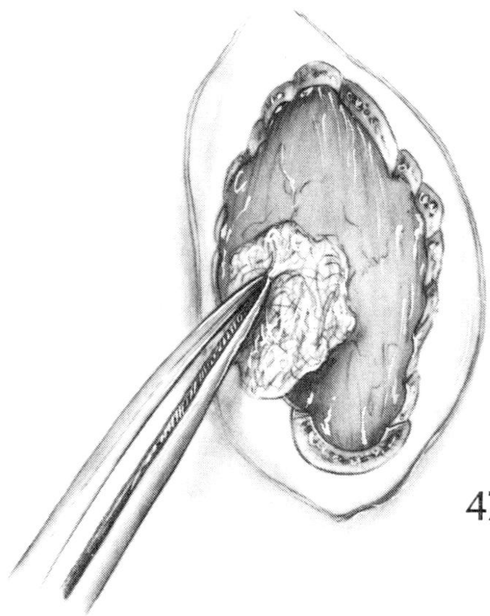

47

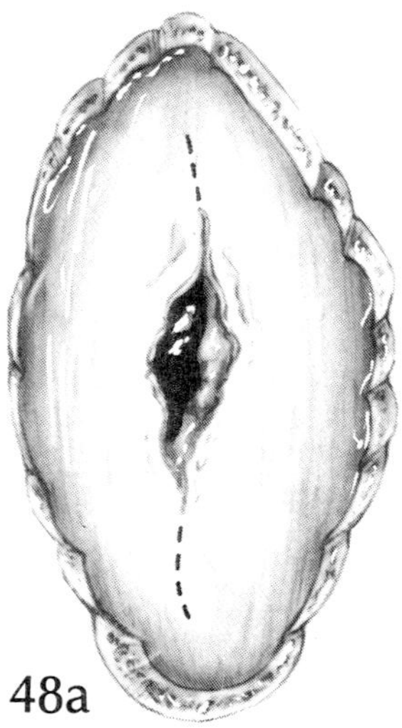

48a

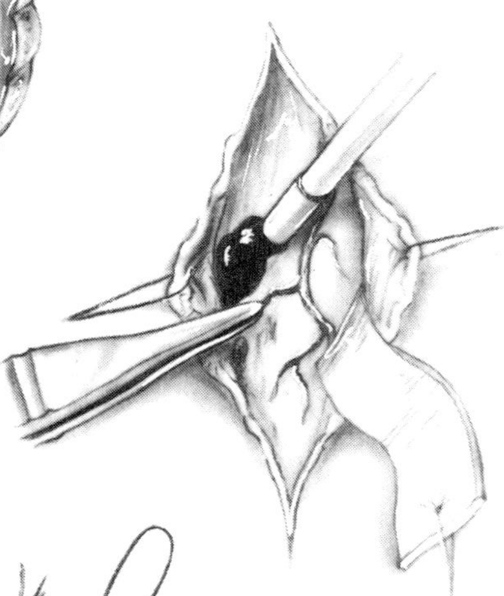

48b

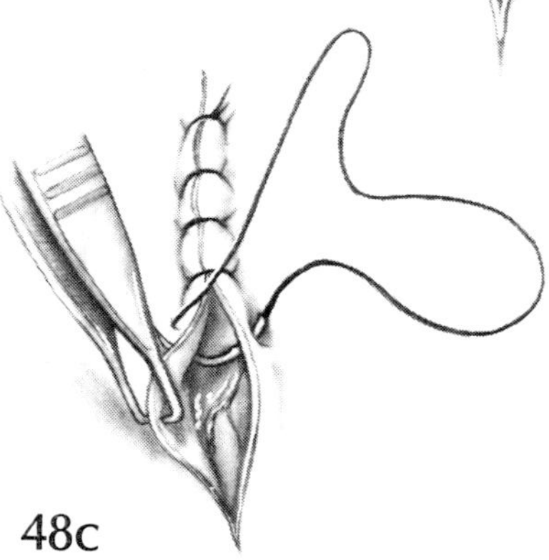

48c

## 48a, b & c

If the dura is torn, its edges are defined (*a*), freed from the underlying brain, and retracted with stay sutures (*b*). It may be necessary to extend the opening to expose the damaged brain adequately; this is cleaned with gentle suction. Devitalized or contused cortex is removed by suction, along with any significant haematoma. At this stage bleeding may occur from cortical arterioles, which will need diathermy to achieve permanent control. The brain is covered with haemostatic gauze and the dura is closed with an absorbable suture (*c*). A graft will be needed if much dura has been lost.

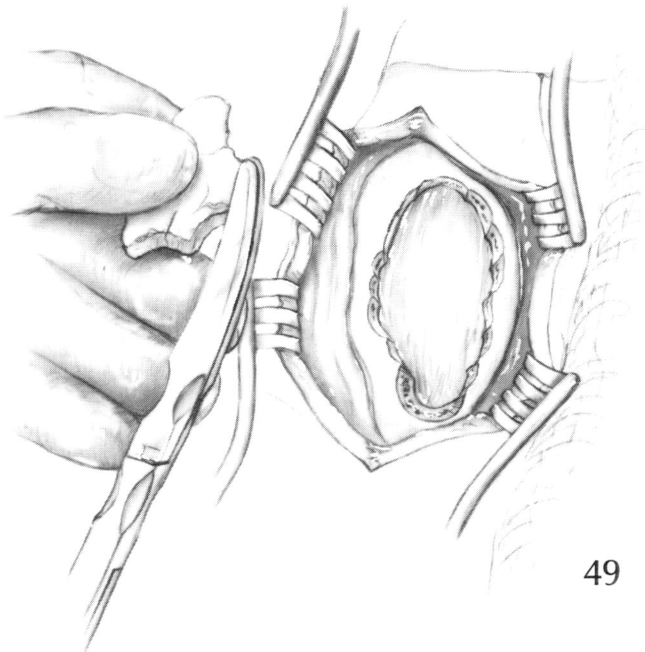

49

# 49 & 50

After cleaning with peroxide or antibiotic solution, the bone fragments are trimmed and one or more large pieces replaced. These are covered with Surgicel and, if possible, a layer of the pericranium is sutured over to stabilize bone fragments.

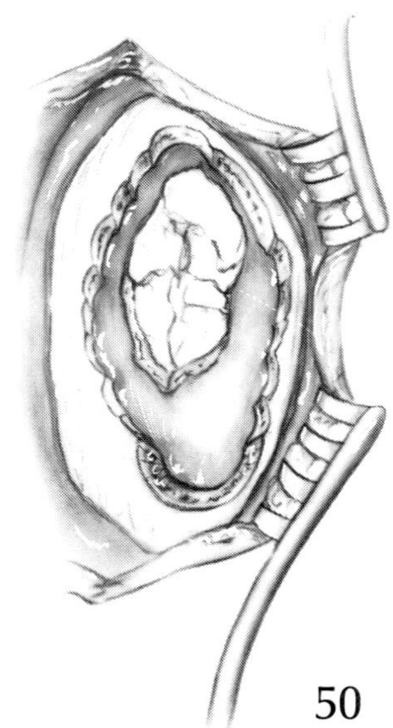

50

## Closure

## 51

The incision is closed using separate layers to the aponeurosis and skin.

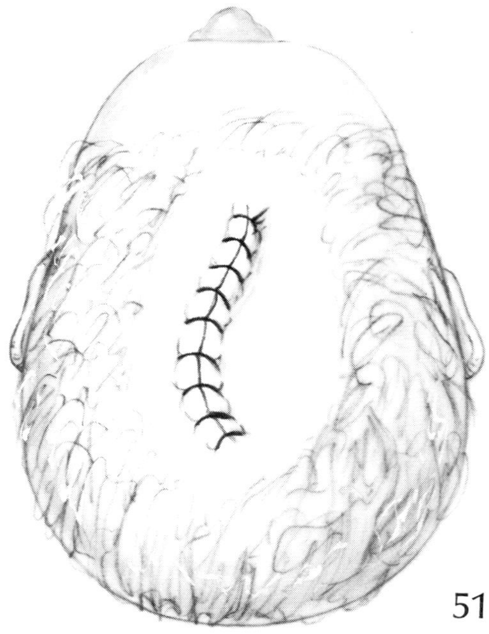

51

# Postoperative care

Neurological and general monitoring are continued as described previously.

The sutures are removed from the skin on the third day. The value of continuing antibiotics and of anticonvulsants is debatable.

# Results

The rate of infection after operation is low, being around 3–5 per cent; delays in diagnosis are the main cause. Overall, late epilepsy occurs in 15 per cent of cases; this is more likely if the dura has been torn, if there are focal signs, if there was amnesia for more than 24 hours, or if there has been an early fit.

## ANTERIOR FOSSA FRACTURE

### Principles

# 52 & 53

The anterior cranial fossa is commonly involved in a fracture of the base of the skull. The injury may be compound into the frontal, ethmoidal, or sphenoidal sinuses or into the nose itself.

The greatest risk is of meningitis, typically due to pneumococcus. An intracranial abscess or an aerocele can also occur. Diagnosis initially depends upon clinical signs such as bilateral orbital haematoma, or cerebrospinal fluid rhinorrhoea. Sometimes the brain plugs the fracture and there is no external leak of cerebrospinal fluid.

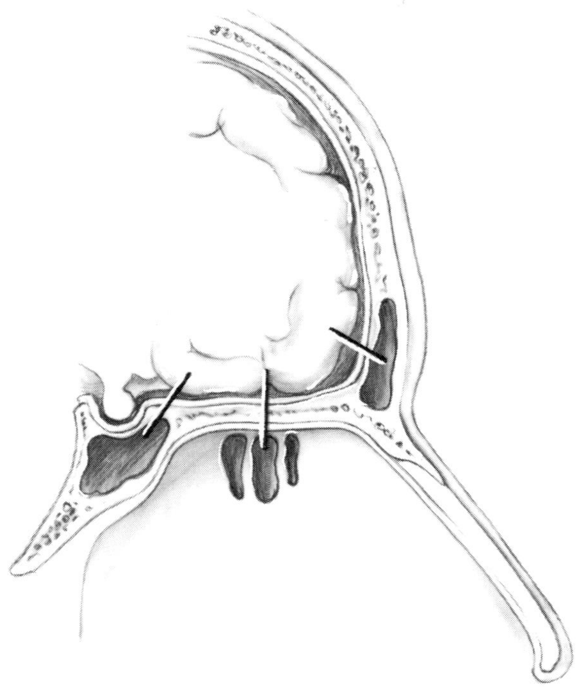

52

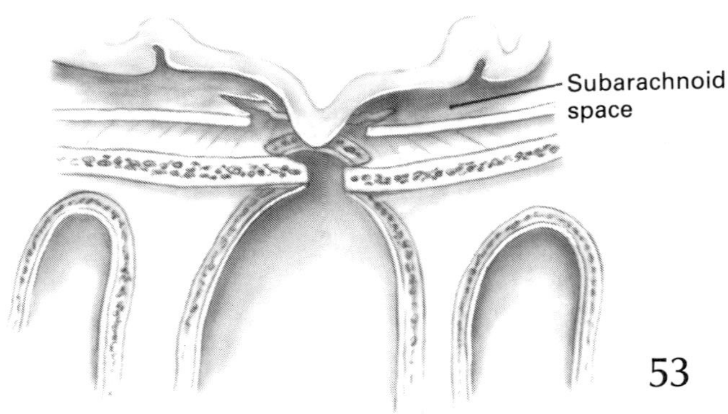


53

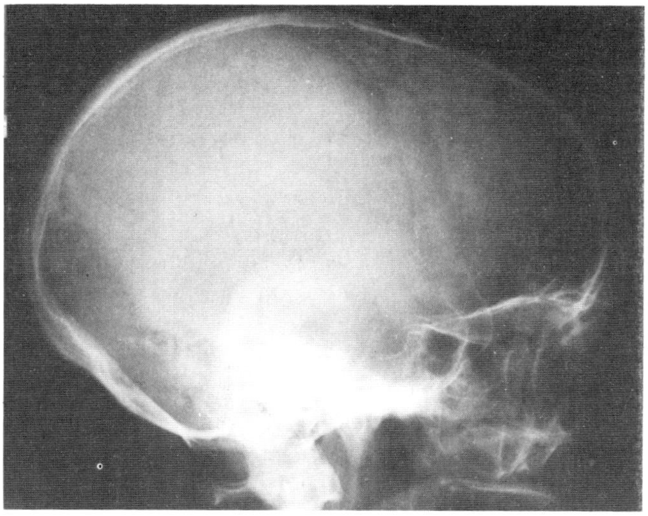

54a

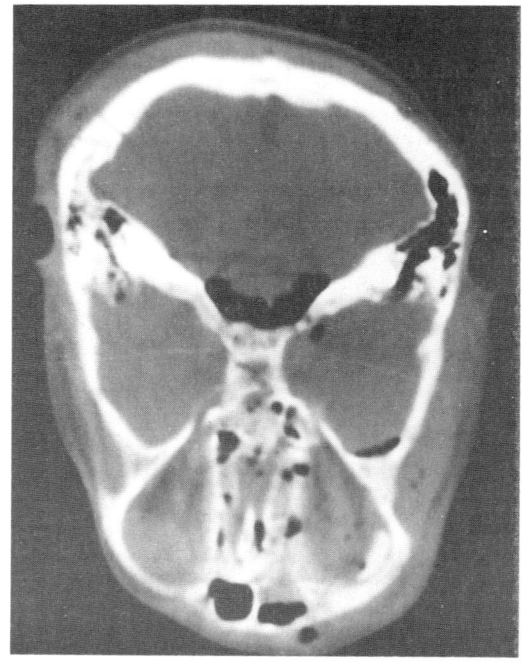

54b

# 54a & b

Skull X-rays may reveal intracranial air or a fluid level in a sinus. *Illustration 54a* is a lateral skull radiograph showing intracranial air in the frontal region. *Illustration 54b* is a CT scan showing air in the subarachnoid space in front of the brain stem and in the middle cranial fossa.

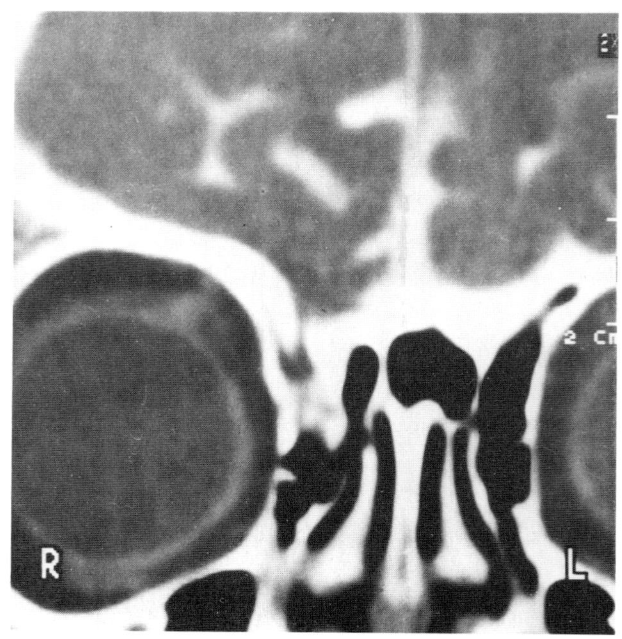


55

# 55

The definitive diagnosis can be made by CT scanning after an intrathecal injection of a non-ionic water-soluble contrast agent.

## Preoperative care

Cerebrospinal fluid rhinorrhoea usually stops spontaneously. Repair is required only if the leak persists for more than 7 days. Operation is also indicated in a patient who has suffered extensive destruction of the anterior fossa, which is usually combined with facial injury. Some patients have a comminuted depressed fracture of the frontal bone which is compound both at the base and the vertex, and which also involves the orbit. In such patients early operation is more difficult owing to brain swelling, and is also associated with a high rate of postoperative infection. This can be particularly troublesome to eradicate if wire is used in the reconstruction. Operation is therefore best delayed for 7–10 days. Scalp laceration should be sutured and the patient treated with penicillin and a sulphonamide; the use of broader spectrum antibiotics is controversial.

# The operation

## 56

### Incisions and exposure

The patient is placed supine with the head in a neutral position. A bifrontal skin flap is turned down.

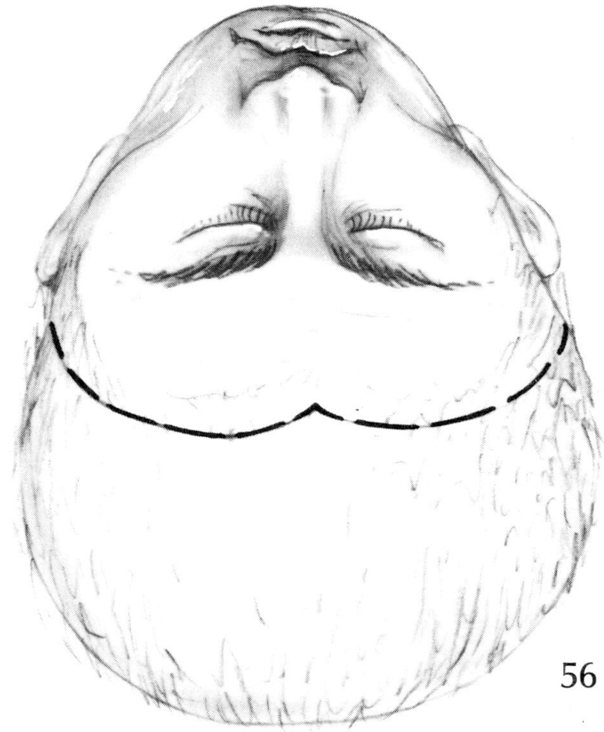

56

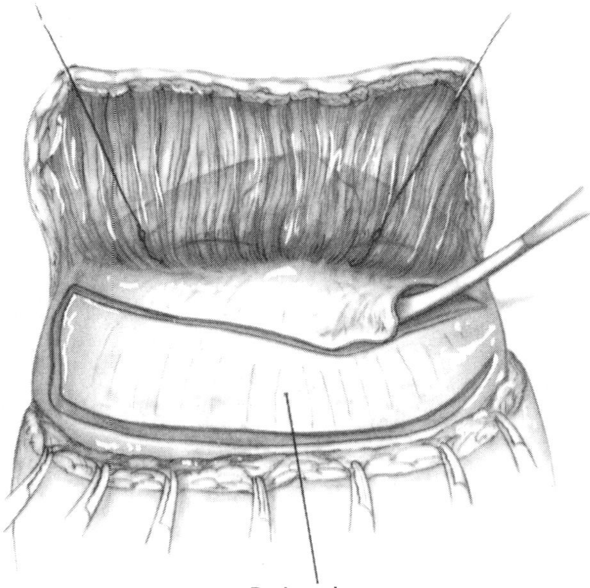


57

## 57

A triangular flap of pericranium is incised with its base along the superior orbital margin. This will be used later to cover the frontal sinus if this is exposed in the bone flap. The flap of pericranium is elevated from the bone and reflected anteriorly and downwards to expose the supraorbital margin. The remainder of the pericranium is incised to form a flap based on the right.

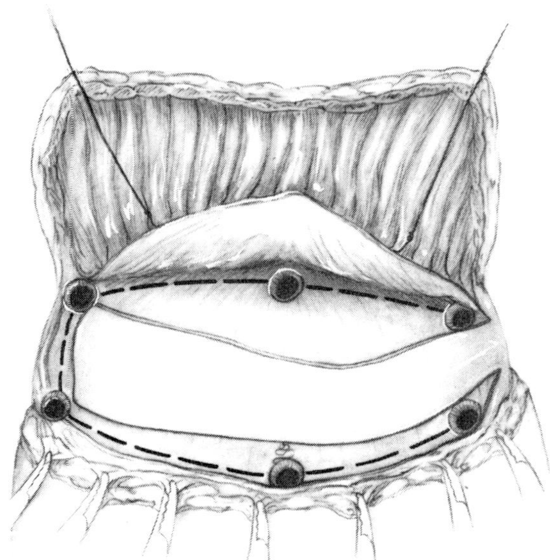

58

## 58

The bone flap must be cut as low as possible, even if this involves going through the frontal sinus. Central burr holes are placed in the midline over the sagittal sinus. If the frontal sinus is entered with the lower midline burr hole, it is sometimes difficult to cut through the posterior wall. In this case a second burr hole in the posterior wall may be necessary.

# 59

The frontal sinus is often opened. Its mucosa should be stripped and the sinus packed with absorbable gelatin sponge covered with penicillin powder.

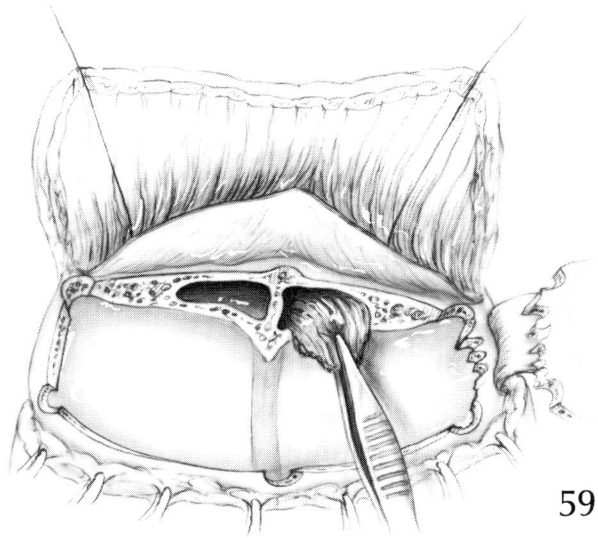

59

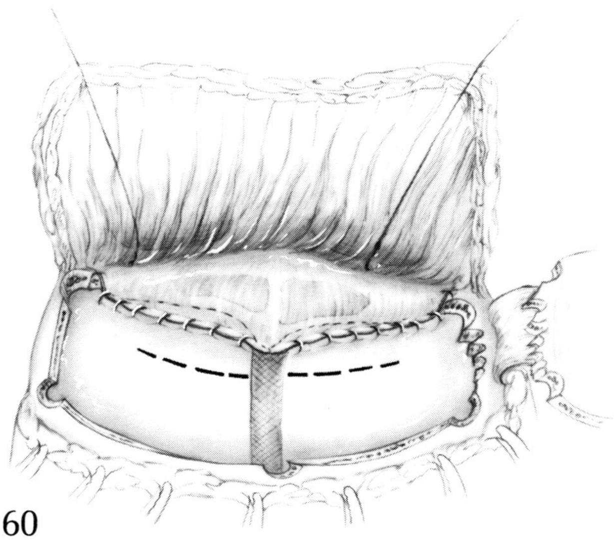

60

# 60

The triangular flap of pericranium cut previously is folded over the frontal sinus and either stitched or glued to the dura.

The dura is opened on both sides of the sagittal sinus.

# 61

The brain is retracted from the sinus and falx cerebri.

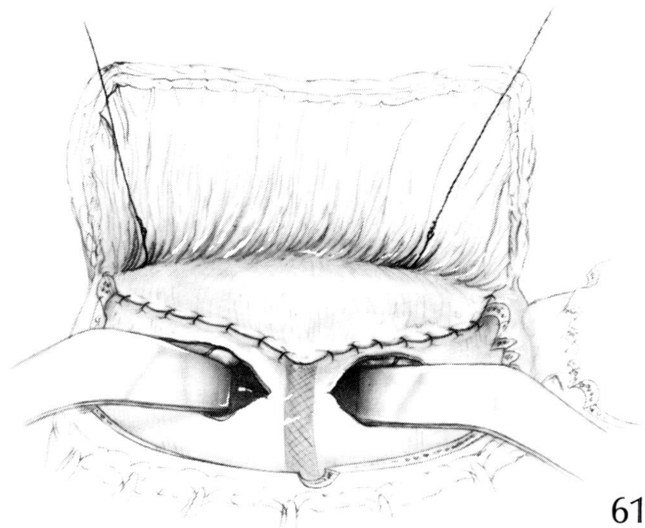

61

## 62

The falx and its lower margin are identified.

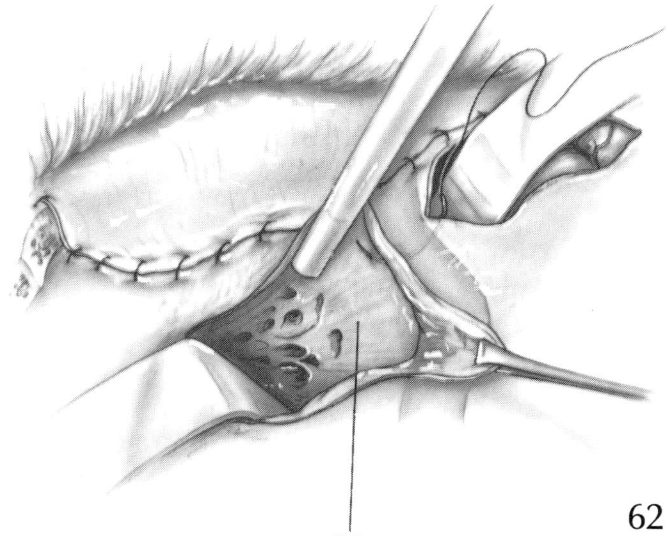


62

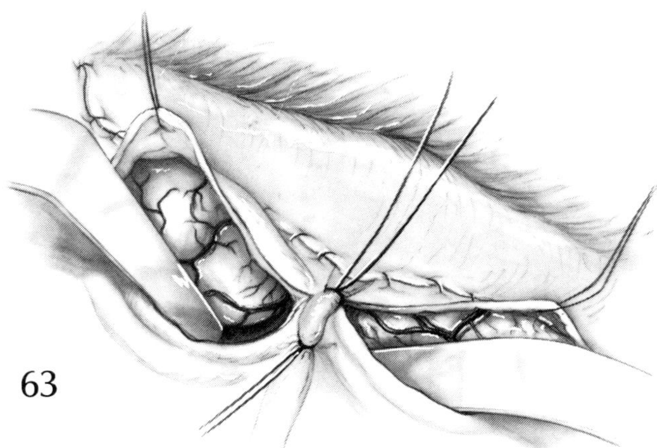

63

## 63

The sinus is doubly occluded with transfixion sutures and divided between the ligatures.

## 64

The incision is carried down through the falx to its free lower margin. Stay sutures are placed in the dura anteriorly and posteriorly, and the dura is retracted.

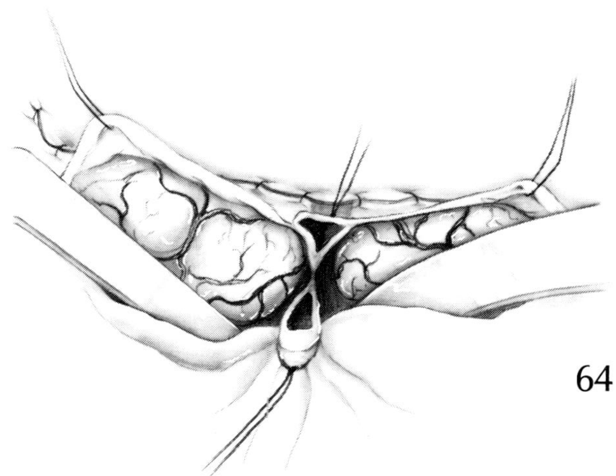

64

# 65

The self-retaining retractors are now repositioned to retract the frontal lobes and expose the floor of the anterior fossa. As a rule, the whole anterior fossa has to be explored bilaterally as far back as the optic chiasm. There may be an exception if CT scanning with intrathecal contrast enhancement has demonstrated a well-localized and strictly unilateral leak.

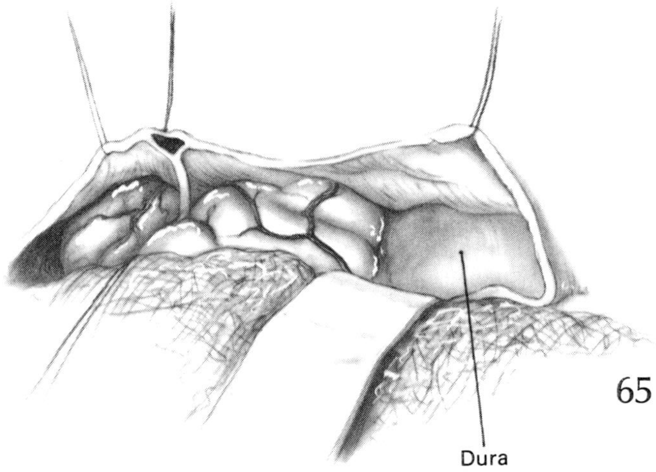


65

# 66

The position of the dural defect and fracture is usually suggested by a brain hernia. Normal dura has to be identified clearly all round.

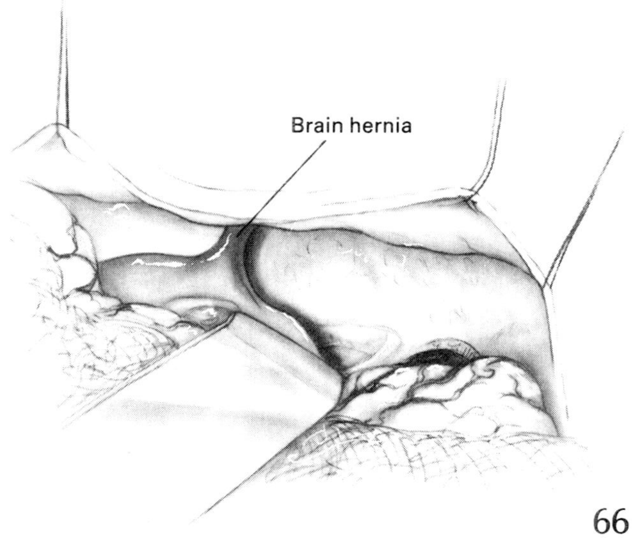


66

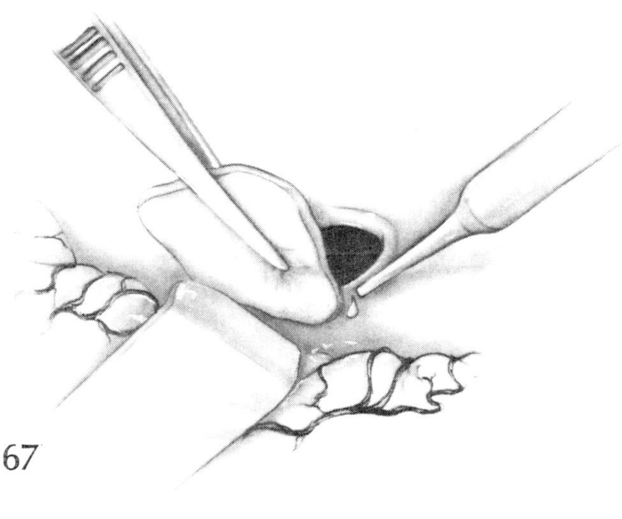

67

## Dural patch

# 67

A patch of either pericranium or, more usually, artificial dura is cut to fit the defect and is glued or stitched into position. The technique for inserting a large patch is to place the edge of the patch along the posterior aspect of the defect, with the rest of the patch pulled back over the frontal lobe. The posterior edge is then glued in position and the patch is gradually moved forward with successive gluing. The dura is then closed.

## Craniofacial injury and anterior fossa fracture

# 68 & 69

If there is an associated comminuted fracture of the frontal bone, the fragments, especially those of the orbital rim, should be individually removed and retained. In order to preserve a series of fragments it may be necessary to cut around them. This is usually achieved by making a lower midline burr hole above the fracture, and positioning the inferior line of the bone flap above the fragments of the fracture.

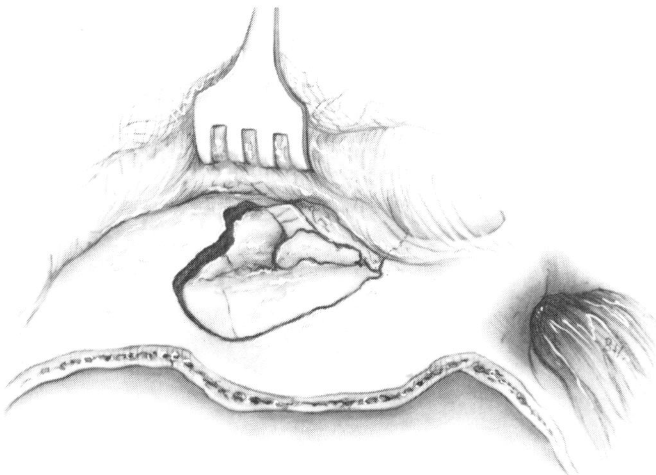

68

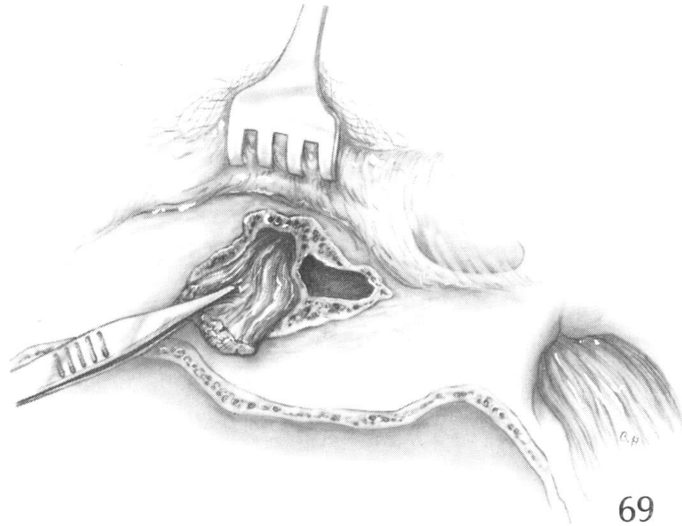

69

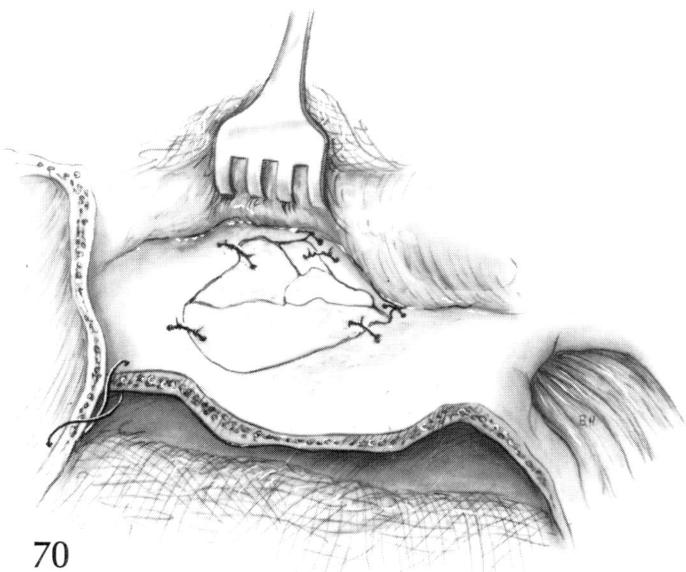

70

# 70

At the stage of closing a comminuted frontal fracture, all the bone fragments are wired back in position and the orbit is reconstituted.

## Postoperative care and results

Standard postoperative monitoring is performed. Antibiotics should be continued for 7 days postoperatively.

With delayed operation, mortality is very low. Preoperative and postoperative intracranial infection occurs in about 5 per cent of patients.

Illustrations by Barbara Hyams

# Trans-sphenoidal hypophysectomy

**D. G. T. Thomas** FRCP, FRCS
Senior Lecturer and Consultant Neurosurgeon, Institute of Neurology, The National Hospitals for Nervous Diseases, London, UK

## Introduction

After the first successful trans-sphenoidal surgery by Schloffer in 1907, several technically varied approaches were rapidly developed to approach the pituitary through the sphenoid from the nose, face or mouth. However, Cushing (1914)[1] synthesized these developments into a sublabial, trans-septal, trans-sphenoidal pituitary approach by employing a bivalve speculum for exposure, together with headlamp illumination during the operation. In the modern era the method has been refined and developed in its application by pioneers like Guiot (1978)[2] and Hardy (1979)[3] with the introduction of peroperative radiology and the operating microscope (see Landolt and Strebel, 1980[4] for a detailed review).

## Preoperative

### Indications

This technique is used for removal of adenomas of the pituitary gland, as well as for ablation of the normal gland. Rarely it may be indicated for surgery of cystic craniopharyngiomas, but it is contraindicated for other sellar and suprasellar masses, including meningiomas, most craniopharyngiomas, optic chiasm gliomas and giant aneurysms.

Endocrine-active pituitary adenomas will usually present with syndromes due to hormonal imbalance, including most commonly amenorrhoea and galactorrhoea due to prolactinomas, acromegaly due to growth hormone-secreting adenomas, Cushing's disease and Nelson's syndrome due to ACTH-producing adenomas. Such patients will usually be investigated jointly with a Department of Endocrinology before any decision as to excisional surgery is made. Selective adenoma removal by trans-sphenoidal hypophysectomy, with sparing of normal residual pituitary function and suppression of abnormal hormone secretion, is often possible in cases of prolactinoma, but is less common in acromegaly and ACTH-secreting adenomas. Where selective hypophysectomy has been unsuccessful, adjuvant therapy with drugs (bromocriptine; Parlodel, Sandoz, Middlesex, UK), radiotherapy or further surgical total hypophysectomy may be indicated.

Pituitary adenomas which are not causing endocrine activity may present with mass effects, usually visual impairment due to suprasellar extension, often in combination with hypopituitarism or with less common features like pituitary apoplexy. In many of these cases, even with large suprasellar extension, partial or subtotal removal may be practical by the trans-sphenoidal route. However, multinodular, irregular frontal, or lateral temporal extensions, as well as any doubt whether the tumour is a pituitary adenoma, may contraindicate this approach and favour a transcranial approach at craniotomy. In general, the trans-sphenoidal procedure is smaller and better tolerated than craniotomy, particularly in the elderly, and its use virtually obviates the risk of postoperative epilepsy.

### Investigations

Both normal and pathological conditions of the endocrine system are now well understood (Lightman and Everitt, 1986)[5], and accurate reproducible radioimmunoassays for pituitary trophic hormones are widely available, permitting rapid assessment of the endocrine status of the patient with a pituitary tumour. This should be done by the endocrinologist both before surgery and during follow-up. Dynamic stress tests can add further to the analysis of pituitary function, particularly in postoperative assessment of surgery for functioning microadenomas, but this is beyond the scope of this chapter. Neuro-ophthalmological assessment with formal perimetry is also desirable, and essential where there is visual failure before surgery and at follow-up.

# 1a & b

Neuroradiology is crucial in the preoperative investigation of the patient. The size and shape of the pituitary gland and the sella are revealed by high resolution CT scanning with sagittal and coronal reformats. Plain skull X-ray and NMR scanning can also contribute in this assessment.

Bony erosion and enlargement of the sella, as well as the slope of its floor, may indicate the probable site of an adenoma within the gland. The presence of soft tissue expansion within the gland at the site of a microadenoma may be shown directly by CT or NMR. Alternatively, in larger tumours these scans reveal the extent, direction and the relationship of suprasellar extensions to the third ventricle. The latter investigations will also indicate the presence of a partially empty sella before surgery. Preoperative plain skull films or the CT scout should also be examined to confirm the pneumatization of the sphenoid before employing this route to approach the pituitary.

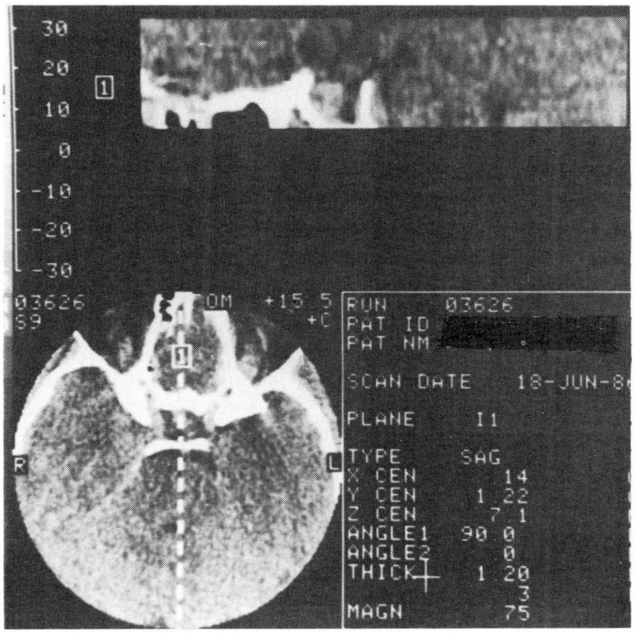


1a

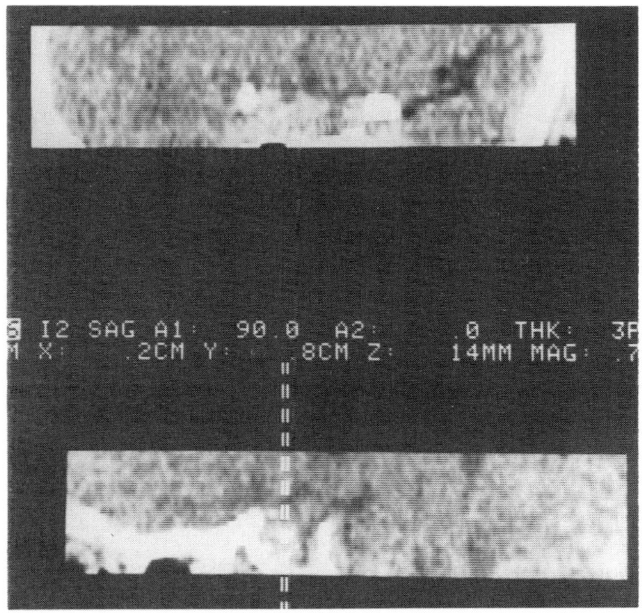


1b

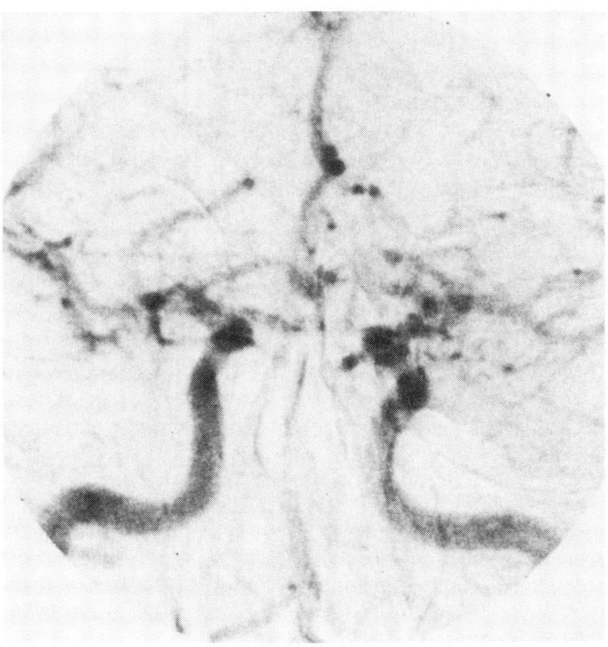

2

# 2

Angiography may be necessary to exclude the presence of an aneurysm on the carotid circulation, as well as to confirm that the carotid arteries do not lie abnormally close to the midline. Usually, digital angiography will be sufficient for this purpose. In cases with significant suprasellar extension, angiography also defines the extent of elevation of the anterior cerebral arteries, as well as sometimes contributing usefully to the differential diagnosis of a pituitary tumour from other suprasellar masses, including aneurysm.

Bacteriology swabs should be taken from the nose and throat before surgery and before commencing prophylactic antibiotic therapy.

## Anaesthesia

General anaesthesia through an endotracheal tube (preferably armoured and with pack *in situ*) and controlled ventilation are essential in order to attain ideal operating conditions. Relative hypotension is desirable to reduce bleeding from the mucosa of the mouth and nose. Continuous monitoring of arterial pressure and of ECG allows alterations in blood pressure and pulse rate to be observed, and corrections made. Although trans-sphenoidal operations are not normally prolonged, a heat-retaining blanket is useful in preventing hypothermia which can delay postoperative recovery from anaesthesia.

## Drug treatment

Antibiotic prophylaxis should be commenced preoperatively. If nose and throat swabs have revealed colonization by specific organisms, appropriate antibiotic therapy is prescribed, and if necessary the procedure delayed until satisfactory clearance of serious pathogens is confirmed by further negative nose and throat swabs. Otherwise, if no growth is found, or only that of commensals, routine prophylaxis may be started the day before surgery, using parenteral penicillin and sulphadimidine, together with local administration of antiseptic cream (Naseptin; ICI Pharmaceuticals, Cheshire, UK).

Steroid cover should be instituted before surgery with dexamethasone 4 mg 6-hourly, together with hydrocortisone 100 mg 6-hourly. As a precaution against peptic ulceration, an F2 antagonist may be administered concurrently with the dexamethasone.

## Position of the patient

The patient is positioned supine with the neck slightly extended and the head rotated a few degrees from the midline towards the surgeon. Elevation of the head end of the operating table to 15° helps to reduce venous pressure. The surgeon stands or sits to the right of the patient's chest, with the assistant and scrub nurse on the opposite side.

The C-arm of the image-intensifier system or, alternatively a portable X-ray tube and film carrier, are placed to provide a strict lateral view of the skull. The alignment of whichever radiological system is used should be checked before the patient is draped. The operating microscope is placed so that it can be introduced from the direction of the crown of the patient's head, interfering neither with the arrangements for lateral screening or X-ray of the skull, nor with the surgeon and his assistant who are able to face one another across the patient's chest. The right hip is slightly flexed and internally rotated with the right thigh supported by a sandbag or pad so that access to a graft of fat, fascia or muscle from this site is facilitated. The instrument table may be placed more caudally, over the patient's feet or on a separate trolley next to the scrub nurse.

The anaesthetist, together with the ventilator and monitoring equipment, will be situated beyond the lower end of the operating table. The skin of the right thigh is prepared and draped routinely and separately from the nose and mouth. The external surface of the nose and mouth is prepared with water-based antiseptic skin preparation, and antiseptic cream is applied to both external nares. The mucosa of the mouth is cleaned and prepared, and the throat pack, which has been placed previously by the anaesthetist around the endotracheal tube, is covered with a further gauze pack soaked in antiseptic. The area of the nose and mouth is covered with plastic-based impermeable drapes and the cloth towels held to this by sutures, to avoid the presence in this region of metal towel clips which may interfere with peroperative radiology. Overhead operating lights are positioned to illuminate the regions of the mouth and right thigh. An operating headlight is also required during the nasal dissection.

Prior to incision of the mucosa, 2–3 ml of 1 per cent lignocaine solution may be injected through the philtrum into the plane between the mucosa and the maxilla in order to lessen bleeding.

# The operation

## The incision

### 3

The assistant retracts the upper lip using two small Langenbeck retractors, so exposing the mucosa of the mouth. An incision (dashed line) approximately 4 cm long is made in the mucosa, and deepened using cutting diathermy to the bone of the maxilla. The incision should be carefully placed in the mucosa in order to leave sufficient tissue adherent to the maxilla to receive sutures during closure, but not too close to the lip, as this may cause troublesome scar tissue.

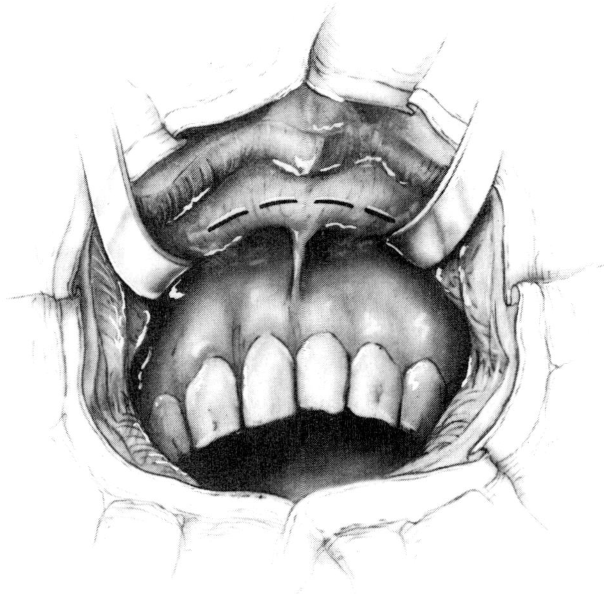

3

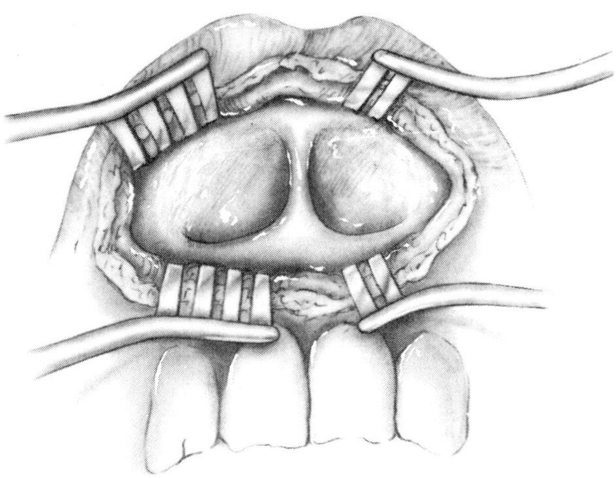

4

## Exposure

### 4

Using a small rugine, the mucosa is reflected to expose the bony floor of the nares bilaterally, together with the midline nasal septum. A plane of cleavage between the nasal mucosa and bone is first started most easily in the floor of the nares 4–5 mm lateral to the midline. Using blunt as well as sharp dissection at the base of the midline septum where the mucosa is generally very adherent, the plane between mucosa and bony maxilla may be developed with the least risk of laceration of the nasal mucosa.

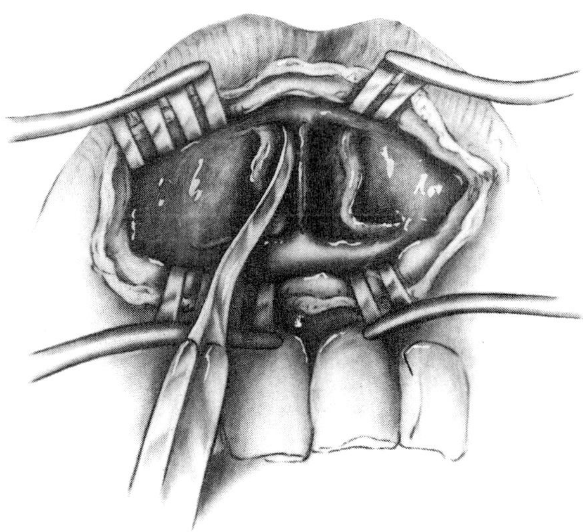

5

### 5

In a similar way, blunt dissection is used to develop a plane between the nasal septum and the mucosa of the nose bilaterally. The septum is seldom exactly in the midline. A hand-held nasal speculum is then used to spread apart the mucosal surfaces which have been freed in this way on both sides of the cartilaginous nasal septum. As dissection proceeds, increasingly longer specula can be inserted, until the bony septum lying posterior to the cartilaginous septum is also exposed.

# 6

At this stage fluoroscopy or check X-ray film may be employed to confirm that the approach is on track for the sphenoid sinus. If there is an error, which at this stage is generally too high an approach, heading towards the ethmoid sinuses and anterior fossa floor, corrections to the trajectory are made.

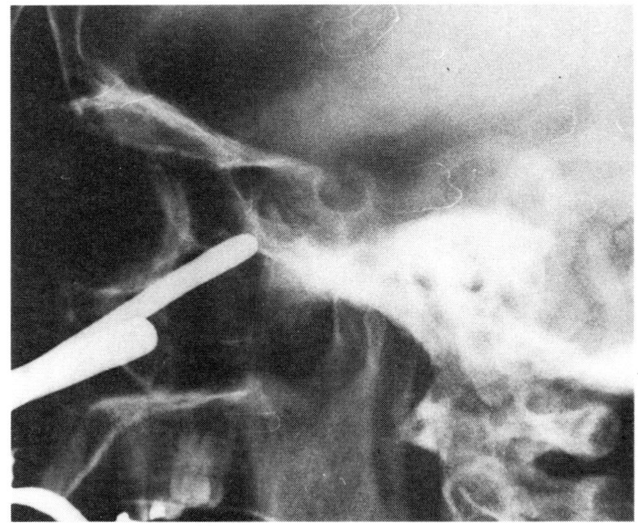

6

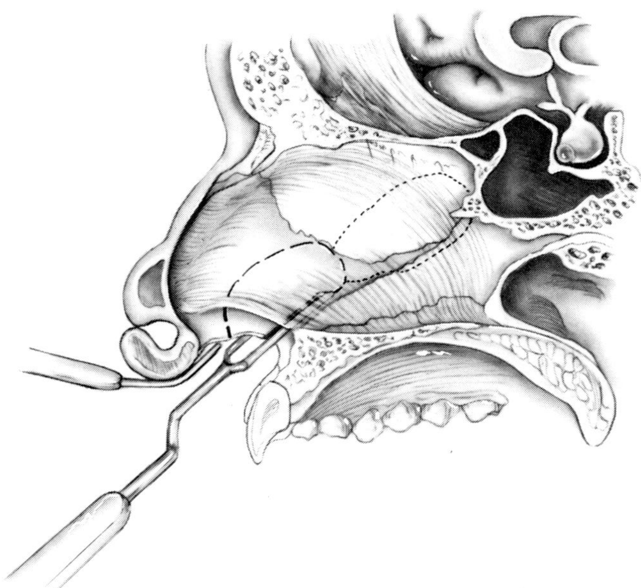

7

# 7

Using a swivelling knife the cartilaginous septum is excised, where possible in a single, large piece which can later be used during closure.

# 8

A self-retaining nasal speculum of a length appropriate to the size of the individual patient is inserted into the nose between the intact mucosal surfaces, and with its lips lying on either side of the bony nasal septum and reaching to the 'keel' of the sphenoid sinus. At this stage the sphenoid bone appears to the surgeon to be shaped like the keel of a boat or the breastbone of a bird. The ostia of the sphenoid sinus will also usually be visualized superiorly and laterally to the lips of the retractor.

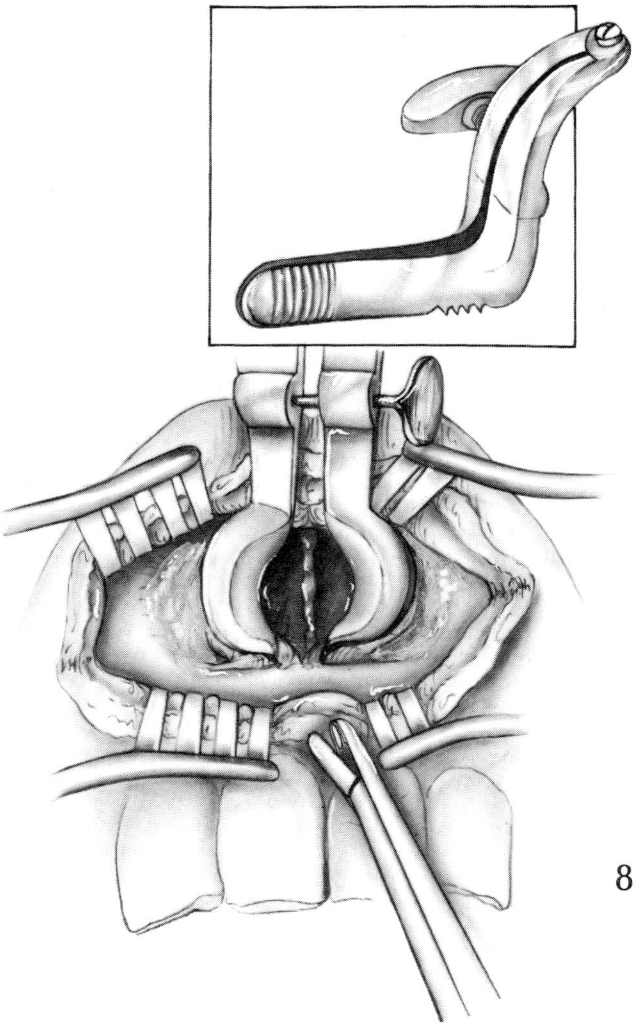

8

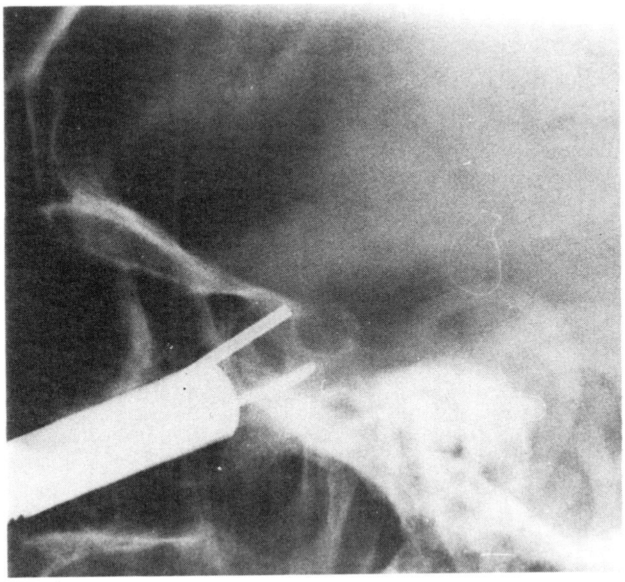

9

# 9

Further X-ray control confirms satisfactory position of the retractor.

The instrument is self-retaining by virtue of the serrations in its surface which abut on the maxilla, and secure fixation may be facilitated by gently striking the retractor with a metal mallet. Subsequent dissection is made easier by positioning the retractor accurately on track and right up to the sphenoid bone, with the nasal mucosa retracted well away from the midline by the tips of the retractor blades. At this stage the operating microscope is introduced.

## 10

Using bone rongeurs and if necessary a small bone chisel, the sphenoid sinus is opened. There is usually asymmetry between the two sides of the sinus, with the midline bony septum tending to deviate to some extent from the midline. The bony septum and the mucosa of the sphenoid sinus are removed piecemeal using rongeurs and suction. If the mucosa is thickened, it is advisable to send a specimen for bacterial culture, as this may represent chronic inflammatory disease and have implications for the choice of further antibiotic treatment. The thorough removal of sphenoid mucosa at this stage lessens the risk of postoperative development of a mucocele.

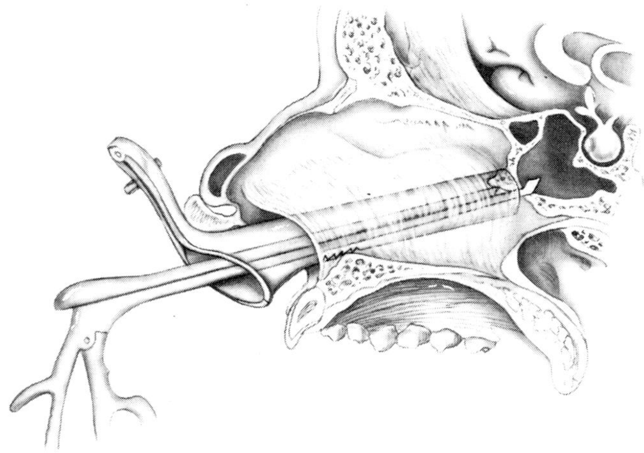

10

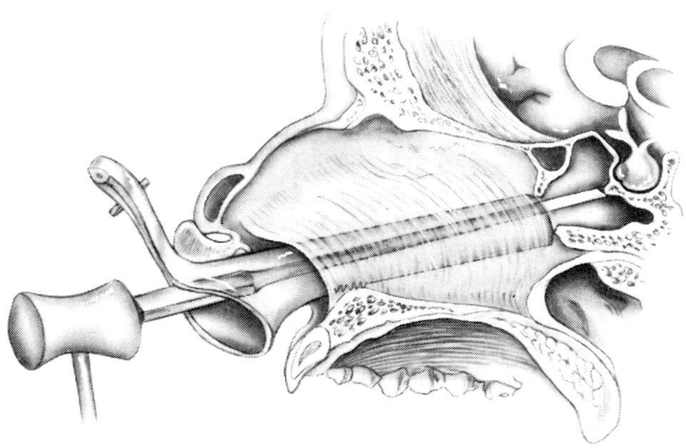

11

## 11

The anterior wall of the pituitary fossa is visualized as the sphenoid is cleared of mucosa. In some cases, particularly of macroadenomas of the pituitary, the bone may be paper thin or even completely eroded with tumour invasion into the sphenoid. In other cases, where the enlargement of the gland is negligible, the bony anterior wall may be thick and hard. In the latter cases a bone chisel with a width of 3–5 mm must be used, with a mallet, to open a window in the anterior wall of the pituitary fossa gently.

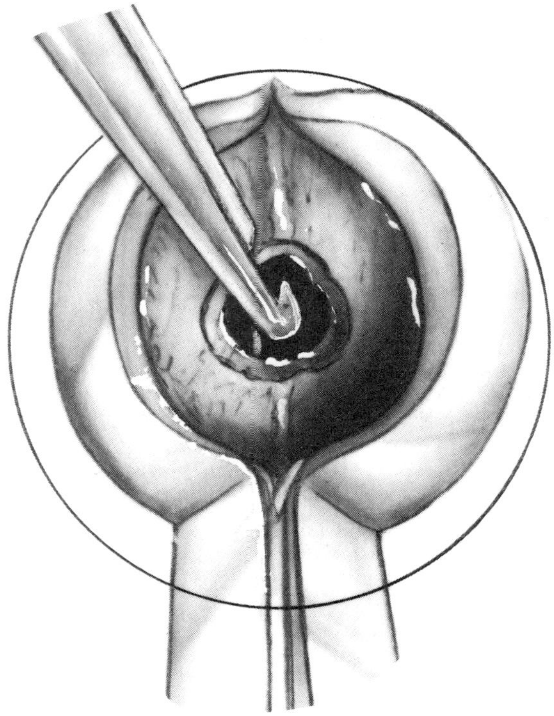

12

# 12 & 13

At this stage, or in the former cases directly, small oblique or right-angled, upcut or downcut bone punches can be used to develop a larger window which exposes the whole width and depth of the pituitary fossa. The opening removal of the wall of the pituitary fossa should be done with great care in order to preserve the dura intact, without small lacerations. Inspection of the gland with the dura intact may indicate enlargement of the gland at a specific site, as illustrated, where there is microadenoma on the patient's right anteriorly and inferiorly within the gland. If possible, a rim of anterior wall should be left intact superiorly, laterally and inferiorly, to facilitate closure with a plug of cartilage later. Peroperative radiology is again useful (*see Illustration 9*).

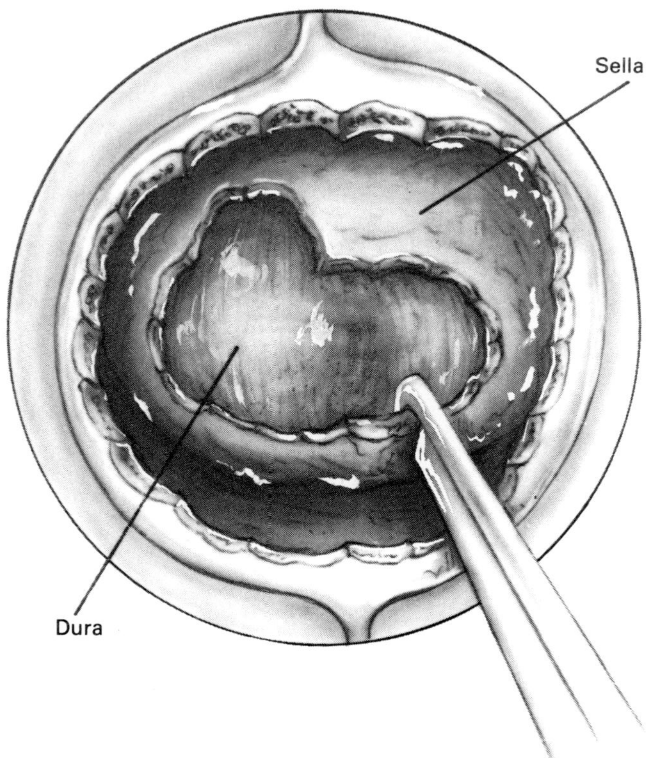


13

# 14

## Incision of the dura

Using pointed diathermy, the dura over the anterior surface of the gland is incised in a cruciate fashion, using a low cutting current. The cutting should be done carefully, without laceration of the gland, in order to allow as much information as possible to be obtained about the probable site of an adenoma within the gland. Inspection is carried out through the microscope and by gentle palpation with a microdissector before artefacts are introduced when the gland is incised.

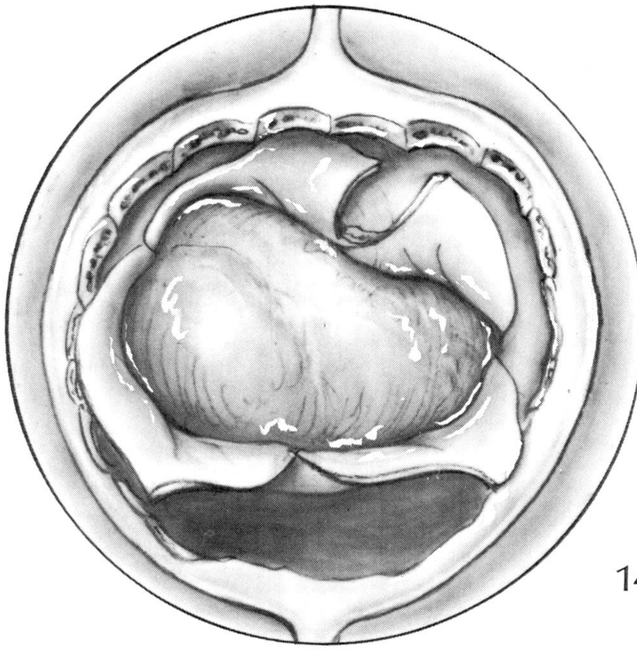

14

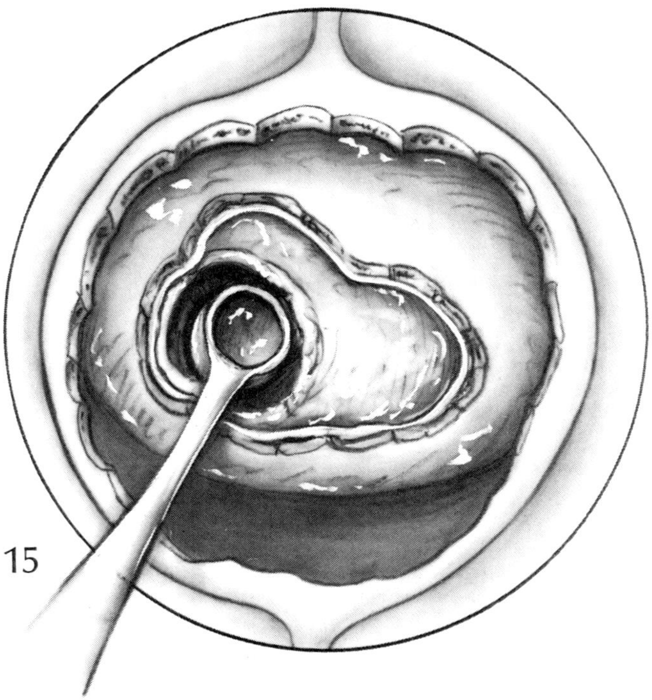

15

# 15

If the tumour is visible, an incision through the thin pituitary capsule allows tumour material to extrude. Small cup and ring curettes together with pituitary rongeurs are used to remove the material, at the same time obtaining biopsies for histology. If the tumour is very soft, a trap on the sucker is useful to collect biopsy material. Complete selective removal of the microadenoma is obtained using suction and curettage, leaving residual normal gland. Provided that there is no cerebrospinal fluid fistula at this stage, 1 ml of absolute alcohol may be instilled in the tumour bed, and left for 60 seconds to sterilize residual neoplastic cells. Generally, adenoma tissue is softer in texture, and grey rather than yellow in colour, compared with normal anterior pituitary. If the adenoma is not visible, the gland may be incised vertically and horizontally with a tenotomy blade, in an attempt to locate the adenoma. Intraoperative histological studies using smear or frozen-section techniques are very valuable in such cases.

# 16

Peroperative radiology will also confirm the site of dissection. In cases of empty sellae associated with adenomas, the lateral walls of the fossa adjacent to the cavernous sinus are inspected with particular care. Review of preoperative CT scans is generally helpful in identifying suspicious areas within the gland (*see Illustrations 1a and b.*)

In cases of larger macroadenomas there is usually no problem in locating tumour tissue. The extent of the partial or subtotal excision to be carried out depends on the tumour's suprasellar expansion and invasiveness within the sella. Irregular multinodular suprasellar extensions, or extensions frontally or into the temporal fossa, cannot be effectively approached trans-sphenoidally. However, relatively large regular midline suprasellar extensions may be partially resected from below. Usually when the dura is incised, soft tumour will be removed using suction and curettage, and the diaphragma sellae will descend progressively. It is possible to show this peroperatively using air or positive contrast in the suprachiasmatic cisterns. Using X-ray control of the placement of curettes and dissectors as well as inspection through the operating microscope, effective decompression and partial removal may be achieved. Lateral extensions into the cavernous sinus can also be partially removed. However, it is important to avoid breaching the dura of the diaphragma sellae above, and of the cavernous sinus laterally. The former leads to troublesome cerebrospinal fluid leakage which may be difficult to control during closure; the latter causes serious venous bleeding, which may be controlled by packing with absorbable gauze, but often with difficulty.

If the pituitary tumour is firm and fibrous, or if the lesion proves to be a meningioma, a chiasmal glioma, or a solid craniopharyngioma, it is better to abandon the procedure and consider reoperation by craniotomy.

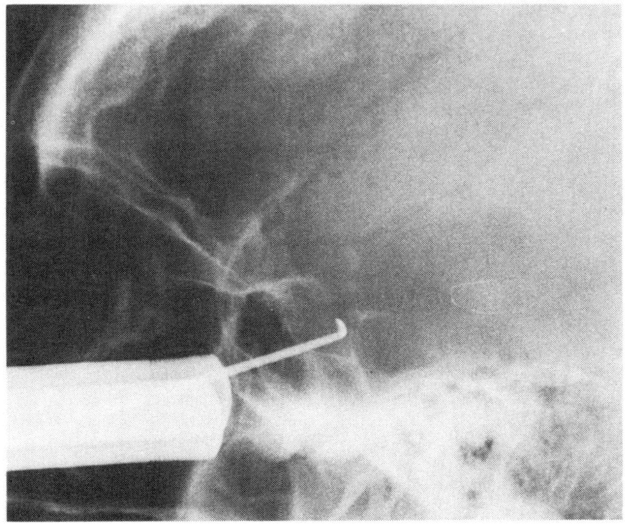

16

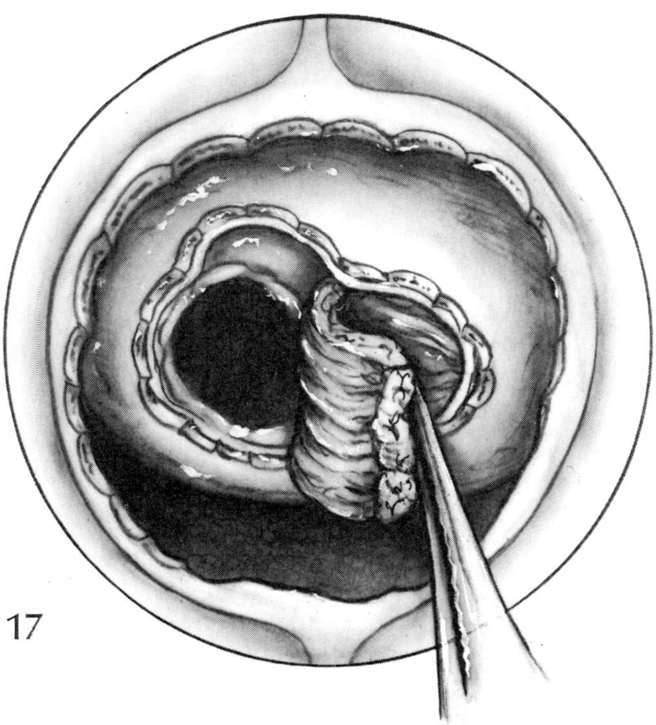

17

## Closure

# 17

A graft is cut from the right thigh to close the sella. This procedure may be done conveniently after tumour removal, allowing a period for haemostasis within the sella which can be packed temporarily with a saline-soaked cotton-wool ball. At this stage it is clear how large a graft is required and of what type. In cases of selective removal of a small microadenoma it is sufficient to take fat only, and generally a small volume is sufficient. In cases where the sella is left largely empty and where there is a large cerebrospinal fluid fistula, it is necessary to obtain fascia lata to line the lower surface of the diaphragma, as well as muscle to fill up the sella and effectively to support the fascia in position. The tissue graft is cut to an appropriate size to fill the defect left in the sella, not only to close any fistula but to prevent later subsidence of the chiasm downwards into a void area.

# 18

The cartilaginous septum excised during the approach to the sphenoid is trimmed slightly larger than the defect in the bony anterior wall of the sella. This cartilage graft is then passed through the sphenoid into the sella using a three-pronged trident instrument, so that the cartilage wedges the soft tissue securely in the sella. A secure watertight seal is required whenever there has been leak of cerebrospinal fluid peroperatively. This is achieved by tamponading the soft tissue in place, and can be further secured by the application of fibrin glue (Tisseel, Immuno, Dunton Green, Kent, UK) over the defect in the sella. If the sella has been extensively destroyed by invasive tumour it may not be possible to achieve closure in this way. In these cases the sphenoid itself may be obliterated by a large muscle and fascia graft held in position by struts of cartilage wedged across the opening in the sphenoid sinus.

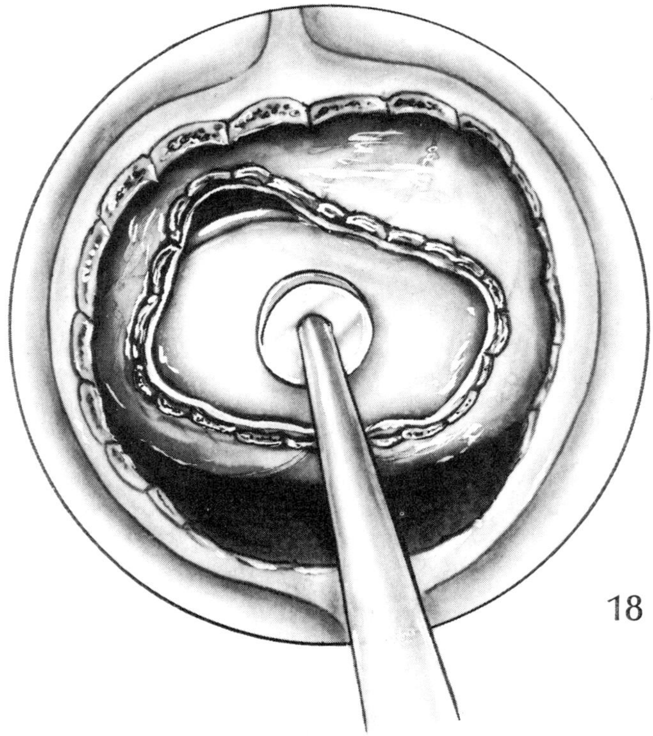

18

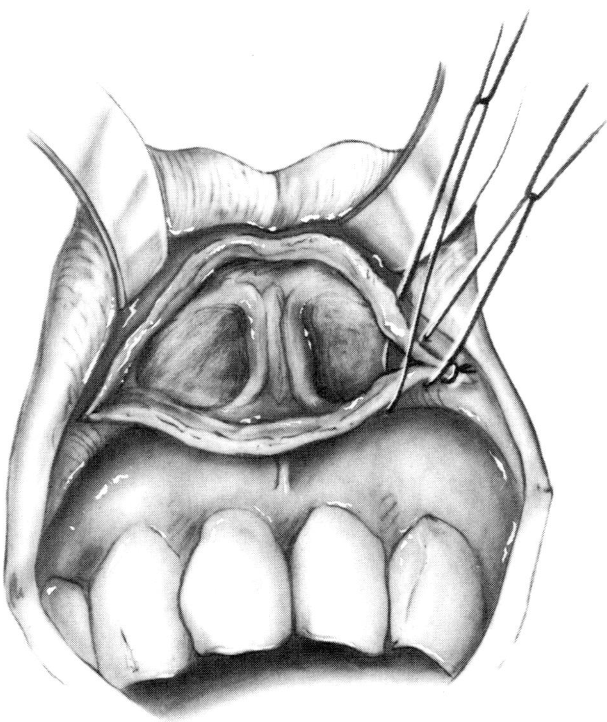

19

# 19

The self-retaining speculum is withdrawn, and after haemostasis has been obtained in the mucosa of the nose and gum, the mucosal incision is closed with interrupted catgut sutures.

# 20

Hand-held nasal specula are inserted into both nostrils. The nose is then packed bilaterally with BIPP-impregnated nasal ribbon gauze, which tamponades the midline mucosal surfaces together in the absence of the excised septum, as well as applying the mucosa to the anterior wall of the sphenoid sinus. Both the leading end and the trailing end of the packing tape should be left projecting from the nose so that no loose pack can pass down into the pharynx and cause irritation. The ends of the right and left side packs may be tied together as a further precaution against migration of the ribbon gauze into the patient's throat.

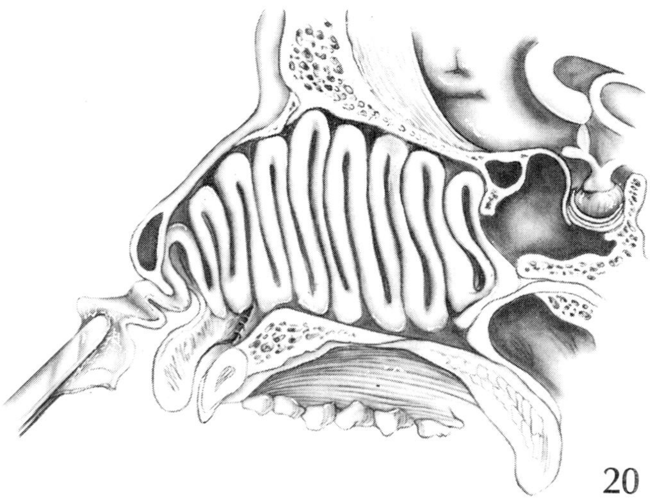

20

## Postoperative care

The patient is extubated with care to remove throat packs, and to avoid drainage of blood from the operative site into the stomach where it may cause vomiting. As soon as the patient is properly awake he may be nursed in the recumbent position, with 10–15° of head-up tilt of the upper part of the body. The nasal packs are removed under light intravenous sedation 5 days postoperatively. After the packs have been removed, the patient is instructed not to blow his nose vigorously for 2 weeks. Instead he should gently wipe the nose with tissues as required. If there has been cerebrospinal fluid leakage peroperatively, lumbar punctures are carried out daily for several days to reduce cerebrospinal fluid pressure. Antibiotic therapy is continued for 10 days postoperatively, or longer if there is a cerebrospinal fluid fistula. Dexamethasone may be tapered off within 2–3 days postoperatively, but hydrocortisone replacement should be only gradually reduced to normal replacement levels of 37.5 mg daily, where it should remain until postoperative endocrine assessment is performed 2–3 weeks after surgery. At this stage the necessity for long-term replacement with cortisone, thyroxine, gonadotrophin or posterior pituitary hormone can be further evaluated.

In the early postoperative period, diabetes insipidus with urine outputs of more than 1000 ml in 4–6 hours may become evident; if this happens, treatment with desmopressin (DDAVP) in intermittent doses may be necessary. Often this is only a temporary state, but sometimes prolonged posterior pituitary hormone replacement may be required. The nasal mucosa will generally have recovered sufficiently for nasal administration to be effective within 3–4 weeks of surgery. The patient can usually be mobilized within 1–2 days, and if necessary may stand to pass urine or use the commode within a few hours of surgery. The catgut sutures in the mucosa of the gum do not require removal. The skin sutures in the thigh are removed at 10 days.

## Complications

Cerebrospinal fluid fistula, with the risk of meningitis, is the most frequent serious risk of trans-sphenoidal surgery of the sella. If it occurs, repeated lumbar punctures or continuous lumbar spinal drainage will often produce spontaneous resolution of the fistula. If this is not successful, radiological investigation with metrizamide-enhanced CT cisternography may be useful in defining the site of the leak. Re-exploration of the sphenoid, either by the sublabial transnasal route, or alternatively via a transethmoidal route through previously untouched tissue, is indicated. In some cases the site of the fistula will be clearly visualized and a fresh tissue graft of fascia and muscle may be applied. In other cases no distinct fistula is visualized, but re-exploration of the sphenoid and repacking of the sella generally results in closure of the fistula. In some resistant cases, further re-exploration of the sphenoid from below, or exploration of the sella via a transcranial route, may be required to identify and seal the leak.

Other rare complications of the procedure include cranial nerve palsies, particularly diplopia owing to involvement of the third or sixth nerves in the cavernous sinus, anterior fossa fracture with anosmia, peroperative or delayed haemorrhage from the cavernous carotid artery, and increased visual field defects owing to changed deformity of the chiasm, for which chiasmopexy may occasionally be required.

### *References*


1. Cushing, H. (1914) Surgical experiences with pituitary disorders. Journal of the American Medical Association, 63, 1515–1525

2. Guiot, G. (1978) Consideration on the surgical treatment of pituitary adenomas. In: Treatment of Pituitary Adenomas, R. Fahlbusch, K. V. Werder (eds.), pp. 202–218. Stuttgart: G. Thieme

3. Hardy, J. (1979) Functional neurosurgery of neuroendocrine disorders. In: Functional Neurosurgery, T. Rasmussen, R. Marino (eds.), pp. 143–153. New York: Raven Press

4. Landolt, A. M., Strebel, P. (1980) Technique of trans-sphenoidal operation for pituitary adenomas. In: Advances and Technical Standards in Neurosurgery, H. Krayenbuhl *et al.* (eds.), pp. 119–177. Vienna: Springer-Verlag

5. Lightman, S. L., Everitt, B. J. (1986) Neuroendocrinology: integrated functions of the central nervous system. In: Neuroendocrinology, S. L. Lightman, B. J. Everitt (eds.), pp. 1–4. Oxford: Blackwell

Illustrations by Barbara Hyams

# Cranioplasty

**Derek S. Gordon** MCh, FRCS
Consultant Neurosurgeon, Royal Victoria Hospital, Belfast, UK

**George A. S. Blair** MDS, FFD
Consultant in Restorative Dentistry, Royal Victoria Hospital, Belfast, UK

Most skull defects result from head injury or from removal of operative bone flaps which have become infected or are involved by tumour. Congenital skull defects rarely close spontaneously and can be repaired in early childhood. The first cranioplasties were performed in the 17th century. In 1600 Fallopius recommended the use of gold plates. Autogenous bone grafting, introduced in the 19th century, became established practice in the management of battle casualties in the 1914–1918 war. In the 1939–1945 war, alloplastic plates became increasingly popular. By 1960 tantalum and methylmethacrylate plates had almost replaced bone grafting in the treatment of large skull defects. In 1964 Simpson[1] introduced titanium, which is now widely used as plates, strips or as wire mesh.

## Indications for cranioplasty

The chief indications for cranioplasty are disfigurement and protection of the brain from injury. A visible skull defect may affect the patient's career prospects. Discomfort and tenderness associated with scar retraction at the edge of a defect are sometimes an indication for cranioplasty. Cranioplasty may relieve headache and dizziness – 'the syndrome of the trephined' – occurring with rapid changes of posture. The patient's age, prognosis and occupation are taken into account.

## Requirements for cranioplasty

*Precision* The compound complex curvature of the skull must be reproduced, especially in the frontotemporal region and at the supraorbital margin. A close fit between the periphery of the prosthesis and the bone surrounding the defect is important.

*Ease of fixation* The cranioplasty material can be inlaid in the defect or onlaid over the edge of the defect. Onlay fixation with screws removes the need to dissect the edge of the defect and to separate the dura from the skull – an important advantage in dealing with large defects.

*Mechanical strength* The material must be resistant to heavy impact loading. The impact resistance of an onlay prosthesis greatly exceeds that of an inlay prosthesis.

*Tissue acceptance* There should be little, if any, postoperative effusion, and experimental evidence should show no late tissue reaction to the material[2].

*Radiolucency* Patients who have had surgical treatment for a tumour may need further neuroradiological investigations if a recurrence is suspected.

*Malleability* A preformed plate may need fine adjustment to achieve a perfect fit.

*Ease of sterilization* The cranioplasty material must be easily sterilized.

## Materials for cranioplasty

Cranioplasty is, in principle, a simple operation, but the diversity of techniques shows that difficulties exist. Most of the materials in common use are suitable for small defects; however, in the treatment of large defects, some materials have decided advantages.

### *Osteoplastic reconstruction*

Bone grafts are difficult to contour for large defects; they are usually inserted by inlay fixation using wire sutures. A bone graft when fused has adequate strength but it sometimes undergoes resorption. Tissue acceptance and radiolucency are good. Small outer skull table grafts are sometimes placed over skull defects which involve the frontal air sinuses. Bone grafts taken from the ilium or ribs leave a painful donor site.

### *Alloplastic implants*

*Acrylic resins* Acrylic resin plates are difficult to contour and attach to the bony margin of large defects. Heat-cured preformed plates need to be thick and bulky to achieve adequate strength and are usually suitable only for inlay fixation. Incomplete polymerization with traces of residual monomer may stimulate wound effusion and reactive changes in the adjacent tissues. Fine last-minute adjustment is impossible.

During the fabrication of autopolymerization plates *in situ* excessive endothermic heat is generated. With a limited polymerizing time it is difficult to mould an accurately fitting plate for all but the smallest defects.

The acrylic resins are radiolucent. Sterilization of the heat-cured plates is often unsatisfactory.

*Metals and alloys* Metal and alloy plates can be contoured accurately, are easily sterilized, and have the advantage of early onlay fixation by screws, giving considerable mechanical strength. The metals and alloys in use include tantalum, stainless steel, titanium and chrome cobalt alloys.

Tantalum sheet has been used extensively, the plates being contoured by a dental die–counterdie swaging technique. It has good tissue acceptance, fine adjustment is possible, but the metal has a relatively high specific gravity and is not radiolucent. Stabilized austenite stainless steel has also been shaped by a swaging technique; it is malleable and, when formed, becomes work-hardened. However, because of the presence of chromium and nickel, adverse tissue reactions are common.

Titanium sheet has been used for over 20 years. Experience with titanium in Belfast started in 1969 using a hydraulic cold forming system[3]. Thin section (0.60 mm) titanium sheet (IMI-115; Imperial Metal Industries, Kyneth, Birmingham, UK) can be formed to a very accurate contour. The plate is radiolucent and has excellent tissue acceptance.

## Initial operation

The difficulties of cranioplasty can be minimized by careful planning at the initial operation. In treating a compound depressed skull fracture it is usually best to suture the scalp laceration and then turn a generous semicircular flap extending at least 2 cm beyond the anticipated edge of the skull defect. Dural repair is essential, augmented if necessary by a graft of pericranium or temporal fascia to prevent adhesions between the scalp and the brain. At this stage a template is cut in dental foil to the shape and contour of the defect and 1 cm over size. In a large defect it is more convenient to take an impression with sterile dental alginate. The thickness of the skull is measured to determine the correct length of the fixation screws. If there has been scalp loss, an advancement or rotational flap may be needed to prevent scalp tension after cranioplasty.

## Preparation of preformed plate

### *Metal or alloy plates*

If an impression of the defect has not been taken at the initial operation, an external impression technique is used[4]. The size and shape of the defect are determined by X-ray. The margin of the defect is palpated and outlined with an indelible pencil. If the margin is difficult to define, small strips of metal are attached to the skin and further X-rays are taken to check the accuracy of the pencil marking. When complex compound curvatures have been lost, for example in the supraorbital region, a dental silicone putty is moulded and placed in the defect to restore the correct contours. An impression of the defect is then taken in dental plaster. After the plaster has set, appropriate landmarks are recorded on the surface of the impression.

If a bone flap corresponding to the defect is available, this can be used instead of an impression. From the impression or the bone flap a model of the defect is cast in plaster of Paris. The indelible pencil mark on the impression will be transferred to the cast and the required contour is then built up with wax. A die is then made in strong dental stone and placed in a high-pressure hydraulic forming chamber[5]. A sheet of titanium (IMI 115, 0.60 mm thick) is placed across the die and moulded to the desired contour by high-pressure oil generated by a hydraulic pump.

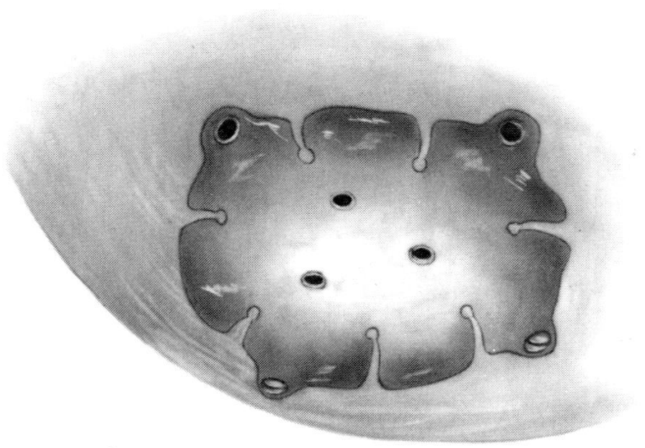

1

1

The formed plate is trimmed until the rim overlaps the margin of the defect by about 5 mm. Projections are left at predetermined sites to receive the fixation screws. Radial slots 2 mm wide are cut between the projections to allow fine adjustment of any part of the plate.

Tissue acceptance is enhanced by anodizing the finished plate in a solution of 80 per cent phosphoric acid, 10 per cent sulphuric acid and 10 per cent water. Anodization changes the colour of the plate from dark grey to gold and prevents the dark shadow which may show through thin exposed skin.

## Timing of cranioplasty

Immediate cranioplasty is occasionally performed using metal strips or preformed plates[6]. More often the operation takes place about 3 weeks after the initial operation. If there has been delayed primary wound healing or when a fracture has involved air sinuses, the operation is delayed for 6 to 12 months.

## Anaesthesia

Small plates can be inserted under local anaesthesia but for larger plates general anaesthesia is preferred. Postoperative antibiotics are occasionally used if there has been infection in the wound. A prophylactic course of antibiotics is rarely necessary.

# The operation

Excision of the original operative scar is seldom required. The incision follows the line between the scar and the intact scalp closely. For frontal defects a coronal incision is most satisfactory. In separating the scalp from the dura, the correct tissue plane is identified by blunt dissection with McIndoe scissors or sometimes by finger dissection. If the dura has not been carefully closed, a cerebrospinal fluid (CSF) leak may appear; it should be sealed with a pericranial graft. A dural defect which has not been covered in the initial operation by a fascial or pericranial graft may have an inadequate layer of false dura which must be repaired. If necessary, the cranioplasty is deferred. Sometimes cranioplasty is delayed because a frontal sinus has been involved by the fracture. If the scalp is dissected carefully, the regenerated sinus mucosa can be left intact. When doubt exists, the plane of dissection can be altered so that the galea over the damaged sinus is left adherent to the sinus mucosa. In some head injuries, especially those caused by missiles, extensive scars may overlie the skull defect. Rotation flaps can now often be avoided by use of the subgaleal expansion balloon, which stretches the adjacent normal scalp to such an extent that it will cover the defect.

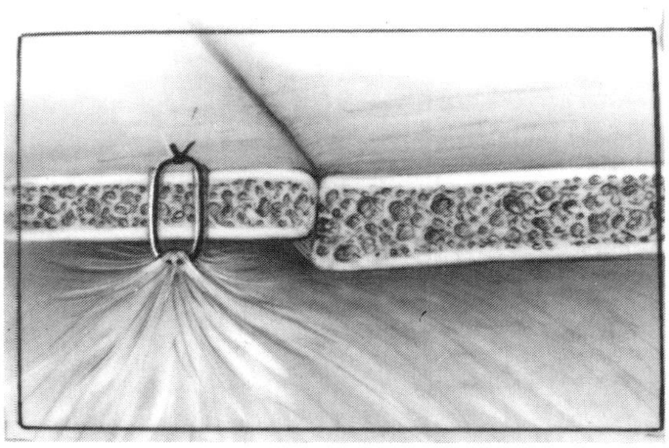

2

## AUTOGENOUS BONE CRANIOPLASTY

### 2

The bone graft is usually obtained by resection of lower ribs with or without their periosteum; for a small defect the outer table of ilium or the outer table of skull is satisfactory. When the bone graft is to be inlaid, the operation involves dissection of the bone edge of the defect and separation of the dura from the undersurface of the skull. A split rib graft may sit firmly when tapped into the prepared defect. Fixation can be augmented by dural sutures or by wire passed through holes in the skull and in the graft.

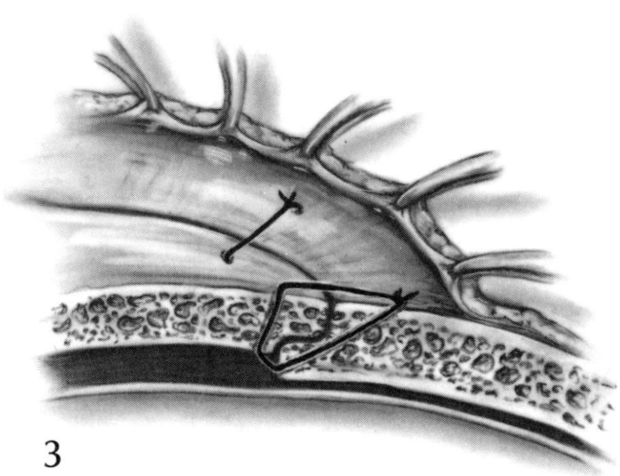

3

### 3

Alternatively, a shelf can be prepared by removing part of the outer table of the skull using a dental bone burr or a chisel. The graft may then be tapped into position. In a large defect contouring is difficult and time-consuming.

## ACRYLIC RESIN CRANIOPLASTY

# 4

A preformed plate is usually inserted as an inlay; if used as an onlay, an acrylic plate is bulky and creates a raised edge. Fixation involves dissection of the edge of the defect and passage of sutures or wire through drill holes in the skull into the extradural space and through holes in the plate. No final accurate adjustment can be made.

The alternative use of acrylic is the autopolymerization technique, in which measured quantities of monomer and polymer are mixed. When the mix acquires a doughy consistency it is applied to the defect. The temperature at the centre of the mass can reach 90°C. The brain must be protected by damp lint and plastic sheeting. Forming the contour of a large defect is difficult; inlay insertion is used with fixation by wire.

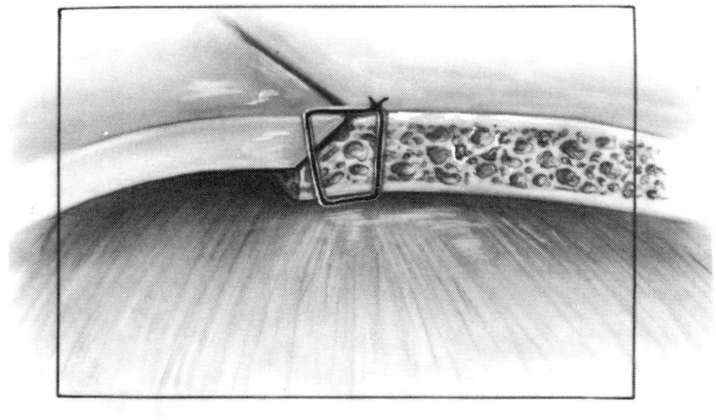

4

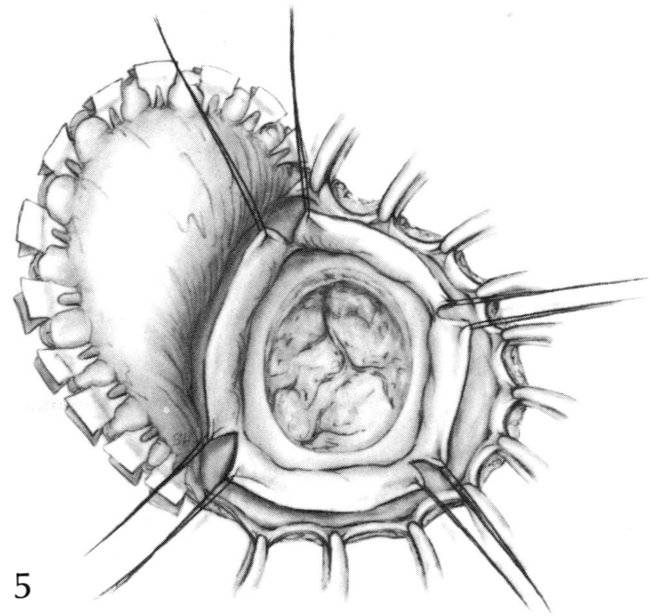

5

## TITANIUM CRANIOPLASTY

# 5

When the scalp flap has been reflected, a circumferential periosteal incision is made near the margin of the defect, followed by small auxiliary radial incisions to allow the periosteum to be reflected 1–2 cm away from the edge of the defect. If the periosteum is very thin, the plate can be applied on top of the periosteum. No dissection of the edge of the defect is necessary. The plate is laid over the defect. Fine adjustment with hawksbill orthodontic pliers ensures a perfect fit.

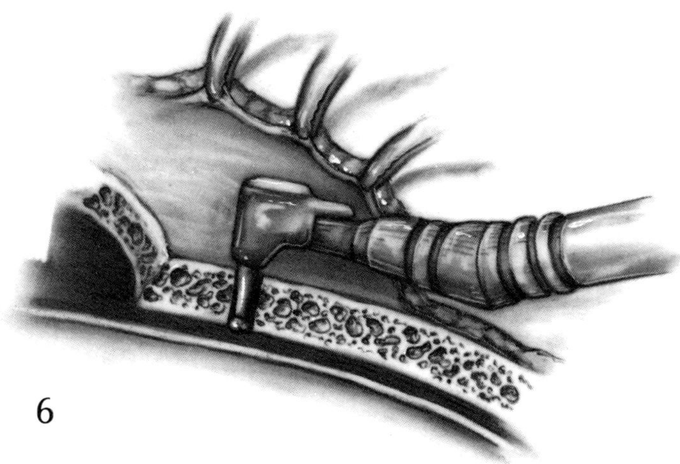

6

# 6

When the skull thickness is not known, an exploratory hole is made with a 5 mm No. 8 dental burr mounted in a right-angled dental handpiece. In adults a 6 mm or 7 mm burr usually just penetrates the inner table of the skull.

# 7

If the defect involves part of the frontal sinus or mastoid air cells, the plate must be so designed that the fixing screws will not enter an air-containing cavity. If the skull defect includes the supraorbital margin, a tongue of titanium is turned back to form a rounded flange which restores the front of the orbital roof.

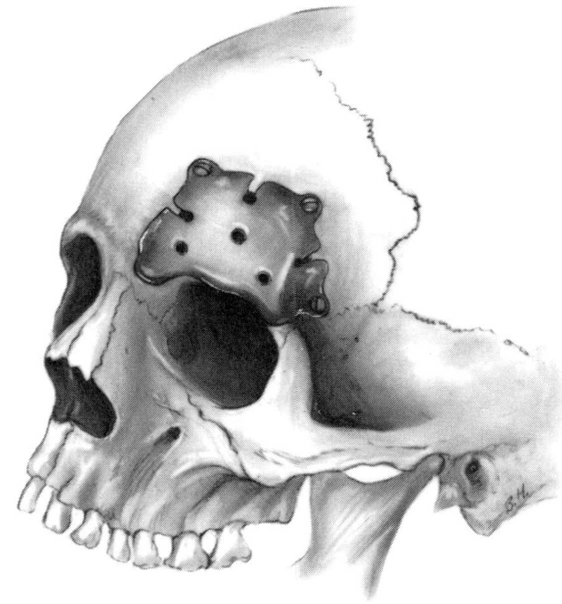

7

# 8

A titanium self-tapping slotted screw (IMI-325 JCH342 – 18,19,20; Down Brothers, UK) is inserted using a titanium-tipped screwdriver. The number of screws varies with the size and shape of the plate. Bone grows into the slot in the screw and prevents any tendency to loosening. Even in a 1-year-old child a 5 mm screw will usually be gripped by the bone[7].

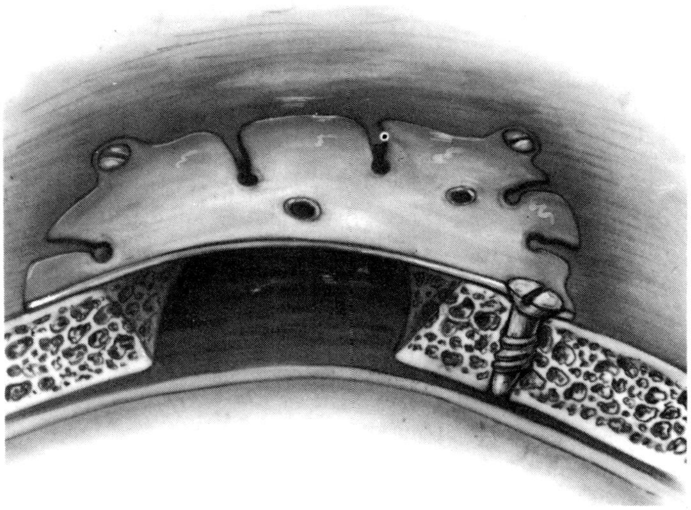

8

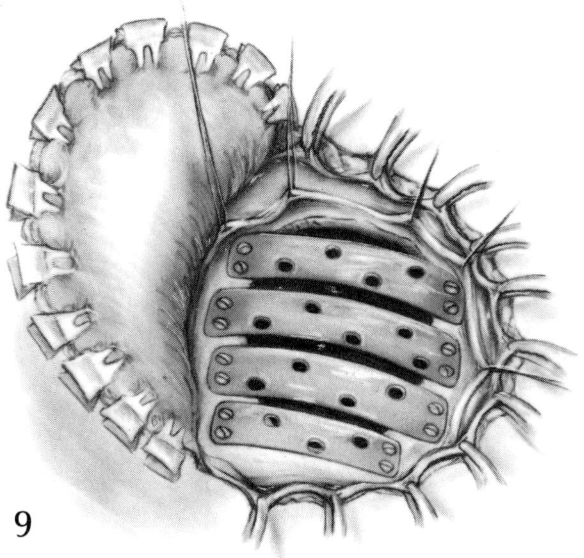

9

## TITANIUM STRIP CRANIOPLASTY

# 9

Preformed strips of titanium (0.60 mm thick) of varying lengths and widths are used for this simple technique. Holes with chamferred edges are drilled at the ends of the strips to receive the fixing screws. The strips are malleable, but when they are bent to the skull contour and fixed at each end by screws they acquire a rigidity comparable to that of the skull. Strip cranioplasty has the advantage of an onlay technique which can be applied easily and without preparation.

# 10

If there are widespread scars, uncovering the whole defect could interfere with the blood supply to the scalp, but it is still possible to insert a metal plate or strip under the scarred area. The scalp is undermined until the full area of the defect is defined. The plate can now be slipped under the intact scalp edge until the bone defect is covered. A 2-mm incision is made over the hole in the projection of the plate. A dental burr inserted through the hole can be used to drill through the skull and a self-tapping screw is then inserted. A single suture will seal the 2 mm incision.

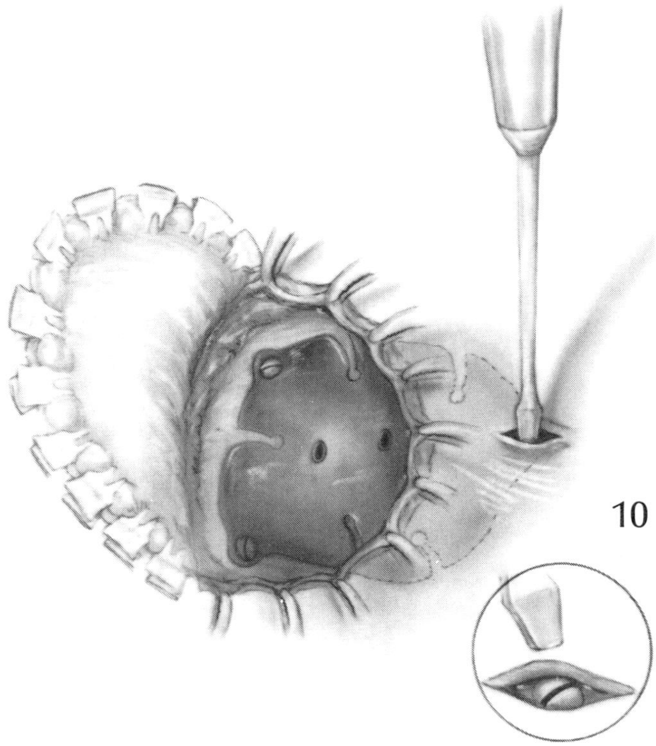

10

# 11a & b

A patient who has had cranioplasty because of tumour involving the skull may need a further operation for tumour recurrence. If necessary, the whole plate can be removed. However, if tumour recurrence is confined to one side of a large defect, only a part of the plate need be removed using a modified Monodex sheet-metal cutter (Patentools Ltd, Brighton, UK). Once the recurrent tumour has been removed, the cranioplasty can be restored using titanium strips or a small preformed plate.

The skin is closed with a single layer of interrupted 3/0 or 5/0 nylon sutures or with metal staples. The vacuum drain can be removed in 1 to 2 days.

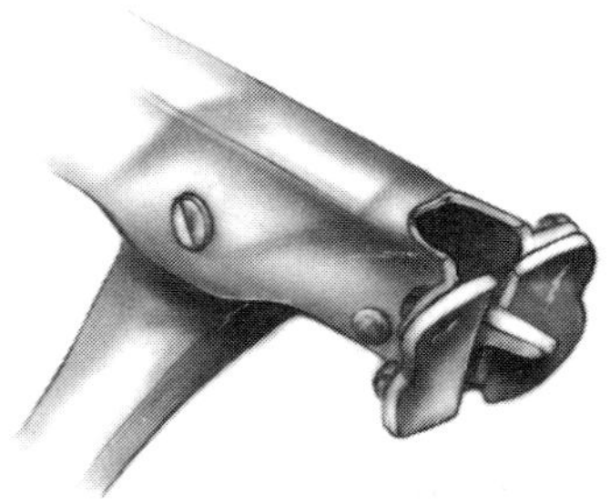

11a

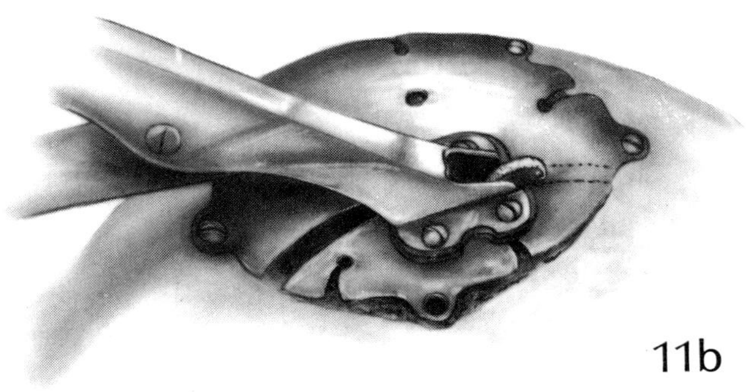

11b

## Complications

Complications are very rare. Extradural haematoma has been reported after an inlay technique involving dissection of the bone edge. Infection can usually be traced to an error of judgement, such as operating too soon after infection, repairing a defect over a sinus before the mucosa has regenerated or inserting a fixation screw into an air sinus.

### *References*

1. Simpson, D. (1965) Titanium in cranioplasty. Journal of Neurosurgery, 22, 292–293

2. Meachim, G., Williams, D. F. (1973) Changes in nonosseus tissue adjacent to titanium implants. Journal of Biomedical Materials Research, 7, 555–572

3. Gordon, D. S., Blair, G. A. S. (1974) Titanium cranioplasty. British Medical Journal, ii, 478–481

4. Beumer, J., Firtell, D. N., Curtis, T. A. (1979) Current concepts in cranioplasty. Journal of Prosthetic Dentistry, 42, 67–77

5. Bahrani, A. S., Blair, G. A., Crossland, B. (1965) Slow rate hydraulic forming of stainless steel dentures. British Dental Journal, 118, 425–431

6. Blair, G. A. S., Fannin, T. F., Gordon, D. S. (1976) Titanium strip cranioplasty. British Medical Journal, ii, 907–908

7. Blair, G. A. S., Gordon, D. S., Simpson, D. A. (1980) Cranioplasty in children. Child's Brain, 6, 82–91

Illustrations by Barbara Hyams and Robert N. Lane

# Intracranial abscess

**John Garfield** MA, MChir, FRCP, FRCS
Consultant Neurosurgeon, Wessex Neurological Centre, Southampton General Hospital; Clinical Teacher in Neurosurgery, University of Southampton, Southampton, Hampshire, UK

## Preoperative

### Clinical diagnosis

Despite advances in methods of radiological diagnosis, especially CT scanning and more recently nuclear magnetic resonance imaging (NMRI), the success of treatment of intracranial abscess still depends on early clinical diagnosis and prompt referral for neurosurgical management. With the decline in chronic suppurative otitis media, due to generally improved standards of living and better primary treatment of acute middle ear infections, there has been some change in the pattern of intracranial abscess and its presentation. The disease is less likely to present in a florid 'classical' way but tends to be more atypical and insidious in onset. Nevertheless, the lynchpins of clinical diagnosis remain the following.

1. A history, or the presence, of a pre-existing focus of infection.
2. Evidence of a focal neurological disturbance.
3. Evidence of raised intracranial pressure.

# 1

*Focus of infection and aetiology*

In the major reported series of intracranial abscess[1–3], chronic suppurative otitis media was the site of infection in up to 60 per cent of all cases and in up to 93 per cent of cases of temporal intracerebral and cerebellar abscess. Paranasal sinus infections, especially frontal and ethmoidal, account for about 10 per cent of cases of intracranial abscess – a decline since earlier large series[4], which showed figures of up to 25 per cent. Although in the past chronic intrathoracic sepsis (bronchiectasis and empyema) was a major cause of metastatic brain abscess[2,5], subacute bacterial endocarditis is now more important, at least in developed countries. Indeed, in the presence of congenital or acquired valvular heart disease, even without positive evidence of endocarditis, a cerebral lesion should be regarded as an abscess until proved otherwise. In up to 30 per cent of cases of intracranial abscess, a source of infection cannot be identified, so that its absence by no means excludes the diagnosis. An important change in recent years has been the occurrence of frontal intracerebral and especially acute subdural abscess after relatively mild and acute frontal or ethmoidal sinusitis, instead of the more traditional features of chronic sinusitis.

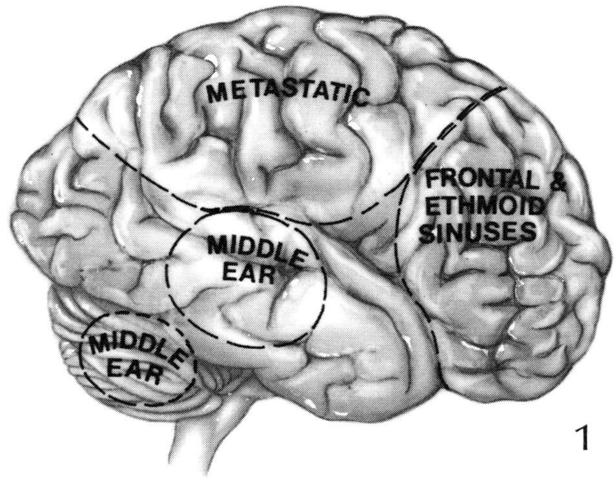


1

*Focal neurological disturbance*

Epilepsy is the common form of focal neurological disturbance, particularly with subdural abscess, and occurs in up to 33 per cent of patients[6]. Surprisingly, epilepsy is more common with frontal than with temporal lobe abscess[7]. With the exception of dysphasia, focal abnormal neurological signs are of little value in localization of supratentorial abscess, although hemiparesis occurs in up to 67 per cent and hemianopia in up to 17 per cent[1].

It must be stressed that any focal neurological disturbance in the presence of a source of infection is enough to warrant urgent intracranial investigation.

*Raised intracranial pressure*

Symptoms and signs of raised intracranial pressure may be mild or absent despite the presence of a large intracranial abscess[1]. Papilloedema occurs in less than 50 per cent of patients and is not related either to site and size of the abscess or to the level of intracranial pressure. Deterioration in level of consciousness is an indication of a severe rise in intracranial pressure and is often a prelude to tentorial herniation or spontaneous rupture of the abscess.

Intracranial abscess is usually associated with increasing cerebral oedema, thus aggravating the rising intracranial pressure, which in itself provokes further oedema so that tentorial or foraminal herniation may be imminent. An abscess may at any time rupture into the ventricular system. Survival after rupture is unusual.

## Clinical differential diagnosis and lumbar puncture

In the absence of a clear source of infection, differentiation between abscess and rapidly growing malignant tumour may be impossible, and therefore the presence of malignancy should never be assumed. In the presence of a source of infection, especially the middle ear, the most important differentiation is from bacterial meningitis and encephalitis. Since neck stiffness may be due to either bacterial meningeal irritation or impaction of the cerebellar tonsils at the foramen magnum, errors in diagnosis could be fatal. Because deterioration following lumbar puncture is a real hazard[2] and in abscess the cerebrospinal fluid (CSF) may be normal[1], lumbar puncture should not be performed in patients with signs of meningeal irritation who have evidence of a focal neurological disturbance or papilloedema.

If a lumbar puncture is done in the mistaken belief that the diagnosis is bacterial meningitis, and the CSF is macroscopically clear and colourless, immediate investigation to exclude an abscess should be instituted without awaiting the results of laboratory examination of the CSF.

## Localization

*Site of sepsis*

Ear, nose or throat sepsis often provides a remarkably accurate guide to the location of the intracranial abscess. The abscesses produced by foci of ear, nose or throat sepsis are usually intracerebral or cerebellar (*see Illustration 1*) but pus may extend widely in the subdural space. Localization by site of ear, nose or throat sepsis is so accurate that when the patient's level of consciousness is deteriorating rapidly it may be used as the sole guide to the placing of a burr hole for aspiration.

### *Electroencephalography (EEG)*

With the advent of more sophisticated radiological methods, there is now little call for EEG in the primary diagnosis of abscess. However, it remains very valuable when there is a strong differential diagnosis of encephalitis, especially herpes simplex encephalitis. If the EEG shows the characteristic unequivocal pattern of that disease, the diagnosis can be accepted without CT scanning. However, if the patient shows signs of rising intracranial pressure and advancing neurological deficit, a CT scan will still be necessary because histological and virological confirmation of encephalitis, with or without internal decompression at craniotomy, may be required.

### *Carotid arteriography*

The use of arteriography has been largely superseded by the non-invasive techniques of radioisotope and computerized scanning. Arteriography may provide accurate localization of temporal lesions, but in other sites the degree of accuracy is low unless the periphery of the lesion is outlined by a pathological vascular pattern[5], which is a relatively rare finding.

### *Air ventriculography*

Although largely superseded by CT scanning, air ventriculography remains a very valuable method of investigation when scanning facilities are not available, and especially in those patients in whom there is no certain clinical lateralization or in whom the clinical diagnosis is of an infratentorial lesion. The dangers of the procedure have been exaggerated in the past. As well as relative accuracy of localization, ventriculography allows inspection of the subdural space and thereby the diagnosis of subdural abscess, and examination of the ventricular CSF. In the presence of acute severe obstructive hydrocephalus due to a posterior fossa abscess, ventriculography with release of CSF from the supratentorial ventricles may prevent fatal tonsillar (foramen magnum) coning. Displacement of the fourth ventricle and aqueduct as visualized by ventriculography allows rapid localization of the lesion, which is then removed.

### *Radioisotope brain scanning*

Isotope (radionucleotide) scanning has been largely superseded by CT scanning, although, when the latter is not available, it should be remembered that in the localization of supratentorial abscess radioisotope scanning has proved reliable in up to 91 per cent of cases[8]. However, an area of increased radioisotope uptake may be due to septic cerebritis before the formation of a true abscess. If there is supporting evidence of a space-occupying lesion, e.g. a displaced calcified pineal gland or a shift of the midline demonstrated by echoencephalography, a positive isotope scan should lead to surgery.

### *Computerized axial tomography (CT scan)*

CT scanning is now the method of choice for the localization of intracranial abscess. It can demonstrate not only the precise area involved by the disease, but also the consistency of the abnormal tissue and whether there is a space-occupying element requiring evacuation[9, 10]. Enhancement by iothalamate aids differentiation from tumour and from oedema with accentuation of the abscess capsule, although the appearances of a cystic glioma are very similar. Sequential CT scanning in the early stages of abscess formation and then in following progress after aspiration of the pus is invaluable and has virtually replaced the injection of radio-opaque material (e.g. Steripaque) into the abscess. However, the limitations of CT scanning must be stressed, in particular the difficulty of differentiating between abscess and malignant tumours, primary or metastatic. Therefore it remains essential to establish the pathology and not to assume that single or even multiple intracranial lesions are necessarily malignant.

Subdural abscess may be very difficult to demonstrate by CT scan. A normal contrast-enhanced scan can never be said to exclude the presence of subdural abscess, either over the convexity of the hemispheres or on the medial surface of the hemisphere, when there may be bilateral or unilateral parafalcine pus. Therefore, when the index of clinical suspicion is high (e.g. when epilepsy occurs in the presence of frontal sinusitis), exploratory frontal burr holes (*see* below) should be made even when CT scan is normal. Alternatively, provided that the patient's condition is stable, the CT scan should be repeated at daily intervals.

## Bacteriology and choice of antibiotics

Earlier reports of bacteriological findings in intracranial abscess[1, 5] showed that staphylococci were as prevalent as streptococci. However, in recent years streptococci, and particularly anaerobic or microaerophilic streptococci, have become predominant[2, 11]. Whereas in the past a proportion of abscesses were thought to be sterile, recent work[12] has shown conclusively that with good bacteriological technique organisms can be grown from most abscesses, and that *Streptococcus milleri* is the predominant and most dangerous organism. The commonest organism after the microaerophilic or anaerobic streptococci is now bacteroides, usually occurring in combination with the streptococcus. Staphylococci are rare and restricted to the few cases of metastatic abscess associated with staphylococcal septicaemia or empyema. Haemophilus may be found in solitary abscesses of unknown cause, while proteus tends to be associated with chronic middle ear disease. The ultimate choice of antibiotic depends on the results of culture and sensitivity determination. However, because of the likely organisms responsible and their probable sensitivities, the antibiotics of choice before the bacteriology is available are penicillin (24 megaunits in 24 hours) and chloramphenicol, both of which penetrate the brain well and enter abscess cavities.

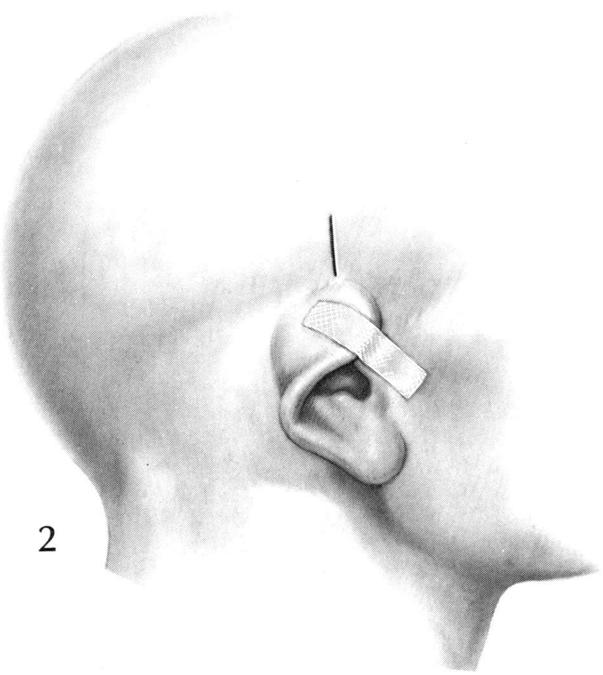

2

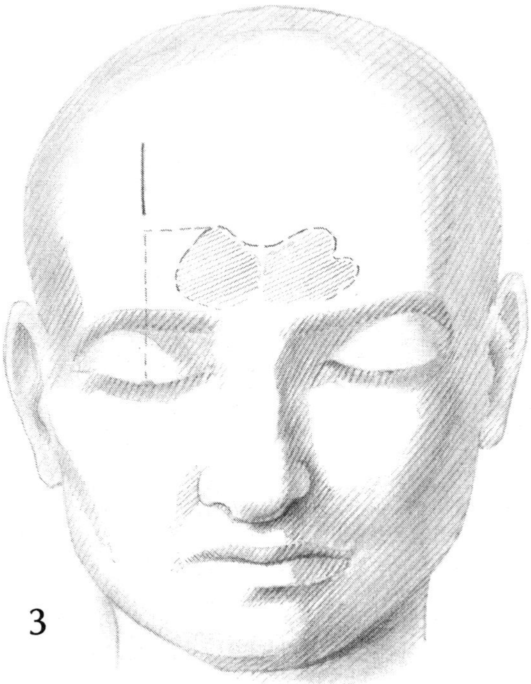

3

## Choice of treatment

Throughout the history of surgical management of intracranial abscess there has been continuous controversy over the different methods employed. The two main forms of treatment have been excision, either as a primary procedure or following preliminary needle aspiration[2, 5, 13], and repeated aspiration[2, 4]. Accurate comparison of these different methods remains difficult, but burr hole aspiration is more widely practised than primary excision. There is no conclusive evidence that primary excision is more effective, provided that aspiration is repeated assiduously and progress is carefully monitored with sequential CT scanning. Recently, the traditional management of subdural abscess by aspiration through multiple burr holes has been reported as less effective than extensive craniotomy[14].

# The operations

Once it has been decided that a supratentorial intracranial abscess is present, the initial surgical procedure is the drilling of a burr hole for needle aspiration.

# 2 & 3

### Position of burr holes

If arteriography, ventriculography or scanning has been used, this will indicate the site for the burr hole. If ear, nose or throat sepsis provides the guide, then the burr hole should be placed accordingly: for an abscess arising from middle ear infection it should be immediately above the root of the pinna; for an abscess arising from frontal sinus infection it should be low frontal, in a line vertically above the centre of the eye, immediately above the upper margin of the frontal sinus as shown radiologically – this usually lies below the hairline. Vertical incisions are desirable because craniotomy flaps may need to be fashioned later. The head is shaved widely round the site and, under local anaesthesia, a standard burr hole is made.

## EXTRADURAL ABSCESS

The commonest site for extradural pus is in the frontal region, where it is related to frontal sinusitis. In this situation, when a frontal burr hole reveals pus in the extradural space, the dura should not be opened but, with a clean set of instruments, a second burr hole should be made 8 cm behind the first to determine the extent of the extradural pus. Even if no pus is found there, the dura is not opened. Finally, a third burr hole should be made in the low frontal position on the other side. If extradural pus is found in any or all of these positions, it should be allowed to express itself. An Adson periosteal elevator may then be inserted gently to depress the dura and encourage further egress of pus. The wounds are then closed and the patient is treated vigorously with antibiotics dictated by the results of immediate bacteriological examination of the pus.

## SUBDURAL ABSCESS: BURR HOLE ASPIRATION

# 4 & 5

If there is no pus in the extradural space, the dura is opened in a cruciate manner. If pus is found in the subdural space, an exploring cannula should on no account be inserted into the brain. The pus should be allowed to express itself and, taking great care, an Adson elevator may then be inserted into the subdural space to depress the brain gently in order to express further pus. When subdural pus is present, a series of burr holes is made (performed in the sequence indicated in Illustration 5, numbers 1–5) to define its extent and aid evacuation. Each hole is made with a clean set of instruments, those on the side opposite to where pus was found initially being made last. Wherever the pus may be found, bilateral posterior parietal burr holes must be included because ventriculography may be necessary later. The wound of a burr hole which does not reveal subdural pus should be closed immediately.

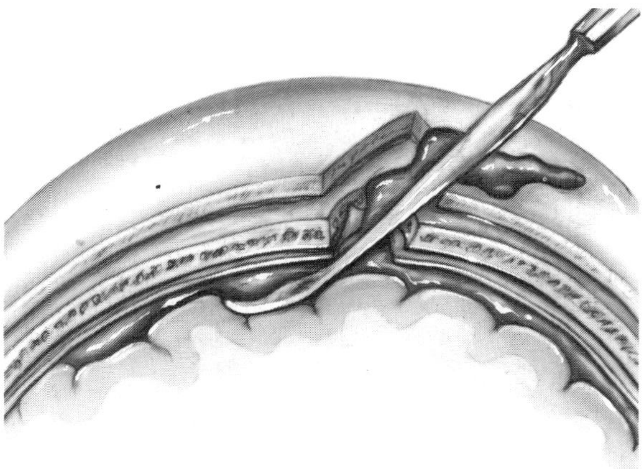

4

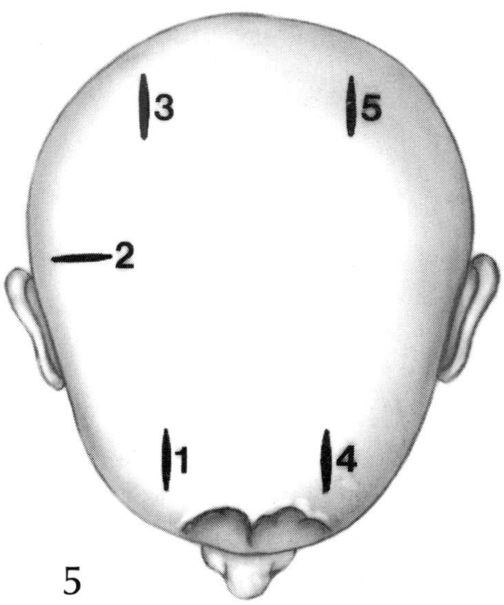


5

Further management requires high doses of systemic antibiotics, and prophylactic anticonvulsants because convulsions are very common after evacuation of subdural pus.

Following the initial aspiration of pus from the subdural space, it is reasonable to tap the space once more after an interval of 24 hours, but it is unusual to obtain more pus. Because of the effectiveness of well chosen systemic antibiotics, instillation of antibiotics into the subdural space is no longer necessary.

### *Craniotomy*

Craniotomy as the primary surgical management is not widely practised but has been advocated[13, 14]. Aspiration, as described, is an essential diagnostic step and allows the organisms to be identified. If CT scanning has shown extensive subdural pus, especially between the medial surface of one or both hemispheres and the falx, an extensive frontoparietal craniotomy approaching the midline may be necessary (*see* chapter on 'Burr holes, trephine and craniotomy', pp. 12–29). If it is not accepted as the primary surgical treatment, craniotomy may still be advisable if the patient does not improve after burr hole aspiration.

## INTRACEREBRAL ABSCESS: NEEDLE ASPIRATION

# 6, 7 & 8

When pus is found in neither the extradural nor the subdural space, attempts are made to aspirate an intracerebral abscess with a graduated blunt brain cannula. The cannula is held gently between finger and thumb and advanced slowly but steadily, without touching the sides of the burr hole so that any sensation of resistance may be clearly felt. In a chronic abscess this resistance will be firm but pliable; the depth is noted and the cannula then advanced in order to pierce the capsule. The stilette is removed and, if pus does not flow spontaneously from the cannula, gentle aspiration with a 10 ml syringe is applied. At all times this aspiration should be slow and gentle, as any abrupt change in the pressure within the abscess may precipitate communication with the ventricular system, or haemorrhage. As soon as any blood appears in the pus or when no further pus is obtained by gentle aspiration, the syringe is removed and 20 000 units of intrathecal penicillin injected. When facilities for sequential CT scanning are not available, 2 ml of Steripaque (barium sulphate suspension) is inserted to the cavity. The cannula is then removed, the wound closed in layers (pericranium, galea and skin) and a head dress applied.

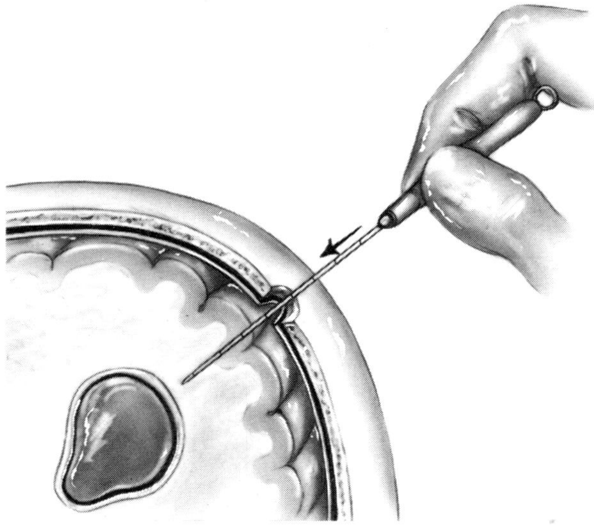

6

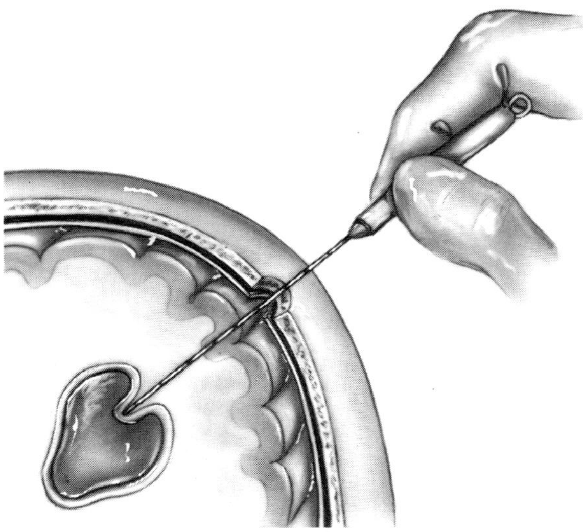

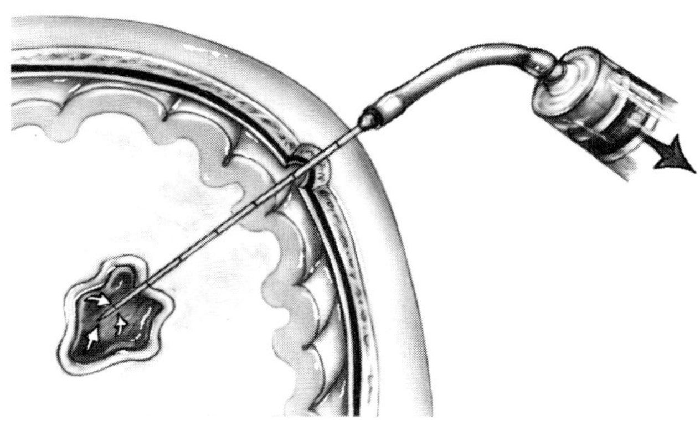

8

## ASPIRATION OF OTOGENIC TEMPORAL ABSCESS

# 9

For aspiration of a temporal abscess arising from middle ear infection, the cannula should be directed low so that the surface of the petrous bone is felt. If the cannula is directed too high it may easily pass over the temporal abscess.

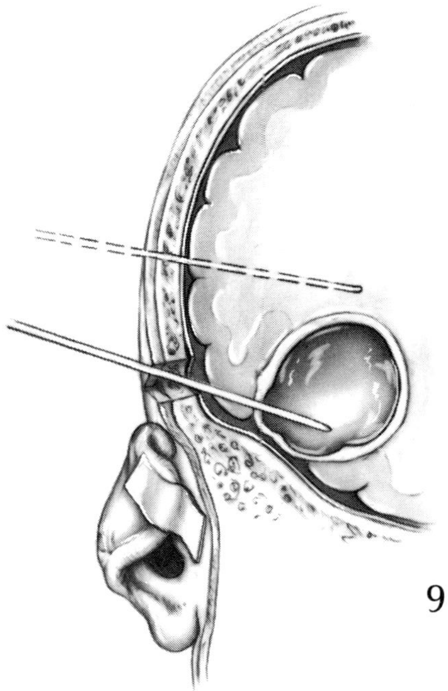

9

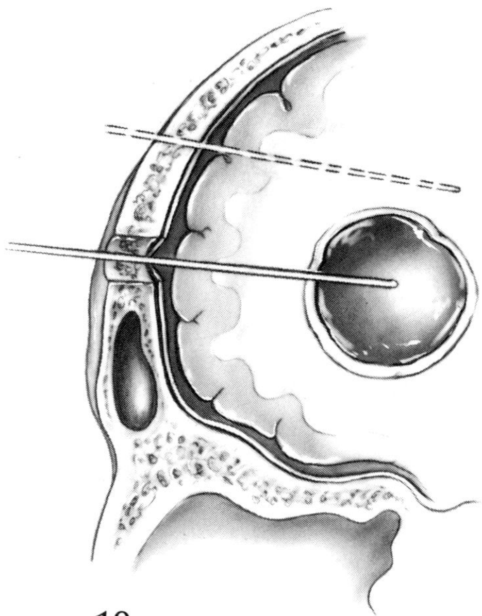

10

## ASPIRATION OF LOW FRONTAL ABSCESS

# 10

In aspirating an abscess arising from the frontal sinus, unless the burr hole is placed low and the cannula directed downwards, the abscess may not be entered.

## Repeated aspiration

# 11 & 12

Following initial diagnostic and therapeutic aspiration, the frequency of further aspirations will be dictated by the patient's clinical state and the results of repeated CT scan, and by the volume of pus obtained at each aspiration. The objective is to shrink the abscess as rapidly as possible, and this may require daily aspirations for the first few days. The brain cannula can be inserted for this purpose through the surgical incision and burr hole without reopening the wound. Even when the abscess has shrunk and no more pus can be obtained, it may take many months before total CT resolution occurs. Indeed, a small area of scarring may remain visible indefinitely. Antibiotics appropriate to the organism identified should be continued for a total of 6 weeks, usually intravenously for the first 3 weeks and orally thereafter. Prophylactic anticonvulsants (e.g. phenobarbitone 30 mg three times daily, or phenytoin 300 mg daily for adults) should be continued for up to 1 year, and indefinitely if fits occur during that period. If CT scanning is not available, the progress of the abscess can be assessed by insertion of 2 ml of Steripaque into the abscess at first aspiration. The radio-opaque substance is taken up preferentially by the abscess capsule so that plain radiographs taken thereafter will demonstrate shrinkage of the lesion.

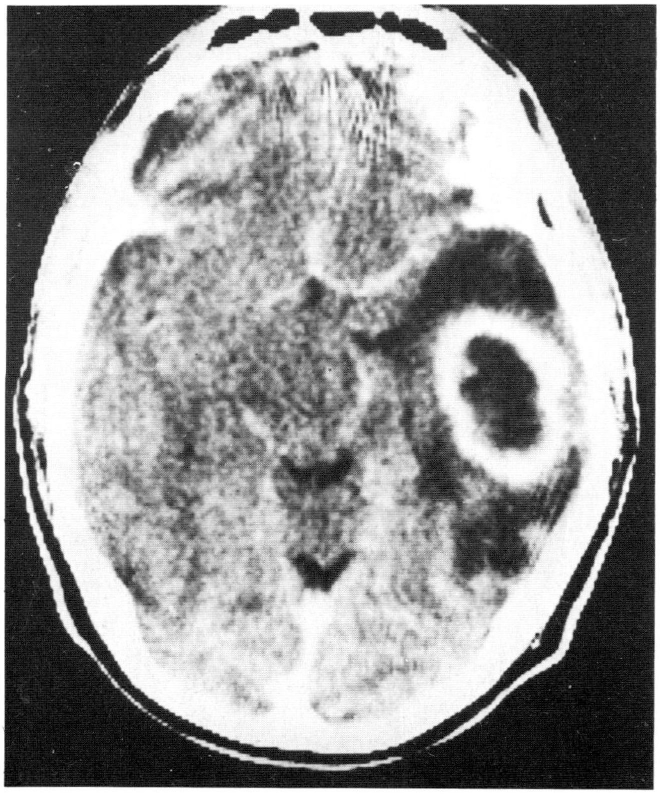

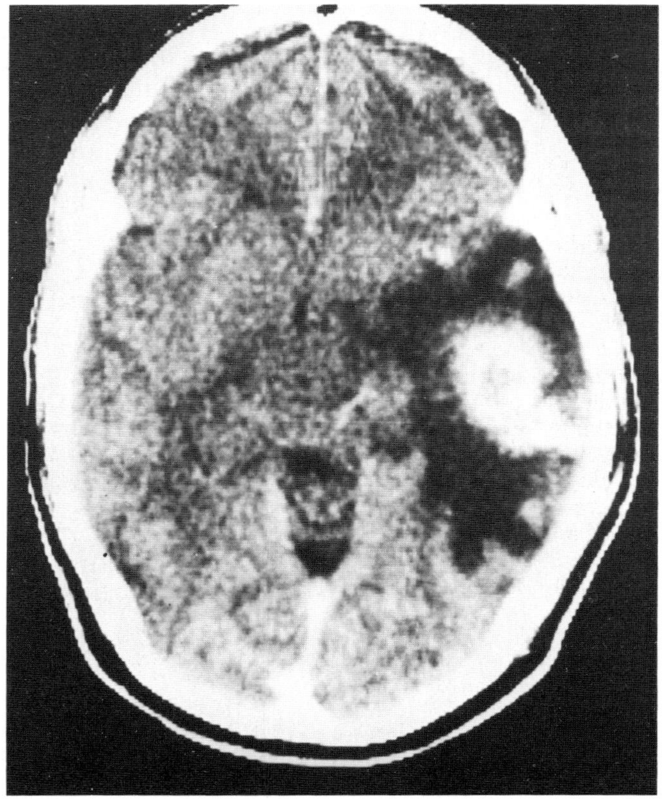

CT *scans showing satisfactory shrinkage of the temporal lobe abscess treated by repeated aspiration*

11

12

## CRANIOTOMY AND EXCISION OF ABSCESS

### Indications

Failure of the abscess cavity to shrink satisfactorily after repeated aspiration is an indication for craniotomy. However, if aspiration has been assiduously repeated and systemic antibiotic cover is adequate, this should rarely arise. Excision should be delayed until sterility has been achieved.

Excision at craniotomy as a first procedure as soon as the diagnosis is confirmed has been advised, but the author does not subscribe to this view. However, if there is deterioration despite aspiration, early craniotomy may be necessary. Craniotomy is usually required for a cerebellar abscess demonstrated by CT scan or ventriculography.

### Technique

# 13 & 14

This differs only in minor detail from the procedure for other supratentorial or cerebellar space-occupying lesions, the initial steps being identical. Antibiotic cover is given. Using very gentle pattie dissection, great care is taken to remove the entire abscess capsule without its rupture. In cerebellar or temporal abscesses arising from middle ear infection there is frequently a fibrous cord attaching the capsule to the superior or posterior aspect of the petrous bone; this must be completely detached from the dura. If sterility has been achieved preoperatively, rupture of the abscess during removal, which is not uncommon even in the most skilled hands, does not affect the outcome adversely. The craniotomy is then closed in the usual fashion without any drain to the abscess bed.

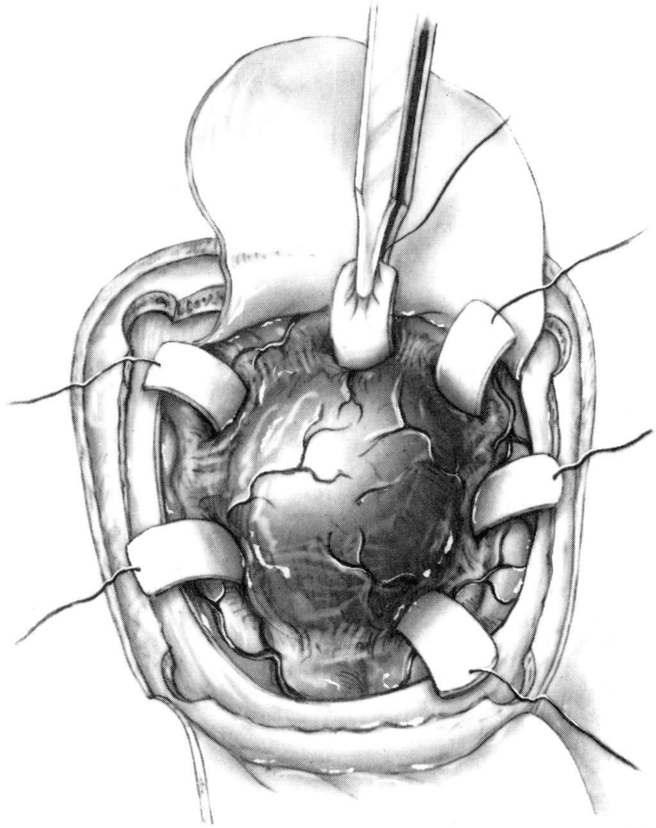

13

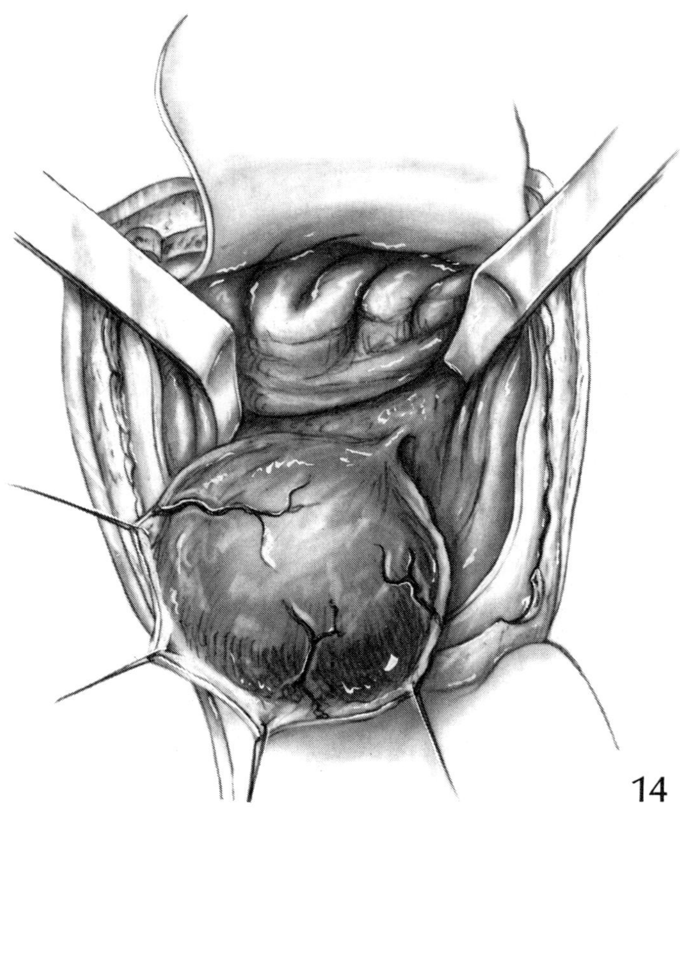

14

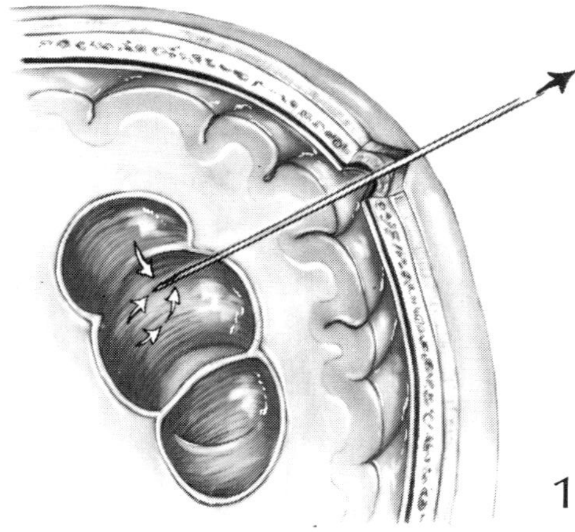

15

## Complications of surgery

### Ventriculitis

Ventriculitis due to leakage of pus from the abscess into the ventricular system usually produces a sudden rise in fever, with tachycardia, an abrupt fall in blood pressure, deterioration in the level of consciousness and neck stiffness. Bilateral posterior parietal burr holes are made without delay, both ventricles are tapped and, if the diagnosis is confirmed, treatment by daily tapping of both ventricles and insertion of the appropriate intrathecal antibiotics and steroids (cortisone 25 mg) is continued until the ventricular CSF cell count is normal. This regimen may well save patients from what in the past was usually a fatal complication.

### Loculation

# 15, 16 & 17

Occasionally, although the initial abscess appears to shrink, CT scan may indicate an adjacent cavity which is not shrinking. This means that loculation has occurred and the aspirating cannula should be redirected. If this fails, excision at craniotomy may be indicated.

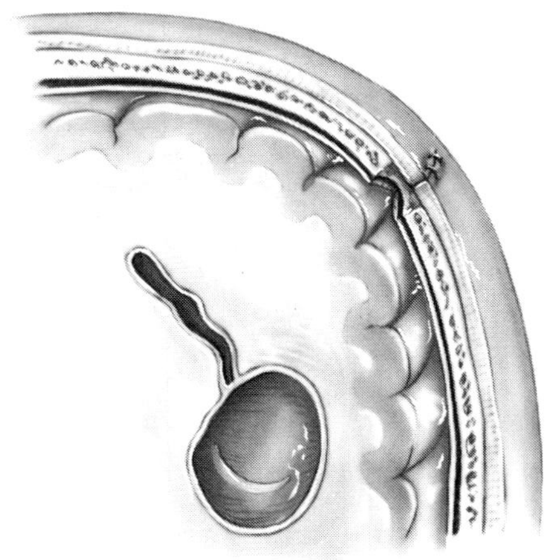

16

### Convulsions

Status epilepticus may follow abscess surgery, particularly after the initial aspiration of subdural pus. If not responding to large doses of anticonvulsants, it is best managed by curarization and controlled respiration.

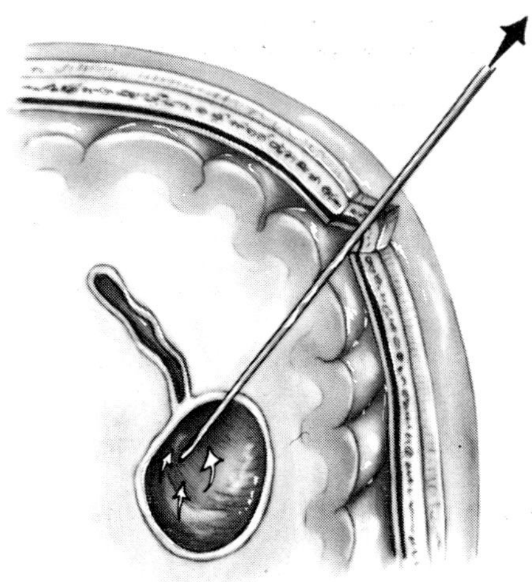

17

## Follow-up

After surgery for intracranial abscess the patient must be reviewed at monthly intervals. Antibiotics should be continued for a minimum of 6 weeks. At the slightest sign of deterioration in terms of headache or neurological deficit, the patient should be readmitted for further radiological investigation. Even when the patient remains well, it is wise to have a scan done after 3 months as occasionally an abscess may recur without producing any neurological deterioration until relatively late in the process.

## Results

During the past 20 years the overall mortality of treated intracranial abscess has declined from about 40 per cent to 10 per cent. A successful outcome depends especially on early clinical and radiological diagnosis, and the patient's level of consciousness when treatment is started. It depends also on the use of appropriate antibiotics based upon improved techniques of microbiology. Early and late epilepsy, particularly with subdural abscess, remain a problem[15–17].

### *References*


1. Bonnal, J., Descuns, P., Duplay, J. (1960) Les abscès encéphaliques a l'ère des antibiotiques. Etude statistique de 547 observations. (Rapport presenté à la réunion annuelle de la Societé de Neurochirurgie de langue Française.) Paris: Masson
2. Garfield, J. (1969) Management of supratentorial intracranial abscess; a review of 200 cases. British Medical Journal, ii, 7–11
3. Shaw, M. D., Russell, J. A. (1975) Cerebellar abscess a review of 47 cases. Journal of Neurology, Neurosurgery and Psychiatry, 38, 429–435
4. Tutton, G. K. (1953) Cerebral abscess; the present position. Annals of the Royal College of Surgeons of England, 13, 281–311
5. Krayenbuhl, H. A. (1966) Abscess of the brain. Clinical Neurosurgery, 14, 25–44
6. Kiser, J. L., Kendig, J. H. (1963) Intracranial suppuration. A review of 139 consecutive cases with electron-microscopic observations on 3. Journal of Neurosurgery, 20, 494–511
7. Pennybacker, J. (1950) Brain abscesses in relation to diseases of the ear, nose and throat. Annals of the Royal College of Surgeons of England, 7, 105–127
8. Suwanwela, C., Posyachinda, V., Posyachinda, M. (1971) Brain scanning in the diagnosis of intracranial abscess. Acta Neurochirurgica, 25, 165–175
9. Blaquière, R. M. (1983) Computer tomographic appearances of intra and extracerebral abscesses. British Journal of Radiology, 56, 171–181
10. Britt, R. H., Enzmann, D. R. (1983) Clinical stages of human brain abscesses on serial CT scans after contrast infusion. Computerized tomographic, neuropathological and clinical correlations. Journal of Neurosurgery, 59, 972–989
11. Garvey, G. (1983) Current concepts of bacterial infections of the central nervous system. Bacterial meningitis and bacterial brain abscess. Journal of Neurosurgery, 59, 735–744
12. De Louvois, J., Gortvai, P., Hurley, R. (1977) Bacteriology of abscess of the central nervous system; a multicentre prospective study. British Medical Journal, ii, 981–984
13. Le Beau, J., Creissard, P., Harispe, L., Redondo, A. (1973) Surgical treatment of brain abscess and subdural empyema. Journal of Neurosurgery, 38, 198–203
14. Bannister, G., Williams, B., Smith, S. (1981) Treatment of subdural empyema. Journal of Neurosurgery, 55, 82–88
15. Legg, N. J., Gupta, P. C., Scott, D. F. (1973) Epilepsy following cerebral abscess: a clinical and EEG study of 70 patients. Brain, 96, 259–268
16. Cowie, R., Williams, B. (1983) Late seizures and morbidity after subdural empyema. Journal of Neurosurgery, 58, 569–573
17. Calliauw, L., de Praetere, P., Verbeke, L. (1984) Post-operative epilepsy in subdural suppuration. Acta Neurochirurgica, 71, 217–223

Illustrations by Barbara Hyams

# Surgical and microbiological management of subdural and extradural abscesses

**A. J. Strong** MA, FRCSE
Consultant Neurosurgeon, The Neurosurgical Unit of Guys', Maudsley and King's College Hospitals, The Maudsley Hospital, London, UK

**H. R. Ingham** FRCPath, DipBact
Consultant Microbiologist, General Hospital, Newcastle-upon-Tyne, UK

## Introduction

Subdural empyema and extradural abscesses are rarer than intracerebral abscess, but, as with the latter condition, early diagnosis is essential for a satisfactory outcome. Since the aetiology, microbiology, and principles of surgical management of extradural and subdural abscesses resemble one another, the two will be dealt with simultaneously, and points of divergence noted where they arise.

### Aetiology

The most frequent antecedent cause of subdural empyema is frontal sinusitis. Less frequently infection of the middle ear is the primary source, and on occasions infection has originated from an apical dental abscess, reaching the subfrontal space via the maxillary and frontal sinuses[1]. It may also complicate basal or anterior fossa fracture or result from haematogenous spread. Rarely, an osteoplastic bone flap may become infected following surgery and, if the dura has been left open, any underlying collection may become infected secondarily. Extradural abscess is almost always associated with frontal sinusitis.

Failure to recognize the condition is the single most important factor in the mortality of subdural empyema, which is still as high as 40 per cent in some series.

## Pathology

# 1 & 2

*Subdural empyema*

Subdural empyema may arise either as a result of direct extension from the ear or frontal sinus of an osteitic process, or indirectly by progressive thrombophlebitis of mucosal veins and spread to dural veins, venous sinuses and cerebral veins[2]. Once the infection reaches the subdural space, pus forms rapidly and may extend widely. Extension of pus varies with the primary source, as shown in the illustrations. With paranasal suppuration, collections are seen at the frontal poles and pus may extend posteriorly over the convexity of the frontal lobe; it may also extend along the falx and the sylvian fissure. Subfrontal extension is rarer. Parafalcine spread may progress posteriorly or under the falx to the opposite hemisphere. With an otogenic source, the collection extends towards the falx and some may reach the posterior fossa, but more commonly the empyema remains supratentorial, accumulating around the occipital pole. There are thus three principal sites in which subdural empyemas localize: the frontal or fronto-parietal region, the parafalcine spaces and the occipital poles.

*Extradural abscess*

Extradural abscess almost always originates from chronic frontal sinusitis. As with subdural empyema, mucosal veins become thrombosed and infected, leading to osteomyelitis of the sinus wall and access of infection to the extradural space. Osteomyelitis may then involve the convexity of the frontal bone, with accumulation of pus in the subperiosteal and subgaleal planes. Why sinusitis should lead to subdural infection more frequently than to an extradural collection is not clear.

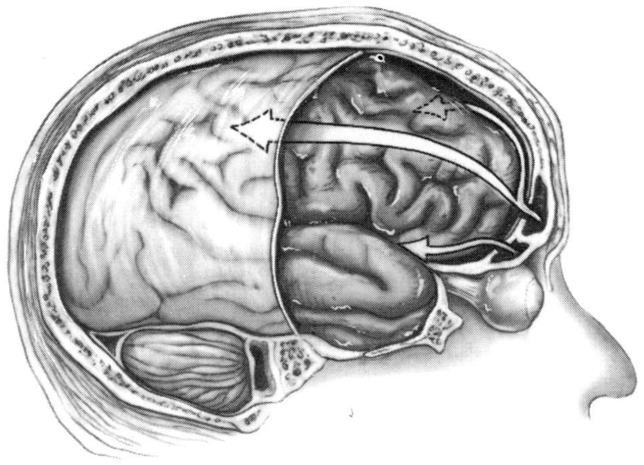

1

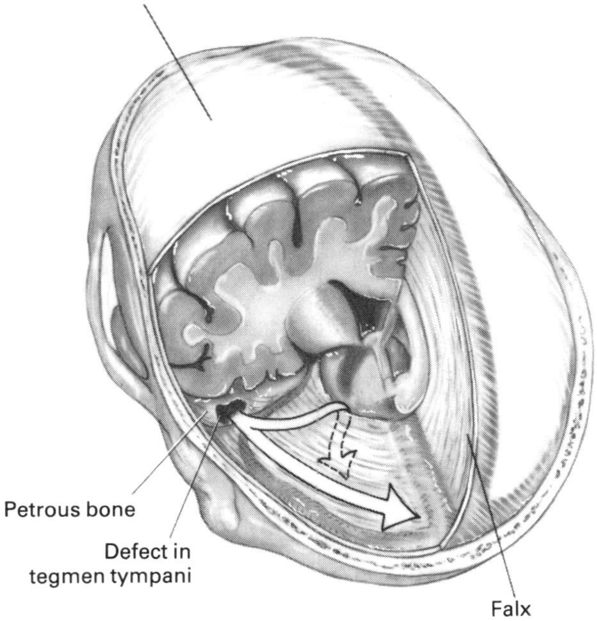


2

## Clinical features

*Subdural empyema*

Where there is a preceding history of sinusitis the presenting history is usually of severe headache, vomiting, pyrexia, disturbance of consciousness, meningism and occasionally frontal or orbital swelling. Focal deficit often develops abruptly, and normally consists of hemiplegia and aphasia, with or without hemianopia. Epilepsy is frequent, often focal, and leads to more rapid deterioration. If subdural empyema is a complication of surgery or trauma, headache is less prominent, and the presentation will be with deterioration of conscious level, other signs of raised intracranial pressure, and progressive focal deficit.

*Extradural abscess*

The effects of acute osteomyelitis determine the presentation. Severe frontal headache is followed by the development in some cases of diffuse, tender swelling over the frontal convexity, together with extension of oedema into the eyelids. Pitting oedema of the scalp over the affected area is a prominent and pathognomonic feature (Pott's puffy tumour).

*Differential diagnosis*

In the case of extradural abscess, local frontal pain and scalp tenderness with oedema in the context of a recent history of sinusitis leave little room for doubt as to diagnosis.

If there is evidence of frontal sinus or chronic middle ear infection, the differential diagnosis embraces extradural, subdural or intracerebral abscess, cortical thrombophlebitis, pyogenic meningitis, cavernous or lateral sinus thrombosis, and sphenoid sinus empyema.

In a patient with progressive loss of consciousness and focal deficit, but without evidence of local sepsis, the following should be considered: herpes simplex or other forms of encephalitis, tuberculous or viral meningitis, and septic infarction from subacute bacterial endocarditis. Conversely, great care must be taken not to miss a covert subdural abscess by mistakenly diagnosing one of the above conditions.

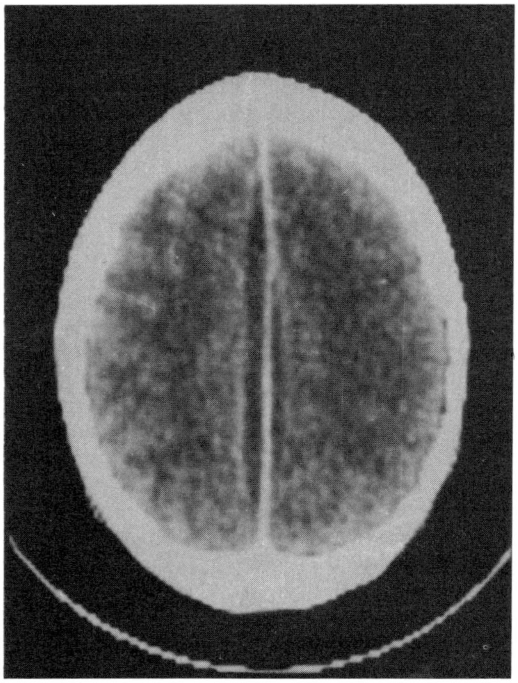

3

*CT scan with contrast enhancement illustrating typical bilateral parafalcine collections in a patient with subdural empyema complicating frontal sinusitis.*

## Investigations

Examination of the peripheral blood will normally reveal polymorphonuclear leucocytosis, and chest and skull radiographs should be taken. Plain skull films may reveal opacification of one or more paranasal sinuses.

Lumbar puncture is contraindicated but, if undertaken to confirm a suspected diagnosis such as bacterial meningitis, will reveal cerebrospinal fluid (CSF) under increased pressure, with a moderate mixed leucocytosis, predominantly polymorphonuclear, and a raised protein but normal glucose concentration. It is usually sterile on culture.

*CT scanning*

# 3

CT scanning is usually very helpful but can be misleading. Some extradural and subdural abscesses will appear as low-density space-occupying lesions with the appropriate midline or ventricular displacement. However, these lesions may be isodense, and bilateral collections over the hemispheres may not be accompanied by a midline shift, as in the case of subdural haematoma. The use of intravenous contrast enhancement is therefore important, and will often delineate a lesion.

# 4

The principal value of CT scanning is in the management of subdural empyema. Development of multiple loculi is common and may be subfrontal or, more commonly, parafalcine. Such secondary loculation is best identified by CT scanning and should be drained surgically. This possibility should always be borne in mind when assessing CT scans routinely.

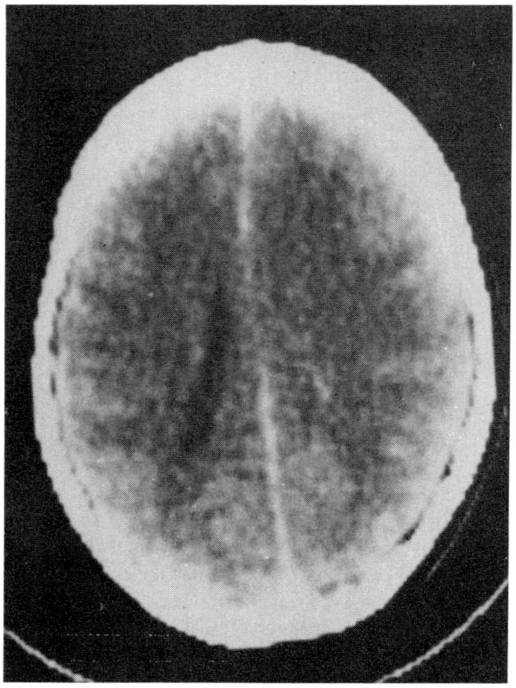

4

*High CT cut in a patient with a right hemisphere surface collection, showing depression of the body of the right lateral ventricle.*

### *Isotope scanning*

Where CT facilities are not available, the principal alternative technique which remains non-invasive is isotope scanning. However, this produces an appreciable false-negative rate. The indicator which has usually been used is $^{99m}$Tc, which reveals areas of disturbed blood-brain barrier function associated with inflammation. Newer indicators conjugated to white cells have not yet been fully evaluated. An advantage of isotope emission scanning is the direct availability of images in the coronal projection, which may be of particular value where conventional CT imaging in the horizontal plane may not reveal bilateral convexity lesions.

### *Angiography*

It should not be necessary to resort to angiography unless the results of non-invasive investigations are equivocal. Angiography will provide the only definitive assessment of the presence of a convexity lesion. The surgeon may contemplate the alternative approach of making exploratory burr holes, but the importance of identifying each potential loculation of pus demands that, where deterioration is not too rapid, all possible information be accumulated before embarking on surgery.

### *Microbiology*

The bacteriology of subdural empyema is determined by the primary pathology. In trauma, surgical or metastatic infections, *Staphylococcus aureus* is common; other species of organisms are much less frequently encountered. With a sinusitis or otogenic source, the flora is more complex. When sinusitis is the primary focus, *Haemophilus influenzae* may be encountered but *Streptococcus milleri* is one of the most commonly reported isolates[3]. This is a non-haemolytic, penicillin-sensitive organism frequently requiring 10 per cent carbon dioxide or anaerobic culture for primary isolation. Strains implicated in subdural empyema almost invariably carry the Lancefield group F antigen and have almost certainly been misidentified in the past as microaerophilic or anaerobic streptococci. Obligate anaerobes such as fusobacteria, bacteroides and anaerobic streptococci are not infrequently found in subdural empyema, their presence being indicated by malodorous pus. Growth of these organisms occurs only in good anaerobic conditions. They almost certainly account for the large number of patients with reputedly sterile empyemas in some previous studies.

The ideal sample for microbiological examination is a quantity of pus in an ordinary glass container examined within the hour. Failing this, at least two saturated swabs of the purulent material should be provided.

# Treatment

Sometimes a patient may present with a suspected, but unproven, diagnosis of either subdural empyema or extradural abscess; the CT scan may be entirely normal or show low-density areas suggestive of cerebritis. Institution of appropriate chemotherapy in such patients may result in an initial improvement in the clinical condition. It is vital that these patients be kept under close clinical and CT review, as there may be rapid, unexpected deterioration due to progression of the infection. The fact that appropriate antimicrobial therapy has now been identified and established for use after surgical drainage does not mean that chemotherapy alone can be relied upon to arrest the progression of the inflammatory process to frank pus formation with its associated rise in intracranial pressure.

## Principles of surgery

The planning of surgery should be guided by four precepts.

1. The identification and adequate drainage of all loculations of pus.
2. The need to avoid, if possible, the establishment of any communication between an infected area and the subarachnoid space or brain parenchyma.
3. Treatment of the primary source.
4. Removal of any potential source of reinfection, in particular an infected bone flap.

## Choice of procedure

When a single large loculus is present over the hemisphere convexity, the choice for the surgeon lies between craniotomy and burr holes. Although burr hole drainage is advocated by some surgeons, we would agree with the majority view of recent publications that this is not generally reliable and that craniotomy is preferable. Parafalcine, subfrontal or occipital loculi must be drained specifically, if necessary by separate access by burr holes or craniectomy.

## CONVEXITY SUBDURAL EMPYEMA

### Burr holes

Burr holes should be made over the frontal and parietal convexities using fresh instruments for each site. The dura is opened and any underlying membrane breached. Pus is collected for microbiological assessment within the hour. After spontaneous flow of pus has ceased, an Adson elevator is used to depress the brain gently around the entire periphery of the opening in sequence in order to allow egress of further pus. A large Jacques' catheter with multiple perforations may be gently introduced into the subdural space for drainage. If pus is present at both sites on the convexity, a temporal burr hole should be made; if pus is found here also, it is probably more extensive than first supposed and craniotomy should be undertaken forthwith. In any event, the opposite convexity should be checked by making frontal and parietal burr holes, again using fresh instruments.

### Craniotomy – general

A wide scalp flap is turned and the bone flap raised and wrapped. The dura is opened according to the surgeon's preference and any underlying membrane breached. Pus is obtained for microbiology as above, and the remainder removed by suction. Any membrane at the deep aspect of the empyema should be dissected with caution in order to avoid breaching the subarachnoid space. A careful check should be made for extension of the empyema beyond the margins of the craniotomy by gentle depression of the brain with a broad retractor. The dura is replaced in position but not resutured, and the bone flap is removed and preserved for later replacement. This provides decompression in the event of secondary brain swelling and also recognizes the considerable risk of infection of the flap if it is replaced primarily. The skin is closed with a single layer of non-absorbable sutures such as polypropylene which are removed after 10 days.

### Craniotomy – specific sites

*Bifrontal convexity*

A large coronal scalp flap is turned and reflected forwards, and a bifrontal osteoplastic flap is turned with or without a midline saw cut, according to the surgeon's preference. The lower margin of the craniotomy should be designed to avoid opening the frontal sinus, but the priority is that it should be low enough to allow inspection of the anterior subfrontal region without the need for significant retraction. The dura is opened towards the midline and the subdural space widely inspected and drained. The parafalcine region should be checked on either side and any collection sucked out. If the frontal sinus is entered, it should be cleared, if necessary in collaboration with the otolaryngologist, and necrotic bone in the posterior sinus wall removed.

*Unilateral convexity*

A large flap should be turned with the medial limb a little across the midline and the lateral limb 1–2 cm anterior to the coronal suture to allow extensive inspection of the convexity and of the parafalcine region. The siting of the horizontal margin has been discussed above in the context of bifrontal flaps. At the end of the procedure, contralateral frontal and parietal burr holes should be made (using fresh instruments) to exclude an undiagnosed collection over the convexity.

*Parafalcine loculi*

Parafalcine loculations frequently extend along the entire length of the falx and may require clearance by two separate routes to effect adequate drainage. The best approach is probably a combination of a small craniotomy at the frontal pole extending well up to the midline to provide a clear view backwards into the parafalcine space, together with separate drainage of the occipital loculus (*see below*).

*Occipital loculi*

An occipital loculus is likely to be secondary to a principal collection or source elsewhere, which is treated as described above. The occipital collection is approached with a vertical skin incision, followed by two burr holes enlarged to a craniectomy centred on the relevant lateral aspect of the sagittal sinus 3 cm above the torcula. The craniectomy is enlarged slightly and a linear incision made in the dura lateral to the sinus. The brain is retracted gently laterally and the parafalcine space entered and drained. If parasagittal veins restrict access, it may be necessary to pass a brain needle through the cortex to enter the space and drain it by aspiration, but this is less satisfactory than drainage under direct vision.

If the occipital empyema is the only collection demonstrated preoperatively, and if it originates from middle ear infection, a temporo-occipital craniotomy should be carried out, sufficient to drain the collection and to allow examination of the petrous dura. Any defect should be sealed; in the presence of infection the use of any graft other than autogenous pericranium is probably unwise. The dura is replaced in position and the bone flap removed and preserved for later replacement.

*Subfrontal loculi*

A unilateral frontal craniotomy is carried out as above, with the anterior margin sufficiently low to provide subfrontal access with minimal brain retraction.

### Drainage at burr hole sites

In general, where a craniotomy has been carried out this should provide adequate primary drainage so that no drain is required. However, in the case of burr holes, a Jacques' red rubber catheter with additional side perforations may be left in position for 2–3 days.

### EXTRADURAL ABSCESS

The lesion is normally bifrontal and associated with well established frontal osteomyelitis. A bicoronal scalp flap is reflected forwards and a bifrontal bone flap cut. The bone flap (including pericranium) is removed, swabs are taken and the flap is then cleaned and preserved temporarily for subsequent use as a template for creation of a cranioplasty[4]. Extradural pus is removed. Drainage of the frontal sinus should be established from below either before or during craniotomy and the sinus mucosa removed. Necrotic bone, for example in the posterior wall of the sinus, should be removed. If the dura is under tension, it should be opened (5 mm) with fresh instruments, both over the convexity and at the frontal pole, to check for subdural empyema. If none is found, the dura is closed with polypropylene. If pus is present, the incision is extended and the procedure for subdural empyema followed.

### PRIMARY SOURCE

The primary source must be treated surgically as a matter of urgency. The frontal sinus must be drained, and in the case of an otogenic source a radical mastoidectomy is carried out.

The possibility of a primary dental source should be considered when the bacterial flora in a frontal empyema proves complex, and especially if the maxillary sinus is opacified on plain radiographs; a dental opinion should be obtained in these cases[1].

In the rare instance of subdural empyema developing after craniotomy, usually when the dura has been left open, the bone flap should be removed and discarded, as replacement even after intervals of 6 months or more is likely to be associated with reinfection of the flap. A cranioplasty with tantalum, titanium mesh or acrylic is therefore preferable[4].

# Postoperative management

## Chemotherapy

Modern techniques enable micro-organisms to be isolated not only with greater frequency but with rapidity[5]. In most cases, an indication of appropriate antimicrobial therapy should be available within 24–72 hours, depending on the infecting organism(s). Until this time, antimicrobial agents appropriate to the likely causative organisms are prescribed. A suitable spectrum of activity is provided by a combination of ampicillin 1–2 g 6-hourly, gentamicin 80 mg 8-hourly, and metronidazole 500 mg 12-hourly. Appropriate modifications to the initial regimen can be made in the light of bacteriological findings. The presence of *Staphylococcus aureus* would indicate the use of one of the isoxazolyl penicillins, such as flucloxacillin in a dose of 1 g 6-hourly, possibly with the addition of clindamycin 300 mg 8-hourly. If adequate drainage of the empyema has been provided and any primary source extirpated, a total duration of treatment of 3–4 weeks should suffice. There is no good argument for the use of locally instilled antimicrobial agents, a desperate measure engendered by the uniformly bad prognosis of the disease when the bacteriology was poorly understood.

## Anticonvulsants

Whether or not seizures have occurred, anticonvulsants are always required, as subdural pus is highly epileptogenic. In the case of cerebral abscess, epilepsy frequently develops only after a delay of 3–4 years; anticonvulsant treatment for either condition should therefore probably be continued for at least 5 years after surgery.

## Steroids

The evidence for a beneficial effect of steroids in patients with intracerebral abscess is equivocal, and there is no clear rationale for their use in subdural empyema.

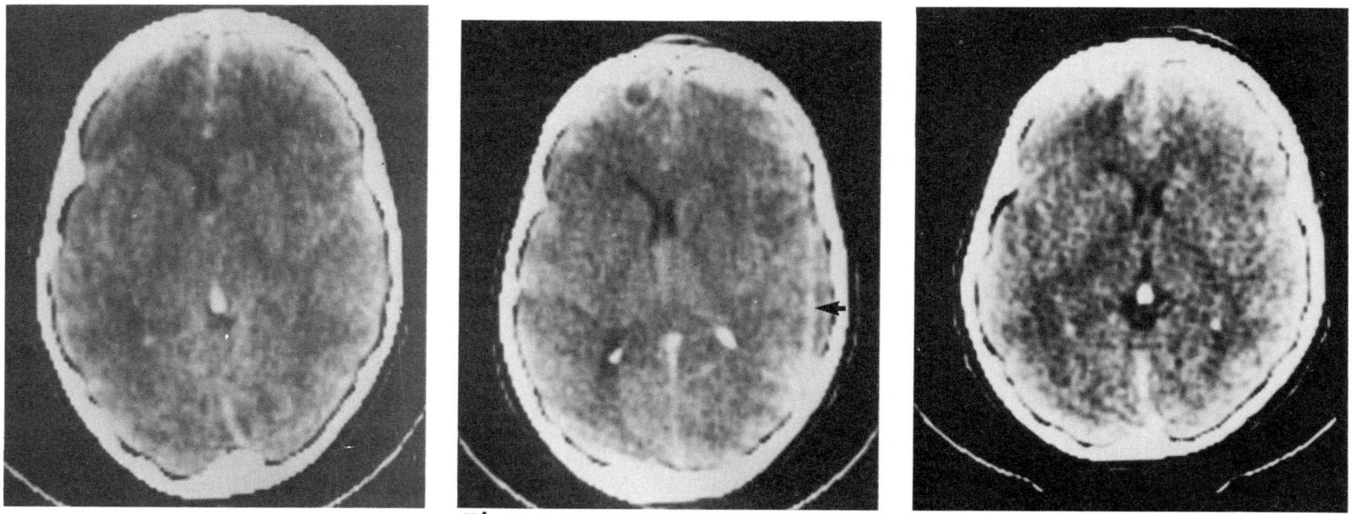

5a 5b 5c

*Sequence of CT scans in same patient as in* Figure 4 *showing* (a) *partial effacement of frontal horn of right lateral ventricle on day of admission;* (b) *development of left frontal ring-enhancing lesion and surface collection with enhancement (arrow) 8 days after admission. The ring lesion was treated conservatively. The surface collection was drained through burr holes;* (c) *showing resolution of left frontal lesion. There was full clinical recovery.*

## Repeat scanning

5

The tendency for fresh loculations of subdural pus to accumulate is notorious; an intracerebral abscess may also develop. In addition to careful clinical observation, CT scanning with contrast enhancement should therefore be repeated at 3–4-day intervals.

However, it should be borne in mind that the finding of a fresh area of ring enhancement in the brain parenchyma during follow-up should be interpreted in the light of clinical progress. Cerebritis may be self-limiting and resolve in response to continued antimicrobial treatment. We have often observed gradual resolution of ring enhancement in parallel with uneventful clinical recovery from cerebral abscess after a burr hole and a single aspiration (together with appropriate systemic antibiotic therapy). The demonstration of ring enhancement during follow-up after drainage of intracranial pus is therefore an indication for careful observation rather than immediate surgery.

## *Acknowledgements*

*Illustration 1* is reproduced by courtesy of Botterell and Drake and the American Association of Neurosurgical Surgeons[6].

We are also grateful to Dr V. McAllister and Mr. R. M. Kalbag for permission to reproduce the CT scans in *Illustrations 3, 4 and 5.*

## *References*

1. Sprott, M. S., Newman, P. K., Hall, K., Welbury, R. R., Ingham, H. R. (1981) Subdural abscess secondary to covert dental sepsis. Postgraduate Medical Journal, 57, 649–651

2. Courville, C. B. (1944) Subdural empyema secondary to purulent frontal sinusitis; a clinicopathologic study of 42 cases verified at autopsy. Archives of Otolaryngology (Chicago), 39, 211–230

3. de Louvois, J., Gortvai, P., Hurley, R. (1977) Bacteriology of abscesses of the central nervous system: a multicentre prospective study. British Medical Journal, ii, 981–984

4. Bannister, G., Williams, B., Smith, S. (1981) Treatment of subdural empyema. Journal of Neurosurgery, 55, 82–88

5. Ingham, H. R., Dutton, J., Sisson, P. R., Sprott, M. S., Selkon, J. B. (1978) An aid to the preliminary identification of non-sporing anaerobes. Journal of Clinical Pathology, 31, 806–807

6. Botterell, E. H., Drake, C. G. (1952) Localised encephalitis, brain abscess and subdural empyema. Journal of Neurosurgery, 9, 348–366

Illustrations by R. N. Lane

# Management of carotico-cavernous fistulae

**Brian E. Kendall** FRCP, FRCR
Consultant Radiologist, Lysholm Radiological Department, The National Hospital, London, UK

Serbinenko[1] was the first to describe a percutaneous transarterial method of treating carotico-cavernous fistulae using a coaxial catheter system for introducing and detaching a latex balloon. This technique, with minor modifications[2], has become a routine method of treatment of arteriovenous fistulae. More recently, another system was described for introducing a silicone rubber balloon which can be detached without the use of a coaxial system. After successful clinical application in the treatment of varicocele and pulmonary arteriovenous fistulae[3], it was successfully applied to carotico-cavernous fistulae[4].

Carotico-cavernous fistulae may be direct or dural. Direct fistulae are due to rupture of the intracavernous segment of the internal carotid artery, which may be precipitated by trauma or occur spontaneously if the vessel is diseased, usually by atheroma with or without aneurysm formation. The clinical effects of the fistula are due to a combination of reduced arterial perfusion and elevated venous pressure in the orbit, causing hypoxia, venous congestion and oedema. Symptoms are pain, bruit, diplopia and loss of vision, and the signs are congestion of the eye, chemosis, proptosis, ophthalmoplegia and decreased visual acuity.

Dural arteriovenous fistula is between meningeal branches of the internal and/or external carotid arteries and veins in the dura adjacent to the cavernous sinus. They may drain directly into the cavernous sinus or one of the adjacent sinuses, particularly an inferior petrosal sinus, which communicates with it. Symptoms are similar but usually milder than with the direct fistula and are much less likely to progress very rapidly.

Distinction between the two types of fistulae is made by selective carotid angiography, best performed by the routine Seldinger technique from the femoral artery.

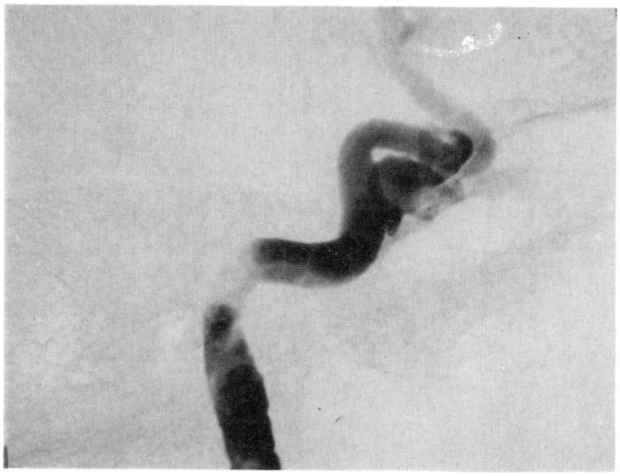

1a

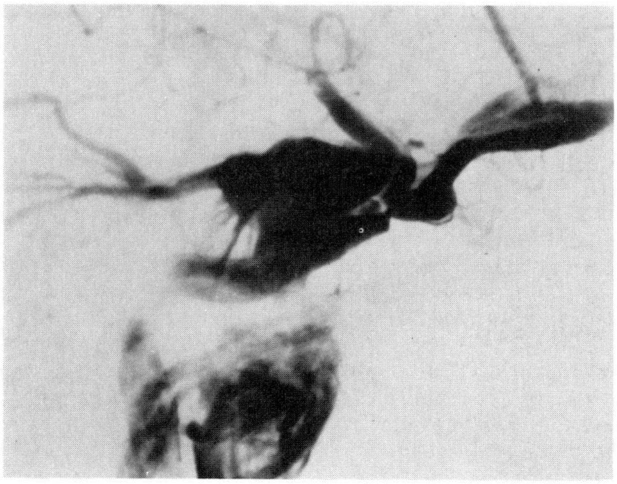

1b

# 1a & b

The rate of flow through direct carotico-cavernous fistulae varies considerably, but it may be so rapid that, when injections are made into the ipsilateral internal carotid artery, early filling of the cavernous sinus tends to obscure the site of the shunt.

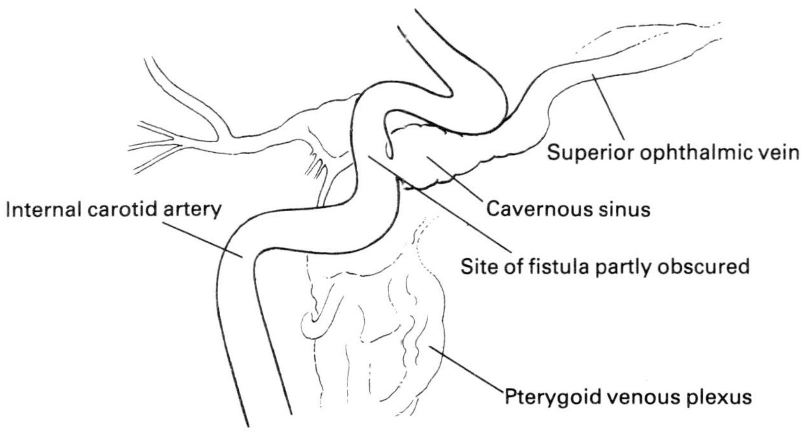


**Figure 1** *Composite diagram of* **(a)** *early and* **(b)** *late phase of internal carotid angiogram*

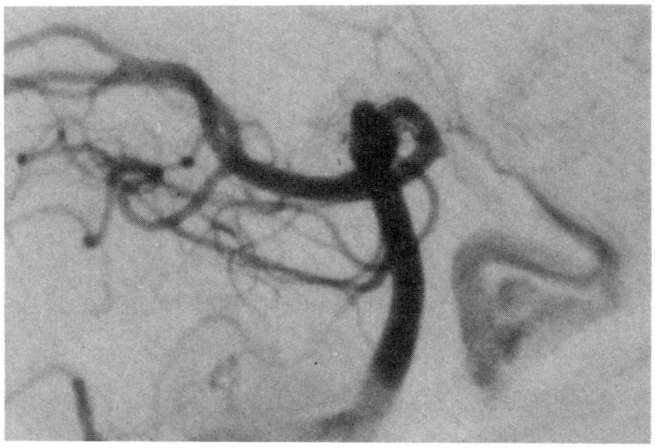

2

2

In such cases there is often reversal of flow in the terminal carotid, and the anatomy of the fistula may be more clearly defined by rapid serial radiography during retrograde filling from the posterior communicating artery while injecting into a vertebral artery.

Other important angiographic features which may influence prognosis include the amount of opacification of the ophthalmic and cerebral circulation occurring from ipsilateral carotid injections, and spontaneously from contralateral carotid and vertebral injections. The effectiveness of cross-circulation during obstruction of the ipsilateral cervical carotid artery is a major factor in determining the feasibility of therapeutic procedures which may require carotid occlusion.

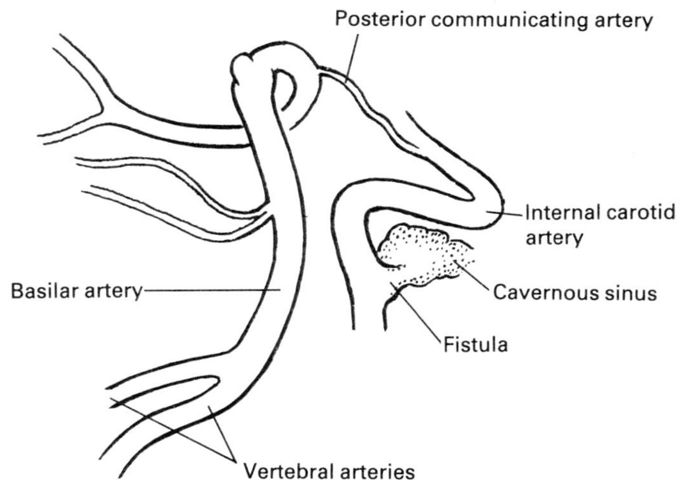


**Figure 2** *Vertebral angiogram*

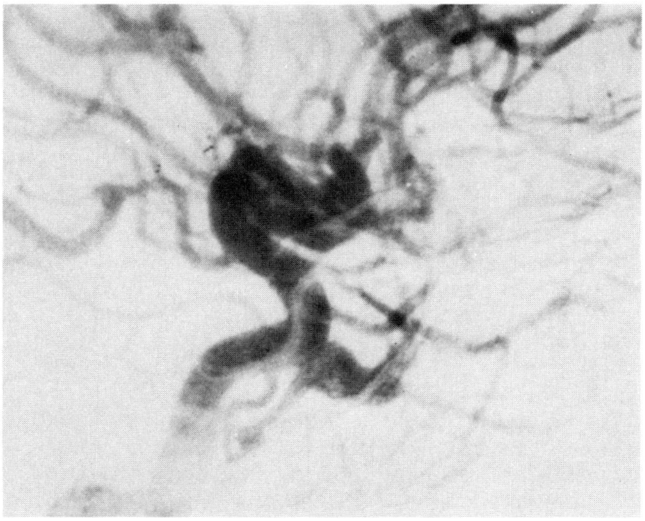

3a

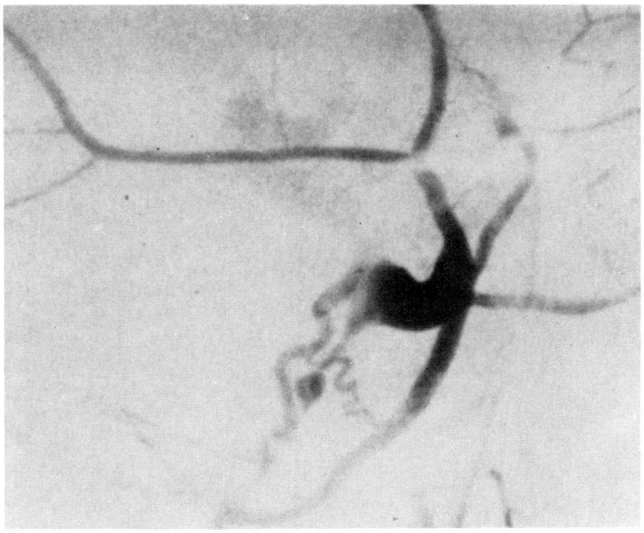

3b

# 3a & b

When a direct fistula is not revealed, the external carotid circulation is studied for connections to a dural fistula.

Spontaneous permanent closure of direct carotico-cavernous fistulae after the acute phase is rare; extrapolating from the large series reviewed by Sattler[5] and Sugar and Meyer[6], it is probably in the region of 2 per cent and most often occurs following controlled carotid compression or angiography[7]. Medical treatment to improve blood flow through the eye by dealing with any factors which reduce the arteriovenous pressure gradient, such as right-sided heart failure, systemic hypotension or polycythaemia, has limited success in a few cases. Generally speaking, the symptoms are progressive and occlusive therapy should be initiated at an early stage.

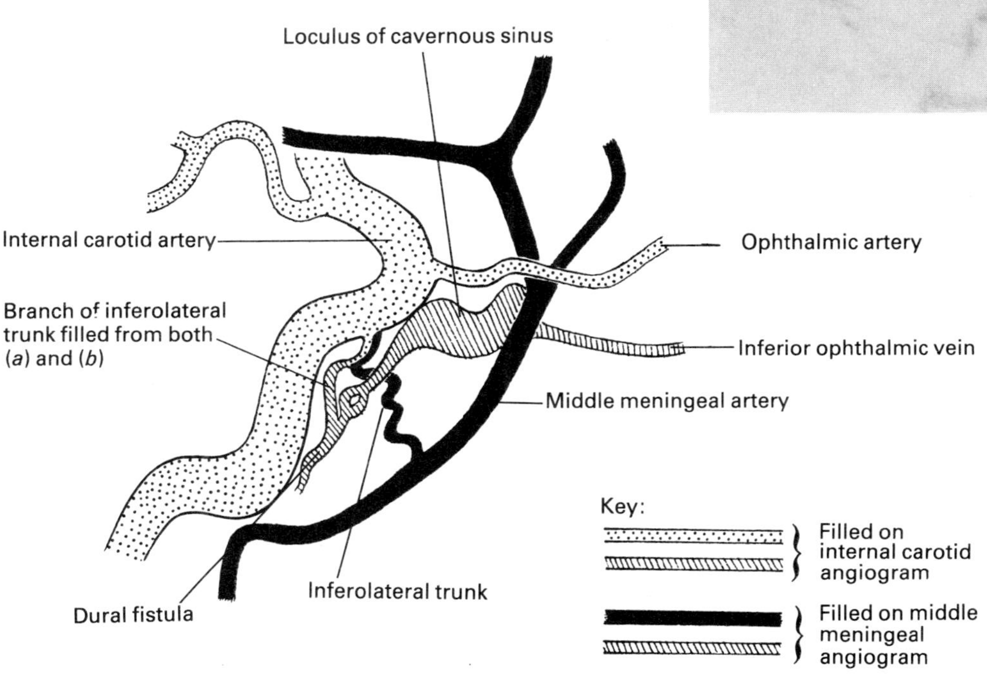


**Figure 3** *Composite diagram of* **(a)** *internal carotid and* **(b)** *middle meningeal angiogram*

# 4a & b

Prognosis is much better in dural fistulae, in which spontaneous closure occurs in about 45 per cent[8] and in which spontaneous remission of symptoms is not uncommon, so that conservative treatment with careful clinical follow-up examinations is reasonable. Embolization of the fistula with small particles of polyvinyl alcohol is indicated if signs of progression, particularly threat to vision, should occur.

The objective of treatment of direct carotico-cavernous fistulae should be to restore the circulatory dynamics to normal by obliterating the fistula while preserving carotid and ophthalmic artery flow and avoiding damage to the nerves in the cavernous sinus. Surgical procedures to occlude the carotid above and below the fistula often failed because of extensive collateral circulation, and also lowered the ophthalmic artery pressure. When such trapping operations are combined with arteriotomy and packing of the cavernous segment of the carotid artery, the fistula is usually obliterated, but carotid flow is lost and ophthalmic flow diminished. Loss of vision was a frequent complication and, even when patients who could not withstand carotid occlusion were excluded, there was still a substantial incidence of hemiparesis. In most direct fistulae, a balloon can be placed on the venous side to occlude the fistula, leaving the carotid flow intact.

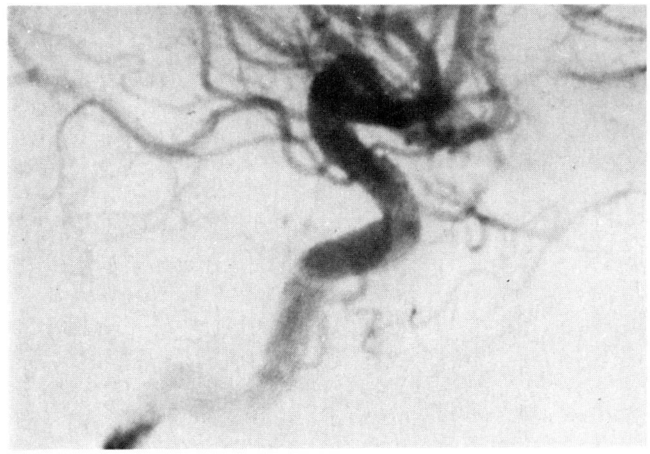

4a

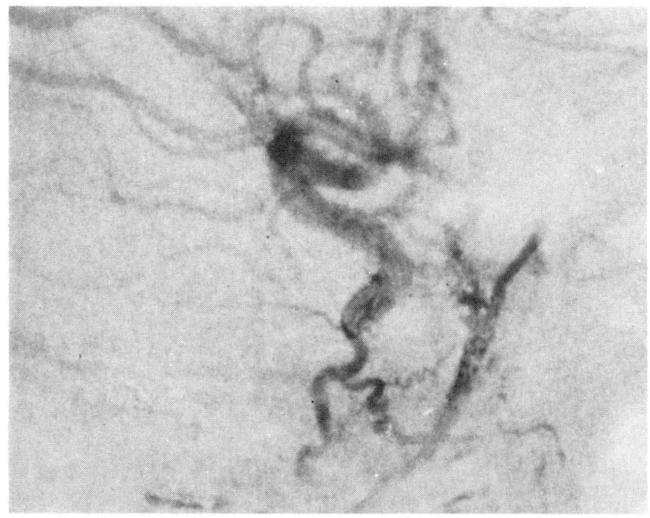

4b

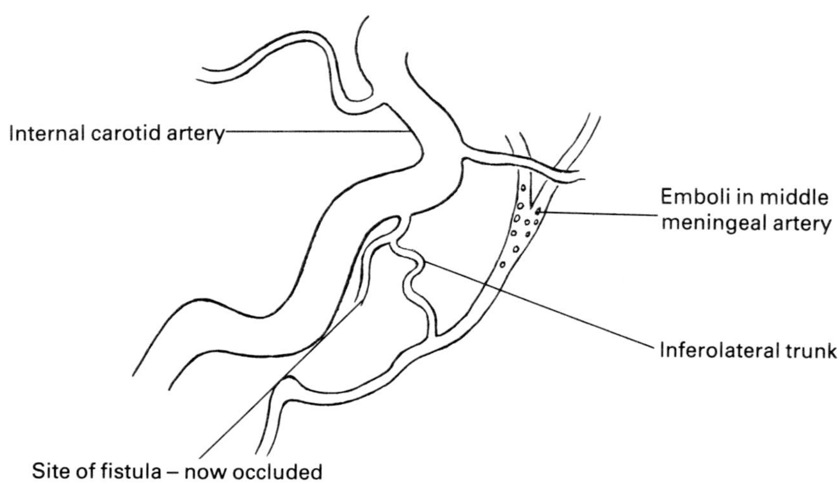


**Figure 4** *Composite diagram of* **(a)** *internal carotid and* **(b)** *middle meningeal angiogram after embolization of fistula with polyvinyl alcohol*

## BALLOON SYSTEMS

### Latex balloon coaxial detachment system

This system is manufactured by Ingenor Medical Systems, Paris, France.

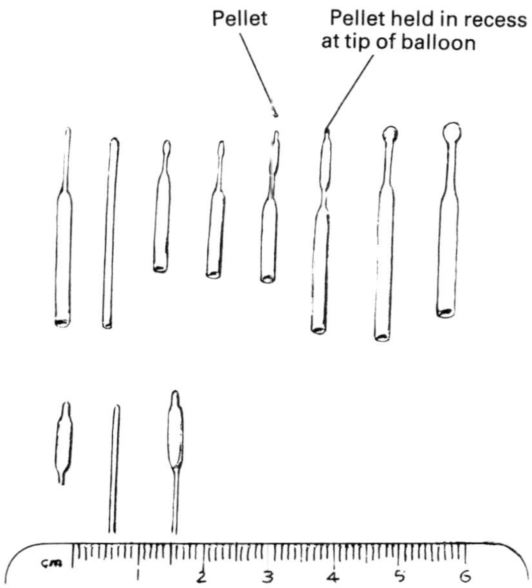


5

**5**

The uninflated latex balloons are 0.8–2.3 mm in diameter and 2.0–5.0 mm in length. They can be made with a small distal recess for insertion of a silver or gold pellet which facilitates observation of the uninflated balloon on the fluoroscopic screen.

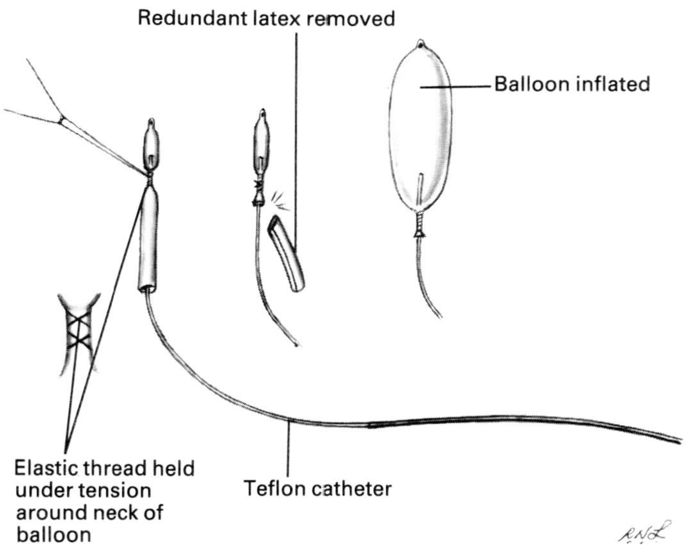


6

**6**

The neck of the balloon is sufficiently tight to grip a thin-walled Teflon (El Du Pont, UK) catheter onto which it is ligated with elastic thread under tension so that the ligature will close the neck of the balloon when it is detached.

Similar balloons can be obtained ready tied, and latex balloons with a self-occluding valve have recently been introduced. The capacity of the balloons varies from 0.1 to 2.5 ml, the inflated diameter from 4.5 to 12.0 mm, and the length from 8.5 to 20.0 mm.

The thin-walled Teflon catheter tubing (0.6 mm external diameter) is supple and can be carried distally in the arterial system by the balloon. The coaxial polyethylene catheter is flexible enough to be advanced over the Teflon catheter but sufficiently rigid when advanced to the level of the balloon to detach it with the Teflon catheter held under tension. It can also be used to advance the balloon against the blood flow, as may be necessary if a transvenous approach to a fistula is practical.

This balloon system has the following advantages.

1. The risk of premature detachment is minimal.
2. The system is self-sealing, allowing it to be used with iso-osmolar contrast medium, which is essential in situations where the degree of distension of the balloon necessary to close the fistula is close to the capacity of the catheter system, or where it is difficult to maintain the balloon in its location so that it could become malpositioned in an interval between removing contrast medium and replacing it with silicone. Also, when multiple balloons are necessary to occlude a fistula, the total volume of the distension balloons in the cavernous sinus could cause pressure on cranial nerves, which would be permanent with silicone-filled balloons but tends to be relieved with contrast-filled balloons as these deflate with time.

The disadvantage of the system is the necessity for a coaxial catheter which may be difficult to advance through a tortuous arterial system.

## Detachable silicone balloon system

Only one such system is commercially available (Becton Dickinson UK Ltd, Cowley, Oxford, UK). It consists of a cylindrical silicone rubber balloon attached to a 150 cm long radio-opaque polyethylene catheter, 0.6 mm in outer diameter, by a stainless steel valve pin. The uninflated balloons are of two sizes, 1 and 2 mm in diameter and 5 and 7 mm in length respectively. The maximum recommended inflation volume is 0.15 ml and 0.6 ml, producing outer diameters of 3 mm and 9 mm respectively. Further inflation will not rupture the balloon, but an overdistended balloon may not remain inflated after detachment for as long as the 30 days which is guaranteed for a balloon which is not so compromised.

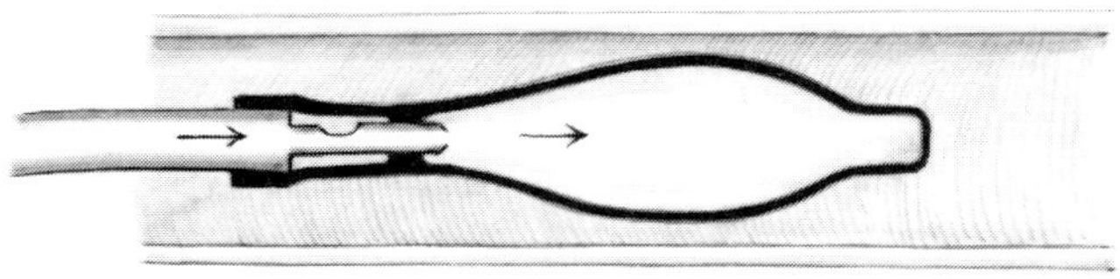

7a

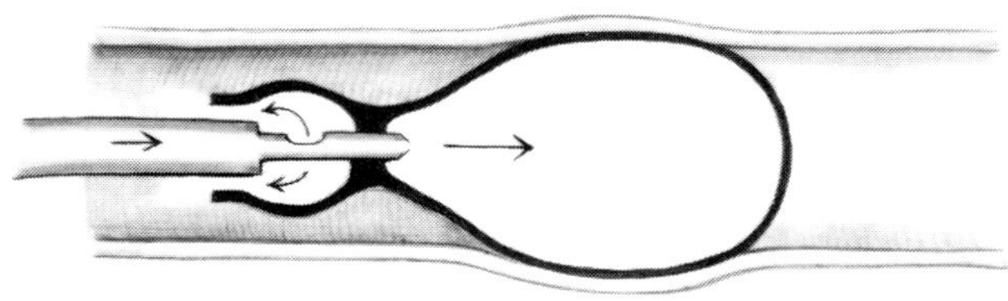

7b

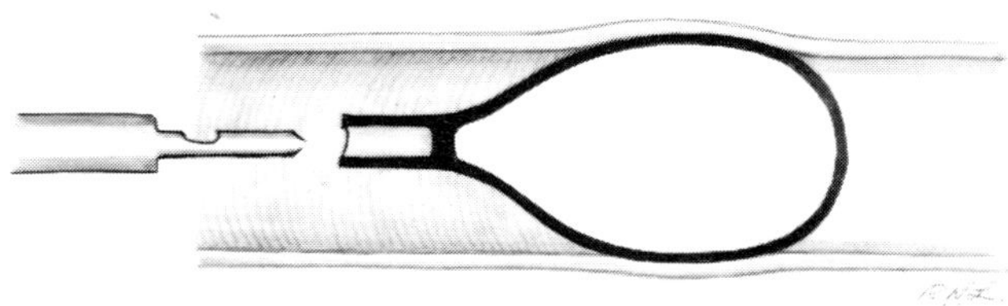

7c

# 7

The valve is fixed in and projects beyond the lumen of the end of the catheter, and both the valve pin and the termination of the catheter are overlapped by the neck of the balloon, which is firmly fixed onto the catheter by the friction between the silicone and polyethylene. There is a side hole in the part of the valve beyond the catheter tip and this acts as a detaching mechanism in the following way. As the contrast medium is injected into the balloon catheter, it preferentially fills the balloon (*a*) until it comes into contact with and is compressed by the walls of the vessel within which it is being inflated. Contrast medium is then forced through the side hole and lifts the neck of the balloon off the end of the catheter (*b*); this allows the catheter to be disconnected by traction (*c*).

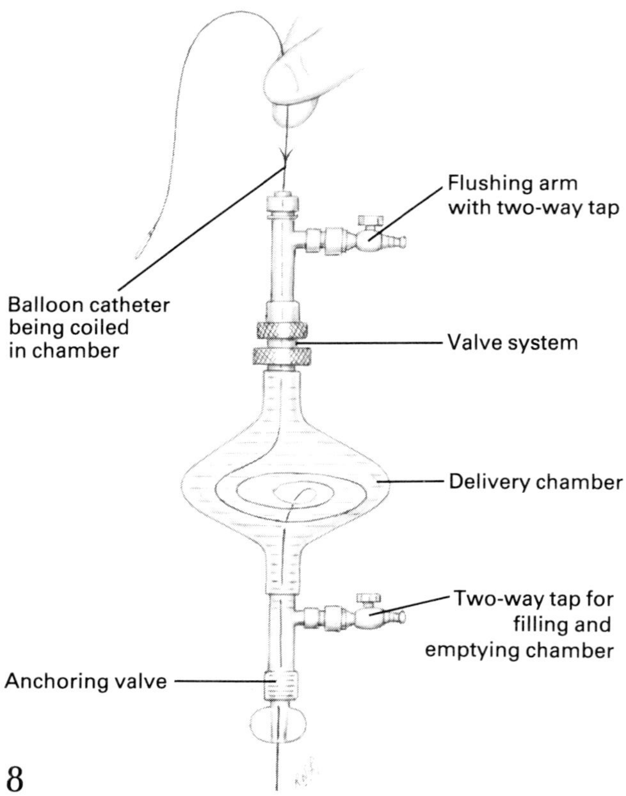


8

# 8

The balloon and catheter have to be washed by a jet of saline through a delivery catheter to the desired position in the circulation from a specially designed pulsion or delivery chamber, in which an appropriate length of the balloon catheter is coiled. The balloon catheter extends through and just protrudes from a connector equipped with a flushing arm and a valve system; this prevents reflux of blood and maintains the balloon in position until the appropriate time for injection into the patient. The distal end of the balloon catheter is anchored by a further valve. The whole system is filled with heparinized saline before being attached to the correctly placed delivery catheter.

# Preoperative investigation

It is desirable to perform diagnostic angiography as a separate study, but in an emergency it is entirely reasonable to proceed directly with the balloon occlusive technique. The patient should previously have been fully assessed for ability to withstand ipsilateral carotid occlusion, since in about 10 per cent of patients it is not possible to occlude the fistula without also occluding the internal carotid artery.

The radiological equipment should be capable of image-intensified fluoroscopy in both anteroposterior and lateral projections. A biplane system is ideal, but a C-arm system is quite adequate.

### Anaesthesia

Procedures from the groin can be performed under local anaesthesia if the patient is cooperative, but puncture and catheterization of the neck, which may be required if femoral catheterization is impracticable, are best performed under general anaesthesia because of the risk of cervical haematoma after removal of the introducing catheter. Many nervous patients also prefer procedures from the groin to be performed under general anaesthesia, and this is permissible unless carotid occlusion becomes necessary. Occlusion should only be undertaken with the patient conscious and cooperating, so that, should it become apparent that neurological symptoms are developing, the balloon can be deflated immediately. If the procedure is being conducted under light general anaesthesia, this should be reversed before the carotid occlusive procedure.

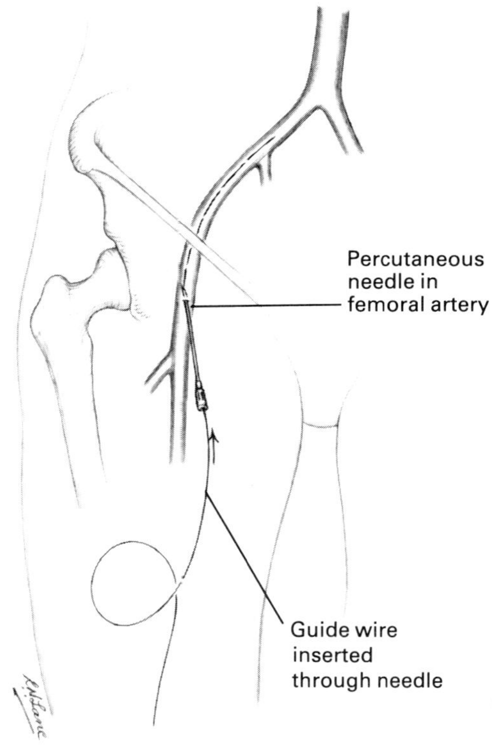


9

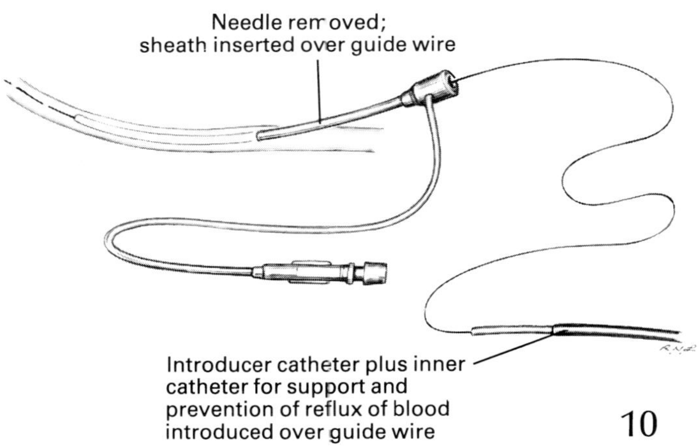


10

# The procedure

### Insertion of introducer catheter

# 9, 10 & 11

This must be of sufficiently large calibre (maximum 8.8 Fr non-tapered) to accommodate the largest balloon which may be required. It is introduced percutaneously through a sheath usually placed in the femoral artery. The catheter must be sufficiently rigid to avoid producing distortion of the lumen at bends or kinks at which the balloon may stick.

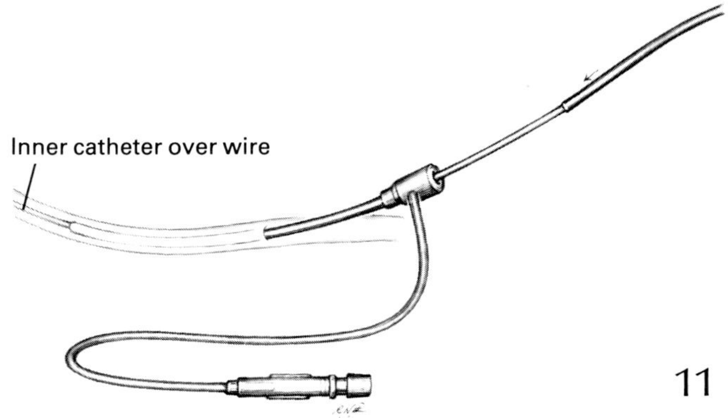


11

# 12, 13 & 14

The catheter tip is usually placed low down in the internal carotid artery to avoid the possibility of inducing spasm by any attempt to manipulate the large catheter more distally.

If arterial tortuosity or severe atheroma precludes catheterization from the femoral artery, direct puncture of the common carotid artery is performed and a sheath of adequate calibre is introduced with its tip in the internal carotid artery.

Lateral carotid angiography is then performed to check the fistula and haemodynamics for any change since the time of the diagnostic angiogram.

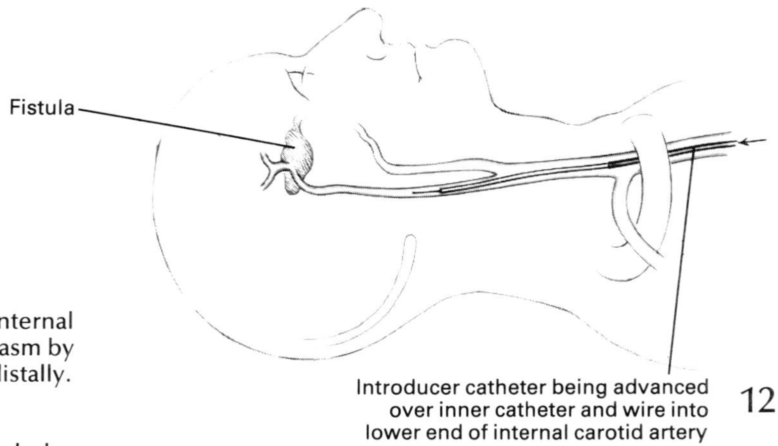


12

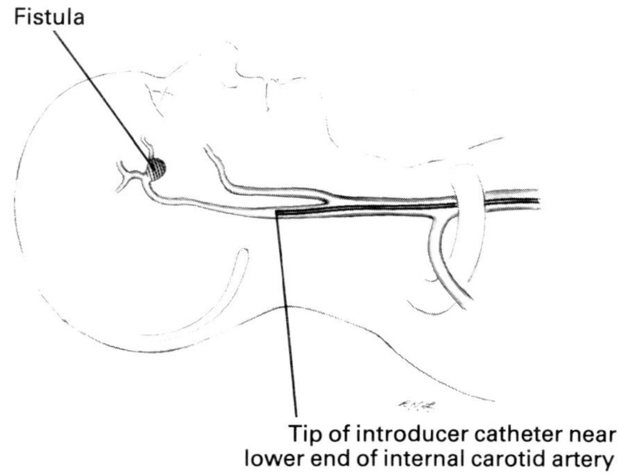


13

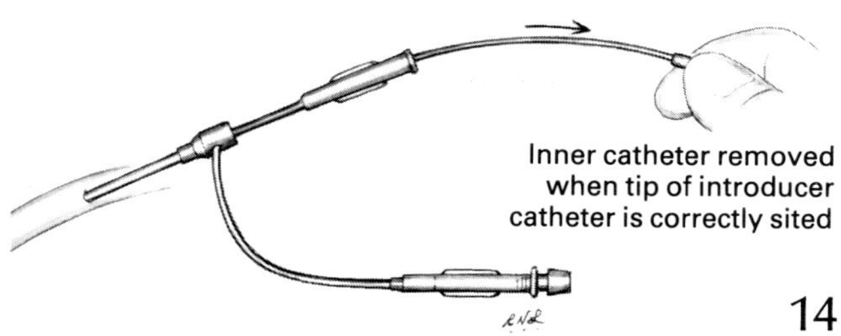


14

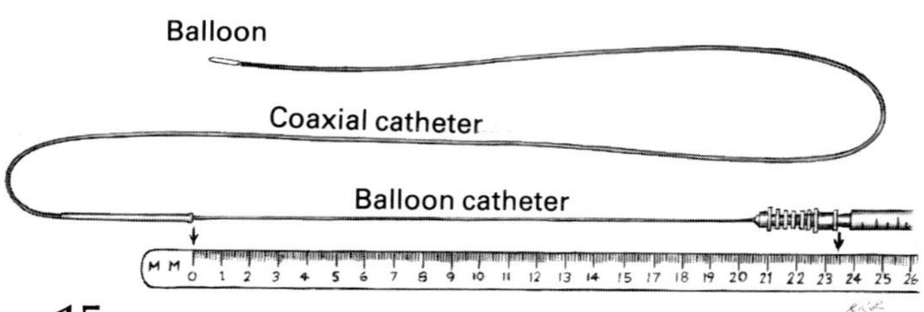


15

# 15

With the latex balloon coaxial system, prior to insertion the coaxial catheter is advanced to the level of the neck of the balloon and the difference in length between the balloon and coaxial catheters noted.

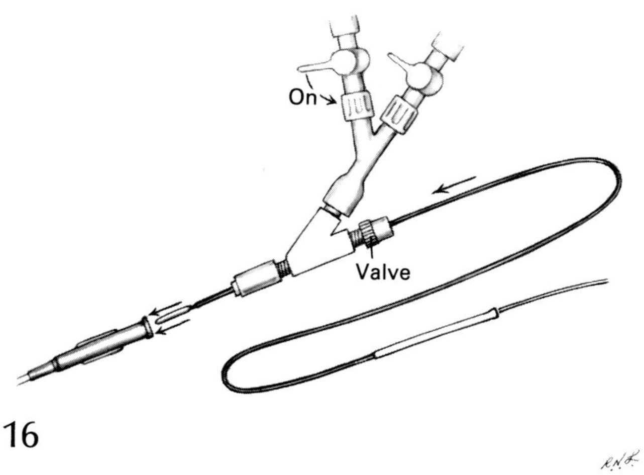


16

# 16

The balloon catheter is advanced into the introducer catheter through the direct limb of a Y-connector, which is equipped with a valve to prevent back bleeding.

# 17

The introducer catheter is continuously perfused with heparinized saline through the side arm of this Y-connector via a further Y-connection equipped with stopcocks, so that control angiography can be performed through this limb.

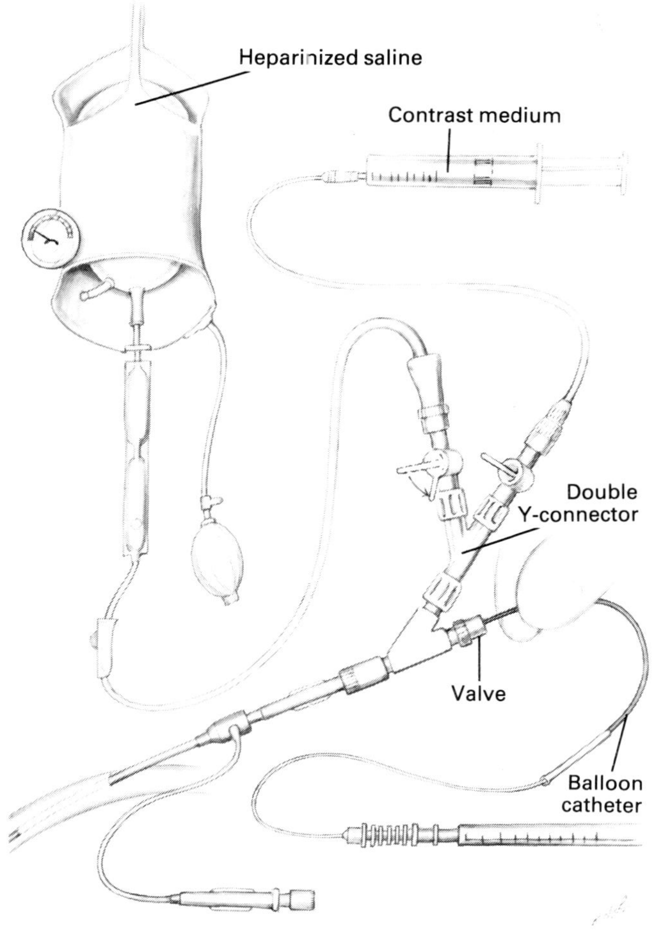


17

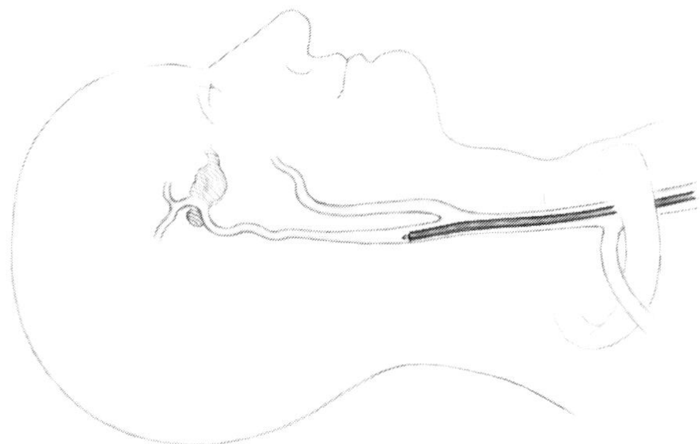

18a

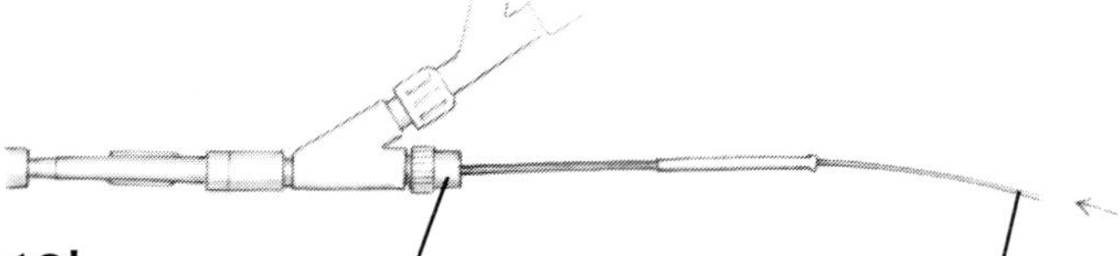


18b

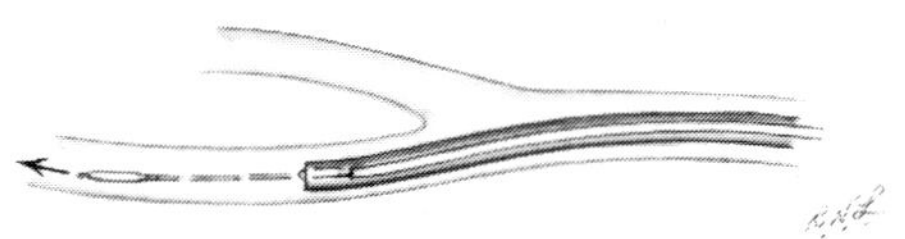

18c

# 18a, b & c

The balloon and coaxial catheters are advanced together until the pellet in the balloon catheter reaches the tip of the introducer catheter (*a*). The coaxial catheter is then fixed (*b*) so that its tip remains within the introducer catheter; in this way the space between the coaxial and balloon catheters is continuously perfused with the heparinized saline, which drips from the tip of the coaxial catheter throughout the procedure. The balloon catheter alone is then advanced through the internal carotid artery (*b* and *c*).

# 19

The balloon catheter is frequently carried by the blood flow as far as the carotid siphon and even through the fistula. If it sticks within the carotid artery below the fistula, it is slightly inflated with iso-osmotic contrast medium, care being taken not to inflate the balloon so much as to occlude carotid flow.

When the balloon is at the level of the fistula it is deflated. If it does not immediately enter the cavernous sinus, as indicated by deviation from the line of the carotid siphon, it is moved backwards and forwards across the origin of the fistula, using minor degrees of inflation with contrast medium as necessary, in the hope of inducing passage through it.

It is usual to begin the procedure with the largest of the balloons which, from examination of the angiogram, are considered to be most likely to occlude the fistula. If the larger balloon fails, it is best, rather than to persist with it, to proceed quickly to progressively smaller balloons. Prolonged attempts are more prone to lead to complications, owing either to premature detachment of the balloon or to clot formation taking place upon it.

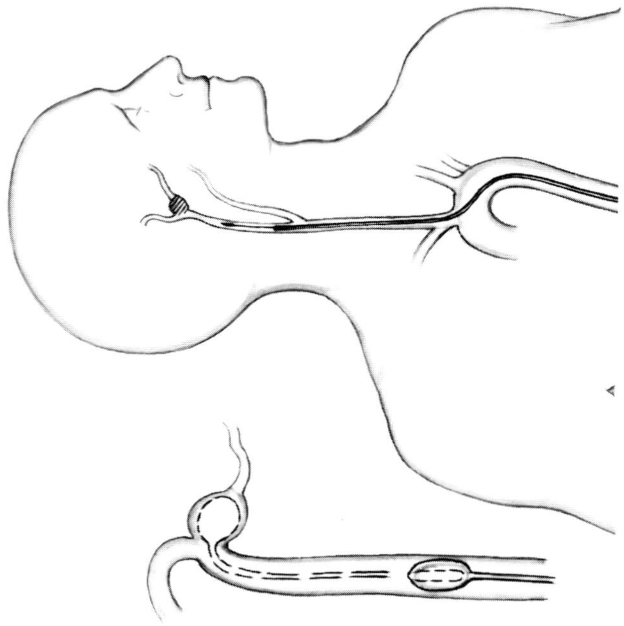

19

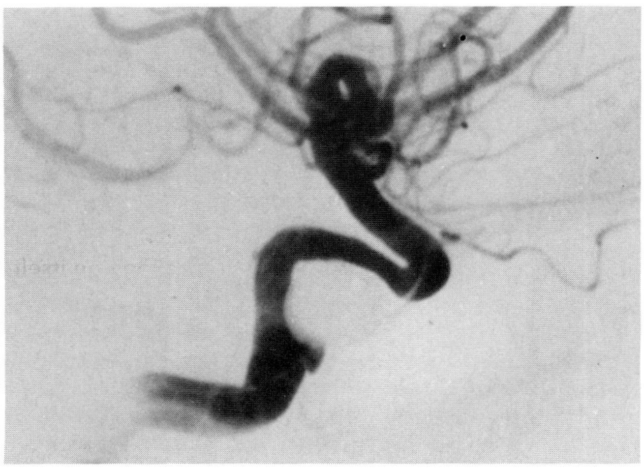

**Figure 20** *Carotid angiogram (same patient as Illustration 1)*

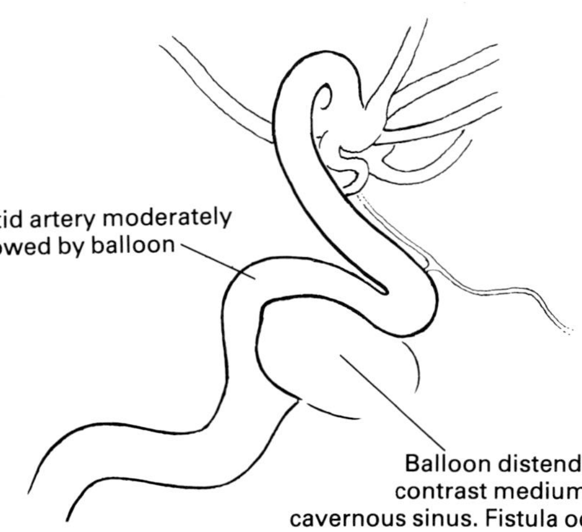


20

# 20

When a balloon has passed through the fistula into the cavernous sinus, it is inflated with a sufficient volume of isotonic contrast medium to occlude the fistula, as confirmed by intermittent injections of contrast medium. If the balloon, when filled to maximum capacity, fails to occlude the fistula, the fully inflated balloon is detached, and a similar procedure followed with further balloons until a final one closes the fistula. The contrast medium is removed from this balloon and replaced with a solidifying mixture of silicones. The silicones maintain permanent inflation of the balloon and reduce the likelihood of later development of a pseudoaneurysm at the site of the fistula.

# 21 & 22

Balloons are detached by advancing the coaxial catheter the measured distance to the level of the balloon, ascertained before introduction of the balloon system (*see Illustration 15*).

Gentle traction is then maintained on the balloon catheter while a firm even push is maintained on the coaxial catheter. A characteristic yield is felt as the balloon detaches.

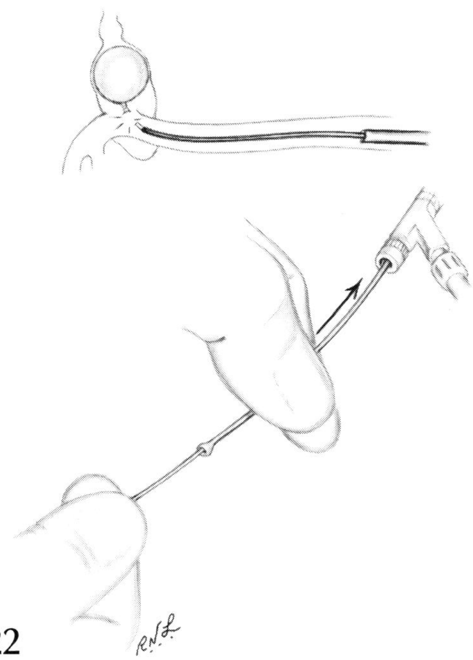

22

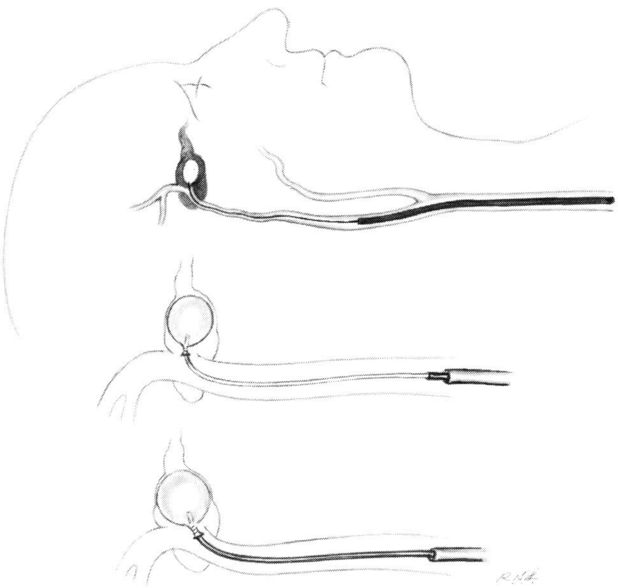

21

## Detachable silicone balloons

# 23

Sufficient catheter is first flushed from the pulsion chamber to extend about 3 or 4 cm beyond the tip of the introducer catheter.

Immediate introduction of larger amounts of catheter is sometimes associated with folding of the balloon on itself, which may cause difficulty with both inflating and deflating. Further catheter is then introduced by coiling loops within the chamber and propelling them individually into the artery. Progress of the balloon can also be facilitated by slight inflation, to overcome sticking. When the balloon is opposite the fistula, the technique of traversing it is similar to that used for the latex balloon.

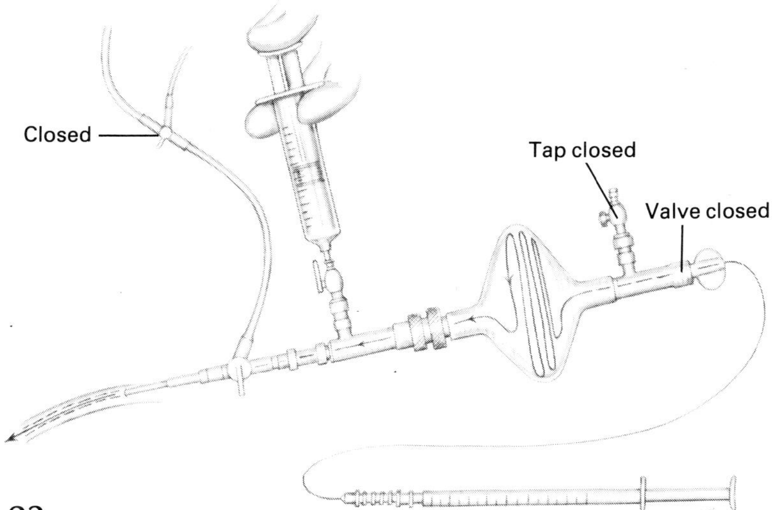


23

# 24a–d

When the balloon is seen to go through the fistula, it is inflated in increments while intermittent injections of contrast medium are made into the internal carotid artery so as to monitor closure of the fistula.

If this occurs when the balloon is wedged between the septa of the cavernous sinus, the increase in pressure within the balloon will open the space between the catheter and neck of the balloon so that it can be detached by gentle tugging. If the balloon is within the cavernous sinus but not fixed, provided that care is taken to ascertain that the balloon is too large to be withdrawn into the internal carotid artery, it can still be detached by tugging and will usually remain within the sinus, trapped between the trabeculae. Further balloons can be introduced and similarly detached until the fistula is closed.

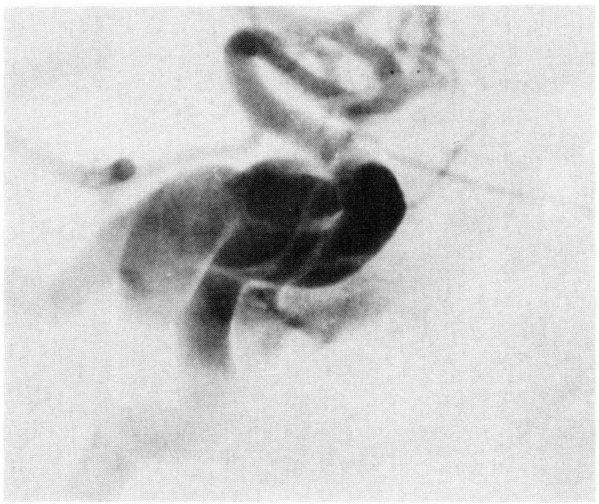

**Figure 24a** *Subtraction of left internal carotid angiogram*

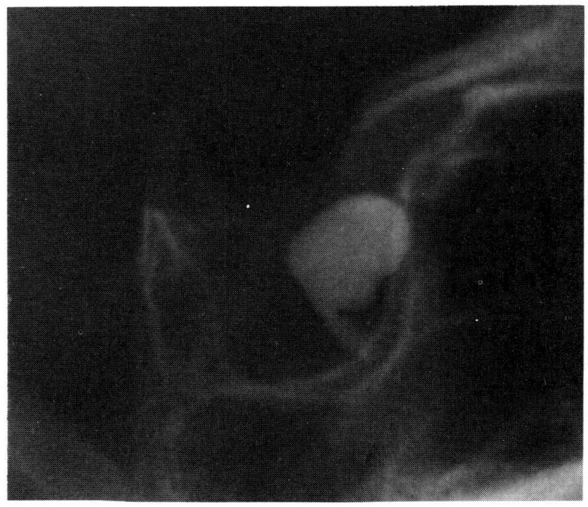

**Figure 24b** *Plain lateral skull X-ray*

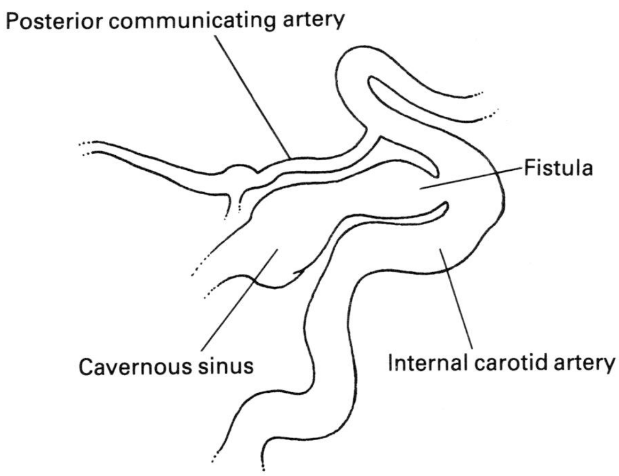


24a

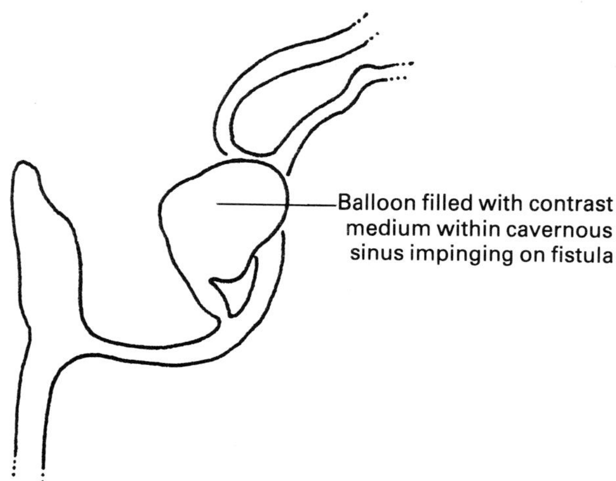


24b

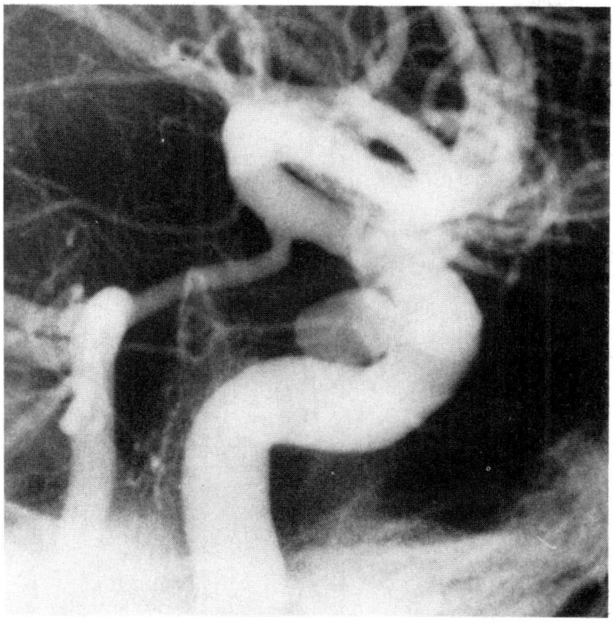

**Figure 24c** *Left carotid angiogram*

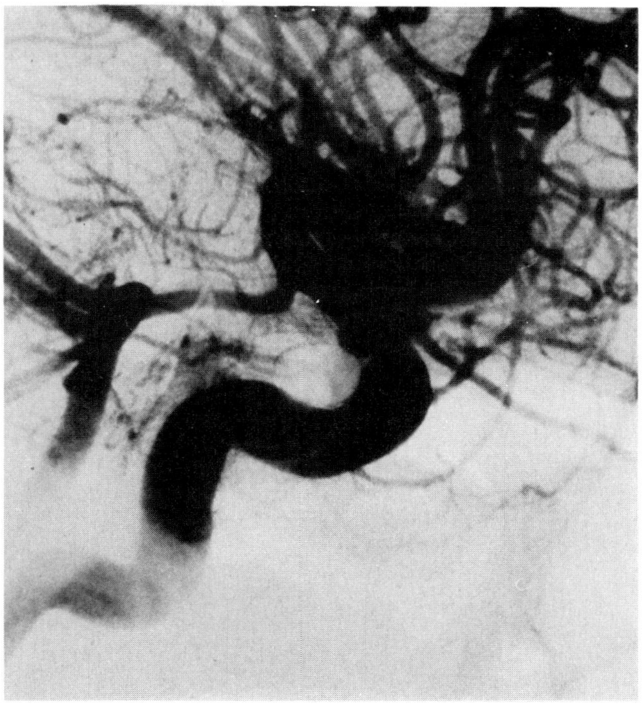

**Figure 24d** *Subtraction print of Figure 24c*

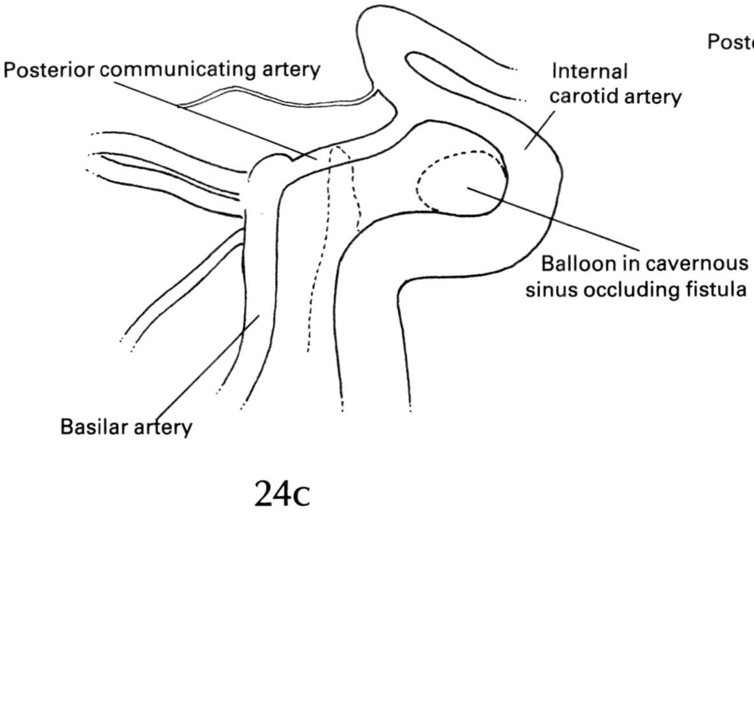


24c

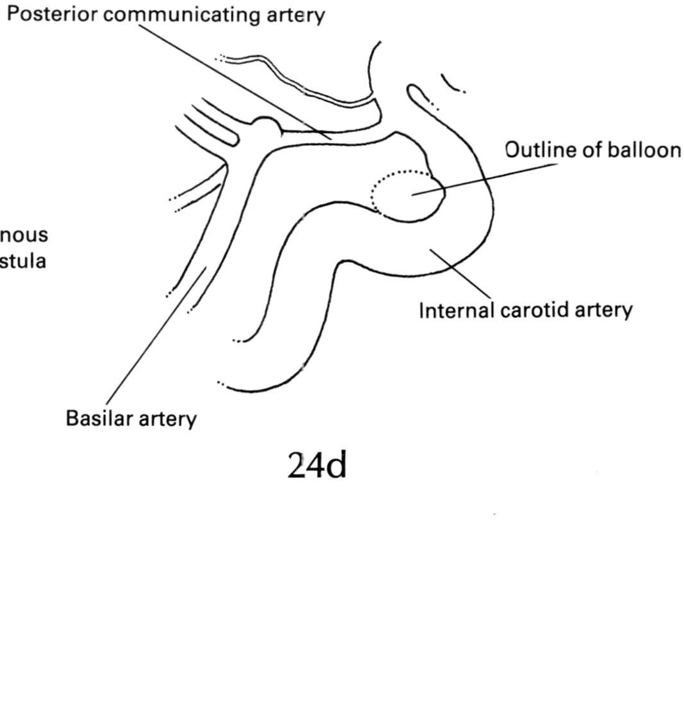


24d

# 25a–f

If attempts to treat the fistula with both the silicone and the latex balloon coaxial systems are unsuccessful, the possibility of occluding the internal carotid artery, together with the origin of the fistula, may be considered.

When both the carotid artery and the fistula are occluded by a balloon detached within the cavernous segment of the carotid, a further silicone-filled balloon placed to occlude the internal carotid artery more proximally will diminish the effects of pulse pressure on the distal balloon, and thus further reduce the remote possibility of displacement of an unprotected balloon.

At the termination of the procedure, angiography is performed. When the fistula alone has been occluded, ipsilateral carotid angiography is sufficient, but if the fistula and the carotid are both occluded, bilateral carotid angiography and if necessary vertebral angiography also (*see Illustration 25f*) are performed in order to document the extent of the cross-flow and to confirm the closure of the fistula.

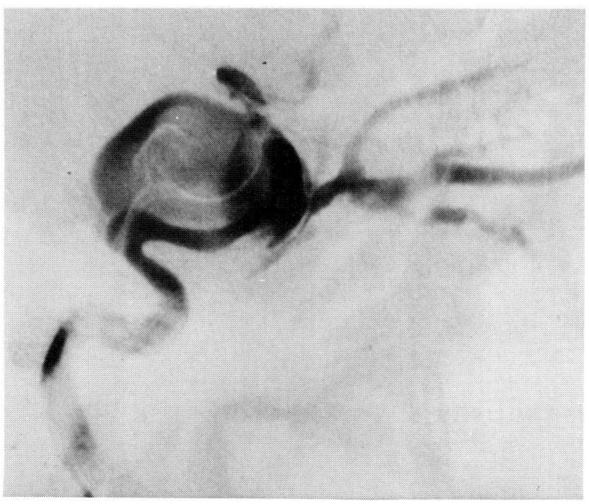

**Figure 25a** *Carotid angiogram early arterial phase*

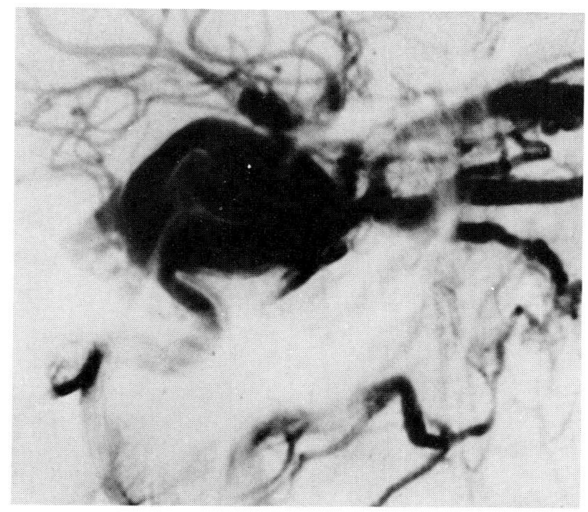

**Figure 25b** *Carotid angiogram later arterial phase*

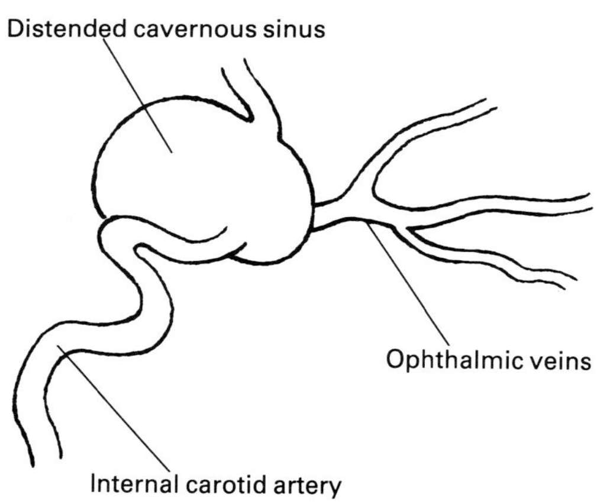


25a

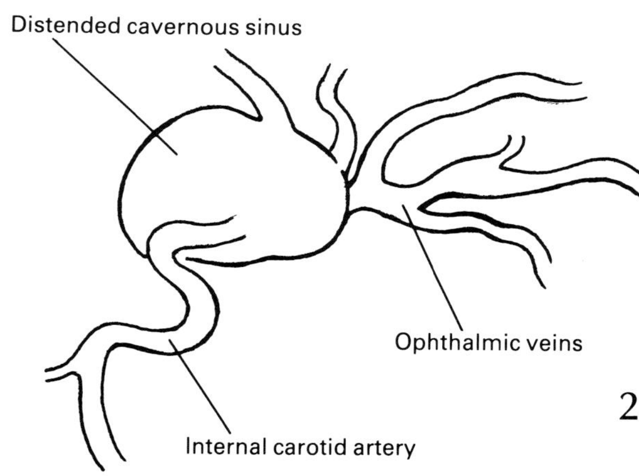


25b

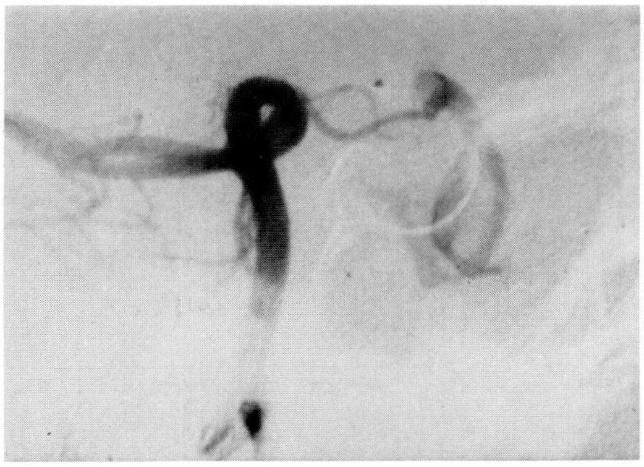

**Figure 25c** *Vertebral angiogram early arterial phase*

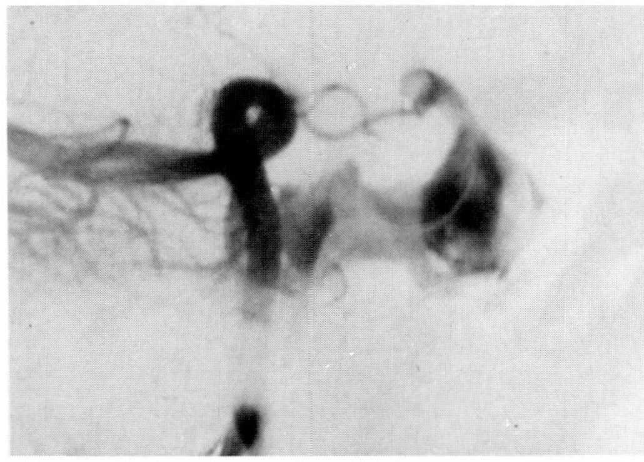

**Figure 25d** *Vertebral angiogram later arterial phase*

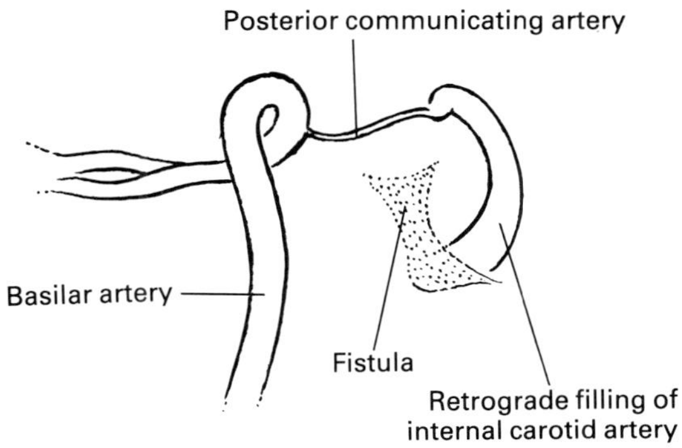


25c

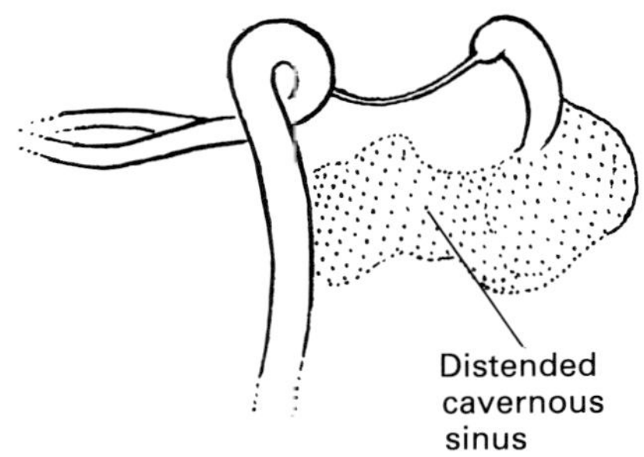


25d

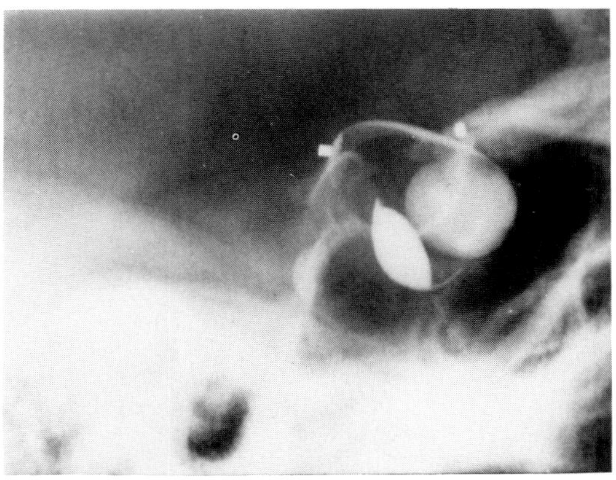

**Figure 25e** *Lateral skull X-ray*

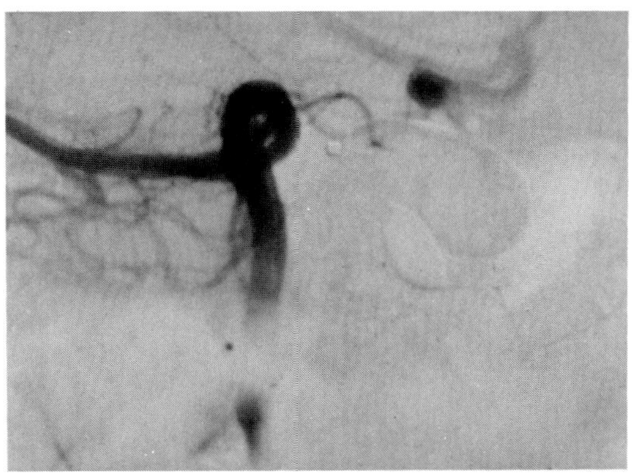

**Figure 25f** *Vertebral angiogram after occlusion of fistula and carotid artery. The subtracted outlines of the balloons are faintly visible*

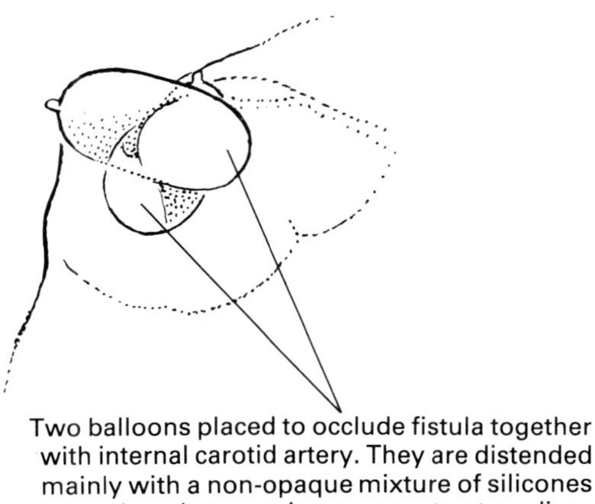


25e

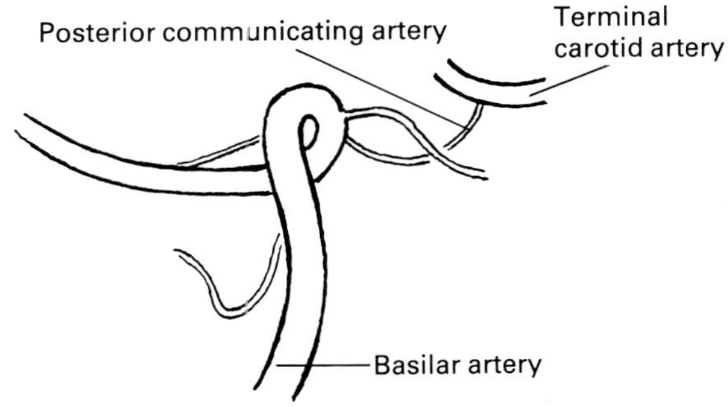


25f

## TRANSVENOUS APPROACH TO CAROTICO-CAVERNOUS FISTULA

# 26a, b & c

A small number of carotico-cavernous fistulae, shunting between the posterior or posterolateral aspect of the internal carotid artery and the cavernous sinus (*a*), can be approached retrogradely by passing a catheter through the internal jugular vein and superior petrosal sinus to enter the posterior part of the cavernous sinus (*b*). The distended balloon lies against the fistula and either occludes or markedly narrows it (*c*). The contrast medium is replaced with the solidifying silicone mixture before detachment. Of five attempts to treat fistulae in this way, three were successful; two developed transient ophthalmoplegia and one cortical venous thrombosis with full recovery.

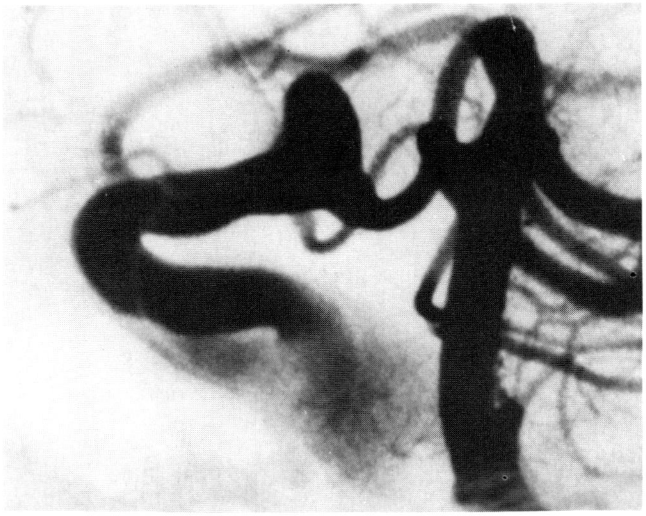

**Figure 26a** *Vertebral angiogram*

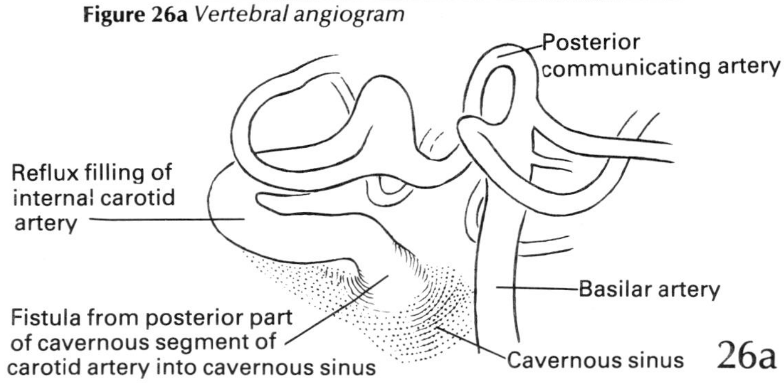


26a

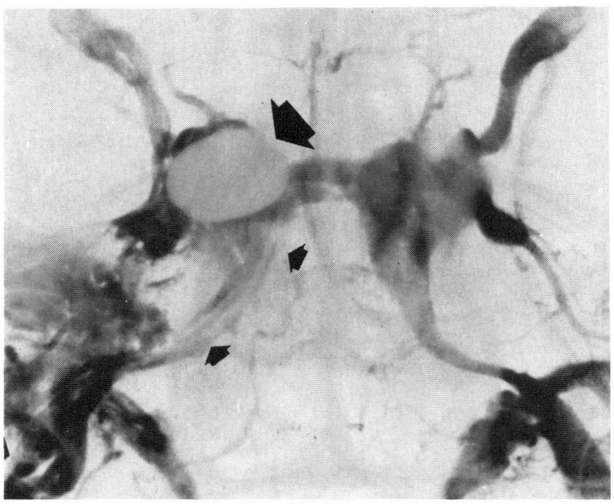

**Figure 26b** *Venogram made through introducer catheter*

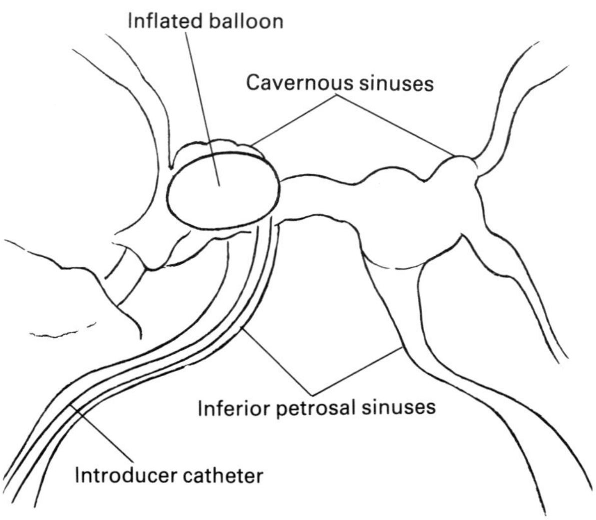


26b

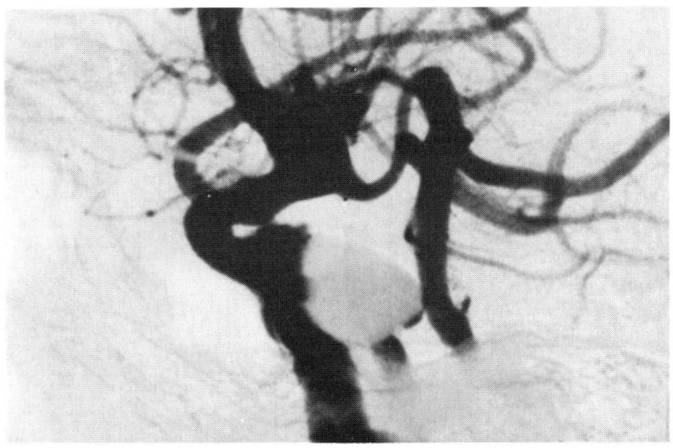

**Figure 26c** *Carotid angiogram after balloon occlusion*

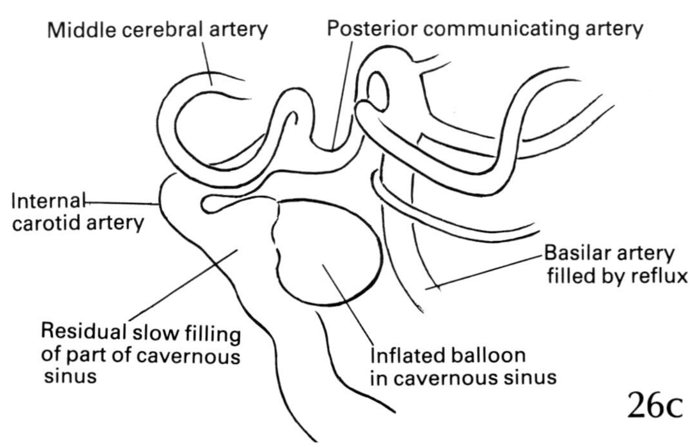


26c

## Postoperative care

Haemorrhage from the catheter site is controlled manually before the patient is returned to the ward. The catheter site and leg pulses are observed in addition to routine neurological observation. Patients in whom carotid occlusion has been necessary are anticoagulated for 5 days. Care is taken to maintain circulation and blood pressure, especially in patients who have undergone carotid occlusion. Any sign of neurological deficit is treated by attempts to increase perfusion, gentle elevation of the blood pressure and maintenance of circulating volume.

Both latex and silicone balloons induce a coating of thrombus which becomes endothelialized within about 3 weeks. Deflation of a balloon after this period is unlikely to cause reopening of the fistula.

## Results of balloon occlusion of carotico-cavernous fistula

A total of 99 cases were treated by the transarterial approach; occlusion was achieved in 88. Two others occluded spontaneously during the procedure and two were narrowed; one of these closed spontaneously at a later date. In 17 of the 88 patients the internal carotid was also occluded at the site of the fistula, and one of these developed an immediate hemiplegia. In one patient, the balloon was dislodged proximally during detachment and the fistula reopened beyond the balloon, occluding the internal carotid artery. This was successfully treated by surgery. One patient developed a clot embolus owing to failure to maintain perfusion of the introducer catheter after the fistula had been closed. This patient developed a transient hemiparesis.

# 27a–d

Routine follow-up angiography was not performed, but in three patients pseudoaneurysms were demonstrated; two of these were symptomatic and required carotid occlusion. Five patients had transient ophthalmoplegia.

The balloon occlusive procedure failed in only seven patients. In two of these it was abandoned because of the occurrence of balloon detachment at an inappropriate site, which resulted in balloon embolization of an intracranial vessel necessitating surgical removal. In four of the patients, occlusion of the fistula could not be achieved without carotid occlusion, which three were unable to withstand. The other fistula was small, presenting with a bruit only, and was not thought to be of sufficient significance to merit loss of a carotid artery.

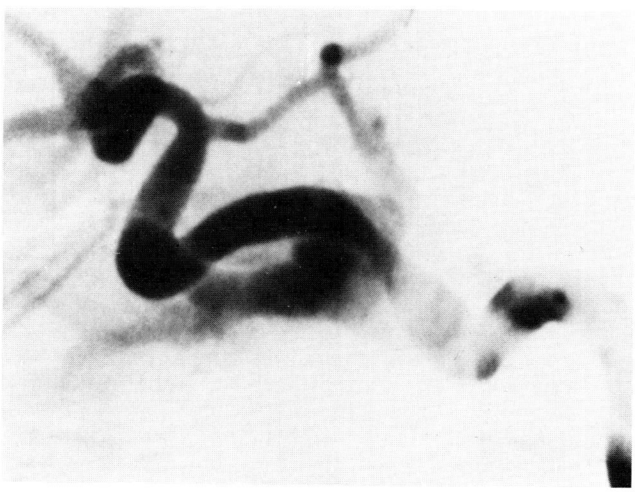

**Figure 27a** *Carotid angiogram before treatment*

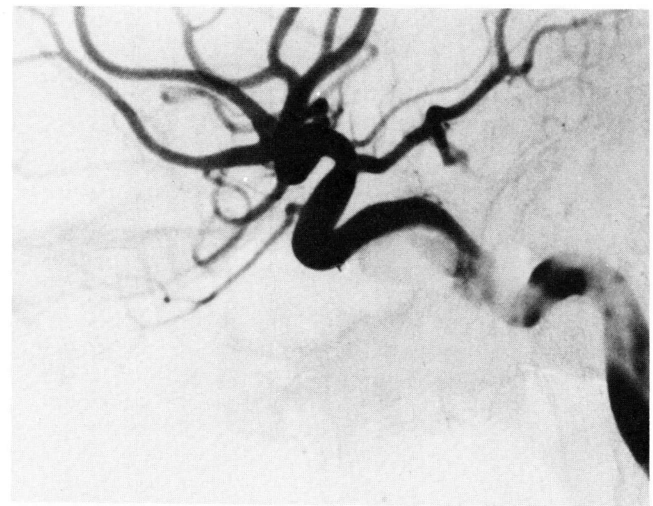

**Figure 27b** *Carotid angiogram after balloon embolization*

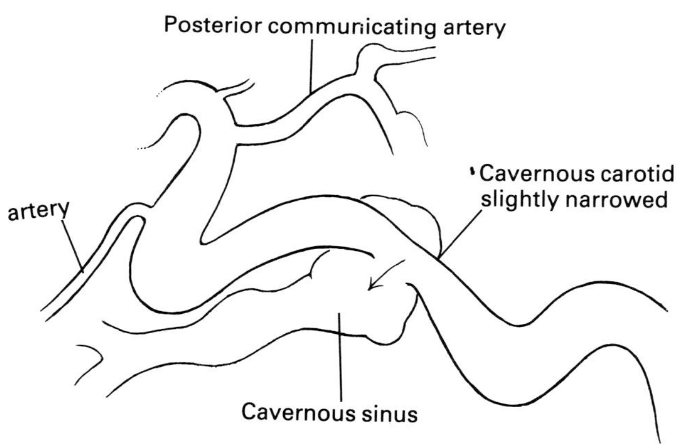


27a

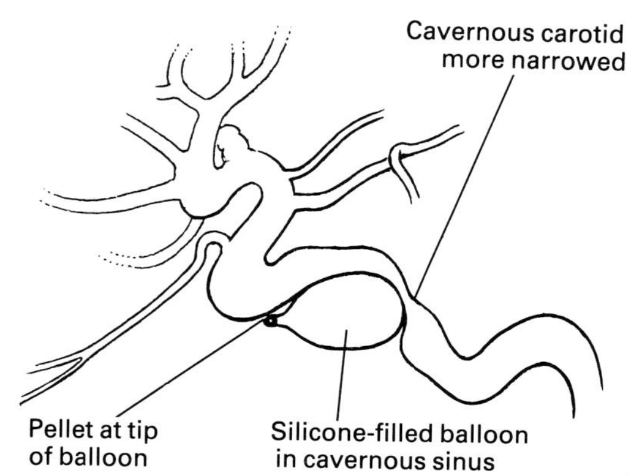


27b

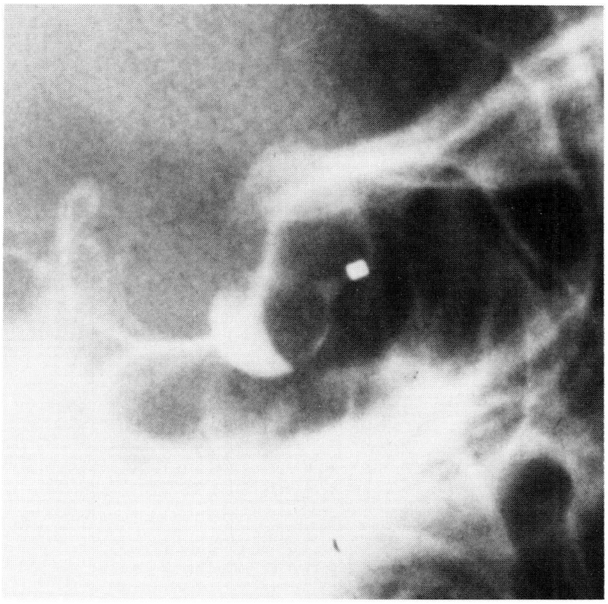

**Figure 27c** *Skull radiograph 1 year after balloon occlusion*

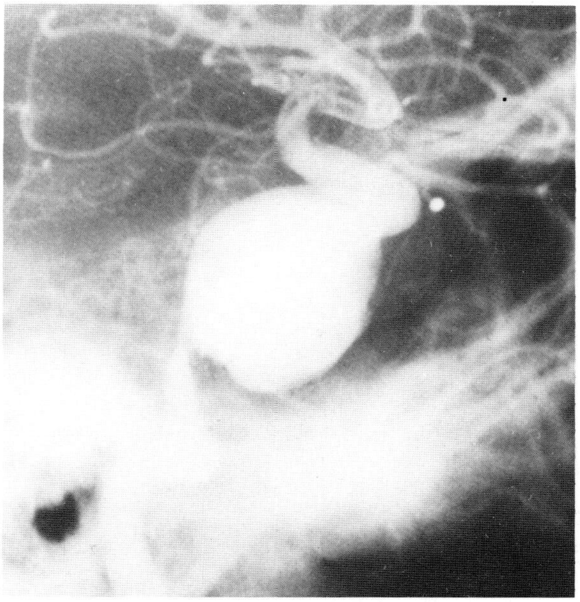

**Figure 27d** *Carotid angiogram 1 year after occlusion*

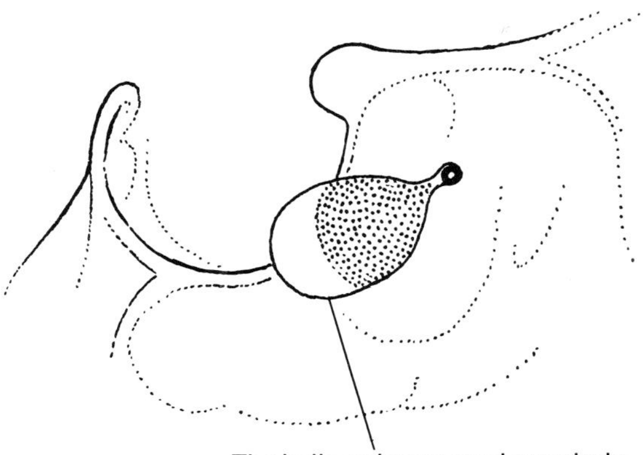


27c

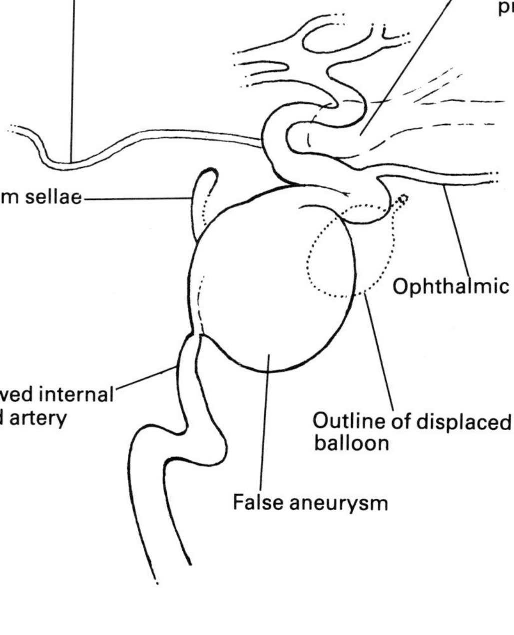


27d

# 28a & b

In the last of the failures, the fistula was at the junction of a primitive trigeminal artery with the carotid artery. Occlusion may well have been possible in this case by a transvertebral and basilar approach, but this was not attempted.

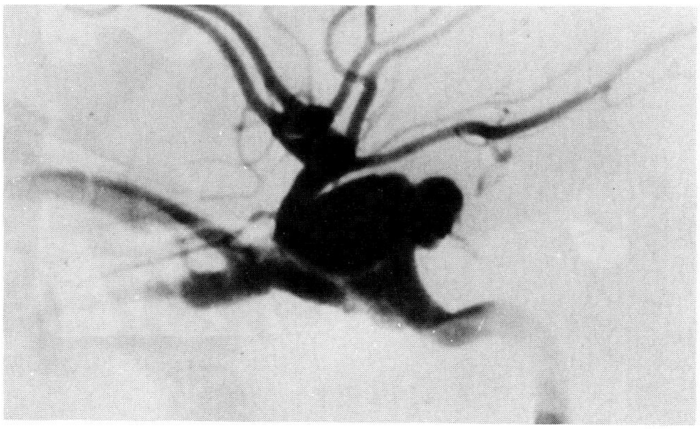

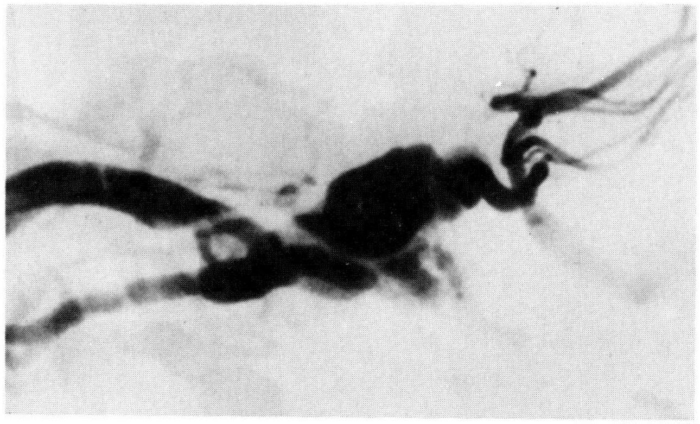

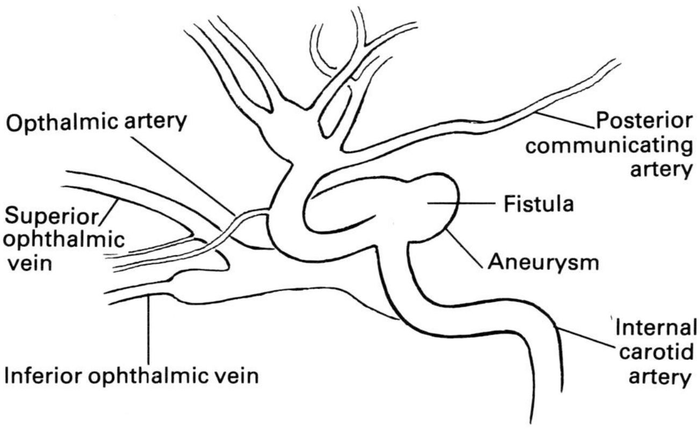


28a

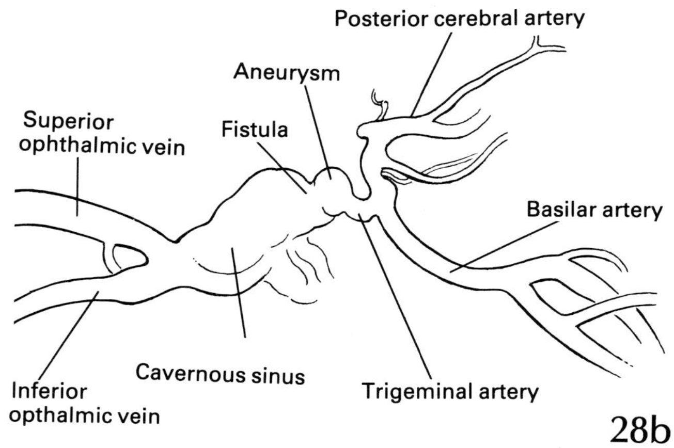


28b

## *References*


1. Serbinenko, F. A. (1974) Balloon catheterisation and occlusion of major cerebral vessels. Journal of Neurosurgery, 41, 125–145

2. Debrun, G., Lacour, P., Vinuela, F., Fox, A., Drake, C. G., Caron, J. P. (1981) Treatment of 54 traumatic carotid-cavernous fistulas. Journal of Neurosurgery, 55, 678–692

3. White, R. I. Jr, Kaufman, S.L., Barth, K. H., DeCaprio, V., Strandbert, J. D. (1979) Embolotherapy with detachable silicone balloons: technique and clinical results. Radiology, 131, 619–627

4. Norman, D., Newton, T. H., Edwards, M. S., DeCaprio, V. (1983) Carotid-cavernous fistula: closure with detachable silicone balloons. Radiology, 149, 149–157

5. Sattler, C. H. (1920) Pulsating exophthalmos. In: Handbuch der gesamten Augenheilkunde, 2nd edn, A. C. Graefe, E. T. Saemisch (eds). Vol. 9 pt. 1, Ch. 13 pt 2. Leipzig: Englemann

6. Sugar, H. A., Meyer, S. J. (1940) Pulsating exophthalmos. Archives of Ophthalmology, 23, 1288–1321

7. Potter, J. M. (1954) Carotid cavernous fistula: five cases with 'spontaneous' recovery. British Medical Journal, ii, 786–788

8. Newton, T. H., Hoyt, W. F. (1970) Dural arteriovenous shunts in the region of the cavernous sinus. Neuroradiology, 1, 71–81

Illustrations by Barbara Hyams

# Treatment of hydrocephalus

**Thomas Herrick Milhorat** MD
Professor and Chairman, Department of Neurosurgery, State University of New York Health Sciences Center at Brooklyn, Brooklyn, New York, USA

## Preoperative diagnosis

The first and most consistent finding in infants with hydrocephalus is an excessive rate of cranial enlargement. As the condition advances, the natural decompression afforded by the immature skull is exhausted and overt symptoms supervene. The most common of these are vomiting, irritability and lethargy. Clinical examination may reveal any or all of the following signs of increased intracranial pressure: enlargement and distension of the fontanelles, diastasis of the cranial sutures, engorgement of the superficial scalp veins, unilateral or bilateral abducent nerve palsy, and a 'setting-sun' sign.

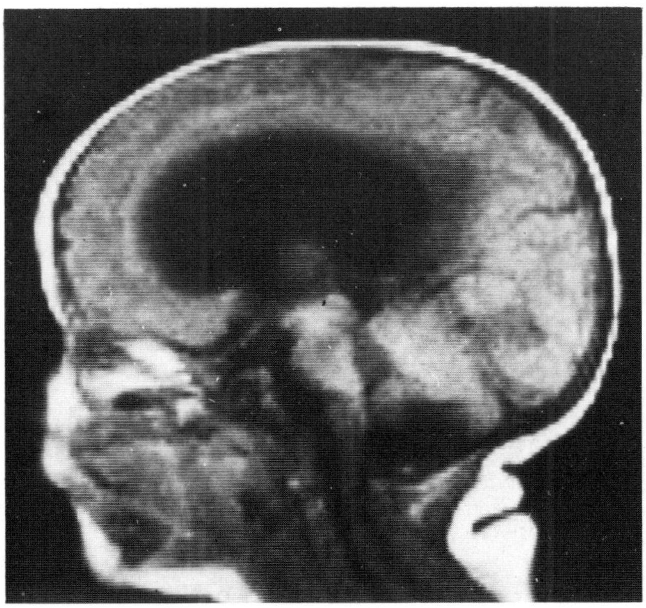

1

### 1

The definitive diagnosis of hydrocephalus requires special tests. This can now be achieved by magnetic resonance imaging (MRI), which not only provides exquisite anatomical images but also avoids the hazards of X-ray exposure. *Illustration 1* is an MRI scan demonstrating hydrocephalus secondary to aqueductal stenosis in a full-term baby. Until MRI scanning becomes widely available, however, CT scanning remains a simple and reliable means of evaluating infants with suspected hydrocephalus. In the initial evaluation of new patients, it is generally advisable to obtain both a contrast and a non-contrast scan so that congenital mass lesions such as tumours and vascular malformations can be ruled out. If these lesions are suggested by CT or MRI scanning, cerebral angiography may be indicated to define vascular anatomy.

Under special circumstances, CT metrizamide cisternography or ventriculography may be helpful in characterizing CSF flow and dynamics. Such information may be necessary to distinguish certain types of communicating and non-communicating hydrocephalus and is also useful in the assessment of shunt patency, intraventricular loculations, and the communicating nature of intracranial cysts and fluid collections. There appears to be little indication nowadays for the time-honoured procedures of air ventriculography and pneumoencephalography.

# The operations

## Direct operations

The preferred treatment of internal (non-communicating) hydrocephalus is a direct operation on the lesion causing the block. This is superior to any shunting procedure, but is rarely feasible in infants, owing to the nature of most congenital obstructions. Of the more commonly performed direct operations in the paediatric age group, the most important include the removal of intracranial tumours, excision or fenestration of intracranial cysts, and suboccipital craniotomy for anomalies of the craniospinal junction. Intracranial shunts, of which third ventriculostomy and the Torkildsen shunt are the best known examples, are rarely successful in infants because the distal subarachnoid pathways are usually obliterated or otherwise incompetent.

### EXTRACRANIAL SHUNTS

An extracranial shunt is the procedure of choice for treating most cases of communicating hydrocephalus, and for those cases of non-communicating hydrocephalus that are not amenable to direct operation or an intracranial shunt. As surgical experience has grown, the mortality of first operations has been reduced almost to zero, and the 5-year survival rate, including patients with all types of hydrocephalus, now approaches 95 per cent.

## Shunt devices

The majority of shunting devices so far developed consist of three separate or integrated components: a ventricular catheter, a connecting flush pump and a distal catheter. A unidirectional flow valve, which is essential for vascular shunts, is usually incorporated into the system to promote cerebrospinal fluid drainage at a relatively constant rate and pressure. Since introduction of the first valve-regulated shunts, a whole new technology has evolved, and rarely a year goes by in which new valves, reservoirs and 'obstruction-proof' catheters are not developed. Despite such innovations, it is the author's opinion that the simpler the shunt the better, and to achieve consistency in surgical technique and follow-up data, he has relied almost exclusively on the Heyer–Schulte system. When it is anticipated that intraventricular inoculations of chemotherapeutic agents or antibiotics will be required, an Ames double-barrel reservoir or a Rickham reservoir attached to a Holter valve is employed.

Because little is known about the biophysics of hydrocephalus, the surgeon must use subjective criteria in choosing among the various valve-regulated shunts, which offer a wide range of flow rates and pressures. In general, high-pressure valves which open at between 60 and 110 $mmH_2O$ are indicated for older children with massive ventriculomegaly to avoid rapid collapse of the ventricular system and attendant complications such as subdural haematoma. Medium-pressure valves (40–60 $mmH_2O$) can be used in the majority of cases of chronic hydrocephalus, and shunts to the peritoneum in premature infants require no valve at all. There is little evidence to suggest that anti-syphon devices significantly reduce the incidence of subdural haematoma, and 'on-off' valves are too fanciful in concept to be recommended here, except possibly when intrathecal drug therapy is required.

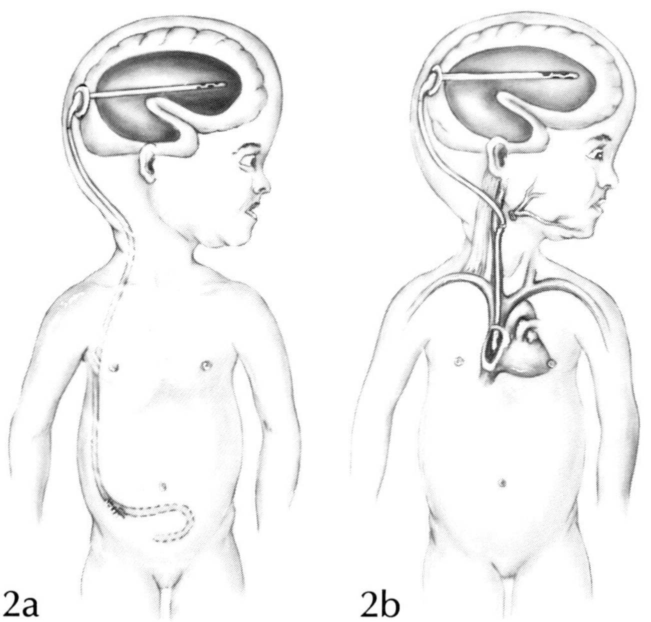

2a 2b

# 2a & b

## Choice of shunt

Through trial and experience, two operations can be recommended for widespread use: the ventriculoperitoneal shunt and the ventriculoatrial shunt. The former, because it is easier to implant, easier to revise, and much easier to lengthen in growing children, has become the preferred procedure with most neurosurgeons. Obstruction and infection are the most common complications of ventriculoperitoneal shunts, and septicaemia and thromboembolism are of additional concern in patients with ventriculoatrial shunts.

## Contraindications

*Infection* Extracranial shunts should not be performed in the presence of sepsis, local infection of the scalp, meningitis or ventriculitis. Indeed, if there is evidence of infection anywhere in the body it is best to postpone these procedures as long as possible. In patients with post-meningitic hydrocephalus, it is usually safe to consider a shunt once the cerebrospinal fluid is sterile and contains no more than 15–20 cells/mm$^3$, the majority of which are mononuclear.

*Subdural effusion or haematoma* The presence of a subdural collection in association with hydrocephalus is a contraindication for ventricular shunting. In such cases the subdural collection should be drained first, so that the dilated ventricular system can expand the cerebral mantle outward. Once the subdural space has been obliterated, a ventricular shunting procedure can be considered.

*Large posterior fossa tumours* In children with large mass lesions of the posterior fossa, upward (transtentorial) herniation is a recognized risk of 'preoperative shunting'. This practice can no longer be recommended and has recently fallen out of favour.

### VENTRICULOPERITONEAL SHUNT

## Preparation

# 3

Operations are performed under general endotracheal anaesthesia with the patient supine and the head turned to the left. An intravenous catheter should be in place, but a transfusion is rarely necessary unless the patient weighs less than 3 kg.

Careful preparation of the skin is the key step in preventing shunt infections. The operative field should be shaved, meticulously washed with antiseptic solutions, and painted with triple applications of povidone-iodine. It is helpful to mark out the proposed incisions with a scalpel, and to employ waterproof drapes that exclude the ear, the axilla, the umbilicus and the groin.

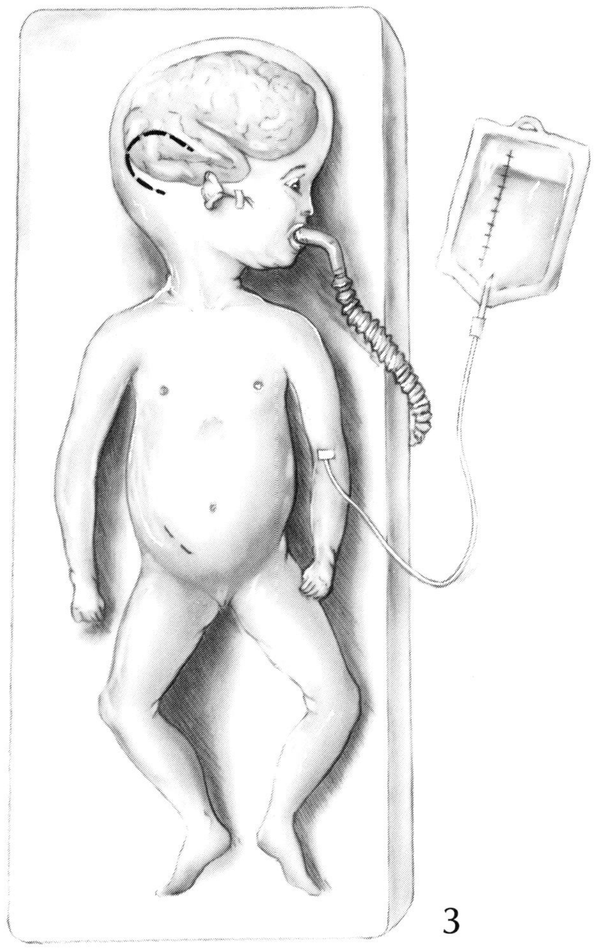

3

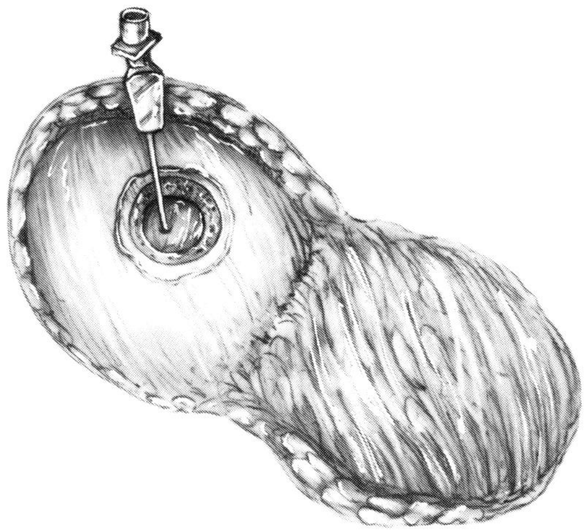

4

# 4 & 5

## Cephalic incision

A curvilinear incision is made above and behind the right ear. An alternative site is the parasagittal area immediately in front of the coronal suture. To avoid unnecessary bone bleeding, the galea is separated from the pericranium and the latter is left attached to bone. A burr hole is made of sufficient size to accommodate the given valve or reservoir. The dura is then coagulated and a ventricular needle is passed into the occipital horn of the lateral ventricle. Once a good flow of cerebrospinal fluid has been established, the needle is removed and replaced with a ventricular catheter attached to a flush pump assembly. The length of the catheter is tailored so that its tip comes to lie in the frontal horn anterior to the choroid plexus, or within the occipital horn behind the glomus of the choroid plexus. After collecting samples of cerebrospinal fluid for chemical and bacteriological analysis, a short piece of tubing is attached to the distal end of the flush pump and temporarily clamped off.

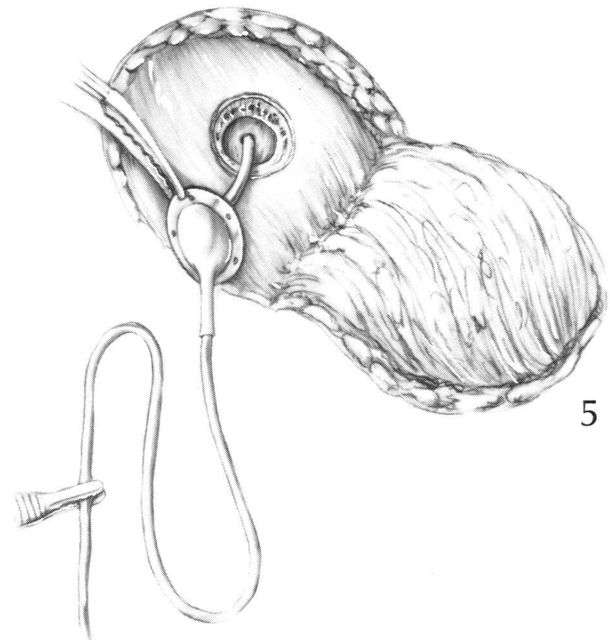

5

# 6, 7 & 8

## Abdominal incision

A small McBurney incision is made in the right lower quadrant. After splitting the abdominal muscles along their fibre lines, the peritoneum is elevated, opened with iris scissors, and secured with fine straight clamps. A four-cornered purse-string suture of 4/0 or 5/0 silk is then placed around the peritoneal opening, and a plain Silastic (Dow Corning, UK) catheter with multiple perforations at its distal end is introduced into the peritoneal cavity. The suggested length of the intra-abdominal tubing is 10 cm for premature infants, 25–30 cm for term infants, and 40–50 cm for children of 2 years of age and older. It is important that the purse-string suture be tied down loosely to permit free movement of the catheter in and out of the abdomen. The patency of the system is checked by injecting saline through the catheter and demonstrating free gravity drainage.

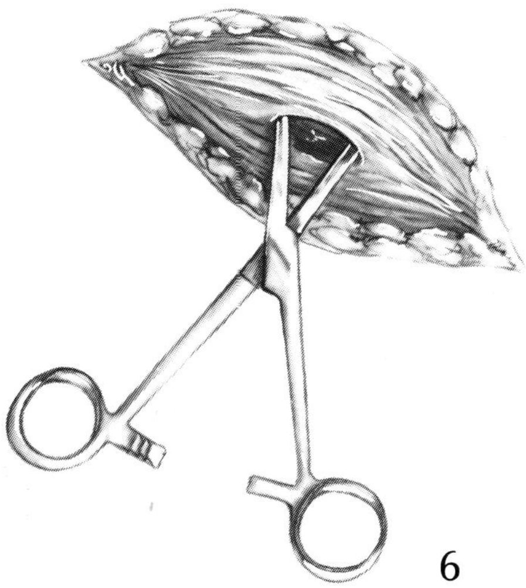

6

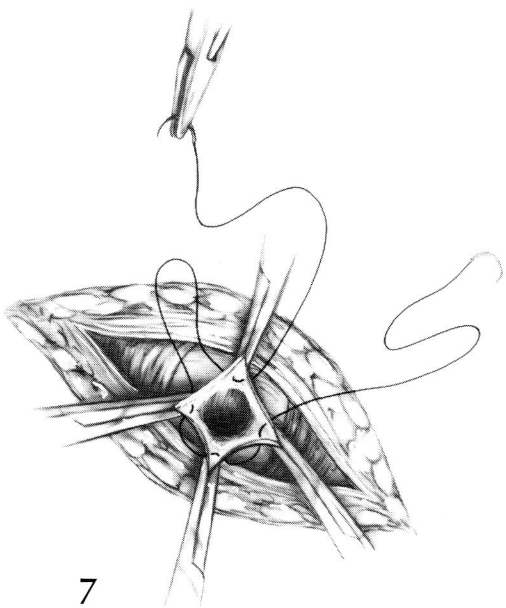

7

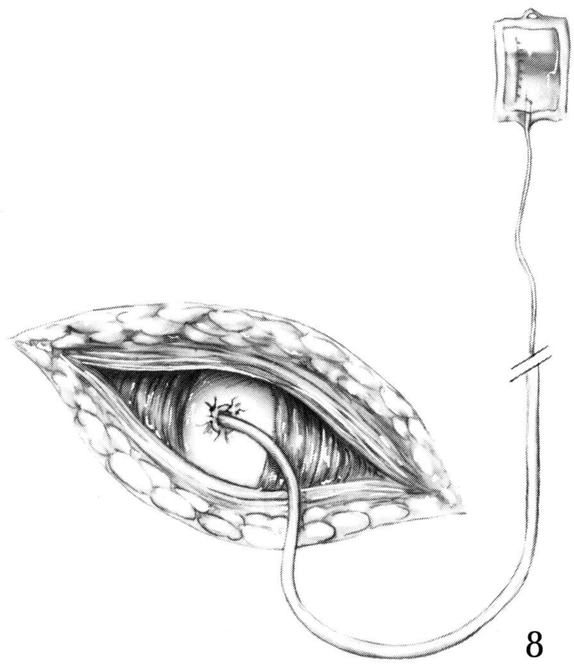

8

# 9

## Connection

The proximal end of the peritoneal catheter is passed up to the cephalic wound through a subcutaneous tunnel just lateral to the nipple line. A connecting incision in the neck is sometimes required in older children. After joining the two ends of the shunt over a plastic connector, all junctions are secured with ligatures of heavy silk. The reservoir of the shunt is then sewn to surrounding pericranium, and extraneous tubing is pulled down to the abdominal wound and passed into the peritoneal cavity. The wounds are closed in layers using 3/0 silk or Nurolon (non-absorbable braided polyamide). It is advisable to reinforce all dressings with waterproof tape. Postoperatively, the patient is kept in an upright position and antibiotics are administered prophylactically for 3 days. Pumping of the reservoir is discouraged except to check shunt patency.

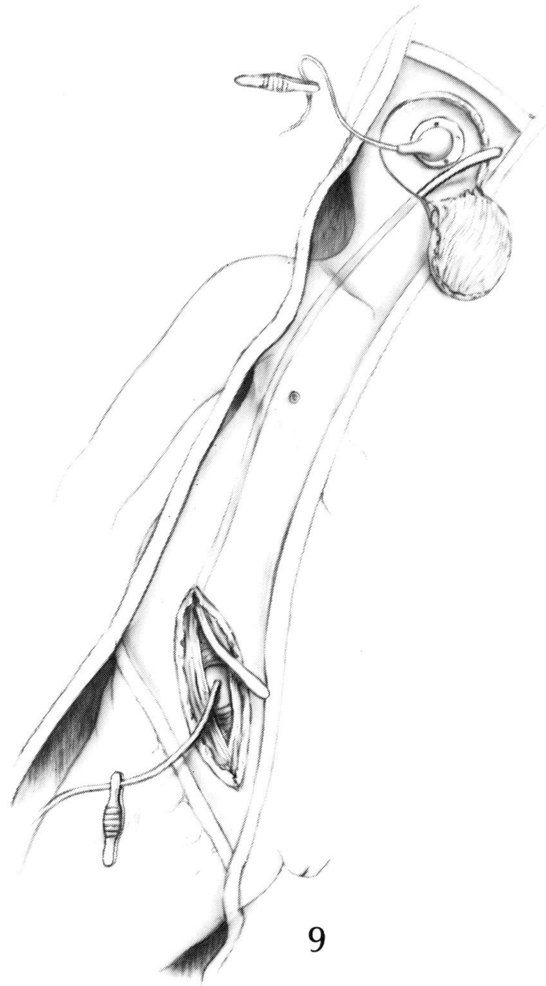

9

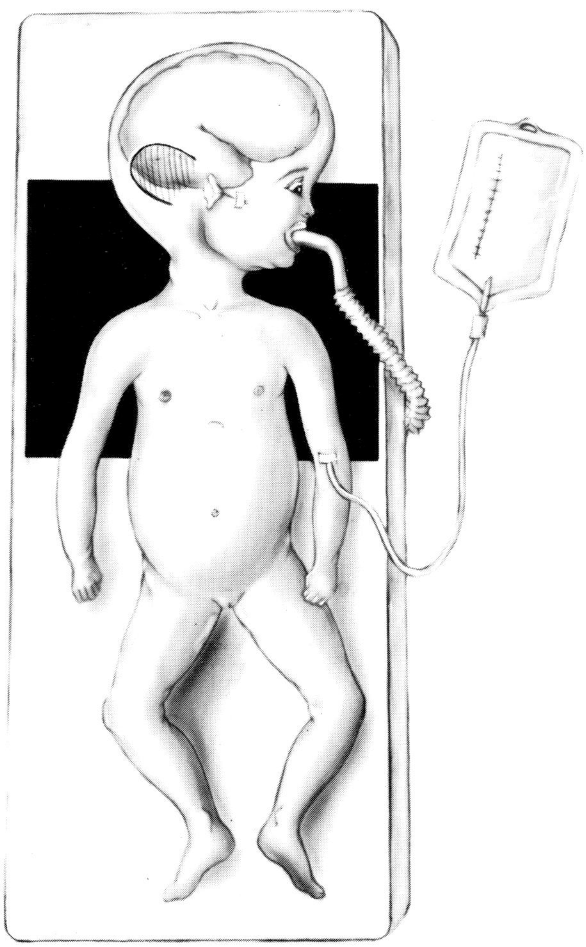

10

### VENTRICULOATRIAL SHUNT

Thromboembolism and central venous thrombosis are well known complications of ventriculoatrial shunting procedures. Although pulmonary vascular lesions probably occur in up to 25 per cent of the cases, the majority are asymptomatic. Presenting symptoms of massive venous thrombosis or embolism include cor pulmonale, shock and even sudden death. Acute pulmonary hypertension should be taken as indication for prompt removal of the shunt and possibly open thoracotomy for purposes of thrombectomy.

# 10

## Preparation

Operations are performed under general endotracheal anaesthesia with the patient supine and the head and neck turned to the left. An intravenous catheter should be in place, and an X-ray cassette is positioned under the patient prior to draping. Implantation of the ventricular catheter and reservoir is carried out as described for the ventriculoperitoneal shunt.

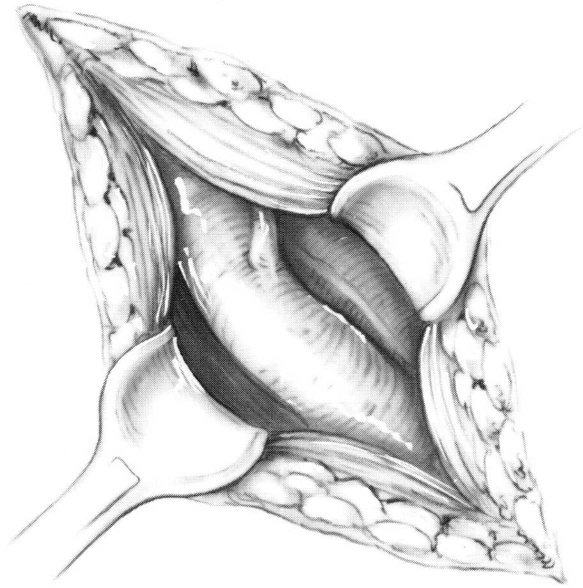

11

# 11 & 12

## Cervical incision

A cervical incision is made along the medial border of the sternocleidomastoid muscle. By a combination of sharp and blunt dissection, the junction of the facial and jugular veins is identified and the vessels are secured with umbilical tapes or heavy ligatures. Whenever possible, it is preferable to introduce the atrial catheter into the facial vein, which can be tied off proximally. Proper positioning of the atrial catheter is monitored under X-ray control after filling the tube with 50 per cent Hypaque (Sterling Research, Guildford, UK). The tip of the catheter should lie at the level of the T6 vertebral body to be in optimal position. After securing the atrial catheter to the vein with a fine silk ligature, the patency of the system is checked manometrically by injecting sterile saline through the catheter. With the Heyer–Schulte slit valve, the pressure should vary from 0 to 40 $mmH_2O$.

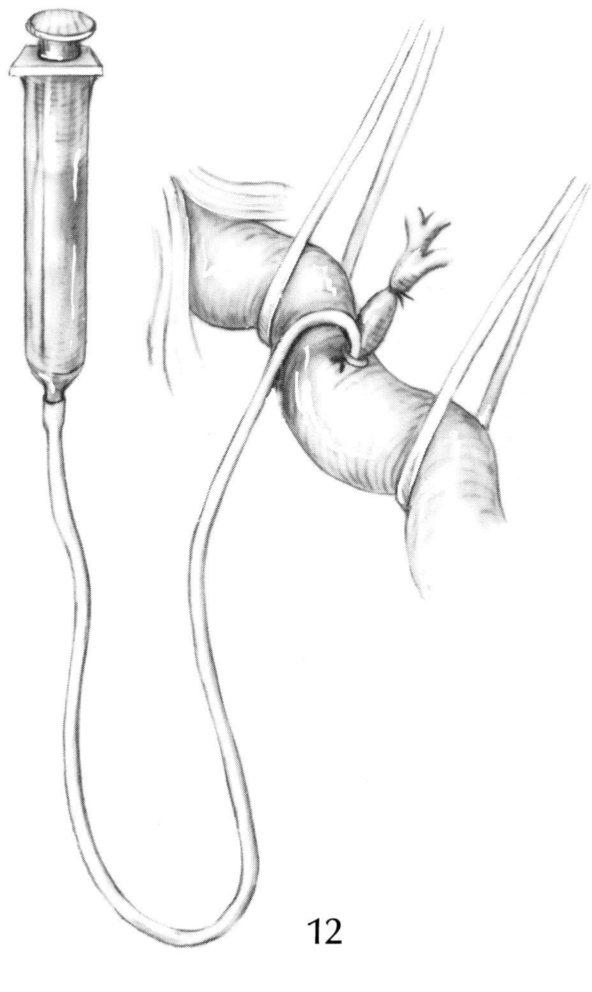

12

# 13

## Connection

The proximal end of the catheter is passed up through a subcutaneous tunnel to the cephalic wound, where it is connected behind the ear to the reservoir. Postoperative care is the same as that described for patients with ventriculoperitoneal shunts.

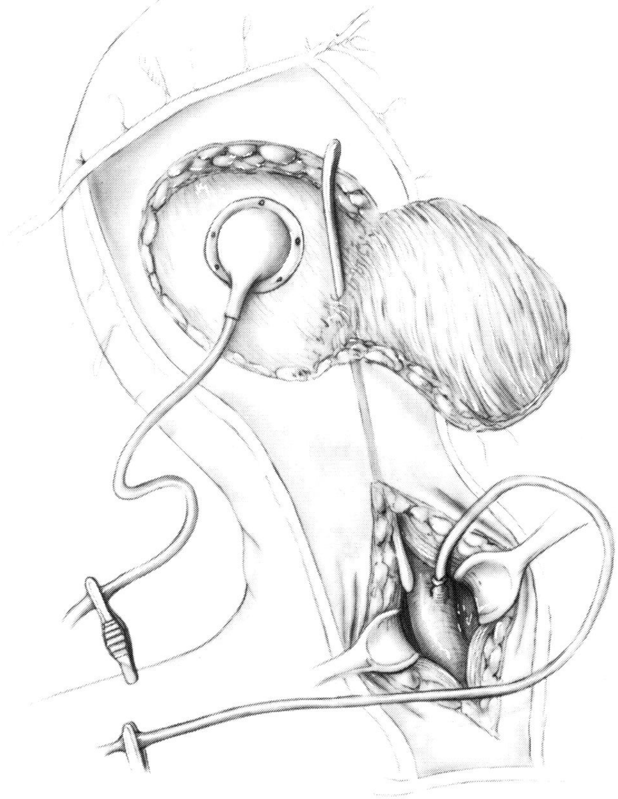

13

# Elective shunt revision

It is generally agreed that planned revisions should be part of the general maintenance of a functioning shunt in a growing child. This is certainly appropriate for most children with non-communicating hydrocephalus, and also for those with communicating hydrocephalus in whom past shunt failure has established the patient's shunt dependency. The aphorism 'once a shunt always a shunt' is very nearly correct if the goal of treatment is to achieve an optimal physiological state. Although the criteria for elective shunt revision have not been fully defined, it is probably best to revise ventriculoatrial shunts when the catheter tip comes to lie at or above the level of the T4 vertebral body. In infants with ventriculoperitoneal shunts, elective revisions are performed at 4–6 years and again at 10–15 years of age.

## VENTRICULOPERITONEAL SHUNT

## 14

The patient is prepared as described for a primary ventriculoperitoneal shunt (*see Illustration 3*). The original cephalic and abdominal incisions are reopened and the shunt system is isolated from investing scar tissue. At the cephalic wound, the flush pump assembly and peritoneal catheter are disconnected. If there is a free flow of fluid from the proximal end, the ventricular catheter and reservoir may be assumed to be functional. Conversely, if there is no flow or inadequate flow from the proximal end, the ventricular catheter and/or reservoir may be assumed to be obstructed and both are replaced.

At the abdominal wound, the peritoneal catheter is extracted from the abdomen and its distal end is tied with a heavy ligature. This ligature is then tied to a new catheter of desired length which is drawn up to the cephalic wound, connected to the flush pump assembly, and temporarily clamped off. Next, the peritoneum is exposed by splitting the rectus abdominis muscle medial to the original site of implantation. This can usually be accomplished without extending the abdominal incision. The distal end of the new catheter is introduced into the peritoneal cavity as described in *Illustrations 6–8*. It is important to pump the reservoir of the shunt to confirm its patency and to empty air bubbles from the system. The wounds are closed and the patient is managed as described for a primary ventriculoperitoneal shunt.

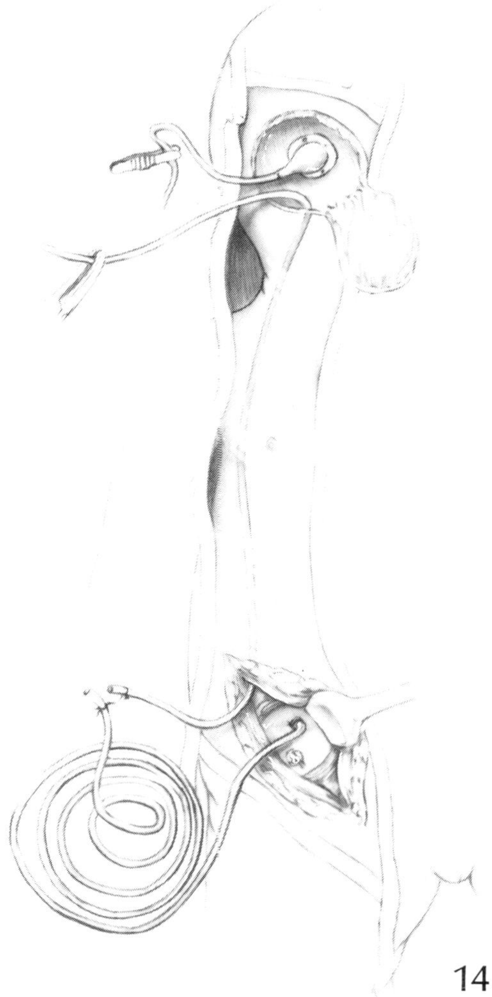

14

## VENTRICULOATRIAL SHUNT

Elective revision of a ventriculoatrial shunt should allow for the possibility that it is often difficult, and sometimes impossible, to reimplant a new atrial catheter into the ipsilateral cervical venous system. The use of the opposite jugular vein is not generally recommended, since the operation is awkward and requires running a catheter diagonally across the neck. It is advisable, therefore, to drape the operative field to include the peritoneum.

# 15

The original wounds are reopened and the shunt system is isolated from investing scar tissue. At the cephalic wound, the atrial catheter is disconnected from the flush pump assembly and occluded with a bulldog clamp. If there is a free flow of fluid from the proximal system, there is no need to replace it. Next, the atrial catheter is unclamped and tested for flow manometrically. If the distal end is patent, the atrial catheter can be lengthened by splicing it to a plain Silastic catheter over a plastic connector. If the atrial catheter is obstructed, it must be replaced.

At the cervical wound, the entry site of the atrial catheter into the facial vein is identified and the securing suture is removed. It is sometimes possible to advance the atrial catheter toward the heart by applying countertraction on the facial vein. If this is impossible, the catheter should be removed and replaced with a new, unspliced catheter which is introduced into the jugular vein just below the original entry site. If the catheter fails to pass, a superior venacavagram can be performed by injecting 5–10 ml of 50 per cent Hypaque through the catheter and obtaining a simultaneous X-ray of the chest. This will help to demonstrate venous anatomy and is useful in excluding a thrombus in the superior vena cava. If there is no evidence of a thrombus, the jugular vein can sometimes be dilated with bougies, or the catheter can be introduced into the external jugular vein or one of its branches as an alternative route to the right atrium. If all such efforts fail, the shunt should be diverted to the peritoneal cavity.

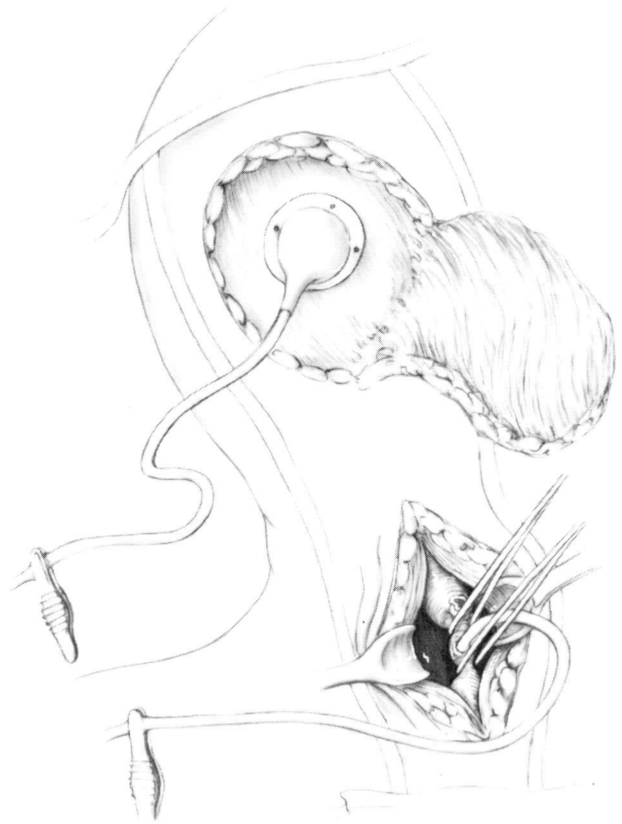

15

## Shunt obstruction

As soon as a diagnosis of shunt failure is made, it is advisable to prepare the patient promptly for surgery. Temporizing measures such as forced pumping or percutaneous irrigation of the reservoir are rarely successful, and ventricular taps to tide the patient over are to be condemned. The specific techniques for revising extracranial shunts have been described above. Operations should allow for two possibilities: firstly, that the shunt may be obstructed at either or both ends regardless of the preoperative findings, and secondly, that if the distal catheter is obstructed, some alternative route of drainage may be required. These considerations should be kept in mind when the operative field is prepared and draped.

## Shunt infection

The development of ventriculitis or wound infection in a patient with an extracranial shunt is an indication for prompt removal of the entire shunt apparatus. Additional indications in patients with vascular shunts include endocarditis, infectious pulmonary embolism, and proliferating glomerulonephritis. Antibiotics should be administered intravenously, and in most cases it is necessary to institute external ventricular drainage to control intracranial pressure and/or to drain the infected ventricular system.

If the organism responsible is sensitive to antibiotics that are poorly transported across the blood–brain barrier, it may be advisable to administer drugs intraventricularly as well as systemically. External ventricular drainage should be continued until the cerebrospinal fluid is sterile and contains no more than 15–20 cells/$mm^3$, the majority of which are mononuclear. At this point it is usually safe to perform an extracranial shunt to some site other than the bloodstream. Systemic antibiotics should be continued for a minimum of 7–10 days postoperatively.

## Choroid plexus papilloma

# 16a & b

The principal exception to the rule that hydrocephalus results from obstruction of the cerebrospinal fluid pathways is the rare case of cerebrospinal fluid overproduction by choroid plexus papillomas. In infants and children, approximately 70 per cent of these tumours arise in the lateral ventricles (90 per cent on the left side), and total surgical excision is followed by permanent relief of hydrocephalus in about 50 per cent of the cases. Since papillomas tend to float freely and are generally suspended by one major vascular pedicle, the surgical goal is to isolate the tumour's blood supply at the outset.

*Illustrations 16a* and *b* show a CT scan and arteriogram of a 2-year-old boy with choroid plexus papilloma of the left lateral ventricle. Note the vascular pedicle in the region of the trigone.

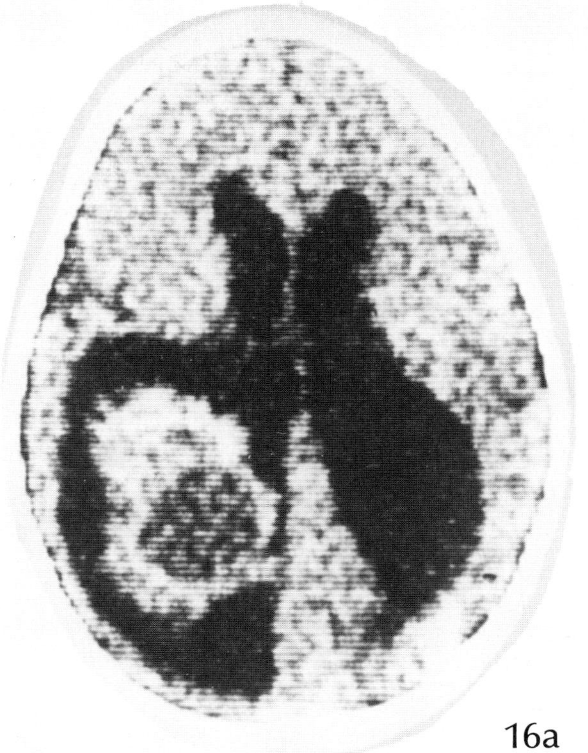

16a

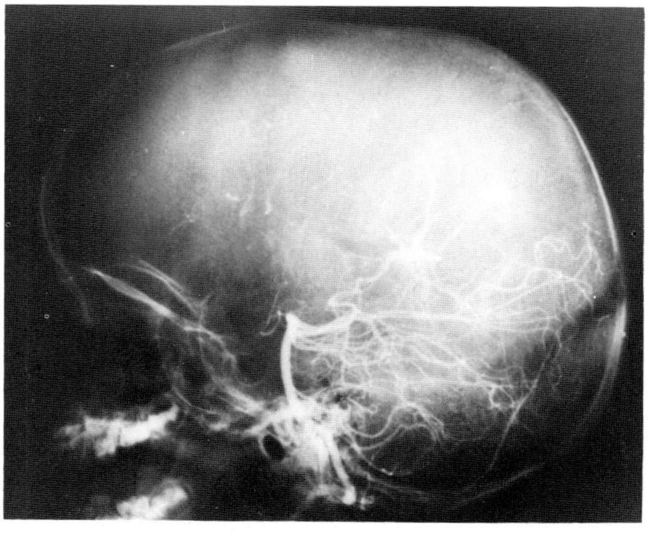

16b

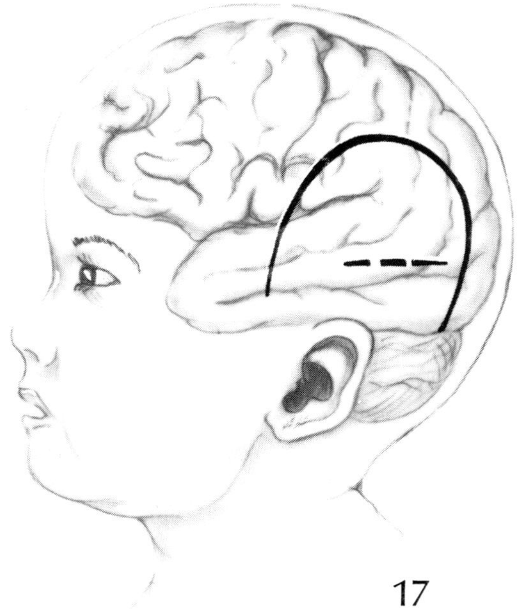

17

## 17 & 18

Tumours arising in the trigone area are approached best through a temporoparietal craniotomy and a linear incision in the middle temporal gyrus that parallels the floor of the lateral ventricle. This provides direct access to the tumour's blood supply, and is far superior to high convexity or posterior incisions which oblige the surgeon to remove this highly vascular neoplasm piecemeal. After exposing the tumour within the ventricle, it is elevated from the ventricular floor and its attachments are identified. With trigone tumours, a minor vascular pedicle may arise from the temporal horn (anterior choroidal supply), but the major blood supply is from the posterior choroidal arteries which enter the base of the tumour as a thick pedicle at the level of the glomus. Once the pedicle has been clipped or coagulated, the tumour shrinks dramatically and can often be delivered in its entirety.

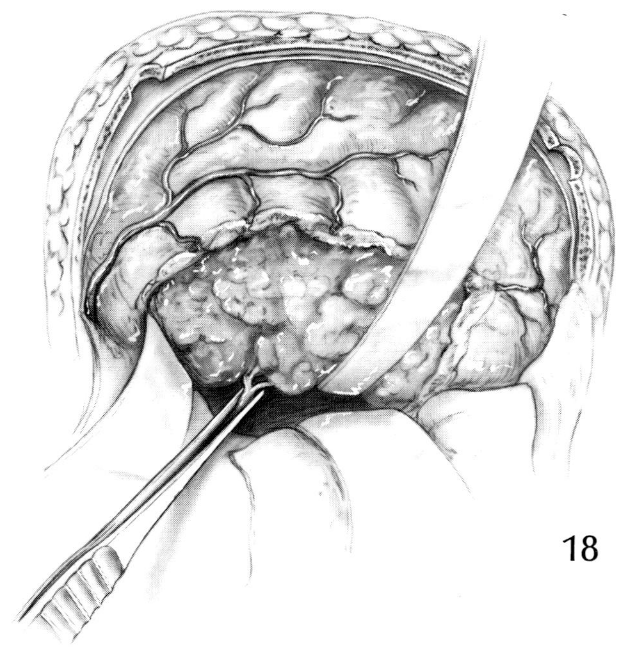

18

Illustrations by Angela Christie

# Syringomyelia and the Chiari malformation

**M. Rice-Edwards** MA, FRCS
Consultant Neurosurgeon, Department of Neurosurgery, Regional Neurosciences Centre, Charing Cross Hospital, London, UK

# SYRINGOMYELIA

## Introduction

Although cystic cavitation of the spinal cord was described over 400 years ago and subsequently named syringomyelia by Ollivier in 1837, it remains an obscure condition. There is no complete agreement about the pathogenesis, classification or even the definition and this forms a poor basis for surgical treatment.

However, syringomyelia is usually considered to be a glial-lined cavity within the spinal cord and it is now generally agreed that there are two main types. The first and by far the most common type has a congenital substrate of a Chiari malformation and a hydromyelic canal. In the second type there is no congenital abnormality and cystic cavitation occurs as a result of acquired conditions: only two causes have definitely been established, following spinal trauma and, very rarely, following widespread arachnoiditis.

The two types of syringomyelia have been called communicating and non-communicating, the communication being with the fourth ventricle but, as shown below, this may be inappropriate and from the practical point of view it is probably easiest to refer to three known causes: (*1*) hydromyelic; (*2*) post-traumatic; (*3*) postarachnoiditic.

Cystic tumours are not considered here and in fact the author's definition excludes them: 'Syringomyelia is a cystic cavity of the spinal cord with a wall free of tumour and mostly lined with glial tissue'.

### Hydromyelia and syringomyelia

Hydromyelia and syringomyelia are not synonymous. The former is a persistence of the fetal state, quite symptomless, in which the enlarged central canal is completely lined with ependyma. In most cases this is associated with a Chiari malformation and a curious observation is that the wall of the hydromyelic cavity breaks down progressively causing glial-lined prolongations, i.e. syringomyelia, into the cord substance until most of the cavity may be lined with glia. Gardner proposed that this was due to hydrodynamic forces from the fourth ventricle; however, the communication between the ventricular system and a syrinx is usually very narrow or even non-existent. For this reason, the author prefers to think that the CSF within the cavity arises from capillaries within the cord or diffuses across the cord from the subarachnoid space and that changes in venous pressure, for instance during coughing, are responsible for the development and expansion of the syrinx. Blocking the central canal at the obex of the fourth ventricle therefore plays no part in the surgical strategy.

### Post-traumatic and postarachnoiditic syringomyelia

In post-traumatic syringomyelia, it is likely that a small haematomyelia or area of necrosis breaks down, forming a small fluid-filled cavity which slowly expands by the same forces that cause the disintegration of hydromyelia. It is also possible that an area of ischaemic necrosis forms the same starting point in the case of severe arachnoiditis although there cannot be any certainty about this.

## Clinical features

The classical signs and symptoms of syringomyelia are well known but are not stereotyped and in any case are usually a mixture caused by both the Chiari malformation and the syrinx. Scoliosis is a classical sign and there is usually wasting of muscles with absent reflexes, a suspended area of sensory loss associated with pyramidal signs and impaired joint position sense in the lower limbs: the classical picture. However, reflexes are sometimes retained, the sensory loss may be restricted to one arm, including impairment of joint position sense (a root entry zone syndrome), or there may be no sensory loss at all. Although the syrinx may extend up into the medulla, the usual cause of medullary symptoms, sometimes called syringobulbia, is more likely to be due to the associated Chiari malformation and, far from being the end stage of a crippling disease, may well be relieved by decompression at the foramen magnum.

In about 2 per cent of patients with traumatic paraplegia or paraparesis and in a small number of tetraplegics, spontaneous pain, pain on coughing or sensory loss ascending above the level of the original deficit heralds the onset of post-traumatic syringomyelia. It occurs after an interval of months or years, the average being about 4 years. The symptoms are typically unilateral at first but progress to both sides with increasing lower motor neurone weakness of the hands and also increasing weakness in the legs of those who are not already paraplegic. Excess sweating above the level of trauma is common.

## Radiology

In the hydromyelic type, plain X-rays may show craniovertebral anomalies and also, in about 20% of cases, an abnormally wide cervical canal.

Myelography should now always be combined with CT scanning. A Chiari malformation or other hindbrain abnormality is present in nearly all cases except those due to arachnoiditis or trauma. The spinal cord is swollen in the majority of cases and CT scanning delayed some 6 hours after the injection may show the dye concentrating within a syrinx even in a cord of external normal dimensions. The investigation of choice is magnetic resonance image scanning which may also show the presence of a cavity even when the cord is small. It is non-invasive and may show the complete extent of the lesion in one sagittal slice.

## Choice of operation

Decompression of the Chiari malformation as described below may lead to shrinkage of a syrinx, possibly due in some way to the resulting changes in hydrodynamic forces in the subarachnoid space at the foramen magnum. In some cases it is difficult to be sure whether it is the Chiari malformation or the syrinx which is the main cause of signs such as pyramidal weakness, and since this operation may be highly effective and is relatively safe it is recommended that this is usually the first course. If a large and very thin-walled syrinx is seen at C2 or C3 in this exposure, it may be incised (syringostomy) in the midline or at the thinnest point. Above 33 per cent of patients will improve (when a Chiari malformation is found in the absence of a syringomyelia, this proportion is greater). No attempt to drain deep cavities should be attempted at this site.

If there is no clinical improvement or the patient relapses and further investigation shows that the cord is still distended, or if it is not thought that a hindbrain anomaly is responsible for the deficit, there are procedures which can be carried out on the syrinx itself. These are as follows.

1. Syringostomy. This involves an incision into the cavity with or without insertion of a tube or wick to ensure communication with the subarachnoid space
2. Syringoperitoneal or syringopleural shunting
3. Division of the filum terminale. Experience so far suggests that the cavity only rarely extends into the filum and this is not an effective means of drainage in most cases.

In the two recognized causes of syringomyelia unconnected with a hindbrain malformation, procedures on the syrinx form the only possibility of surgical correction. Syringoperitoneal shunting may have some slight benefit over a simple syringostomy and this is described below.

The mere demonstration of a syrinx should not be taken to be an indication for a drainage procedure as decompression of the cerebellar tonsils may suffice. In no case is there any merit in draining a syrinx within a collapsed or atrophic cord. There is also little indication for operation when the clinical condition remains the same, which it may for many years. However, if there is relentless deterioration and good evidence that this is due to progressive expansion of the spinal cord, an attempt to drain the syrinx should be undertaken. Nevertheless, in only about 33 per cent of cases will there be substantial improvement over and above that achieved by posterior fossa operation, although in cases of post-traumatic syringomyelia the results are better.

## SYRINGOPERITONEAL SHUNT

# 1

The patient is positioned prone, as for decompression of the Chiari malformation. The site of the laminectomy will be governed by the radiological findings but in most cases the fattest part of the cord will be in the lower cervical or upper dorsal segments. It is best to avoid inducing any further deficit in the arms and to choose the upper dorsal cord when possible.

The laminectomy, usually of four segments, proceeds in a standard fashion. Sometimes the spinal canal is abnormally wide and the laminae thinned. In any case, a wide laminectomy is made by removing the bone laterally with a Kerison punch. The bone edges are waxed and the muscle temporarily covered with lintine so as to prevent blood entering the subarachnoid space.

The dura is opened in the midline and the arachnoid incised. The syrinx may come almost to the surface and present as an area of grey discoloration and it is best to search for this with an operating microscope. The thinnest part of the cord substance is chosen for the syringostomy; this will often be at the dorsal root entry zone but it may also be within one dorsal column or in the midline. The site of the cord incision will also be influenced by the clinical signs. If proprioception is already grossly impaired in one foot the surgeon will feel more confident in incising the dorsal column on that side. If the cord is swollen but there is no sign of a syrinx near the surface, a midline incision between the dorsal columns is appropriate. However, first the syrinx is confirmed by passing a fine needle into the cord, avoiding surface vessels, and aspirating fluid which should be clear and colourless.

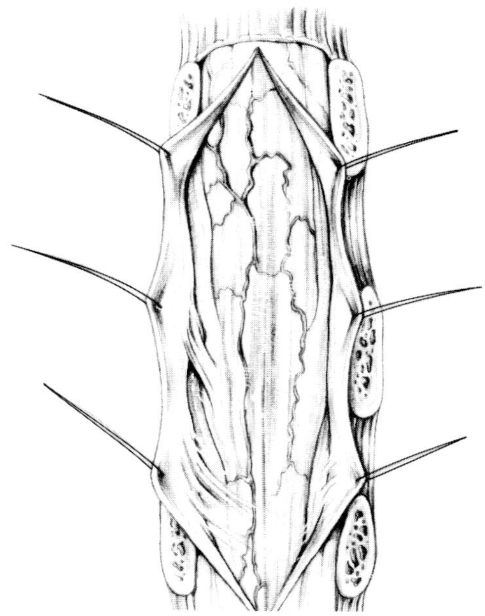

1

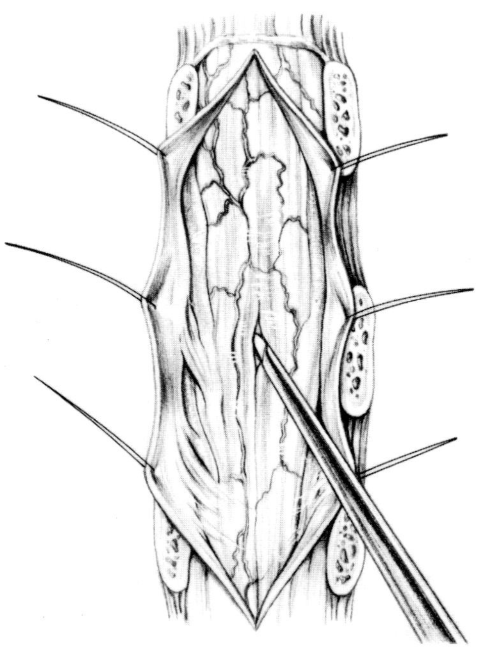

2

# 2

Once the position of the syrinx is confirmed, an incision is made in the cord. This is best made cleanly with a small sharp scalpel or a diamond knife. A laser beam tends to cut a broader trough and is not recommended. Any small vessels which are cut are coagulated with bipolar diathermy.

# 3

The surgeon may now have a limited view into the cavity which has a smooth white appearance and may be partially septated.

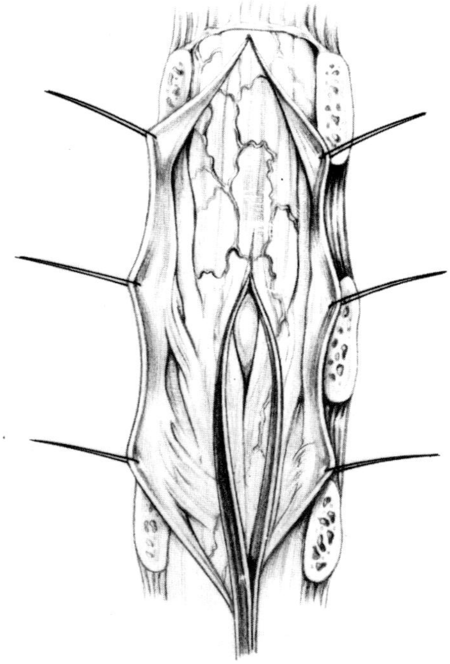

3

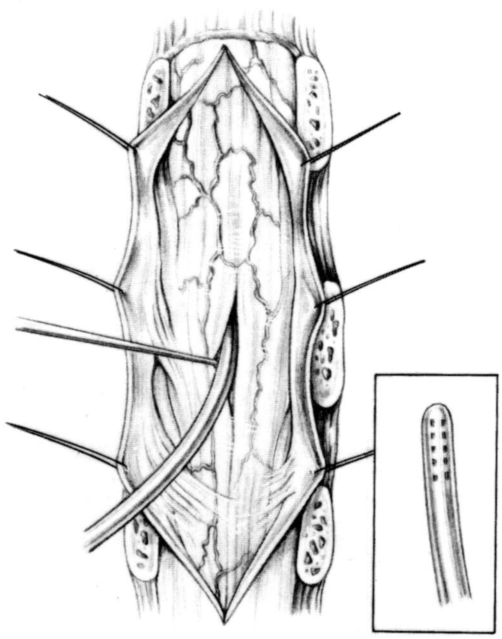

4

# 4

The incision need only be long enough to accommodate a piece of polythene tubing which may be the ventricular end of a Pudenz ventriculoperitoneal shunt system. Alternatively, the author has used a Hakim ventricular catheter with the fins trimmed, but this is rather broad. The T-shaped tube described by Wilson is a logical design and this will soon be commercially available.

## 5

The tube is passed a few centimetres upwards or downwards into the syrinx and the dura is closed snugly around the tube, which may be connected to distal tubing over a connector which is sutured to the dura or to the muscle with silk. This is important in order to stop the tube slipping; otherwise, the dura is closed snugly round the tube with absorbable sutures.

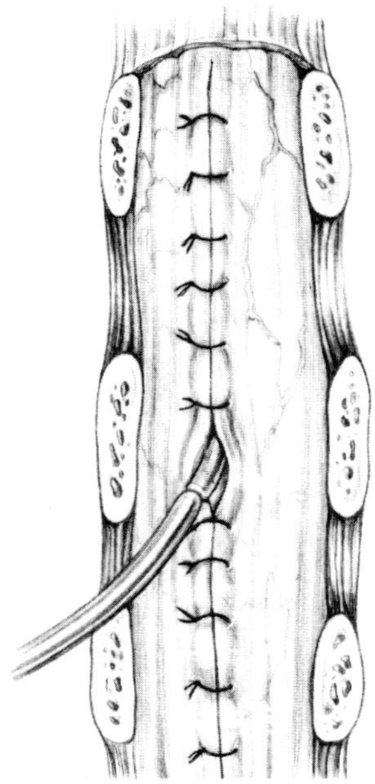

5

## 6

The distal tubing is passed subcutaneously to a flank incision. The laminectomy wound is then closed in standard fashion and one layer of sutures is also used to close the flank wound temporarily while the patient is repositioned on the operating table on the right side. The usual precautions regarding pressure points are taken, with a pad being placed in the axilla and soft padding under the flexed lower knee.

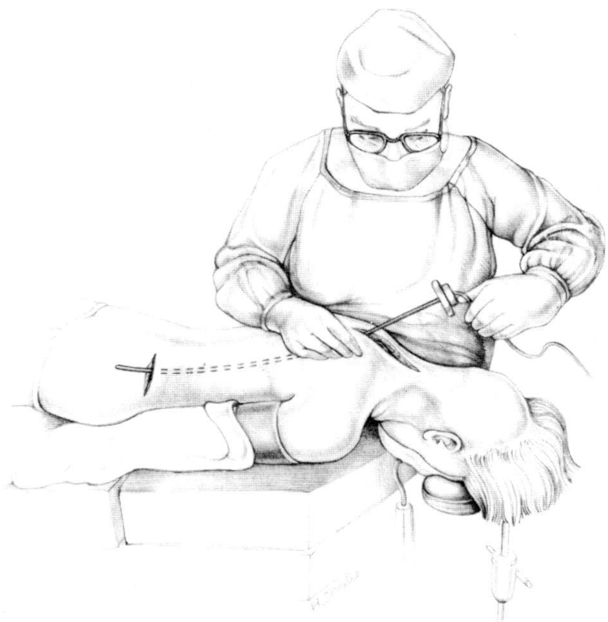

6

## 7

After draping, the flank incision is opened and a second incision made in the upper quadrant of the abdomen; the distal tube is passed subcutaneously and then into the peritoneal cavity. About 10 cm of distal tubing are planned for the intraperitoneal part. No valve is used in the system. The peritoneum and muscle layers are closed with absorbable sutures.

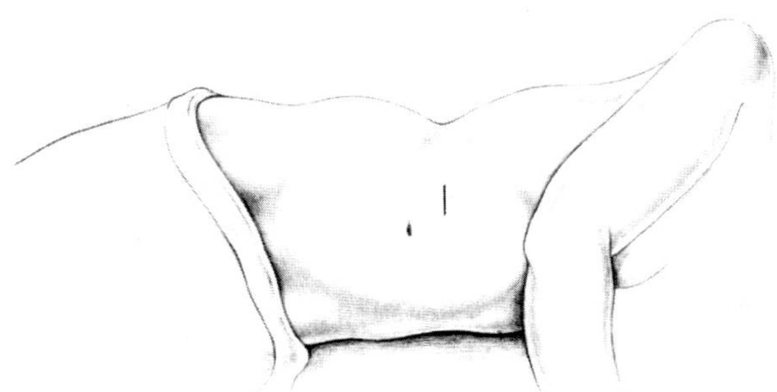

7

# THE CHIARI MALFORMATION

## Introduction

In 1895, Chiari described four types of hindbrain anomaly, of which only two are compatible with life. Chiari's type I is an abnormal prolongation of the cerebellar tonsils through the foramen magnum and type II is a more severe abnormality in which the tonsils and the cerebellar vermis protrude.

Arnold briefly described an example of Chiari's type II. His pupils then referred to the Arnold–Chiari malformation but it is simpler to refer to Chiari's types I and II as well as being a fitting tribute to his detailed work.

Although not a firm rule, type II tends to present in infants with spinal dysraphism and hydrocephalus, whereas the less severe type I does not. Instead, it may be the cause of symptoms in adults; either the sole cause or in association with syringomyelia, in which case either the Chiari malformation or the syrinx or both may be responsible for a progressive neurological deficit.

The Chiari malformation may be responsible for the following.

1. Cough headache or persistent occipital pain.
2. Ataxia with nystagmus.
3. Oscillopsia associated with downbeat vertical nystagmus.
4. Difficulty with swallowing.
5. Progressive limb deficits due to pyramidal or posterior column impairment.

There may be a combination of these abnormalities and a mistaken diagnosis of multiple sclerosis is sometimes made.

Plain X-rays are usually normal, although there is an associated bony anomaly at the foramen magnum in approximately one-third of cases. The diagnosis can be made by myelography with supine screening of the foramen magnum and nowadays this is combined with CT scanning. Magnetic resonance image scanning is also used and is equally reliable, although in this case it is medullary rather than cortical bone which is shown and the malformation, if anything, tends to be overestimated. This may be quite a good thing because in the past, the reverse has been the case. It is the author's experience that classical cough headache in which headache only occurs on coughing, stooping, straining or bending, is invariably associated with an abnormality of the foramen magnum of some type, usually the Chiari malformation. On three occasions, I have operated on patients with classical cough headache in the face of virtually normal myelography, only to confirm a mild but significant degree of tonsillar ectopia, and in each case the symptoms have been relieved by decompression. We have not, as yet, encountered this experience since the advent of sophisticated scanning techniques.

The malformation appears to cause neurological impairment owing to impairment of CSF hydrodynamics (cough headache) or direct compression of the medulla and spinal cord. Improvement or cure of symptoms can be expected after decompression in nearly all cases of cough headache and in approximately 80 per cent of patients with other deficits.

# The operation

## 8

The author's preference is for the prone position, the head resting either in a horseshoe (in which case it must be ensured that there is no pressure on the eyes) or in a Gardner frame. The minor inconvenience of the venous pressure being raised in the prone position is far less serious than the risk of air embolism from very large spinal veins if the patient is sitting up.

The patient is ventilated and normotensive. The head is well flexed and the head of the table tilted upwards about 20 degrees. The thigh is prepared for taking a fascia lata graft.

The skin incision is made from above the exion to the spinous process of C5 or thereabouts, and the scalp dissected away from the exion to give wide exposure to the upper insertion of the cervical muscle.

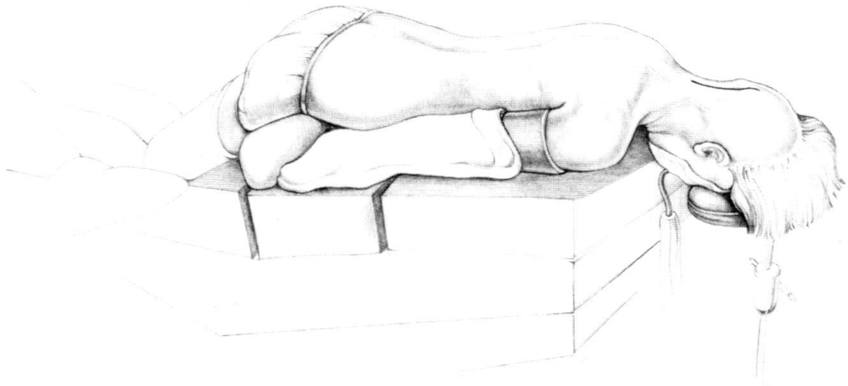

8

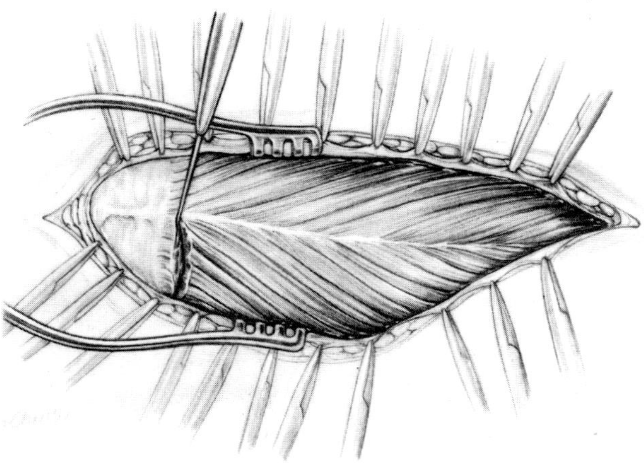

9

## 9

The skin is retracted with subcutaneous haemostats and a T-shaped incision is then made with cutting diathermy. It does not matter which limb is cut first but in *Illustration 9* the cross-bar is being made just below the muscle insertion into the superior nuchal line, leaving a fringe above for effective closure. This cut is made down to the occipital bone.

The longitudinal incision is made in the ligamentum nuchae (easily seen where it is cut through in the cross-bar incision) and the muscle on each side is held apart with self-retaining retractors. The midline incision is deepened down to the occipital bone and the tip of C2 exposed.

# 10

The muscle is stripped back from the occipital plate, using either a sharp separator or diathermy current according to the adherence of the muscle to the bone. The muscle is then separated from the spinous process and lamina of C2 and C3, and, knowing the depth of the C2 lamina, it is now easier to cut down in the midline to the arch of C1. However, care must be taken as the Chiari malformation is associated with bony abnormalities at the foramen magnum in approximately one-third of cases. Most commonly, the posterior arch of C1 may be abnormally high, being adherent or even fused to the foramen magnum and C1 may not be appreciated as a separate structure immediately. Occasionally there is basilar invagination, in which case the foramen magnum may be a little awkward to reach. Most dangerous of all, there may be a bifid posterior arch. This raises the risk that cutting diathermy could be used within this defect without appreciating the abnormality. Always look carefully at the X-rays before starting the operation.

Once the posterior arch of C1 is identified, the muscle is separated from it using a smooth or sharp Adsum elevator. Blunt-nosed scissors are used to divide the muscle from the margin of the foramen magnum and C1 laterally, for it is at this position that it is possible to encounter the vertebral artery. The author has, in over 50 cases, not ruptured or even identified it and accidents should easily be avoided by taking small snips with blunt-nosed scissors.

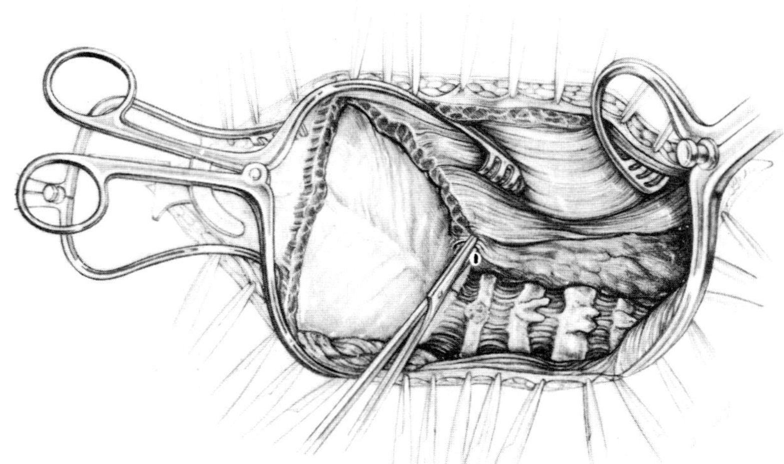

10

# 11a & b

Initially, two burr holes are made, one on either side of the midline of the occiput (*a*), as high as possible, because it is easier to work down than up. The bone is removed across the midline (*b*) and then down to the foramen magnum. There will be considerable crowding of tissues in the presence of a Chiari malformation and the removal of the foramen magnum itself and the arch of C1 should be performed carefully with small rongeurs such as the Pennybacker or the Jensen, without putting the tips under the bone. The bone removal is taken far out laterally, and again, if care is taken to use small rongeurs and to remove bone only without pulling on soft tissues, it is unlikely that damage to the vertebral artery will occur. The lamina of C2 is then removed widely. It is in these lateral areas that large extradural veins may be ruptured, but bleeding may be controlled by light pressure on a pattie and they are usually fairly easy to coagulate.

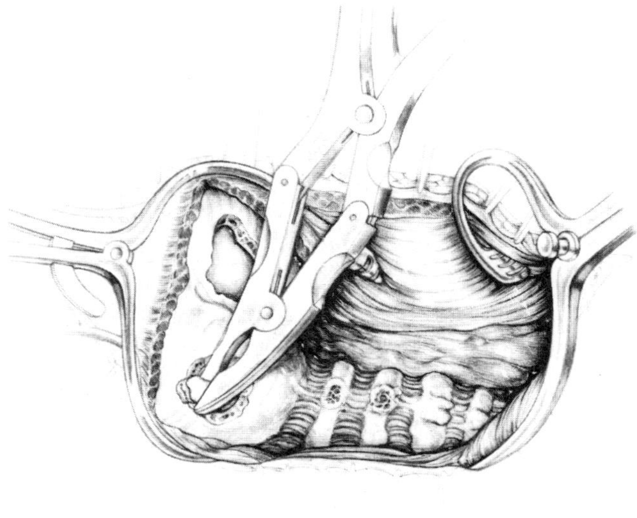

11a

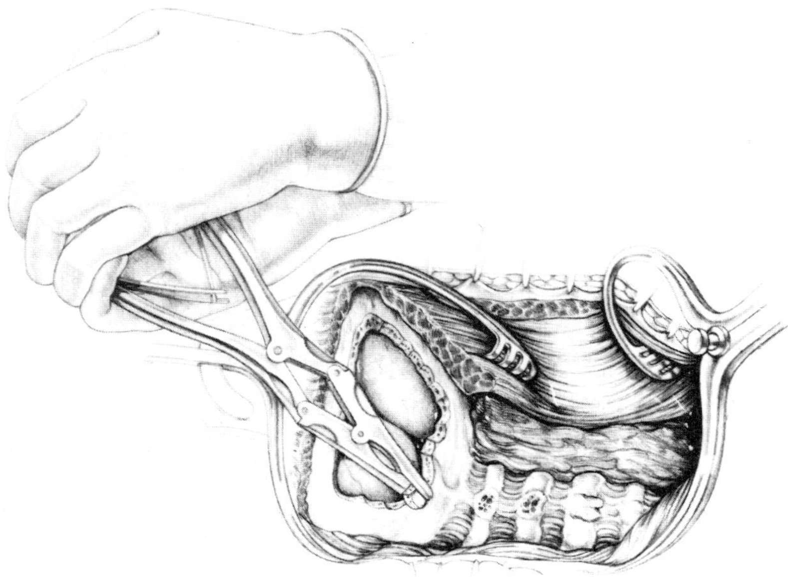

11b

# 12

The dura is opened in a Y-shaped manner, starting over the cerebellar hemispheres on each side and cutting down towards the foramen magnum, but meeting in the midline just above it. Joining the two cuts involves dividing the cerebellar sinus which is variable in size. Sometimes it is insignificant and sometimes quite large. It is usually easy to occlude the sinus with tantalum clips, but occasionally if the sinus is large and the venous pressure high, there may, for a moment, be profuse bleeding and the easiest way to deal with this is to occlude the sinus above and below, quite boldly with haemostats, and then to occlude the sinus with sutures.

The dura is then divided downwards to one or other side of the occipital sinus, across the marginal sinus, which can also be occluded with tantalum clips, and the remains of the atlanto-occipital membrane, and then on down to the spinal dura. Sometimes, and particularly when there is any degree of basilar invagination, there may be a thickening of the dura at the foramen magnum which may extend forward as a shelf. It is easier to make a fresh incision in the spinal dura and to work upwards, joining up with the first incision at the foramen magnum.

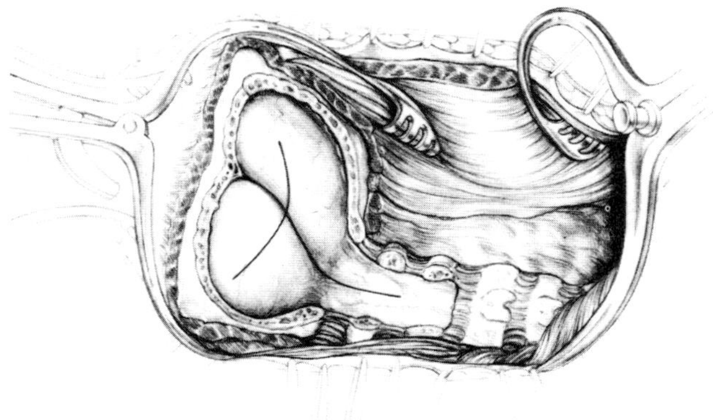

12

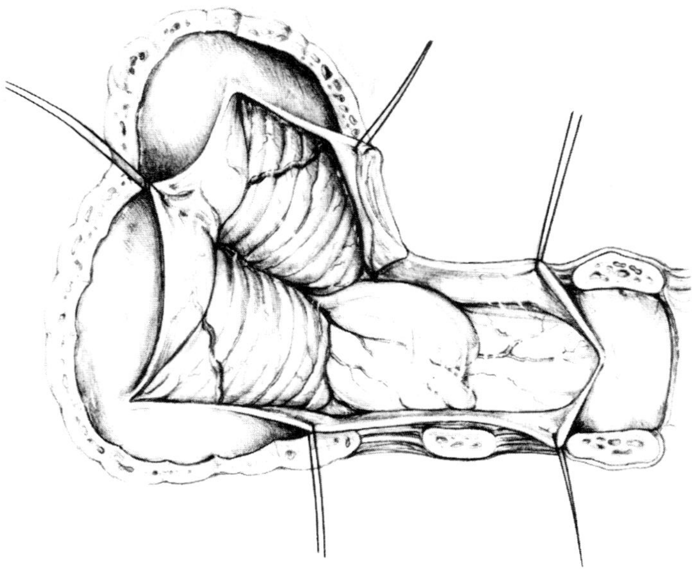

13

# 13

The dura is now held apart with stay sutures and the anatomy viewed through the arachnoid. It is not necessary to open the arachnoid, and indeed, it is a good idea to keep it intact to prevent blood from staining the CSF. Occasionally the arachnoid is so thick that nothing can be seen, and then a small incision can be made in the arachnoid to confirm the appearance of the tonsils, which protrude below the level of the foramen magnum. They do not usually have the normal bulbous shape, but tend to be long and tapered, sometimes white and gliotic at the tips and they may be markedly asymmetrical. The posterior inferior cerebellar artery may or may not be seen looping below the tonsils, and the C2 nerve roots may or may not take an abnormal upward course, depending on the degree of descent of the medulla and spinal cord.

It is not necessary to part the tonsils to inspect the fourth ventricle, nor is it necessary to amputate them. The purpose of the operation is merely to decompress them and that has now been achieved.

## 14

It is not usually possible to reappose the dura over the tonsils, illustrating that compression has been present and the dura is therefore left open at this point, the defect being made good by a graft of fascia lata taken from one or other thigh. This is wonderful material to work with and has very little risk of complication.

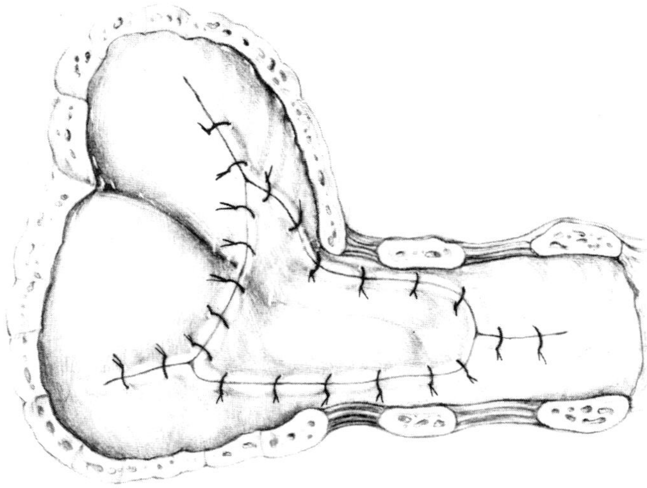

14

## 15

The divided ligamentum nuchae forms a triangle with the apex at the foramen magnum, the two short sides following the line of the occipital and spinal dura and the long side being superficial. First suture the apex of this triangle and then the two short sides and finally the long side where there is room for a second layer. The short limb of the T is easily apposed by one layer of muscle sutures and gives a good, strong, watertight closure. The subcutaneous tissues are closed with fine sutures with clips or silk to the skin. Absorbable sutures are used for all deep layers.

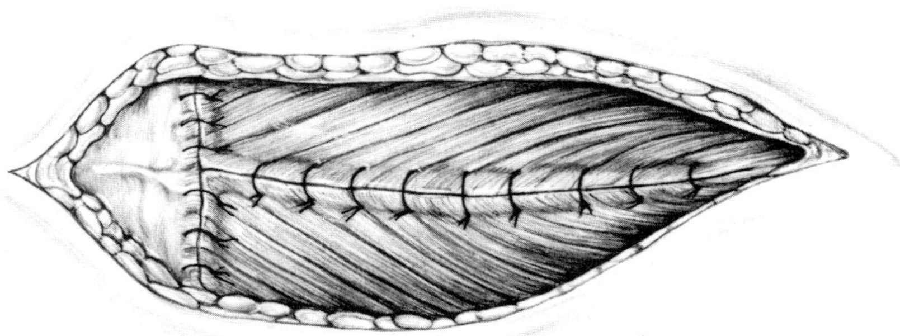

15

Illustrations by J. M. P. Booth

# The principles of microsurgery as applied to aneurysm surgery

**M. G. Yaşargil** MD
Professor and Director, Neurosurgical University Clinic, Kantonsspital Zürich, Switzerland

**R. D. Smith** MD
Department of Neurosurgery, Louisiana State University Medical Centre, New Orleans, Louisiana, USA

**J. L. Firth** FRCP(Ed)
Consultant Neurosurgeon, Regional Department of Neurosurgery and Neurology, University Hospital, Nottingham; Royal Infirmary, Leicester; Harlow Wood Hospital, Mansfield, UK

## Introduction

The operative treatment of cerebral aneurysms is a field which has received keen interest from neurosurgeons in the last 50 years. While it has been recognized that a patient can be protected from further intracranial haemorrhage by exclusion of an aneurysm from the circulation, the results have frequently been disappointing despite a variety of operative procedures. The application of microsurgical techniques to the field of aneurysm surgery has increased our understanding of the complexities attending successful treatment of an aneurysm and has contributed to the development of useful operative techniques and instrumentation in this field. The basic principles of microneurosurgery and their specific application to aneurysm surgery will form the substance of this chapter. The specific steps in the treatment of aneurysms in particular locations will be described in subsequent chapters.

## Concepts of microneurosurgery

### ANATOMICAL PERSPECTIVE

#### Subarachnoid space

Increased attention to the subarachnoid space has disclosed an orderly compartmentalization with recognizable cisterns enclosed by fenestrated arachnoid membrane walls and traversed by arteries, veins, nerves and connective tissue trabecula. Appreciation of the fine anatomy of the subarachnoid space allows the neurosurgeon to maintain proper orientation, preserve delicate structures, avoid strangulation of small vessels by connective tissue strands and develop proper tissue planes when working in the confined areas at the base of the brain.

#### Vascular anatomy

Only quite recently has the importance of tiny perforating arteries to the diencephalon and brainstem and their liability to injury during aneurysm surgery been emphasized. Furthermore, the multiple variations and anomalies of the circle of Willis which are found more frequently in patients with cerebral aneurysm must be recognized and considered if vital arteries are not to be injured during operation. The operating microscope has allowed these structures to be studied *in situ* under essentially physiological conditions and different patterns to be recognized.

#### Aneurysm development

Although the importance of well performed angiography cannot be minimized, it is recognized that the exact morphology and anatomical relationships of an aneurysm can only be fully appreciated at the time of operation. The operating microscope is extremely helpful in this definition. An aneurysm originates within the subarachnoid space and, as it grows, develops reduplications of arachnoid over the fundus. This apposition of arachnoid allows potential planes to be developed between the aneurysm and its parent arteries as well as between the aneurysm and neighbouring perforating arteries and cranial nerves. By staying within the proper subarachnoid planes, the surgeon is able to preserve delicate structures in the vicinity of the aneurysm and at the same time develop a suitable neck to allow placement of a clip.

## APPROACH AND EXPOSURE

### Craniotomy

A narrow binocular base, axial illumination, bayonet instruments and magnification allow an approach through a small craniotomy. A three-dimensional concept of the anatomy at the base of the brain is important when designing a craniotomy. A few millimetres of bone removed from the base of the skull can be translated into considerable operating space under the operating microscope. Having learned to operate in a tunnel-shaped field, the surgeon will find that relatively extensive manoeuvres, reaching across the entire base of the brain or the entire width of the falx, can be performed with minimal damage to normal tissues.

### Retraction

Microsurgical technique emphasizes support rather than retraction of tissues. Three deleterious aspects of brain retraction must be weighed against the need for wider exposure.

1. Distortion of perforating vessels at their origins, as they traverse the subarachnoid septa and as they enter the brain, particularly the brainstem – often remote from the operative site.
2. The possibility of cerebral ischaemia beneath the retractor when perfusion pressure is marginal. This may be implicated in postoperative cerebral oedema when normal blood pressure returns.
3. In aneurysm surgery, injudicious retraction may avulse the fundus of the aneurysm, notably when it is embedded in the cortex or adherent to the base of the skull.

With microsurgical techniques, an operating microscope and a properly fashioned craniotomy, it should be possible to perform most operations for aneurysm with only a few millimetres' retraction of the cortex.

### Brain resection

Brain resection is generally avoided with microsurgical techniques, or limited to very small resections of the gyrus rectus (3–5 mm) and the evacuation of haematomas. The surgeon must learn to work in a few millimetres' space and not depend on wide exposures. Resection of brain leads to oozing of blood which obscures landmarks in the subarachnoid space, disorientating the operator. With microsurgical techniques every effort is made to preserve normal structures.

## ATRAUMATIC HANDLING OF TISSUES

### Dissection

Opening of the thinner arachnoid sheets is accomplished with gentle spreading of the tips of a fine forceps or the bipolar coagulation forceps. Any thickened bands of arachnoid or adhesions should be divided sharply. One must avoid avulsion of connective tissue by blunt dissection and traction. This distorts small vessels and may rupture them from their parent arteries. Vessels should be manipulated by gentle retraction or held by connective tissue attachments rather than directly grasped. When vessels are sutured, the edges are stabilized internally with forceps rather than grasped.

### Haemostasis

The lighting and magnification of the operating microscope allow accurate coagulation of small bleeding points as soon as they develop. Bipolar coagulation is essential to give precision and avoid heating of neighbouring structures. Small veins should be desiccated over a few millimetres' length before being divided so that they do not retract and begin to bleed again. It is most important that all small venous and arteriolar bleeding is immediately controlled to avoid blood infiltrating the subarachnoid space.

# Operating microscope

## Magnification

The actual magnification achieved depends on the focal length of the objective and the magnification power of the eyepieces. In practice a 300 mm objective and 12·5× eyepieces have been found most satisfactory. Tables are available (Carl Zeiss, Germany) for calculation of actual magnification against objective, eyepiece and lens changer settings. Although motorized variable magnification and focusing systems are available, these have been found less useful at the operating table.

## Binocular vision

The importance of an operating microscope is less that of simply making structures seem larger than to provide the surgeon with well-lighted binocular vision into a deep narrow space. In principle, the light reflected from a structure is focused by the objective and observed through the eyepieces and tube which form a telescope. The size of the field to be observed is determined by the Galilean lens changer. Stereoscopic vision is thus limited by the width of field passing from the objective to the lens system (16 mm) rather than the interpupillary distance (60 mm). In essence this gives the surgeon the feeling that he is working within the operating field rather than above it, and adds a new perspective to deep brain structures.

## Lighting

The problem of providing enough light at higher magnifications is not completely solved. In addition to the normal tungsten lamp, which must be cooled by suction, a fibreoptic light source directed through the microscope will provide optimal illumination.

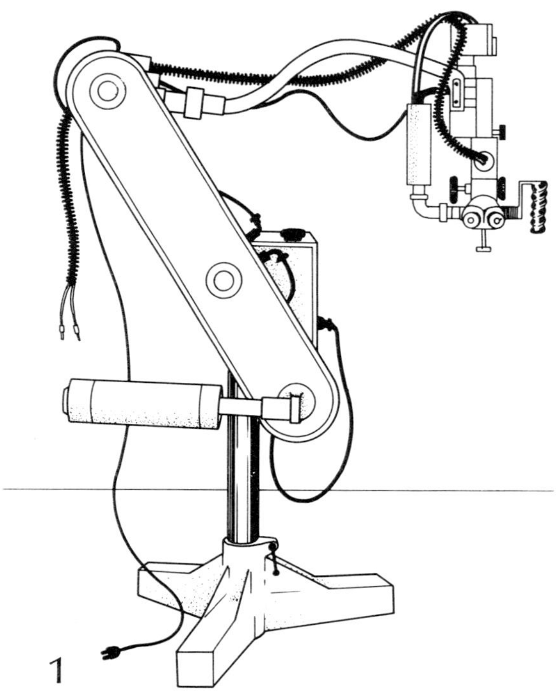

1

1

## Balanced microscope stand

The optical benefits of the operating microscope have, to some degree, been offset by the necessity to reposition the instrument constantly to gain maximum advantage. A microscope stand has therefore been developed which is counterbalanced to make the microscope head essentially weightless. Position is maintained with an electromagnetic braking system released by a mouth switch. This allows both movement and focusing to be controlled by head movements of the surgeon, leaving his hands free. Angular movements of the microscope head require release by a pistol-grip hand switch.

### ACCESSORIES

## Observer tubes

An observer tube allows assistants to follow the progress of the procedure if television monitoring equipment is not available.

## Television camera

Continuous television monitoring permits assistants, anaesthetists, nurses and visitors to participate actively in the procedure, increasing their understanding and their efficiency. In addition, videotapes provide a permanent record of the procedure. Improved colour television monitoring is anticipated.

## Photographic and movie cameras

Important anatomical and pathological findings can be recorded for teaching purposes.

# Microsurgical instrumentation

Although high quality instruments are necessary for successful microsurgical technique, they do not replace the need for sound anatomical knowledge and progressive laboratory experience. Familiarity with new instruments and with the altered perspective of the operating microscope should be gained by continuous laboratory exercise in atraumatic handling of tissues, suturing of small vessels and performing procedures at some depth in a narrow operating field.

The basic requirements for instruments in microneurosurgical procedures are that they are small enough to allow atraumatic manipulation in a confined space, that they are shaped so that they do not obscure the surgeon's view of the operating field through the microscope, and that they can be securely but comfortably handled. Surgeons will vary in their preferences and no definite rules can be made about the most suitable instruments for a given procedure. Most important is that the surgeon has a wide enough range of instruments so that he can work efficiently despite variable anatomical and pathological situations.

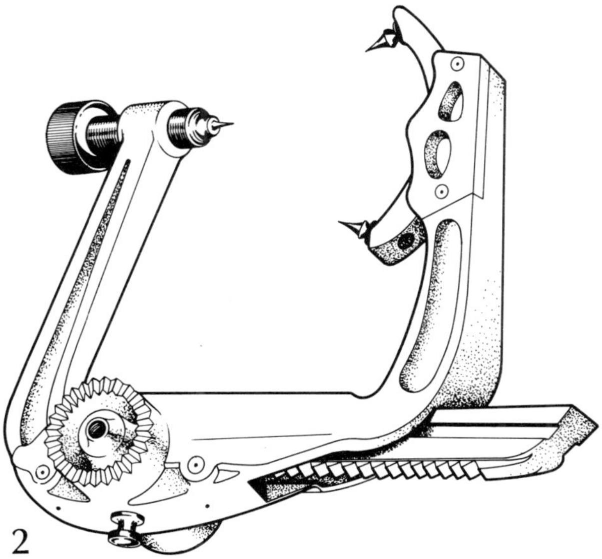

2

## 2

### Head fixation

As procedures must be carried out within very confined spaces and retractors are mounted to the operating table, absolute stability of the head is essential. Three-point skeletal fixation (Mayfield-Kees) is preferred.

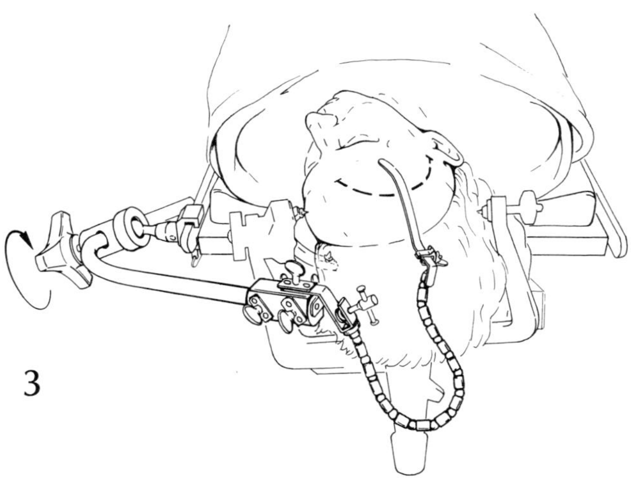

3

## 3

### Retractors

Hand-held retractors cannot provide the stability and gentleness required in microsurgery. Consequently, various types of self-retaining retractors have been developed. The type used at the University of Zürich is a malleable retractor blade attached to a tension-adjustable linked retractor arm. This is mounted to a side rung of the operating table. The retractor allows considerable variability in placement, is secure and provides controlled pressure in retraction.

### Dissection instruments

A variety of forceps, scissors, dissectors, hooks, ligature passers and probes may be required. Bayonet handles are particularly important in keeping the surgeon's hands away from the visual axis of the microscope. Size, balance, strength and compliance are all factors in instrument selection.

## Bipolar coagulation

Bipolar coagulation has played a major part in the development of successful microsurgical techniques. Small vessels can be coagulated and divided without heating effect to parent vessels or adjacent neural structures. A series of coagulation forceps is required, varying in length, tip width and curve or shape of the tips. It is very important that the tips of the forceps are kept absolutely clean and moist to prevent sticking and charring of tissue during coagulation.

## Suction

Wall suction has been found unsatisfactory for microsurgical procedures because the force of suction is too great and too difficult to control. An electric pump suction apparatus is recommended. This should be used at a pressure that does not allow small vessels and nerves to become trapped in the sucker. The judicious use of cottonoid sponges and early control of all small bleeding points eliminates much of the need for vigorous suction.

## Microsutures

Monofilament 10/0 and 11/0 sutures with curved 3 and 5 mm round atraumatic needles are used to repair and anastomose vessels less than 1 mm in diameter. Manipulation may be performed with fine forceps or with specially constructed needle holders. Needle holders that have a catch lock are generally not recommended as they tend to spring the needle through or away from the tissue on release.

## Surgical clips

### *Haemostatic clips*

These are malleable clips applied by compression of the clip onto the vessel. Clips must be large enough to include the entire vessel when it is flattened and should close evenly so that the vessel is not pushed ahead of the clip.

# 4 & 5

### *Aneurysm clips*

For occlusion of the aneurysm neck or occlusion of a large vessel, a spring-loaded clip must be strong enough to withstand the opening force of arterial pressure, yet not traumatize the wall of the vessel so that multiple applications may be made. A variety of sizes, shapes and angles will be required.

### *Temporary clips*

These clips open wider than aneurysm clips but have less closing force. They are used in anastomosis of small vessels, temporary occlusion of arteries in operations for arteriovenous malformations and temporary occlusion of an aneurysm or parent vessels to permit further dissection of the neck.

## High-speed electric drill

For microneurological uses such as removal of the sphenoid ridge, clinoid processes or posterior wall of the internal auditory meatus, drills should be high-speed, low-torque, long-throw, of slim proportions, angulated, and capable of clockwise or counterclockwise rotation. Air-powered drills generally do not fulfil all these requirements. Suction and irrigation are used during drilling procedures.

## Mirrors

Small mirrors in which angulation can be controlled by spring-loading in the handle are useful for examining small corners directed away from the view of the surgeon, e.g. beneath the anterior clinoid process, the interpeduncular fossa and within the internal auditory meatus.

## Operator support

Comfort and performance are improved by an arm support or ledge adjacent to the operating field. A mobile, hydraulically operated stool is a welcome aid in longer procedures.

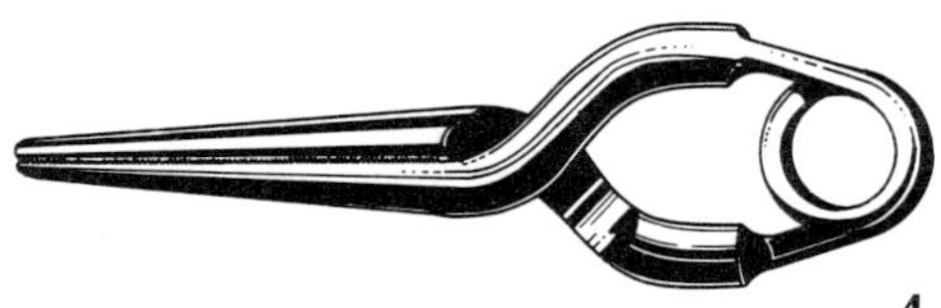

4

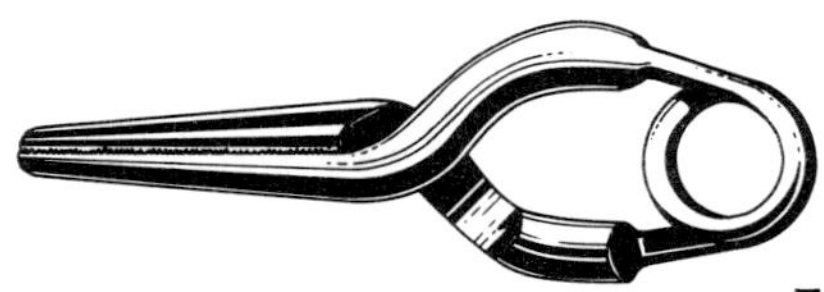

5

# Microsurgical aneurysm operations

## RATIONALE

The goal of operation is to exclude completely and selectively the aneurysm from the normal circulation, maintaining the continuity of the parent vessel and avoiding injury to adjacent vessels and neural structures. As with all demanding procedures, the surgeon must have a clear plan in mind and at the same time be prepared to alter it in the face of unexpected complications and to salvage as much as possible in adverse circumstances. Good angiography and preoperative preparation are prerequisites to successful surgery. Microsurgical techniques offer the following advantages in the operation of cerebral aneurysms.

1. Subarachnoid approach with minimal retraction.
2. Recognition of small perforating vessels and anomalies of the arterial tree.
3. Clear definition of the neck of the aneurysm.
4. Precise haemostasis.

Detailed anatomical knowledge and confidence in executing microsurgical procedures allow the surgeon to devote his full attention to the specific problems encountered in each case.

## APPROACH

Large craniotomies often lead to over-vigorous retraction and expose the brain to drying and mechanical injury while not really improving visualization at the base of the brain. Most aneurysms of the internal carotid artery, middle cerebral artery, anterior cerebral artery complex and upper basilar artery can be treated through a standard frontotemporosphenoidal craniotomy in which the sphenoid ridge and orbital roof are drilled down to provide better exposure of the circle of Willis. Skin and muscle are turned as a single flap to avoid injury to the frontalis branch of the facial nerve. Distal anterior cerebral artery aneurysms are approached parasagittally, and posterior fossa aneurysms subtemporally or suboccipitally depending on their location.

After opening and retraction of the dura, the approach is generally through the subarachnoid space. In addition to providing an organized method of exposure, dissection of the subarachnoid space allows release of cerebrospinal fluid, providing further brain relaxation and working room. The parent vessels are exposed so that temporary clips may be applied to them if necessary. In cases where intracerebral haematomas are superficial, these may be partially evacuated to provide additional space. Systemic blood pressure is lowered at this stage.

## EXPOSURE

Before attempting dissection of the aneurysm neck, it is important to expose all adjacent vessels and brain structures so that they can be protected, and temporary clips applied where necessary. Each location has its particular anatomy and requires identification of all relevant structures. Thickened bands of arachnoid stabilizing vessels and cranial nerves in the subarachnoid space are divided sharply and traction is carefully avoided.

The neck and proximal part of the fundus will be related to adjacent vessels and nerves by arachnoid and arachnoidal adhesions. Vessels which appear to issue from the aneurysm are most often applied to the aneurysm by arachnoidal adhesions and can be separated from its wall by developing a plane between adjacent arachnoid membranes. The operating microscope is particularly useful in clarifying this situation. Adhesions around the neck of the aneurysm should be spread slightly and then sharply divided. The surgeon should not attempt to tear these adhesions with a blunt hook or dissector.

In some situations, limited subpial cortical resection (3–5 mm) is required, especially in the gyrus rectus and less often in the mediobasal temporal and laterobasal frontal lobes. Resection should be limited to a few millimetres, bleeding points meticulously coagulated and the pia left attached to the fundus of the aneurysm until after the neck has been clipped.

## CLIPPING

The variability in size, shape, atherosclerosis and thrombosis of an aneurysm precludes any set method of aneurysm clipping. The following methods have proved useful in particular situations.

1. If the neck of the aneurysm is narrow, regular and reasonably long, a clip is applied primarily and adequate placement ensured.
2. If the neck of the aneurysm is wide, short or irregular, a neck is developed with bipolar coagulation. The tips of the coagulating forceps are placed across the neck of the aneurysm and gently squeezed while short bursts of current are applied (setting of 25 on Malis unit). The forceps are frequently released to assess shrinkage and prevent sticking. The method is limited by atherosclerosis, thrombosis and thin portions of wall.

   An initial (pilot) clip is then applied to the aneurysm, which is opened and coagulated. The increased mobility of the aneurysm may allow a permanent clip to be precisely placed or pressure is applied to the fundus of the aneurysm with a sucker on a cottonoid sponge to deflate the aneurysm while a clip is applied with the opposite hand. The clipped aneurysm can then be held with ring forceps while the clip is slightly opened and adjusted to its final position.

   A silk ligature can be used either to reduce the size of the neck to allow clip placement, or as definitive treatment. The ligature should be passed indirectly beneath the parent vessels rather than directly beneath the aneurysm neck to avoid capturing perforating arteries with the ligature and to minimize the chance of premature aneurysm rupture.
3. If the neck is atherosclerotic or the aneurysm contains significant thrombus, a clip is placed low on the neck, the aneurysm is opened and endarterectomy or thrombectomy performed. The aneurysm is then held closed with forceps while the clip is adjusted or replaced. Temporary clips are placed on the parent vessels, and the aneurysm is then opened and evacuated and a clip placed across the neck. In an occasional case where the neck is too macerated to accept a clip, repair of the vessel may be performed with 10/0 sutures.

   With extensive thrombosis of a large aneurysm, considerable thrombus may need to be removed before the neck can be completely defined.
4. Stepwise (staging) elimination of aneurysm sac. Aneurysms with adherent or inaccessible bases should first be clipped at the most proximal accessible portion to prevent rupture during manipulation, according to the philosophy 'first place the lasso around the neck of the aneurysm, then tame it in the desired fashion'. Following further dissection along the base, the clip can be repeatedly advanced or a second clip applied proximal to the first, which can then be removed, and the freed corners coagulated again. With one or two clips this process is repeated in a stepwise fashion until the neck is completely obliterated, and segments of the aneurysm bulging inferiorly are included within the clip. Sequential bipolar coagulation of the fundus beyond the clips can be used to prevent haemorrhage from friable areas during the clip advancement, or two or more clips can be advanced over one another. Coagulation and excision of the fundus prior to final clip positioning can sometimes provide additional working space.

After clipping, the fundus of the aneurysm is normally resected, although adhesions to delicate structures such as the oculomotor nerve may necessitate leaving a segment of the fundus *in situ*. Placement of the clip is inspected to ensure that parent vessels are not compromised and that no small perforating arteries are enclosed in the clip. The surgeon should not settle for less than perfect clip placement. To strengthen the parent vessel adjacent to the clip, a piece of muscle is wrapped around the base of the clip and held in place with a drop of acrylic bonding agent.

## CLOSURE

Blood pressure is restored to normal and haemostasis is achieved. Any residual haematoma is removed with copious saline washings. A 4 per cent solution of papaverine is applied to the major vessels to relieve spasm, and the sympathetic plexus may be stripped from the adventitia. The dura is closed, the bone flap replaced and the subgaleal space drained for 24 hours.

## INTRAOPERATIVE COMPLICATIONS

### Haemorrhage

Rupture of the aneurysm may occur at any time during the operation, from the time of anaesthesia until the neck is securely clipped. If the aneurysm ruptures in the initial stages of the operation, the surgeon can only work quickly to come down to the aneurysm and attempt to control the bleeding. More commonly the aneurysm will rupture when traction is applied to the brain, when the neck is being dissected or when attempts are made to place the clip or pass the bipolar forceps tips around the aneurysm. If the aneurysm ruptures on the fundus, bleeding can frequently be controlled with application of a cottonoid pattie and continued low-pressure suction directly over the site of rupture. Large suckers tend to increase the size of the perforation in the aneurysm and to damage adjacent delicate structures. If the bleeding point can be brought into the sucker, a temporary clip may be applied with the other hand. If the tear is at the junction of the aneurysm and its parent artery, temporary clipping of the parent vessels will almost certainly be required.

### Aneurysms not amenable to simple clipping

An aneurysm whose neck is partially extradural and those which involve two parent artery branches at the base may not allow complete occlusion by clipping. Attempts may be made to fashion a neck with bipolar coagulation but in other cases one must settle for partial occlusion by a clip and muscle and acrylic glue on the remaining part.

### Small sessile aneurysm

Frequently, during operation for a major aneurysm, the surgeon will encounter small aneurysms or thin blebs on the parent vessel wall. It is occasionally possible to create a neck with bipolar coagulation, but application of the current may cause the aneurysm to invaginate into the parent vessel. If it does not reappear after 5 minutes, it is best covered with muscle and acrylic bonding agent and left.

Illustrations by J. M. P. Booth

# Anterior communicating arterial aneurysms

**M. G. Yaşargil** MD
Professor and Director, Neurosurgical University Clinic, Kantonsspital Zürich, Switzerland

**R. D. Smith** MD
Department of Neurosurgery, Louisiana State University Medical Centre, New Orleans, Louisiana, USA

**J. L. Firth** FRCP(Ed)
Consultant Neurosurgeon, Regional Department of Neurosurgery and Neurology, University Hospital, Nottingham; Royal Infirmary, Leicester; Harlow Wood Hospital, Mansfield, UK

## Introduction

The anterior communicating artery is one of the more common sites of intracranial aneurysms (30 per cent). Aneurysms at this location are associated with a relatively high preoperative and postoperative morbidity and mortality because of their proximity to vital diencephalic centres. The chapter on 'Principles of microsurgery as applied to aneurysm surgery', pp. 146–153, has outlined the general application of microsurgical principles to the treatment of cerebral aneurysms. This chapter will deal with the specific anatomical and operative problems associated with anterior communicating arterial aneurysms and will discuss results and complications that may be expected to accompany operative treatment.

# Surgical anatomy

## SUBARACHNOID SPACE

## 1

The regular compartmentalization of the subarachnoid space allows the surgeon to follow an orderly pattern of dissection and to maintain his orientation through the somewhat altered perspective of the operating microscope. The key landmark to the area of dissection for anterior communicating arterial aneurysms is the junction of the several cisterns in the anterior parasellar area. This point lies above the bifurcation of the internal carotid artery just lateral to the optic chiasm. From this point the carotid cistern (containing the carotid artery and the origins of its branches) extends anteriorly to the anterior clinoid process. The sylvian cistern (containing the middle cerebral artery) extends back into the sylvian fissure. The olfactory cistern with the olfactory tract is above on the basal surface of the frontal lobe. More medially the lamina terminalis cistern (containing the anterior cerebral arteries and their branches, and the anterior communicating artery) and the chiasmatic cistern (containing the optic nerves, chiasm and the pituitary stalk) are midline structures. These cisterns share common walls at the above described confluence of cisterns and these walls are somewhat reinforced at this point. The interpeduncular cistern, whose anterior wall reaches from the medial surface of one temporal lobe to the other, lies beneath the carotid and chiasmatic cisterns and contains the posterior communicating arteries and their branches, the oculomotor nerves and many components of the basilar artery circulation. The crural cistern runs medial to the sylvian cistern and contains the anterior choroidal artery.

The configuration of the anterior subarachnoid cisterns is shown diagrammatically in surgical perspective.

Care must be taken with thickened bands of arachnoid which cross the origins of the middle cerebral and anterior cerebral arteries, and course from the olfactory area to the mediobasal temporal lobe and dorsal surface of the optic nerve, respectively. These must be sharply divided lest retraction of the frontal lobe should compress these arteries or avulse perforating arteries arising near their origins.

Systematic opening of the cisterns allows release of cerebrospinal fluid and provides increased working room and brain relaxation. When the brain remains tense, perforation of the anterior wall of the interpeduncular cistern will provide further release of cerebrospinal fluid. This release of fluid generally obviates the need for ventricular puncture or opening of the lamina terminalis, and will markedly enhance the relaxation obtained by removal of 15–20 ml of cerebrospinal fluid by lumbar puncture.

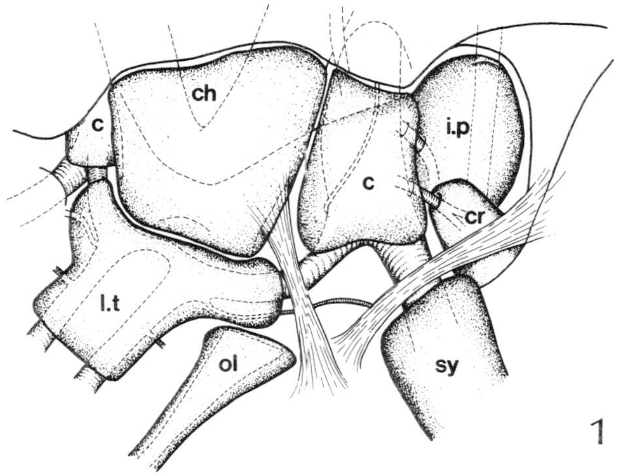


1

C, carotid cistern; ch, chiasmatic cistern; cr, crural cistern; i.p., interpeduncular cistern; l.t., lamina terminalis cistern; ol, olfactory cistern; sy, sylvian cistern.

## ANTERIOR CEREBRAL–ANTERIOR COMMUNICATING ARTERY COMPLEX

### Anterior cerebral artery (A1)

The anterior cerebral artery turns medially from the internal carotid artery bifurcation to pass over the optic nerve or optic tract and beneath the anterior perforated substance. Perforating arteries generally arise in groups of two or three and tend to turn laterally immediately after leaving the main arterial trunk so that they may be adherent to the anterior cerebral artery in their first few millimetres.

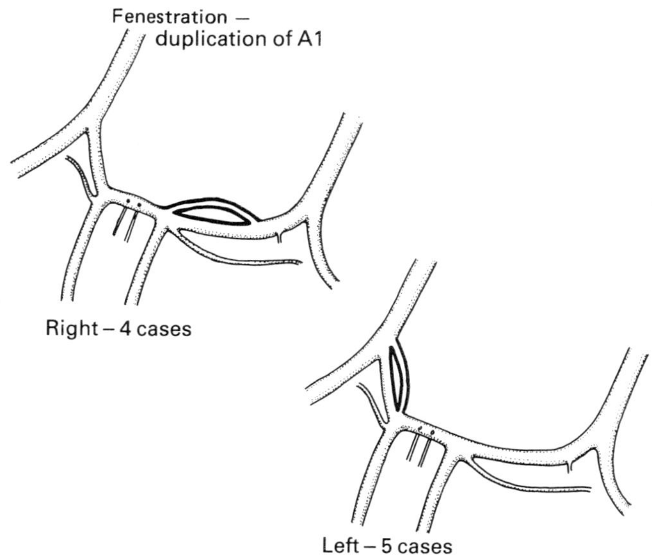


2a

# 2a & b

*Anomalies*

In 80 per cent of patients, the A1 segments are not equal in size, with the left side larger in 50 per cent of cases. Duplication (fenestration) of an A1 segment was noted in nine of 375 patients (2.4 per cent) and aplasia of the artery in another nine. Hypoplasia is distinguished from arterial spasm by the opposite A1 being large, with stout perforating arteries originating proximally on the artery and a pink rather than whitish colour.

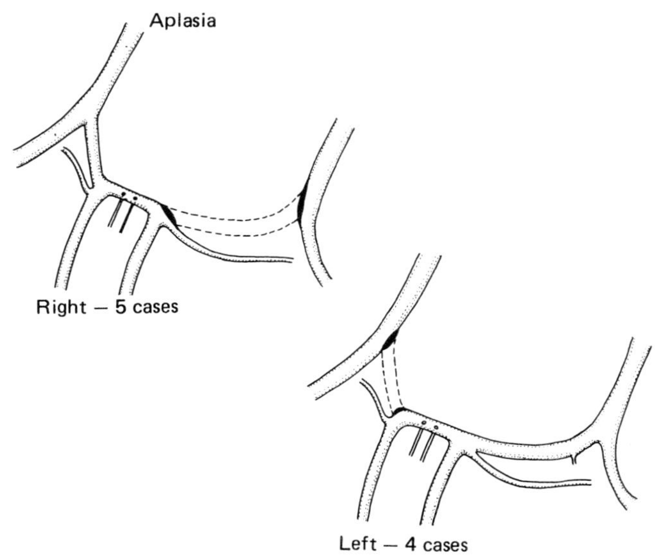


2b

## Anterior communicating artery

Two or three arteries, one of fairly large size, arise from the posteroinferior wall of the anterior communicating artery to run to the hypothalamus and septal areas. These arteries arise from the side of the larger A1 or in the middle of the anterior communicating artery when the A1 segments are equal.

*The recurrent artery of Heubner* generally arises from the corner of the anterior communicating artery and A1 segments and runs laterally to the anterior perforated substance beneath the A1. It may be adherent to the A1 over its first centimetres. When A1 is hypoplastic, an artery with a similar course arises in the midportion of the A1 and the recurrent artery of Heubner is also hypoplastic.

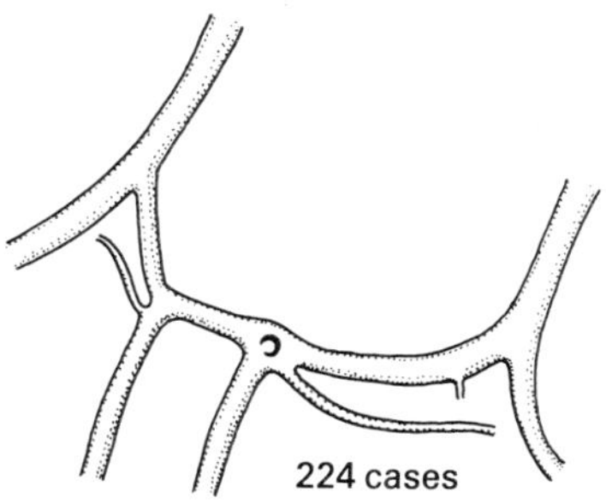


3a

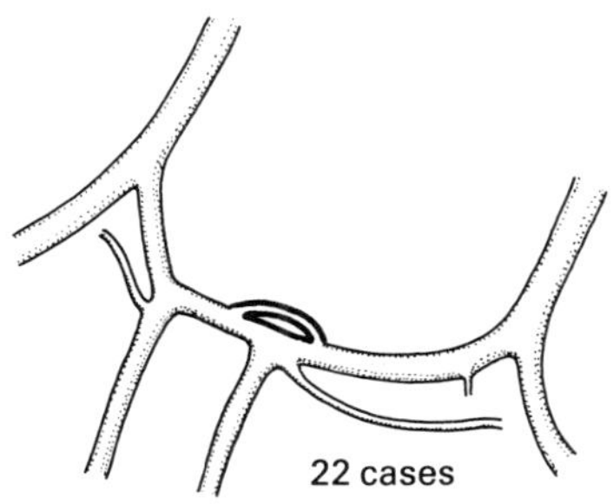


3b

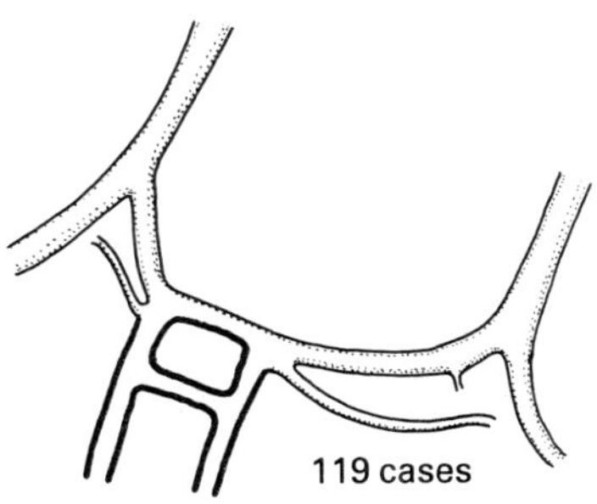


3c

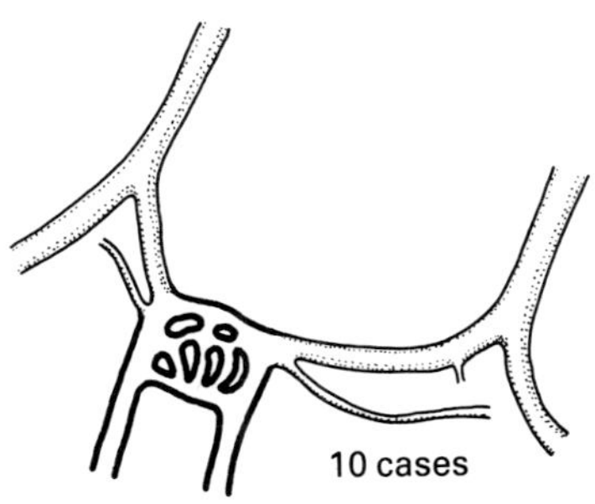


3d

# 3a–d

*Anomalies*

The anterior communicating artery may be duplicated (141 of our 375 patients) or be a network of small channels (10 of 315 patients). A total of 151 of the 375 patients with anterior communicating arterial aneurysm thus showed anomalous construction of the anterior communicating artery (40 per cent).

## Pericallosal artery (A2)

From the A2 segment arises first a small branch which runs to the olfactory tract, then the fronto-orbital artery arising about 5–10 mm from the anterior communicating artery, and more distally frontopolar arteries. Variations are common and the fronto-orbital and frontopolar arteries, as well as the Heubner artery, may arise from a common trunk or each may be represented by more than one artery.

# 4

*Anomalies*

Two of the 375 patients had a single A2, while 36 (9.6 per cent) had three A2s.

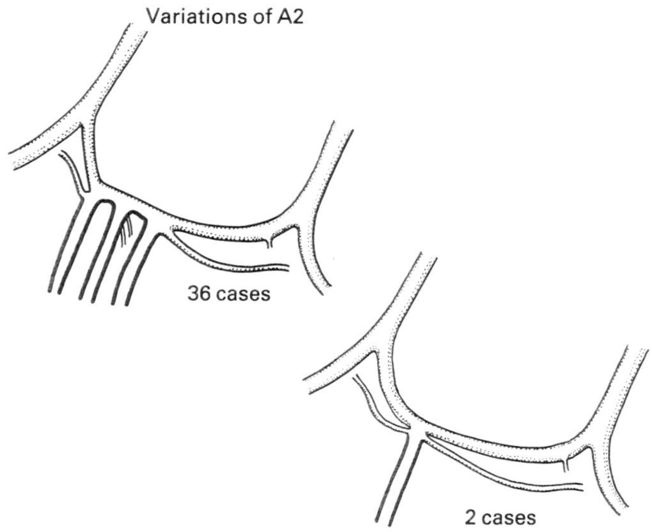


4

## ANEURYSMAL ANATOMY

# 5a, b & c

In 305 (81.3 per cent) of the 375 patients, the aneurysm arose from the junction of the large A1 segment and the anterior communicating artery. In 51.5 per cent this was on the left side (*a*) and in 27.7 per cent on the right side (*b*). In 18.7 per cent the A1 segments were equal and the aneurysm arose in the middle of the anterior communicating artery (*c*). In 2.2 per cent the aneurysm arose from the hypoplastic side (*a* and *b*). Hypothalamic arteries show the same relationship to the parent arteries and therefore usually occur directly beneath the aneurysm and are attached to its posteroinferior wall.

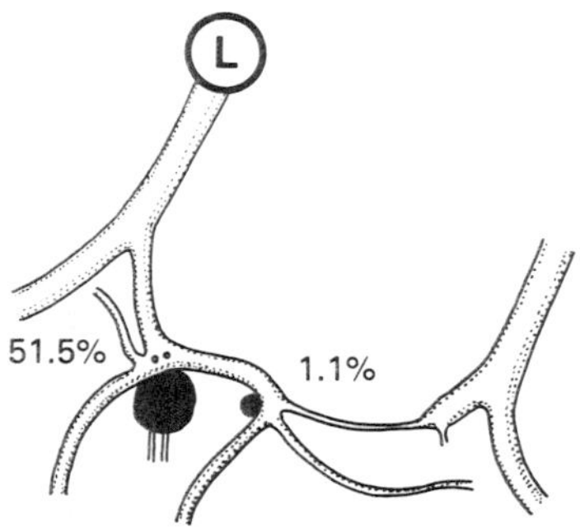


5a

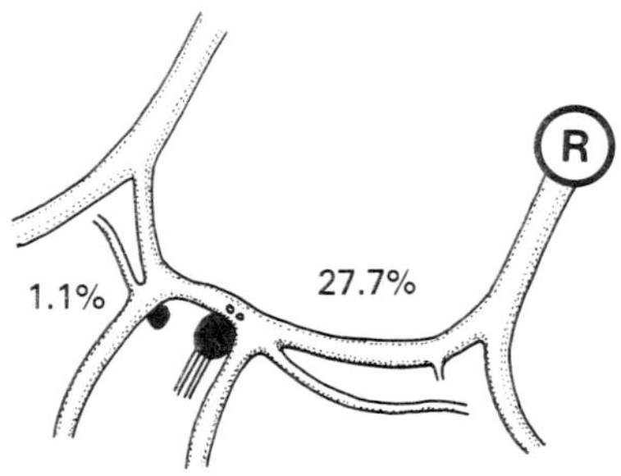


5b

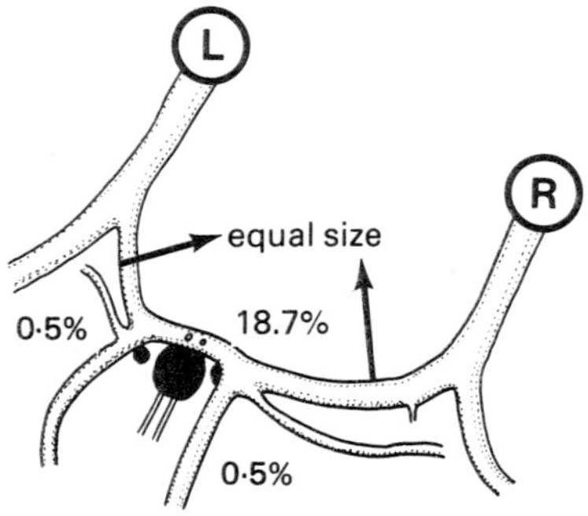


5c

6

In 34.4 per cent (129 of the 375 patients) the aneurysmal fundus was directed posterosuperiorly into the interhemispheric fissure. In 22.7 per cent (85 cases) the fundus was directed superiorly; in 14.1 per cent (53 cases) inferiorly, towards the lamina terminalis; and in 12.8 per cent (48 cases) forward toward the limbus sphenoidalis to overlie the optic chiasm. In the latter position the aneurysm may be adherent to the dura over the anterior sella. In 16 per cent (60 cases) the projections have been multidirectional (complex). The different positions require some variation of operative technique which will be discussed below.

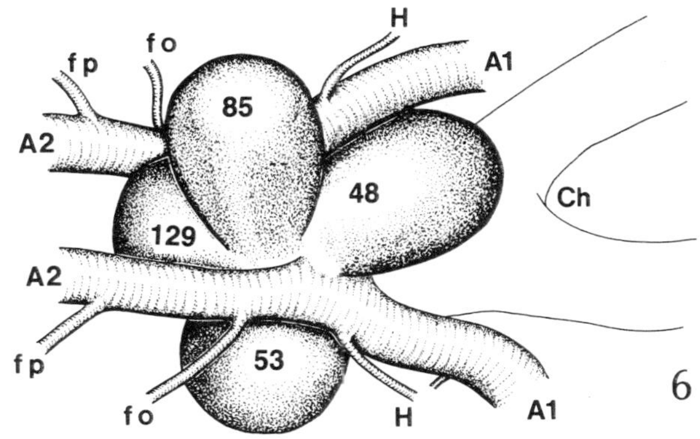


6

Ch, optic chiasm; fo, fronto-orbital artery; fp, frontopolar artery; H, recurrent artery of Heubner.

## Configuration of aneurysm

The aneurysm may be simple, with a more or less spherical shape and narrow neck, or complex, with a multilobed fundus showing different degrees of thinning and a neck which is wide and irregular. A daughter aneurysm close to the neck of the primary aneurysm may be hidden by the fundus of the latter and give rise to difficulties in attempting to place a clip. Atherosclerosis and thrombosis add additional complications to dissection and clipping.

## Relationship to adjacent structures

The recurrent artery of Heubner and the small arteries to the olfactory tract are generally not adherent to the aneurysm. Fronto-orbital arteries are almost invariably adherent to the fundus. The A2 segments are attached to the wall of the aneurysm over a variable length. The hypothalamic arteries are relatively loosely applied to the inferoposterior surface of the aneurysm. When directed forward, the aneurysm may be adherent to the optic chiasm and anterior sella.

# Preoperative

## Investigations

### *Angiography*

Angiography remains the single most important diagnostic method employed in the evaluation of intracranial aneurysms. In ideal circumstances, catheter angiography by the transfemoral route is recommended. A three or four vessel study should be performed because of the approximately 20 per cent incidence of multiple aneurysms. Cross-compression may provide useful information about the integrity of the anterior circle of Willis. Oblique views are essential in studying anterior communicating arterial aneurysms and stereoscopic, subtraction and magnification techniques allow the relationship of the aneurysm to adjacent vessels to be better appreciated.

### *Computerized tomography*

Computerized tomography may add substantially to the preoperative and postoperative treatment of patients with subarachnoid haemorrhage. This non-invasive technique indicates the presence of intracerebral and intraventricular haematoma, show areas of infarction and demonstrate the presence of hydrocephalus. This information is particularly valuable in the assessment and treatment of patients in poor condition following haemorrhage.

## Timing of operation

### *Clinical status*

The patient's preoperative status is primarily graded by his level of consciousness. Patients who are awake (grades I and II) are taken to operation as soon as possible, while patients who are drowsy or comatose (grades III–V) are given time to recover. The presence of an intracranial haematoma generally requires early operation, while the presence of heart disease, diabetes or hypertension may be an indication to delay operation until the medical problems are under control. Patients with acute hydrocephalus may require ventricular shunting or drainage before definitive aneurysm treatment. An arbitrary waiting period for alert patients has not been used in this department.

### *Radiographic vasospasm*

The authors do not consider the presence of vasospasm on angiography in an otherwise alert patient a contraindication to operation. Patients with diffuse generalized and severe spasm on angiography usually show alterations of level of consciousness and operation is delayed.

## Pharmacological aspects

### *General medications*

All patients are begun on corticosteroids (dexamethasone 16 mg/day) and anticonvulsants (diphenylhydantoin 300 mg/day) when first seen. Dexamethasone is tapered off in the postoperative period, while diphenylhydantoin is continued for 12 months. The patient is mildly sedated and given antihypertensive agents to attempt to keep his blood pressure in the normal range. Significant lowering of the blood pressure is not attempted in the preoperative period.

### *Brain relaxation*

Patients are given 20–50 g of mannitol intravenously 30 minutes before the skin incision. The $P\text{CO}_2$ is kept at about 30 mmHg throughout the procedure. Lumbar puncture may be performed and about 20 ml of cerebrospinal fluid removed. Removing this amount does not collapse the subarachnoid cisterns and provides a little more room to remove bone from the base of the skull before opening the dura. Subsequent release of cerebrospinal fluid from the basal cisterns will generally provide adequate brain relaxation.

### *Intraoperative hypotension*

Nitroprusside is used to lower the systemic blood pressure to about 70 mmHg in normotensive patients and to two-thirds of normal in hypertensive patients during exposure and clipping of the aneurysm. Blood pressure is returned to normal before closure.

# The operation

## THE APPROACH

## 7

### Position of patient

The patient is placed supine on the operating table and the three-point skeletal fixation device is applied to the skull with the two-pronged arm opposite the side of the craniotomy. Right-handed surgeons will prefer an approach from the right side unless there are additional aneurysms or intracranial haematomas on the left which require attention at the same procedure. For left-handed surgeons, the situation is reversed. The head is rotated to the left about 30° and the neck extended with the head slightly elevated to make the malar eminence the highest point of the operating field. Sterile attachments for the self-retaining retractors are fixed to the operating table so that they may be draped with the patient.

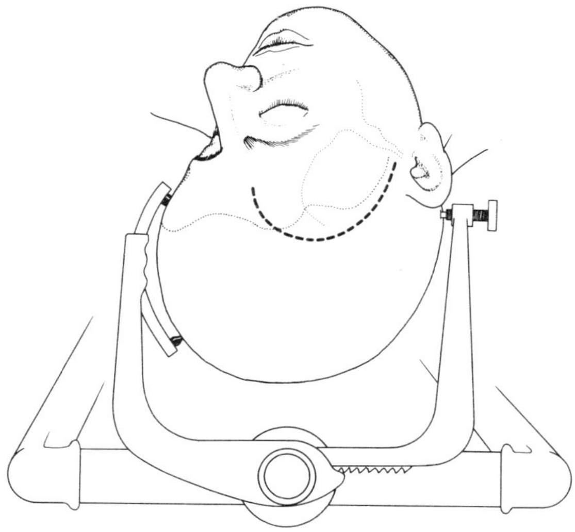

7

### Frontotemporosphenoidal craniotomy

## 8

*Skin and muscle incision*

The skin incision is begun anterior to the ear over the zygoma and continued just behind the hairline to the forehead (*see Illustration 7*). The skin and galea are elevated only for a width of about 1 cm on each side of the incision to allow placement of skin clips on the flap and Dandy haemostats on the galea below the skin margin. A plane is then developed between the layers of the superficial temporalis fascia, and the skin and temporalis muscle are reflected separately using an interfascial temporalis flap. This approach spares postoperative paralysis of the frontalis muscle secondary to injury of the facial nerve branches. The temporalis muscle is released from the medial aspect of the zygomatic arch, stripped deeply from the temporal fossa and reflected posterolaterally to visualize the pterion completely (*see Illustration 9*).

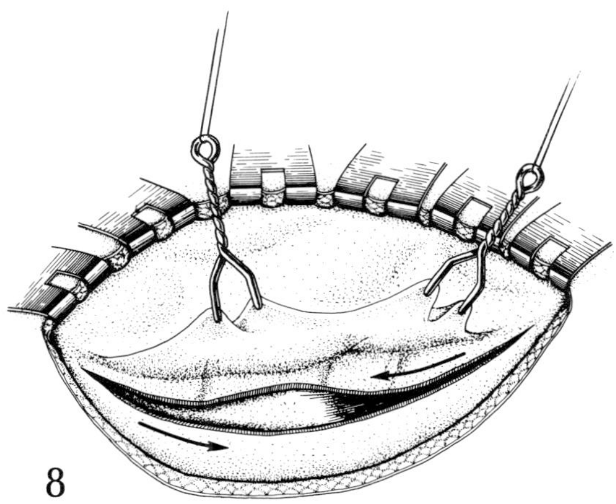

8

*Bone flap*

# 9

Four burr holes are then made: the first is made on the zygomatic process of the frontal bone; the second is on the superior orbital ridge 2.5 cm anterior and superior to the first; the third is on the temporal line 2.5 cm posterior to the first; and the fourth is in the temporal fossa just posterior to the sphenotemporal suture. This diamond-shaped bone flap is freed with a Gigli saw except between the first and fourth burr holes, where a groove is cut with the electric drill to allow the bone flap to fracture across the sphenoid bone.

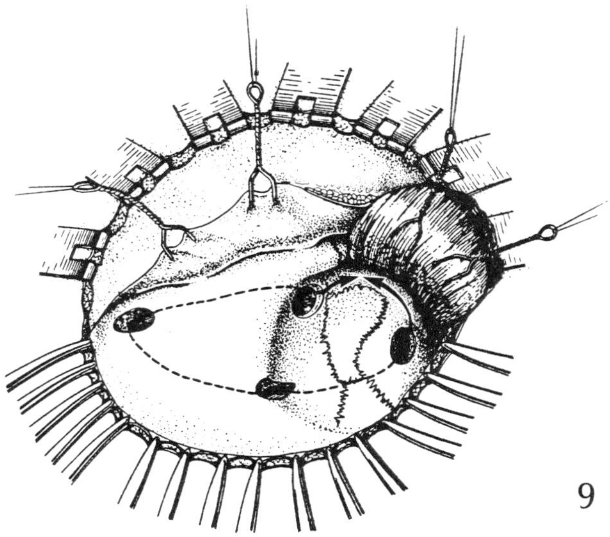

9

# 10

The bone flap is now removed and the microscope brought into the operating field. With gentle retraction to the dura over the frontal lobe, the sphenoid ridge and orbital roof are drilled smooth until the orbitomeningeal artery is encountered. This artery is coagulated and divided. (The dotted line indicates the bone extensions, which should be flattened by electric drill.)

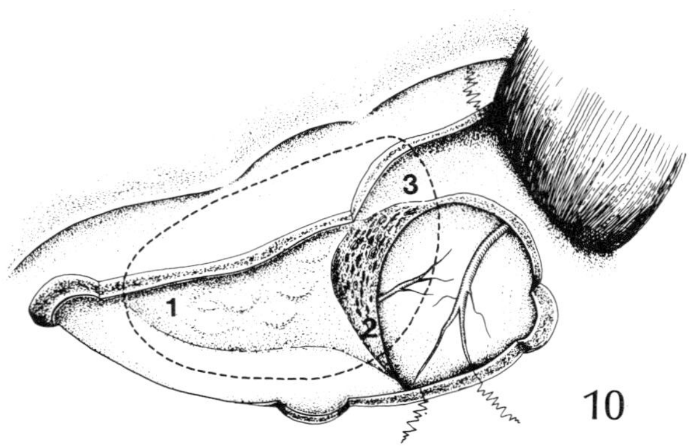


10

1, Orbital roof; 2, sphenoidal wing (medial); 3, sphenoidal wing (lateral)

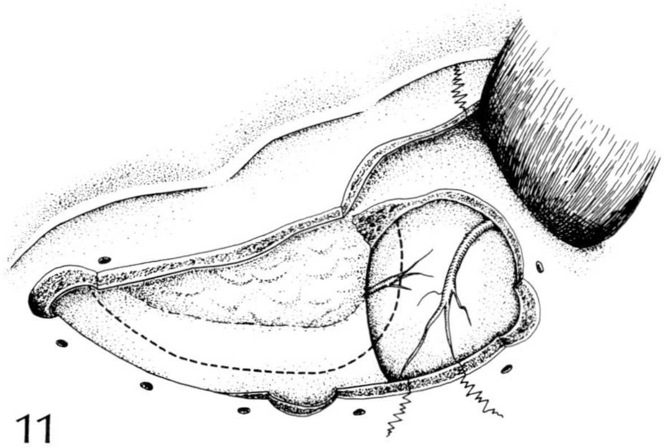

11

# 11

*Dural opening*

The dural incision (dotted line) extends from the anterior burr hole in a semicircle around the exposed orbital roof. The dura is retracted by suturing it to small drill holes in the bone and to the retracted temporalis muscle. The superior portion of exposed dura is normally not opened.

## 12

### Entering the subarachnoid space

The mediobasal aspect of the sylvian cistern is opened on the frontal side of the superficial middle cerebral veins. The middle cerebral artery (M1) is followed to the internal carotid artery bifurcation, where the thickened fibres over the origins of the anterior and middle cerebral arteries are divided. The carotid cistern is opened and a small but constant artery from the dorsal wall of the carotid artery to the dura over the anterior clinoid process is divided. If the brain remains tense, the interpeduncular cistern may be opened either laterally to the carotid artery or between the carotid artery and optic nerve to allow release of cerebrospinal fluid. Retraction is then gently applied to the laterobasal frontal lobe.

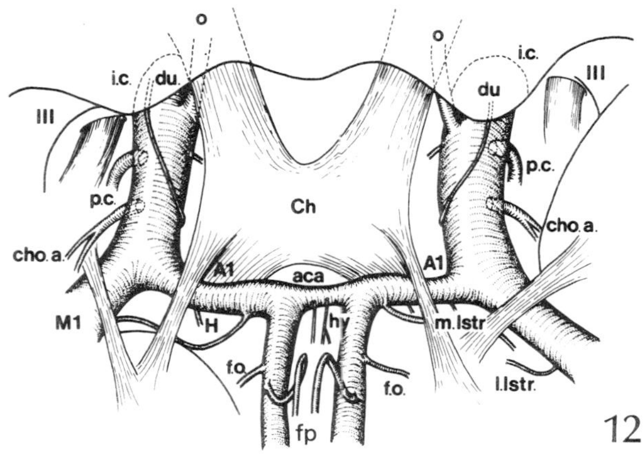


12

Ch = chiasm; o = orbital artery: du = dural branch; i.c. = internal carotid artery; p.c. = posterior communicating artery; cho. a = anterior choroidal artery; M1 = middle cerebral artery; A1 = anterior cerebral artery; aca = anterior communicating artery; hy = hypothalamic branches; fo = fronto-orbital artery; fp = frontopolar artery; H = Heubner artery; l.lstr. = lateral lenticulostriate arteries; m.lstr. = middle lenticulostriate arteries. III = oculomotor nerve

### Problems during approach

#### *Frontalis branch of facial nerve*

This structure was frequently injured when separate skin and temporalis muscle flaps were developed. Turning the skin and muscle as a combined flap seems to have eliminated this problem.

#### *Limited exposure*

It is important that enough of the sphenoid ridge and orbital roof are drilled away. Each millimetre of bone removed provides a significant increase in working space beneath the operating microscope.

#### *Closed sylvian fissure*

In some cases the sylvian fissure cannot be easily opened because of thickening of the arachnoid or close apposition of the frontal and temporal lobes. For dissection of anterior communicating arterial aneurysms, opening the sylvian fissure is not critical and must be weighed against possible injury.

#### *Bridging veins*

A small bridging vein from the superficial middle cerebral vein to the sphenoparietal or cavernous sinus may need to be divided to allow retraction. In some cases the vein can be dissected from the pia to obtain adequate length to avoid injuring it.

## EXPOSURE

### Ipsilateral A1 segment

The lamina terminalis cistern is opened and the ipsilateral A1 segment followed medially. Care must be taken to avoid striate perforating arteries running somewhat laterally to enter the anterior perforated substance. Heubner's artery is identified beneath the anterior cerebral artery. The surgeon should at this time be considering where a temporary clip might be applied should premature rupture of the aneurysm occur or should the artery be damaged during dissection. The size of the artery and its potential collateral flow are evaluated. Not infrequently the A1 segment will bow back to lie considerably posterior, beneath the basal frontal lobe. In this case it is not necessary to dissect the artery completely to the anterior communicating artery. Rather, the initial segment and perforating arteries should be dissected in case temporary clip placement is necessary, and attention then turned to the opposite side.

### Contralateral A1 segment

The dissection is then continued across the optic chiasm to the opposite side of the lamina terminalis cistern, where the contralateral A1 segment is exposed. If the fundus of the aneurysm is directed forward over the optic chiasm, dissection of the contralateral A1 segment will not be possible and must be delayed.

### Anterior communicating artery complex

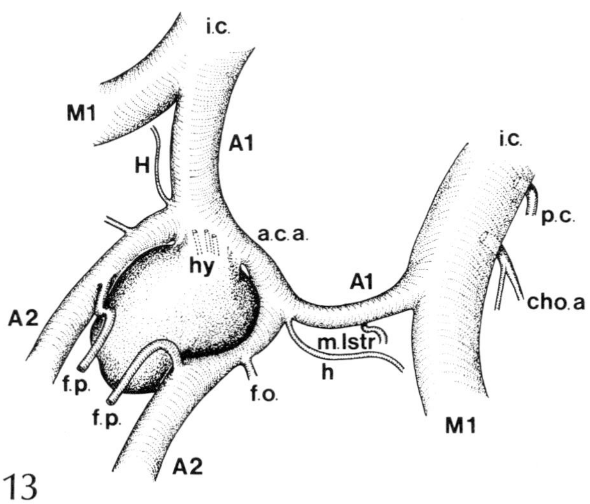


13

## 13

The goal of the surgeon is to identify the five pairs of normal bilateral arteries – both A1 segments, both recurrent arteries of Heubner, both A2 segments, both fronto-orbital and both frontopolar arteries – and the hypothalamic branches and a third A2 segment, if present, before attempting dissection of the aneurysm neck. Anomalies tend to fall into regular patterns as described above. With proximal control gained by exposure of both A1 segments, the surgeon moves his dissection distal to the anterior communicating artery. It may be possible to visualize the A2 segments simply with medial retraction of the laterobasal frontal lobe following release of cerebrospinal fluid from the basal cisterns. More often, however, it will be prudent to perform a 3–5 mm subpial resection of the ipsilateral gyrus rectus to avoid applying too much torque to the aneurysm by additional retraction (for key *see Illustration 12*).

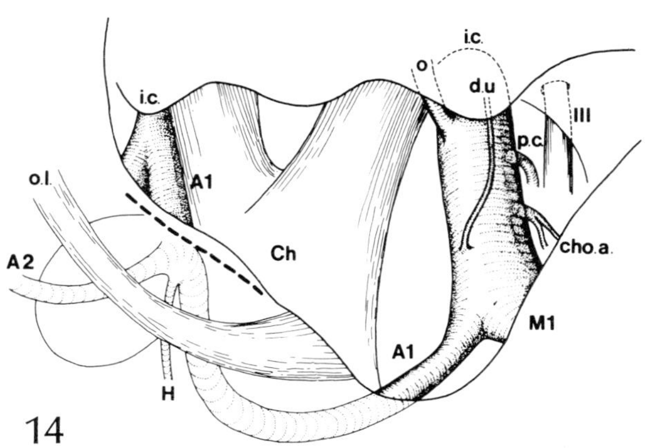


14

## 14

This dissection of gyrus rectus is directed towards the junction of the anterior communicating artery and the A2 segment and should leave the pia attached to the aneurysm wall. In this way the surgeon comes above the fundus of the aneurysm, where both A2 segments can be visualized. Dissecting proximally, an attempt is made to free the fronto-orbital arteries from the area of the aneurysm neck. In cases where the aneurysm fundus is directed forward, the surgeon can follow the A2 segment proximally to free the distal corner of the A1 segment and anterior communicating artery (for key *see Illustration 12*).

## Anterior communicating artery

The neck of the aneurysm may now be prepared by gentle spreading and sharp division of adhesions. An attempt is made to mobilize the neck of the aneurysm enough so that it can be gently elevated to allow inspection of the hypothalamic arteries beneath. These are dissected from the aneurysm wall and protected with a small cottonoid sponge. The neck of the aneurysm is gradually freed from the anterior communicating artery and the adjacent A2 segment until it is well defined over its first 3–4 mm.

## Problems during exposure

### *Arterial anomalies*

Constant regard must be given to the possibility of anomalous configurations of the anterior cerebral–anterior communicating artery complex. A third A2, duplication of the anterior communicating artery and partial duplications of the A1 segment can be easily overlooked. Failure to recognize these may lead to their inadvertent coagulation, rupture or clipping.

### *Recurrent artery of Heubner*

This artery may be closely adherent to the A1 segment near the anterior communicating artery and torn during dissection of the A1 segment.

### *Fronto-orbital arteries*

These may be so adherent to the wall of the aneurysm that their dissection is not feasible. If small, a fronto-orbital artery is better sacrificed to mobilize the aneurysm than to be saved at the cost of avulsing the aneurysm from the parent arteries.

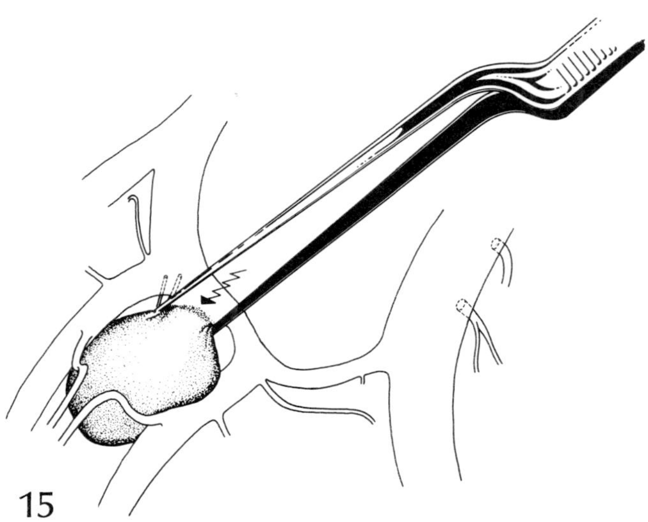

15

### *Haematoma*

When haematoma is present in the basal frontal lobe or gyrus rectus area, it is partially removed to allow increased working room and to facilitate dissection.

### *Haemorrhage*

Premature rupture of the aneurysm at this stage may yield to gentle compression with a sponge and sucker. If not, temporary clips are applied to the A1 segments and the aneurysm is quickly dissected until a temporary clip can be placed across the fundus. If a tear has occurred at the junction of the aneurysm and its parent arteries, temporary clips are applied to the A1 segments while the rent is closed with a clip or repaired with microsuture.

# CLIPPING

## Simple aneurysms

When the neck of the aneurysm is narrow and well defined, a clip is placed across the base and then slowly closed. The surgeon must ensure that the clip includes the whole aneurysm neck, does not compromise the parent vessel and does not include a perforating artery between the blades. Following placement of the clip, the fundus of the aneurysm is resected and the surgeon again ascertains good clip placement.

## Complex aneurysms

General methods of eliminating broad-based, irregular, atherosclerotic or thrombotic aneurysms, are discussed in the chapter on 'Principles of microsurgery as applied to aneurysm surgery', pp. 146–153. The following points apply specifically to anterior communicating arterial aneurysms.

## 15

To shrink the neck by bipolar coagulation, the forceps tips are passed between the A2 segments far enough posteriorly so that the entire aneurysm neck will be between the tips when the forceps is squeezed. Care must be taken that the tips do not damage the hypothalamus or pituitary stalk during coagulation. As mentioned previously, hypothalamic arteries are best protected by a cottonoid sponge during this manoeuvre.

# 16

If temporary clipping is required to complete resection of thin-walled aneurysms or to perform endarterectomy, thrombectomy or suture repair, clips should be placed medial to the perforating arteries so that their flow is not compromised.

In passing a ligature it is important that the ligature lies between the aneurysm neck and the hypothalamic arteries to avoid these arteries being included in the ligature when tied. This restricts the practicality of a ligature in anterior communicating arterial aneurysms rather.

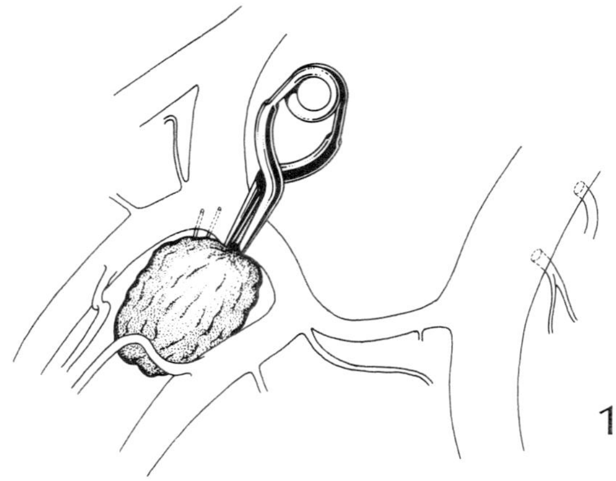

16

# 17

After clipping, the fundus is excised to permit inspection of the clip and to assure complete occlusion of the aneurysm.

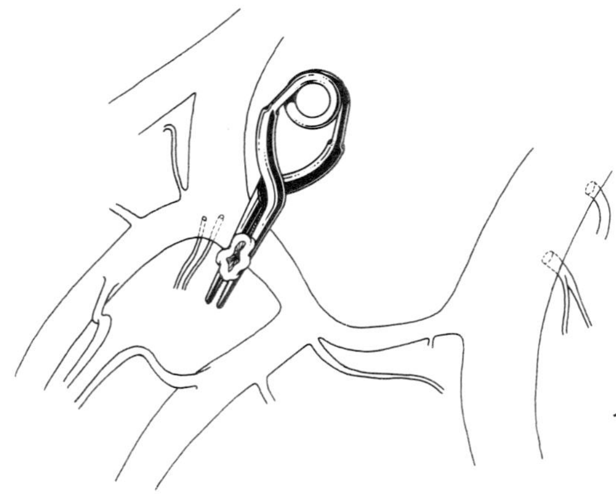

17

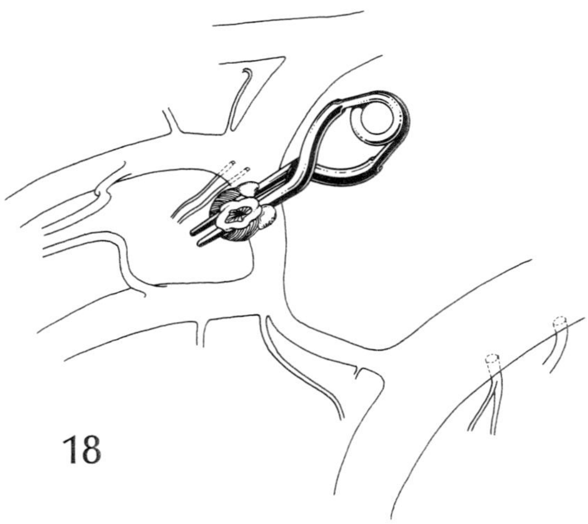

18

## Reinforcement of clip

# 18

Despite good clip placement across the neck of the aneurysm, the wall of the parent artery immediately below the clip represents a potential area of weakness in that it may already be somewhat attenuated by growth of the aneurysm so that it will be forced against the clip with each pulsation. A piece of muscle is therefore routinely placed directly beneath the clip on the parent vessel and held in place with a drop of acrylic bonding agent.

### Problems during clipping

*Irregular base*

The base of the aneurysm may be so diffuse that while a clip will close part of it another part bulges in a different direction. In this situation the remaining aneurysm neck can be wrapped in muscle and fascia and coated with an acrylic bonding agent. It is possible that improved techniques and increased experience will allow primary repair of the involved vessel by microsuture techniques.

*Twisting and tension on parent vessels*

While clipping of the aneurysm must completely occlude the aneurysm, it must not compromise the parent arteries by either stenosis, twisting or tension. The neck of the aneurysm should be further developed to allow better clip placement.

*Haemorrhage*

Rupture of the aneurysm during application of the clip is usually controlled by either advancing the clip or using a wider opening temporary clip on the fundus. If rupture occurs during bipolar coagulation, it may be that one forceps tip is not across the aneurysm neck and has perforated the aneurysm, or that the aneurysm has burst from a sudden increase in pressure from squeezing and heating. Control of bleeding should be attempted with low pressure suction while a temporary clip is applied to the aneurysm. Large suckers tend to damage the aneurysm and surrounding structures further. If bleeding is not controlled, temporary clips to first the larger and then the smaller A1 segment are indicated.

**CLOSURE**

### Alleviation of mechanical spasm

A 4 per cent solution of papaverine is applied to all major vessels to relieve the spasm associated with mechanical stimulation. This need not wait until the aneurysm has been clipped if spasm is noted, but is routinely done before closure. Following application of papaverine to the vessels the periadventitial sympathetic plexus becomes quite clearly defined and can be carefully picked from the arteries to give further protection from spasm.

### Haemostasis

After the aneurysm has been clipped, the anaesthetist allows the systemic blood pressure to return to normal. During this time, small bleeding points are coagulated. Common sources of oozing include small bridging veins, the venous plexi over the optic nerves and, on the lamina terminalis, an avulsed olfactory bulb, the small dural artery from the dorsal wall of the internal carotid artery and tiny pial venules on the gyrus rectus and from beneath the retractor. Following meticulous haemostasis all haematoma is washed from the subarachnoid space with copious quantities of saline, and residual intracerebral haematoma is removed if present. Areas of damaged pia are covered with Surgicel (Ethicon, UK).

### Wound closure

The dura is fixed to the bone margin with 4/0 silk tack-up sutures and the dural incision closed with a running suture. The bone flap is replaced and held in position with 2/0 silk sutures and the soft tissues are closed in layers. The subgaleal space is drained for 24 hours.

### Problems during closure

*Additional aneurysms*

Many patients have small blebs and areas of thinning of the arterial wall. Although the exact fate of these lesions is not known, they are generally covered with muscle or shrunk with coagulation. Others have multiple clinically significant aneurysms. An attempt is then made to treat all those aneurysms which are accessible by this approach at the same operation. Aneurysms of the opposite middle cerebral artery and those low on the opposite internal carotid artery are generally not amenable to treatment at the same operation.

*Burr holes*

Some cosmetic defect may be produced by the two anterior burr holes. These may be filled with bone shavings to provide a more normal contour.

*Cerebrospinal fluid rhinorrhoea*

Any small drill hole in the frontal sinus must be repaired with bone wax and acrylic to prevent cerebrospinal fluid rhinorrhoea.

## Postoperative care

The head is elevated 10–20° in the early postoperative period and progressive ambulation is encouraged. Uncomplicated cases are discharged at the end of the first week.

## Results

The results of intracranial operation in 375 patients are summarized in Table 1. Preoperative grading is as follows:

Grade 0a : unruptured aneurysm, no neurological deficit.

Grade 0b : unruptured aneurysm associated with neurological deficit.
Grade Ia : asymptomatic following subarachnoid haemorrhage.
Grade Ib : alert and orientated, no meningism, but focal, pronounced neurological deficit following subarachnoid haemorrhage.
Grade IIa : alert, but with headache and meningism following subarachnoid haemorrhage.
Grade IIb : as IIa but with focal neurological deficit following subarachnoid haemorrhage.
Grade IIIa : lethargic, confused, disorientated, combative following subarachnoid haemorrhage.
Grade IIIb : as IIIa but with focal neurological deficit.
Grade IV : semicomatose, responding to pain but not to voice following subarachnoid haemorrhage.
Grade V : comatose; pupils not reactive to light.

Postoperative results were grouped as follows:

Good : returned to same employment with no or minimal neurological defict.
Fair : returned to more limited employment because of moderate neurological deficit.
Poor : required supportive care because of severe neurological deficit.
Died : died within 30 days of operation or died of causes related to cerebral aneurysm.

Surgical results have been grouped according to preoperative grade since this more than any other single factor determines the outcome. In addition, different medical and technical problems are encountered in the separate preoperative groups.

**Table 1 Surgical results in anterior communicating arterial aneurysms**

| *Grade* | *Number* | *Good* | *Fair* | *Poor* | *Operative death* | *Death from other causes* |
|---|---|---|---|---|---|---|
| 0a | 2 | 2 | 0 | 0 | 0 | 0 |
| 0b | 2 | 0 | 1 | 0 | 0 | 1 |
| Ia | 82 | 82 | 0 | 0 | 0 | 0 |
| Ib | 0 | 0 | 0 | 0 | 0 | 0 |
| IIa | 150 | 146 | 1 | 0 | 1 | 2 |
| IIb | 66 | 60 | 3 | 1 | 1 | 1 |
| IIIa | 28 | 20 | 1 | 1 | 1 | 5 |
| IIIb | 27 | 18 | 5 | 2 | 2 | 0 |
| IV | 17 | 0 | 0 | 9 | 0 | 8 |
| V | 1 | 0 | 0 | 0 | 0 | 1 |
| *Total* | 375 | 328 | 11 | 13 | 5 | 18 |

## Grade 0b patients

One patient died; this was a 61-year-old man who presented with a visual field deficit suggestive of a chiasmal lesion, without history of subarachnoid haemorrhage. Carotid angiography unexpectedly showed a small aneurysm on the anterior cerebral artery. His operation was uneventful and postoperatively he remained in good condition. At the end of the second week he suddenly died from a pulmonary embolus. The autopsy did not divulge the aetiology of the optic nerve atrophy.

## Grade Ia patients

Of the 82 patients in grade I at the time of operation, all are well and working. Recovery was delayed in two of these patients, both of whom developed hydrocephalus postoperatively and required shunt procedures.

## Grade II patients

Of the 216 patients who were in grades IIa and b preoperatively, 206 have returned to their normal lives. Nineteen required ventricular shunting in the postoperative period. The two patients in grades IIa and b who died were both in their fifties and both died from delayed ischaemic complications. The three other deaths occurred in patients aged 63, 50 and 41 who had had uncomplicated operations for aneurysms on the left corner and midportion of the anterior communicating artery respectively. All three had smooth postoperative recoveries. The first patient died at home 5 weeks later, the second after 2 weeks just as he was to be discharged, and the third 3 weeks later. The cause of death in all cases was pulmonary embolism.

## Grade III patients

Of the 55 patients in grades IIIa and b, 38 have made good recoveries, six remain somewhat impaired but are self-sufficient, and three require supportive care. Eight patients died. Four of these were doing well after surgery but experienced rerupture of the clipped aneurysm with a fatal outcome. One patient died of pulmonary embolism. The sixth patient, a 54-year-old man, developed subdural haematoma. Following removal of the haematoma, the patient remained in a state of akinetic mutism with a left hemiparesis. He died 5 months after operation. Two of the grade IIIb patients with intracerebral haematomas had a fatal outcome. Both patients died from bacterial meningitis.

# 19a–e

Seven patients suffered recurrent subarachnoid haemorrhage following aneurysm clipping. The aneurysms, although arising from different parts of the anterior communicating artery, all bulged inferiorly and somewhat anteriorly, displacing the hypothalamic arteries. The aneurysms could be neatly dissected from the A2 segments and the neck was well prepared, but, despite many adjustments in clip position and every operative trick to eliminate the base of the aneurysm completely, in each case a small portion of aneurysm remained. To avoid sacrificing the hypothalamic arteries, the residual aneurysm was covered with muscle held in the clip by an acrylic bonding agent.

Three patients died at home, between 4 and 6 weeks after operation, of recurrent subarachnoid haemorrhage. Autopsy revealed that in each case the residual portion of aneurysm had enlarged and subsequently ruptured, causing intracerebral and intraventricular haematomas. The fourth patient survived recurrent haemorrhage at home and was readmitted in poor condition. Angiography showed no aneurysm, but there was severe spasm of the entire circle of Willis. Re-exploration proved that the aneurysm had ruptured again below the clip. The clip was moved to a better position, but the patient died a few days later.

In three cases, re-exploration of the aneurysm and application of a staging technique was successful.

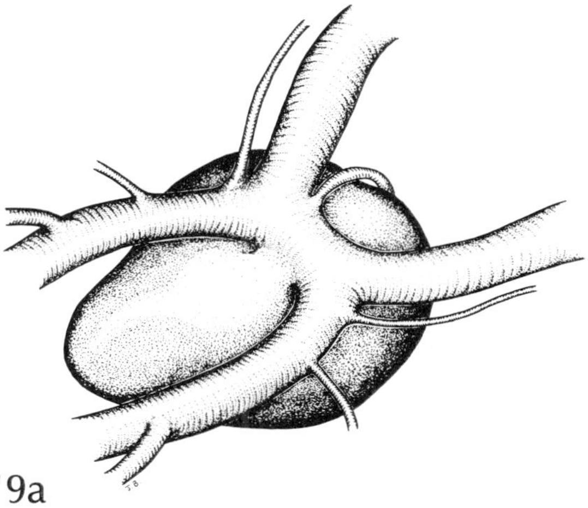

19a

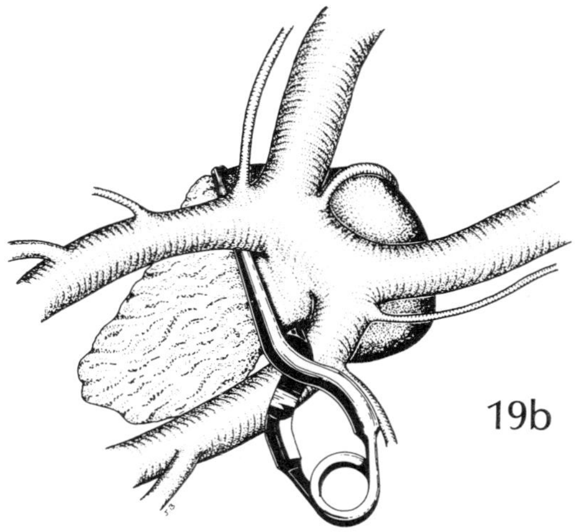

19b

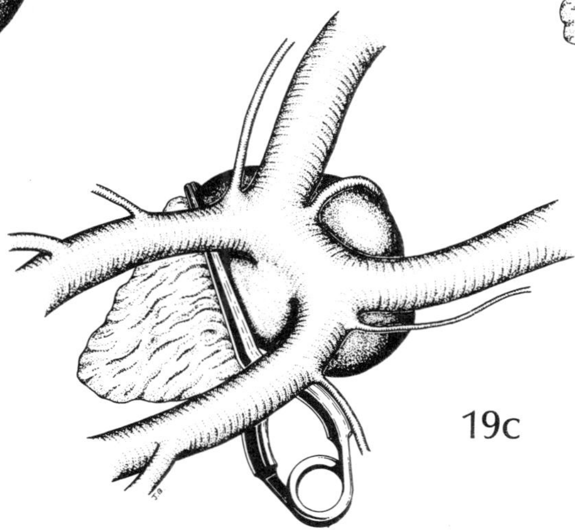

19c

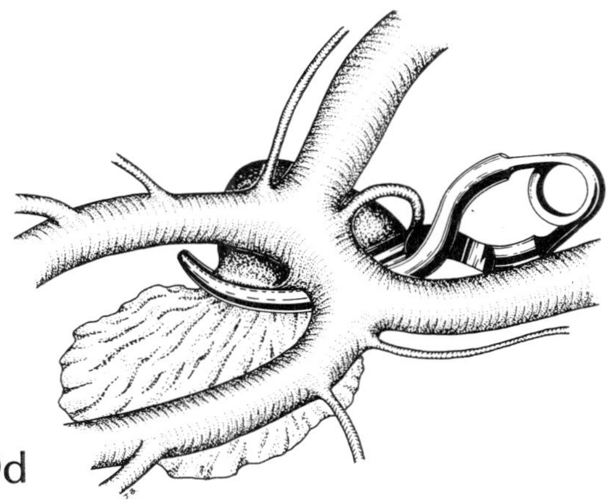

19d

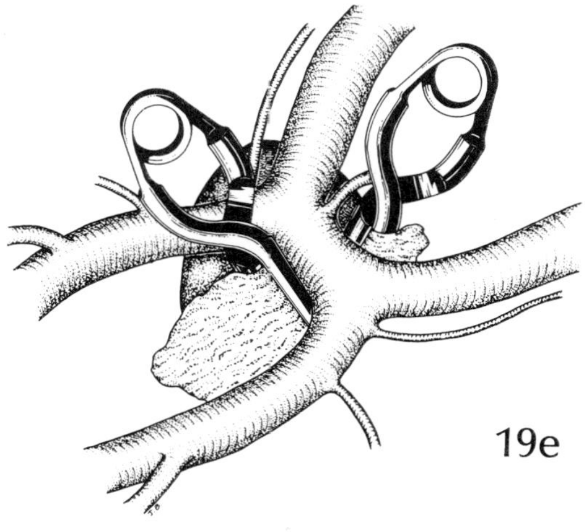

19e

### Grade IV and V patients

None of the 17 patients in grade IV at the time of operation made a worthwhile recovery. Thirteen of these patients had intracerebral haematomas. Nine (six with haematomas) remain in poor condition and eight (seven with haematomas) have died.

The one patient undergoing operation in grade V also died.

## SUMMARY

A total of 375 patients underwent operation for aneurysm of the anterior communicating artery between 1967 and 1980. Overall, 328 patients had a good result (87.5 per cent). In 286 (76.3 per cent) the postoperative course was entirely smooth and the patients were home in less than 4 weeks. In another 42, more time for recovery, ventricular shunting or other procedures was required before the patient could return to normal life. In 39 of these patients, delay was a result of inherent pathological processes, while in three operation played a part in slowing recovery.

Of the 23 patients who died, nine were moribund at the time of operation. Another four died of pulmonary embolism in the postoperative period. One patient fell from bed and suffered brain contusion. Of the remaining nine patients, four experienced rerupture of a previously clipped aneurysm, one suffered hypothalamic damage at operation, one developed cerebral infarction postoperatively, one developed a subdural haematoma, and two died of infection. This represents an operative mortality of 9/375 (2.4 per cent) and a gross mortality of 23/375 (6.1 per cent).

# Complications

### Intracranial haematoma

Five patients developed epidural or subdural haematomas in the postoperative period and one developed an intraventricular haematoma after the aneurysm ruptured again. Two additional patients developed subdural hygromas.

### Hydrocephalus

Approximately 12 per cent of patients required ventricular shunting. Various radiological procedures, including cisternography and computerized tomography, were used in evaluation of these patients. The clinical syndrome varied from lethargy to accentuation of focal neurological deficits.

### Seizures

Eight patients (2.1 per cent) developed transient and another eight permanent seizures in the postoperative period. All aneurysm patients are routinely begun on diphenylhydantoin preoperatively and this is continued through the postoperative period. Seizures were controlled by antiepileptic medications.

### Infection

About 1 per cent of patients had minor wound infections. One patient developed meningitis and in another an infected bone flap ultimately led to brain abscess. Patients in poorer condition frequently developed urinary tract infections, pneumonia or thrombophlebitis.

### Cerebrospinal fluid rhinorrhoea

One patient developed rhinorrhoea from an unrecognized opening into the frontal sinus.

### Psycho-organic syndrome

Thirty patients (8 per cent) showed changes in personality and mental function. In 6 per cent of cases this syndrome was present preoperatively and in 2 per cent it was first noted in the postoperative period.

### General medical complications

Pulmonary embolus, myocardial infarction and gastrointestinal haemorrhage occurred in some patients.

### *Further reading*

Yaşargil, M. G. (1984) Microneurosurgery. New York: Thieme Stratton, vol. 1, pp. 92–129 and vol. 2, pp. 162–231

Illustrations by Robert N. Lane

# Aneurysms in the middle cerebral artery

**Roberto C. Heros** MD
Associate Professor of Surgery, Neurosurgery, Harvard Medical School; Director of Cerebrovascular Surgery, Massachusetts General Hospital, Boston, Massachusetts, USA

Middle cerebral artery (MCA) aneurysms account for approximately 20 per cent of all intracranial aneurysms. About 80 per cent of these aneurysms arise in the area of the main bifurcation of the MCA. The majority of the rest arise from the main trunk of the MCA, either in relation to one of the perforating vessels or in relation to an early branch, such as an anterior temporal or a frontotemporal branch. A few aneurysms arise from one of the secondary divisions of the MCA or more distally from one of the cortical branches. In the latter case it is important to consider the possibility of a mycotic aneurysm since true berry aneurysms are uncommon in these distal locations.

## Clinical features

The majority of MCA aneurysms present with subarachnoid haemorrhage. A few giant aneurysms in this location, however, present with clinical symptoms related to mass effect. Temporal lobe epilepsy is an occasional presenting symptom with these aneurysms, and headaches and papilloedema may occur as a result of increased intracranial pressure if the aneurysm reaches a massive size. Ischaemic symptoms such as transient ischaemic attacks and strokes due to intra-aneurysmal thrombosis with distal embolism or occlusion of one of the branches or the main trunk of the MCA occur occasionally with these aneurysms. Although ischaemic symptoms from unruptured intracranial aneurysms are in general very rare, they do occur more commonly with MCA aneurysms than with aneurysms in other locations.

Rupture of an MCA aneurysm results in a syndrome which is usually indistinguishable from that associated with subarachnoid haemorrhage from rupture of aneurysms in other locations. With MCA aneurysms, however, specific local symptoms are seen more frequently than with other aneurysms. About one-third of patients with a ruptured MCA aneurysm have primarily unilateral headache, which is then always on the side of the aneurysm. Focal neurological deficits also occur more frequently with rupture of MCA aneurysms than with rupture of aneurysms elsewhere. These focal deficits are usually due to intracerebral haematomas which, again, are more commonly seen with MCA aneurysms. These haematomas, particularly when they occur in the temporal lobe, frequently require emergency evacuation because of the mass effect and incipient herniation. Because the haematoma is often peripheral, these patients tend to respond well to evacuation, in contradistinction to patients with haematomas caused by aneurysms in more central locations, which do not usually lend themselves to safe surgical evacuation or have already resulted in extensive damage to central structures.

## Patient selection and timing of surgery

Patients with unruptured, asymptomatic MCA aneurysms which have been diagnosed as a result of neuroradiological procedures obtained for other reasons should be considered for surgery if the aneurysm is more than 7 mm in diameter and the patient is in good medical condition. It is now clear that the surgical morbidity and mortality in these cases justifies such an aggressive approach since the natural history of unruptured aneurysms indicates that they bleed at a rate of approximately 3 per cent per year. Giant aneurysms that become symptomatic should also be considered for surgery. Operations for these lesions can be very complicated, but in view of their very poor prognosis a surgical attempt, even though sometimes attended by considerable morbidity, seems fully justified in the majority of the cases. The specialized surgical techniques sometimes required to manage giant aneurysms will not be dealt with in detail in this chapter.

The controversy about whether to operate early or late in intracranial aneurysms remains unsettled. MCA aneurysms, however, because of their relatively peripheral location, are probably the one type of intracranial aneurysm that should be considered for early surgery, even by those surgeons who generally delay operation for more centrally located aneurysms. With MCA aneurysms, retraction need not be extensive and many can be approached through the superior temporal gyrus, which requires essentially no brain retraction (*see* later). In addition, there is commonly a haematoma in the temporal lobe, which again facilitates exposure without retraction after the haematoma has been evacuated. As indicated earlier, many of these haematomas produce symptoms from their mass effect and thus require early surgical evacuation. In these cases, it is imperative to deal with the aneurysm at the same time, as in our opinion the danger of leaving an unclipped aneurysm after the haematoma has been evacuated is too high. Again, exposure is easy after evacuation of the haematoma. When the patient is drowsy and there is no significant temporal haematoma, we assume that the intracranial pressure is elevated and prefer to delay operation, particularly if the aneurysm seems to be relatively complex from the surgical point of view. We also prefer to delay operation in giant aneurysms since the surgical manoeuvres required to deal with them may be complex. It should be pointed out that by 'early' most surgeons mean within the first 72 hours after subarachnoid haemorrhage. It usually takes that long for vasospasm to develop and it appears that surgery is well tolerated at this stage. If the patient is first seen after 3 days, it is best to wait until at least day 10, when the risk of vasospasm begins to subside.

# The operations

There are three basic surgical approaches to MCA aneurysms. The first involves opening the sylvian fissure from medially and following the MCA from its origin distally towards the aneurysm; the second involves opening the sylvian fissure peripherally and following the MCA branches proximally towards the aneurysm; in the third the aneurysm is approached by subpial dissection after resection of a portion of the superior temporal gyrus.

## MEDIAL SYLVIAN APPROACH

All aneurysms of the main trunk of the MCA should be approached in this way. This is also the best approach to other aneurysms when the main trunk of the MCA is relatively short (less than 15 mm).

### Position of patient

The patient is placed in the supine position with the head turned about 45° to the opposite side and tilted slightly backwards.

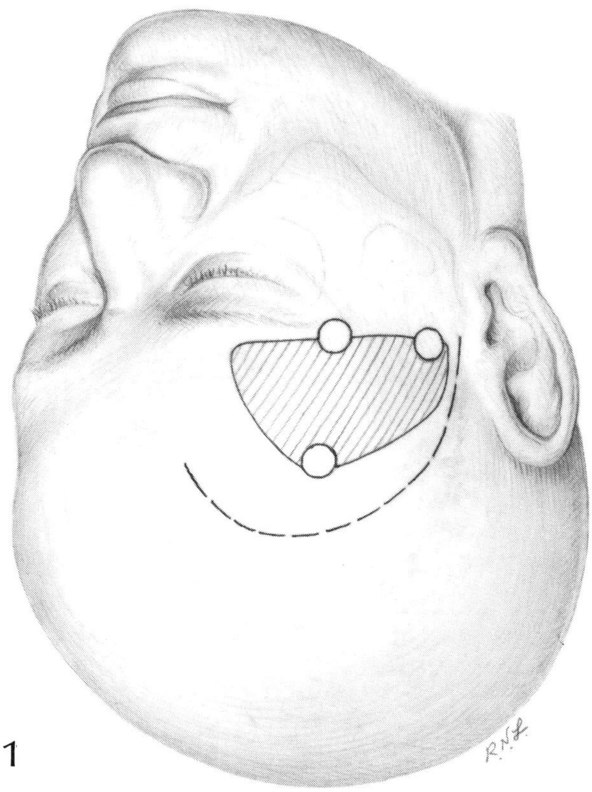

1

1

### The incision

A large curvilinear incision is made, starting at the level of the zygoma just in front of the tragus and then curving gently upwards and forwards to just beyond the hairline at about the level of the pupil in the sagittal plane. By starting the incision just in front of the tragus, both the facial nerve branch to the frontalis muscle and the main trunk and frontal branch of the superficial temporal artery can be spared. The muscle is turned down with the skin flap without being detached, except at its anterior insertion, which is very slightly separated from the fascia from within, just enough to allow retraction of the muscle down towards the temporal region to facilitate exposure of the area of the pterion. Again, by turning the flap in this manner, injury to the frontalis branch of the facial nerve is avoided. Three burr holes are then made: the first at the zygomaticofrontal recess (the 'keyhole'); the second directly posterior to it, on the other side of the pterion in the temporal bone; and the third on the frontal side of the superior temporal line, but far enough back to be behind the hairline so that it does not result in a cosmetic deformity. In older patients in whom the dura is difficult to separate, a fourth burr hole may be placed more frontally. (This can be covered with a plastic button at the end of the procedure to improve cosmetic appearance.)

Once the dura has been separated thoroughly, usually with a Penfield III type of dissector (Codman, USA), a free bone flap is cut with a high-speed craniotome. It is important to cut the flap for at least 1.5 cm in the frontal side of the pterion as low as possible against the floor of the anterior fossa before turning back to join the superior burr hole. The pterion is then flattened completely, using rongeurs and a high-speed drill. The keel of the lateral wing of the sphenoid bone is rongeured or drilled away down to the area where it becomes completely flat, which may require separating the dura almost all the way down to the anterior clinoid process. In this way, a completely flat approach to the base of the brain is obtained. The dura mater is then opened in a crescentic fashion, with the flap based inferiorly. The inferior aspect of the dura is tented upwards and held with sutures tied to the temporalis muscle. At this point, a hand-held retractor can be used to elevate the frontal lobe gently and allow cerebrospinal fluid (CSF) to drain from the medial cisterns. CSF usually flows spontaneously, but occasionally it is necessary to make a small opening in the medial arachnoid on one or other side of the optic nerve in order to achieve free flow (*see Illustration 2*). After 4 or 5 minutes of this manoeuvre enough brain relaxation is almost invariably obtained. A self-retaining retractor is then placed under the frontal lobe and, using a hand-held retractor, the temporal lobe is retracted gently, enough to see the draining veins from the tip of the temporal lobe which need to be cauterized and divided in order to allow retraction of the temporal lobe. The self-retaining retractor on the temporal lobe is then placed and the microscope is brought into the field.

# 2

The initial arachnoidal opening over the optic nerve and carotid artery is shown. The sylvian fissure is placed on stretch by retractors on the frontal and temporal lobes, which are opened much as the pages of a book. Frequently there is a vein crossing from the frontal to the temporal lobe medially and this should be cauterized and divided. In some cases the arachnoid plane in the medial aspect of the sylvian fissure is not easily definable. We do not hesitate then to resect a minimal amount of brain on either the frontal or the temporal side in order to gain access to the deeper portion of the sylvian fissure. Once the carotid bifurcation is exposed, the MCA is followed distally towards the aneurysm. It is important not to disturb the posterior superior aspect of the MCA since the small perforating vessels arise from this area. The artery should be followed along its anterior inferior surface and any occasional early branch carefully preserved. By progressively opening the retractors and gradually inserting them deeper and deeper into the sylvian fissure, the MCA can be followed with little difficulty.

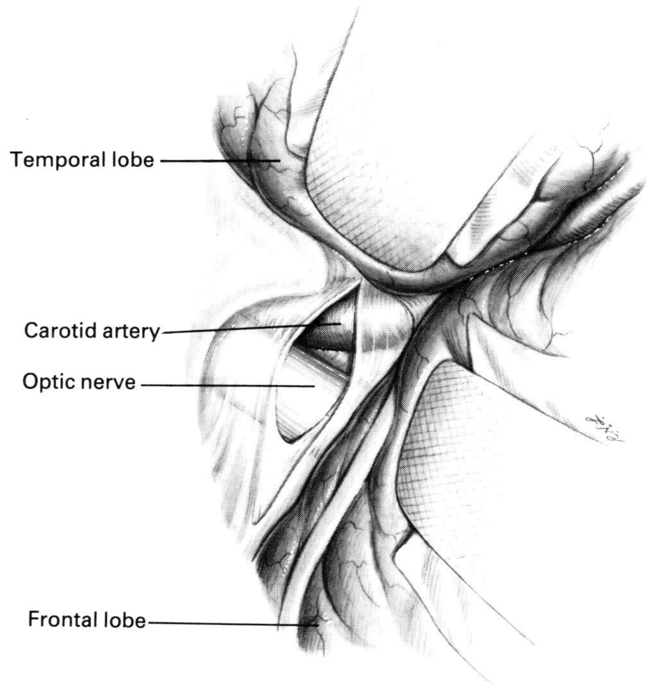


2

3

In patients with relatively small aneurysms of the bifurcation where the main trunk of the MCA is relatively short, it is usually an easy matter to separate each division from the aneurysm. We feel that in aneurysms of the bifurcation of the MCA it is necessary to dissect the entire aneurysmal complex. In our experience, angiographic appearance does not reliably predict the position of the divisions. An early branching of one of the divisions can occur behind the aneurysm and, if the aneurysmal complex is not dissected completely, this branch can be inadvertently clipped. Also, particularly in cases where the main trunk is short, important recurrent perforators to the lateral lenticulostriate area arise from the main divisions, and one of these could easily be included in the clip if the aneurysm is not dissected out completely. Usually we leave a small amount of brain adherent to the aneurysm in the area of rupture and proceed to dissect all the way around until the aneurysm can be moved freely in any direction so that it can be viewed from behind. It is necessary to move the microscope from side to side to inspect the posterior aspect of the aneurysm to best advantage.

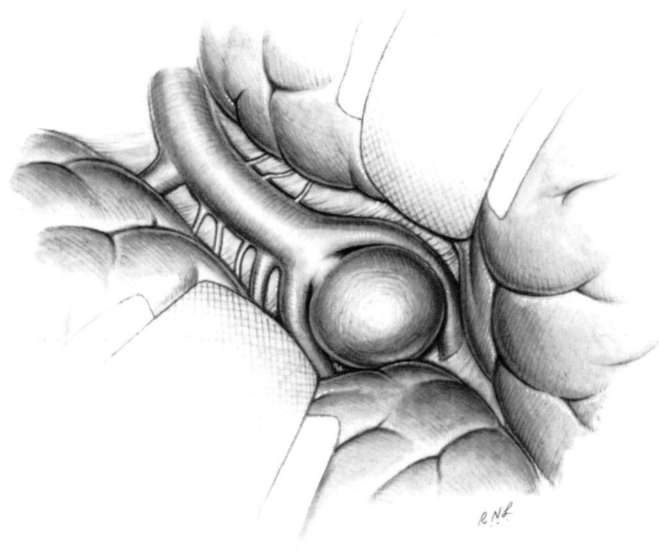

3

In some of the larger aneurysms of the MCA it may appear that one of the divisions comes from the aneurysm itself. Before the era of the operating microscope, such aneurysms were frequently wrapped or glued. This is almost never necessary today, except in cases of giant MCA aneurysms where the base of the aneurysm is so broad that the divisions originate at some distance from the area where the main trunk expands into the aneurysm. In ordinary non-giant aneurysms, what appears to be a division arising from the aneurysm can, by careful inspection under the microscope, almost invariably be shown to be simply a case of a very adherent division which, with careful sharp dissection, can be separated from the aneurysm right down to the neck. Fortunately, the aneurysmal wall is usually fairly hard at the base so that these divisions can be separated with safety from the aneurysm. Occasionally, however, a small tear is produced in this very dangerous area of the neck. This can usually be handled by tucking a bit of Surgicel (Ethicon, UK) into the area of the tear down towards the neck and then applying a clip over this, the clip itself pushing the Surgicel down against the crutch of the neck. During the last 5 years, we have not found a single aneurysm of less than giant dimensions in which a surgical neck capable of accepting a clip could not be developed. Once the neck is developed and the aneurysm has been thoroughly inspected all round, one of the standard aneurysm clips is applied. The aneurysm can then be punctured with a small needle to ensure that clipping has been adequate.

Early in our experience, we used systemic hypotension with mean pressures of about 60–65 mmHg when approaching these aneurysms. During the last 2 years we have made increasing use of temporary clipping, using one of the specially designed low-pressure clips in the middle cerebral trunk for periods of up to 10–15 minutes, but usually not more than 3–4 minutes during the final critical stages of dissection and clipping. We now prefer to use temporary clipping in order to soften the aneurysm and facilitate clip application whenever there is ready access to the afferent artery, which is almost always the case in MCA aneurysms. The temporary clip should be applied as distally as possible to preserve flow through the perforating vessels during the time of temporary clipping.

# 4

Aneurysms of the main trunk of the MCA usually arise in relation to one of the perforating lenticulostriate vessels on the posterior superior aspect of the middle cerebral trunk. The perforating arteries can be quite adherent to the base of these aneurysms, particularly on the proximal aspect of the base. All that is necessary is to separate these perforators enough in the area of the neck of the aneurysm to pass a clip between them and the aneurysm. It is important to inspect the neck circumferentially to make sure that there are no other perforators adherent to the posterior aspect of the aneurysm. It is not necessary in these cases to dissect the entire aneurysmal complex since the dome of the aneurysm is usually adherent to the frontal lobe and the only important vascular structures are at the neck of the aneurysm. However, particular care is required with frontal retraction, as this can result in rupture because the dome is usually embedded in the deeper aspect of the frontal lobe.

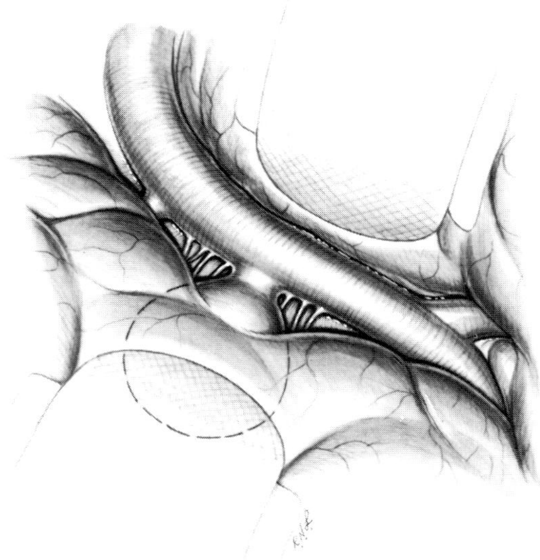

4

## LATERAL SYLVIAN APPROACH

In the more peripherally located aneurysms, which constitute the majority of middle cerebral aneurysms, many surgeons prefer to open the sylvian fissure peripherally and then find the distal divisions and dissect proximally towards the aneurysm. The position, incision and bone flaps are the same as for the medial sylvian approach. This approach has the advantage of facilitating exposure of the distal anatomy of the aneurysmal complex, which is usually the most difficult aspect of the case. The major disadvantage is that the surgeon reaches the aneurysm before achieving proximal control. This problem can be minimized, however, if, as soon as the aneurysm is seen, a bit of brain is left covering the aneurysm before continuing the dissection around the aneurysm to expose enough of the distal trunk of the MCA to achieve proximal control. The distal aspect of the sylvian fissure is sometimes not easy to define, particularly in cases of recent haemorrhage. A helpful manoeuvre is to pick a relatively large cortical vessel and follow it medially towards the fissure.

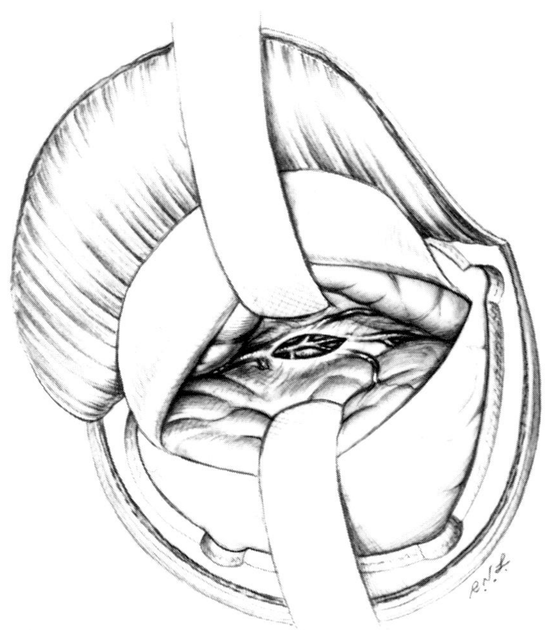

5

# 5

The arachnoid of the sylvian fissure is opened distally with a sharp hook or knife, and self-retaining retractors are then used on the frontal and temporal lobe to open the fissure. The retractors are gradually inserted deeper until a distal branch is found, which is then followed to the aneurysmal complex. The dissection of the aneurysm is as described above. Again, it should be emphasized that the entire aneurysmal complex should be dissected. As mentioned earlier, opening the fissure from distally facilitates this because the distal divisions, which constitute the complex aspect of the anatomy, are identified earlier and can be dissected with ease.

With this approach, there is a tendency to apply excessive frontal retraction since the aneurysm is usually located in a horizontal plane which is higher than that of the lateral aspect of the sylvian fissure. Great care must be taken to avoid such excessive retraction in the frontal operculum, particularly in left-sided aneurysms, because Broca's area is located directly under the frontal retractor. Some surgeons, myself included, therefore prefer to approach these aneurysms through a small resection of the superior temporal gyrus.

## SUPERIOR TEMPORAL GYRUS APPROACH

We approach the majority of aneurysms of the MCA through a small resection of the anterior aspect of the superior temporal gyrus. It must be emphasized that the superior temporal gyrus approach is not suitable for aneurysms of the main trunk of the MCA or for aneurysms that arise at the point of origin of an early branch of the MCA. It is also not suitable for aneurysms located at the bifurcation in cases where the main trunk of the MCA is relatively short. In all of these instances, the medial approach should be used. The position used for this approach is similar to that for the medial sylvian approach, except that the head is turned slightly more (60°) to the contralateral side. In order to facilitate this, a roll is frequently placed under the ipsilateral shoulder.

## 6

### The incision

The incision is started at the level of the zygoma just in front of the tragus, as discussed for the medial sylvian approach. The only difference here is that the incision curves slightly backward over the ear before starting the swing forward to a point just in front of the hairline and about in line with the pupil in the sagittal plane. The muscle is turned down with the skin flap as described earlier. The bone flap is also cut as for the medial sylvian approach except that the cut is extended farther back into the temporal bone, both posteriorly and inferiorly, in order to expose more of the temporal lobe. The pterion and lateral aspect of the sphenoid ridge are removed as for the medial sylvian approach. This step is important because only by flattening the pterion completely can the anterior aspect of the sylvian fissure be exposed, which allows dissection of the aneurysm and clip application from an anterolateral direction if this appears to be preferable. If the pterion is not removed completely, the surgeon is forced to work only from behind, underneath the overhanging bone, which may be a significant handicap.

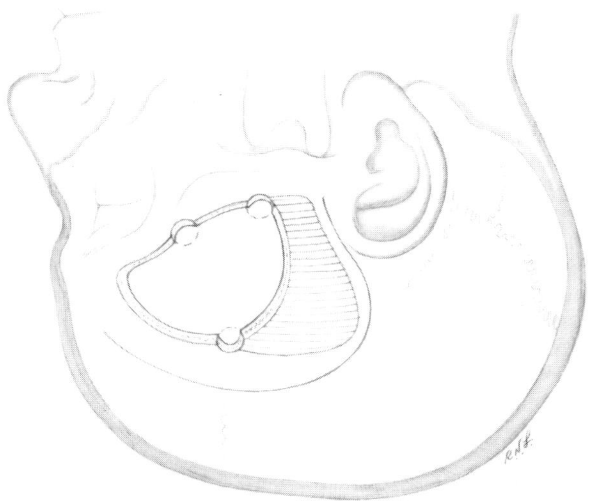

6

# 7 & 8

The dura mater is opened inferiorly in a crescentic fashion, with a perpendicular posterior cut along the sylvian fissure. With this approach, it is not necessary to open the medial cisterns to drain CSF since the initial exposure is achieved by brain resection and, once the sylvian fissure is reached medially, enough CSF drains spontaneously to achieve adequate exposure.

The incision in the brain is made just below the sylvian fissure in the superior temporal gyrus, for a length of 2–3 cm. It extends all the way to the front of the exposure and runs backwards parallel to the sylvian fissure. With suction and bipolar coagulation, the incision is extended medially into the vertical segment of the sylvian fissure over the insula. Here, one of the divisions can usually be identified through the pia. We prefer to follow this division forward by subpial dissection down to the aneurysmal complex, as shown. Once the aneurysmal complex is reached, the proximal aspect of the main trunk of the MCA must be identified. This may be done from behind or from in front of the aneurysm, depending on the projection of the aneurysm as well as its configuration. It is important, however, to do this as soon as the aneurysmal base is reached, before the entire aneurysmal complex is dissected, in order to achieve proximal control and to be able to place a temporary clip if necessary. It can usually be done safely by leaving some brain adherent to the dome of the aneurysm and retracting only its base sufficiently to see the most distal aspect of the MCA.

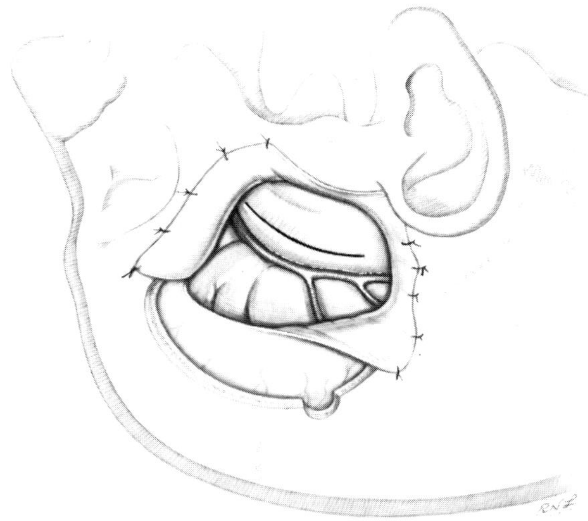

7

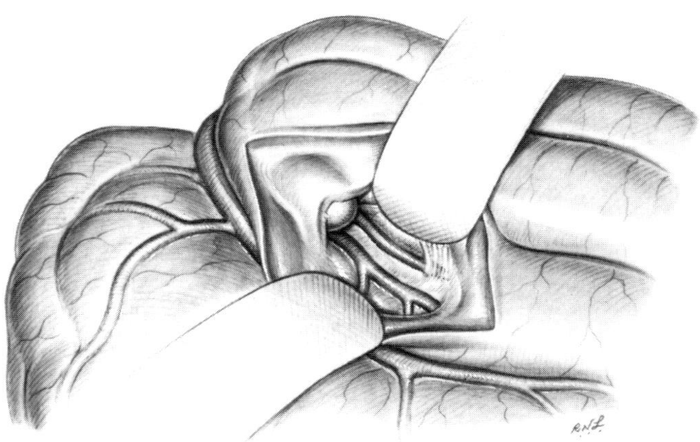

8

9

Once distal control of the MCA is achieved, dissection of the entire aneurysm can be carried out with safety. Again, it cannot be emphasized too strongly that the only way to ensure safe clipping of these aneurysms is to dissect the entire aneurysmal complex to prevent inadvertent occlusion of one of the branches. The separation of the main divisions from the neck of the aneurysm and the preparation of the neck for clipping have been described above.

The advantage of this approach is that it allows much easier access to the distal anatomy, which is usually more complicated. In addition, the clip can be applied from any direction, whichever is best in the case of a particular aneurysm. The most important advantage is that resecting brain in this non-critical area of the brain obviates the need for vigorous frontal retraction, which, as indicated earlier, can result in some expressive aphasia due to damage to Broca's area in left-sided aneurysms. The main disadvantage of this approach is that the aneurysmal complex is reached before proximal control is achieved. This, however, has not been a problem in our experience since, as soon as the aneurysm is seen, the dissection can be continued around the neck to expose the proximal MCA before the entire aneurysmal complex is exposed. It is also probable that most surgeons find this approach slightly more difficult than the medial approach since the anatomical landmarks are not as constant. With experience, however, this can be overcome. In addition, this approach may result in a slightly higher incidence of late epilepsy, although this has not been a problem in our experience.

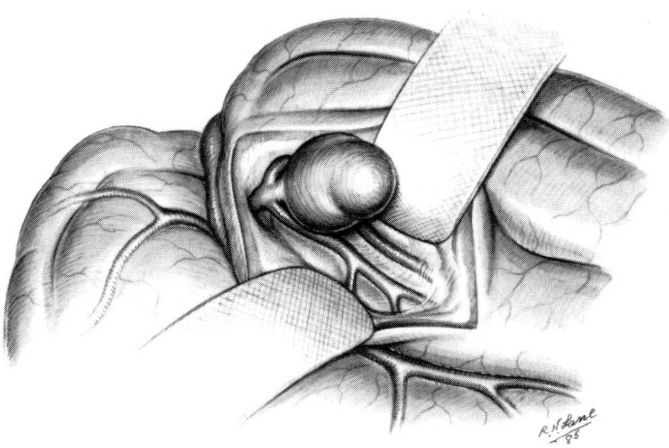

9

# Results

A total of 78 patients with MCA aneurysms have been operated on by the author, or under his supervision, at the Massachusetts General Hospital from 1983–1987. In this series there was a slight bias towards giant aneurysms, which represented 15 of the 78 cases (*see Table 1*). Almost all of these presented with symptoms related to mass effect rather than subarachnoid haemorrhage. Two were found incidentally. Of those with symptomatic giant aneurysms, two died and two had a poor result, which confirms the view that surgery of these lesions is difficult and dangerous. The fact that the majority of the patients with non-giant aneurysms who were in good preoperative condition remained well is a reflection of the fact that in this series the majority of the patients were operated on late. These are strictly surgical results and not 'management' results. We have not tabulated our figures for total management morbidity and mortality, but have undoubtedly lost several patients during the preoperative period because of rebleeding and vasospasm. During 1987 we have been operating on more patients and so far this has not resulted in increased morbidity, probably because we have only been operating early on patients who were in good clinical condition or who had a temporal haematoma. Undoubtedly, as we continue to operate on more of these patients early in an effort to improve total management morbidity, we will see a deterioration in our surgical results.

**Table 1 Middle cerebral artery aneurysms**

| *Preoperative grade (Hunt)* | *Number of cases* | *Surgical result* | | | |
|---|---|---|---|---|---|
| | | *Good* | *Fair* | *Poor* | *Dead* |
| 0,1,2 | 56 | 51 | 3 | 1 | 1* |
| 3 | 13 | 4 | 6 | 2* | 1 |
| 4 | 5 | 1 | 2 | 1 | 1* |
| 5 | 4 | 0 | 1 | 0 | 3** |
| Total | 78 | 56 | 12 | 4 | 6 |

* Cases of symptomatic giant aneurysms.
** All three had massive intracerebral haematomas

Illustrations by John W. Desley

# A surgical approach to aneurysms of the internal carotid artery

**Thoralf M. Sundt Jr** MD
Professor and Chairman of Neurosurgery, Department of Neurosurgery, Mayo Clinic, Rochester, Minnesota, USA

## Introduction

The surgical techniques described in this chapter have evolved from experience in the surgical management of over 1400 intracranial aneurysms. Of these, 525 were aneurysms of the internal carotid artery, and 40 per cent of these were either giant (more than 2.5 cm in diameter) or globular (1.5–2.5 cm in diameter). Because they comprise such a large portion of the author's experience and because they pose special technical problems, considerable attention will be directed toward the management of such large aneurysms. The techniques discussed are those which the author has found helpful and useful, and most of the data are based on personal experience or the experience of his colleagues and close associates at the Mayo Clinic. A list of selected references to the work of others in this field is given at the end of this chapter.

# The operation

## Position of patient

The patient is placed on the operating table with the head turned slightly to the side opposite the aneurysm. The head should be almost neutral and not hyperextended.

1

## Instruments

The fixation arm for the Yasargil retractor is mounted on the operating table and adjusted so that the non-contracted malleable portion of the retractor follows its natural course between the point of attachment of the arm and its support point or fulcrum (arrow). It is essential that the surgeon learn how to use the Yasargil retractor. In virtually all cases only one blade of the self-retaining retractor is required. Proper alignment with the malleable arm, which should stretch without torsion when loosened, permits the surgeon to control the retractor with minimal tension in the arm when contracted so that minimal movement occurs when the arm is loosened or tightened. The retractor blade should not be too stiff, yet should be firm enough to give the feeling of tension necessary to hold the cerebral tissue gently away from the operative field. Used properly, the retractor should serve only as a retaining device and not as a retractor, as the brain should fall away from the area of exposure by gravity and with only minimal pressure.

A malleable needle is used throughout except in unusual circumstances. In the author's experience, controlled spinal fluid drainage is preferable to mannitol, which, except for aneurysms arising near the caput of the basilar artery, is usually not necessary to allow adequate access to the base of the brain.

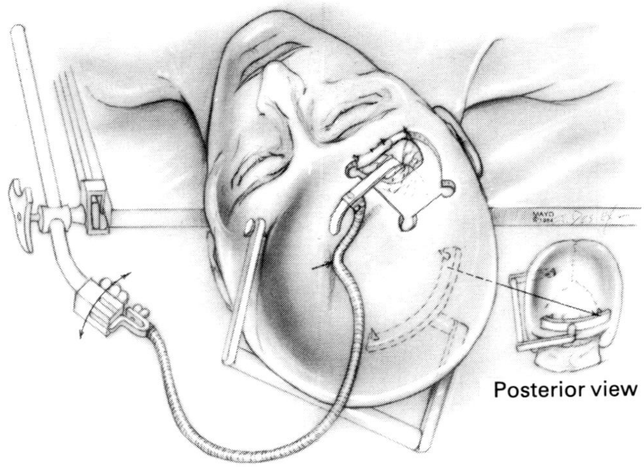


1

## Craniotomy

2

A frontal temporal craniotomy (modified pterional approach) can be achieved by either turning a portion of the temporalis muscle with the scalp flap anteriorly or turning the scalp flap separately from the temporalis muscle, as was initially described by Yasargil (see chapter on 'Anterior communicating arterial aneurysms' pp. 154–170). Although the latter gives slightly better exposure, the difference is not as significant as might be supposed, unless the brain is quite tight. Turning the scalp and muscle as a single flap is faster and, as pointed out by Rhoton (see chapter on 'Operative approaches to the lateral ventricles (supratentorial intraventricular tumours)', pp. 288–326, offers better protection to the frontal branches of the facial nerve. (Turning the scalp flap separately from the muscle can result in partial palsy of the frontalis branch of the facial nerve but this is usually reversible. In the author's experience, this method is less likely to cause atrophy of the temporalis muscle.) Whichever method is chosen, the frontal burr hole should be placed as close to the floor of the frontal fossa as possible and the burr hole directly over the keyhole (*see below*) or slightly inferior to it. The osteotomy between the keyhole burr hole and the posterior temporal burr hole can be made with the air drill (*see Illustration 4*), saving as much bone as possible to provide a firm floor for the temporalis muscle for cosmetic reasons.

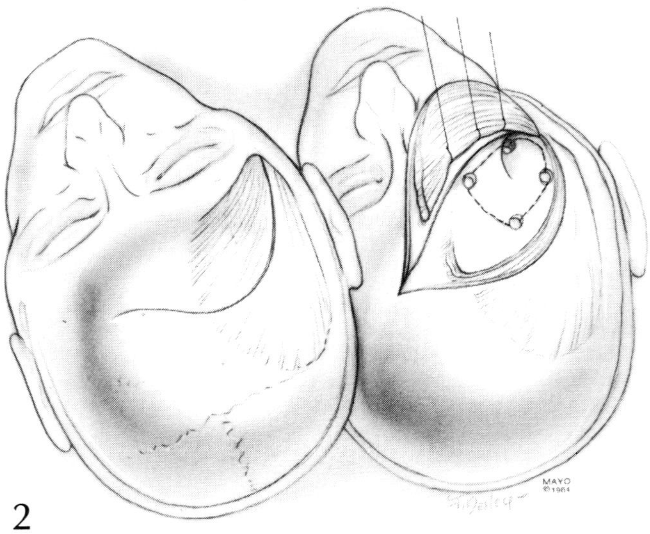

2

# 3

The scalp incision for both methods is the same. In cases in which the temporal artery might conceivably be required for a bypass procedure, the posterior branch should be spared; if this is inadequate, the anterior branch of the superficial temporal artery should be dissected off to be available in case of an emergency. Fortunately, this is seldom necessary in saccular aneurysms.

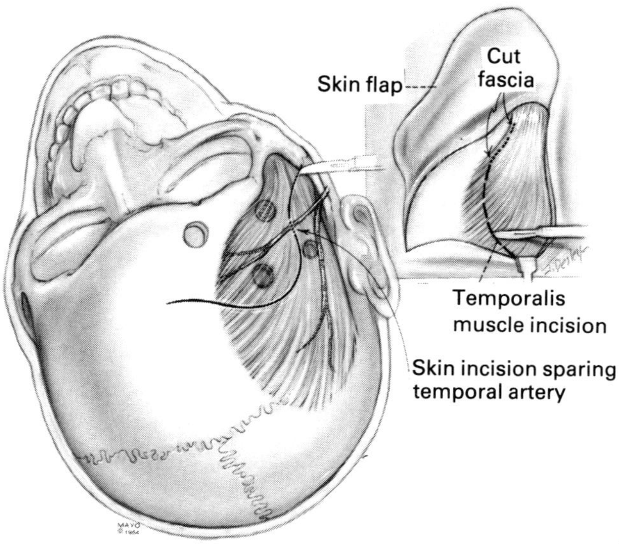


3

# 4

Whether the classic pterional approach or its Rhoton modification is chosen, it is essential to preserve the blood supply to the temporalis muscle. Atrophy of the temporalis muscle is not only a cosmetic deformity but leads to temporomandibular joint arthritis and postoperative headaches. Indeed, the commonest cause for headaches, in the author's experience, after surgery in this area is pain related to the temporomandibular joint; by carefully preserving the integrity of the temporalis muscle much of this pain can be prevented.

Once the muscle has been turned and the bone exposed, the burr holes are positioned. As indicated above, the frontal burr hole should be as low to the floor of the frontal fossa as possible to avoid a lip of bone interfering with the line of vision through the operating microscope. Exposure of aneurysms of the internal carotid artery with minimal brain retraction demands that the approach be along the floor of the frontal fossa and that there be no interference with the light source. Careful examination of skull X-rays usually permits the surgeon to place the burr hole slightly lateral to the frontal sinuses. If the frontal sinus is entered, it can be sealed with a flap of galea, and a spinal fluid leak can usually be prevented. The burr hole in the keyhole area should be placed just inferior to the pterion to allow some exposure of the temporal lobe for the dissection in the sylvian fissure. Wide exposure of the temporal lobe is not necessary, as it will remain undisturbed. Only the anterior superior margin of the temporal lobe needs to be seen so that the appropriate plane of dissection can be identified in the sylvian fissure.

The burr holes should be connected with a Gigli saw and not a craniotome, as the dura is frequently adherent to the bone in this area and a dural tear along the margin of the craniotomy must be avoided at all costs. The burr hole inferior to the pterion and that in the posterior area just below the sylvian fissure are connected with a high-speed neurotome (small air drill) in order to preserve as much temporal bone as possible in this region. This maintains the natural configuration at the floor of the temporal fossa and will restore the superficial appearance of the temporal area to its normal dish.

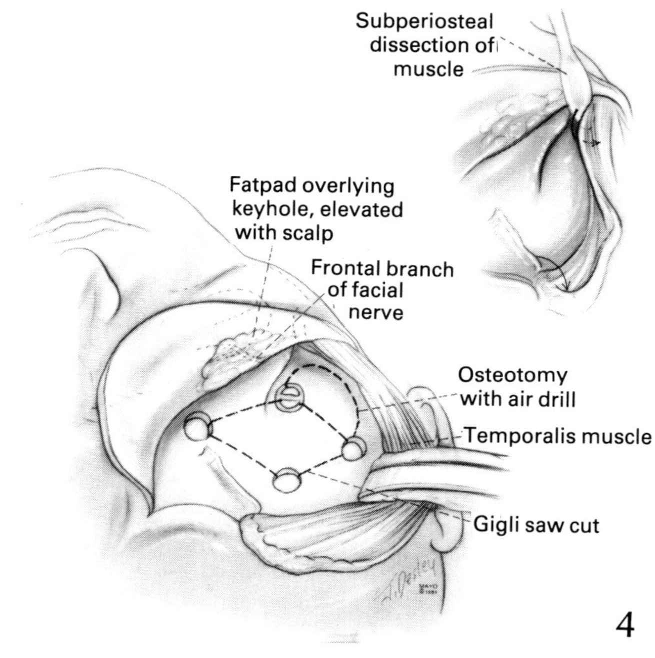


4

## 5

Once the craniotomy has been elevated, the dura is opened about 1.5 cm from the anterior margin of the craniotomy. The dural incision extends from the floor of the frontal fossa across the sylvian fissure and somewhat into the sylvian area. Small tack dural suture holes should be drilled before opening the dura, as soft tissue, including branches of the middle cerebral artery, could be sucked into the intake source when the air drill is used. The tack suture placed in the sphenoid wing after its lateral resection is particularly important. It permits the surgeon to tack the temporal dura to the frontal dura, thus removing much of the obstruction to vision that results from excessive dura overlying the sylvian fissure.

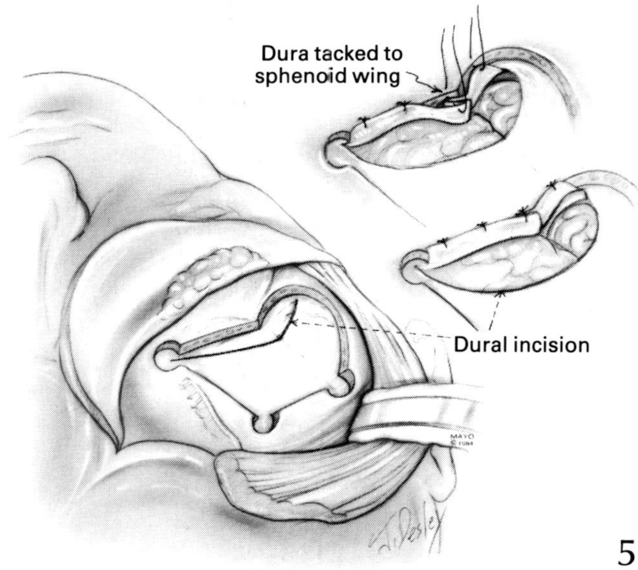


5

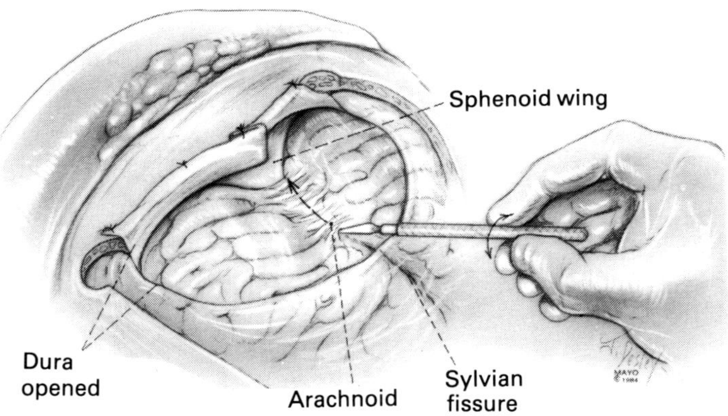


6

## 6

The arachnoidal plane of the sylvian fissure may be easy to develop or, as is typical in young people, be difficult to identify. The tip of a No. 11 blade knife is probably the best instrument to identify the correct plane and to incise the arachnoid. The plane can then be developed with bipolar forceps.

# 7

Allowing the forceps to open separates the arachnoid and identifies bleeding points, which are coagulated in virtually the same manoeuvre. Using bipolar forceps and microscissors, the arachnoidal trabeculations in the sylvian fissure are divided and small venules coagulated. It may be necessary to divide some large veins in the fissure as well. Fortunately, venous drainage in this area seems to be quite ample and in the author's experience there have been no known cases of venous infarction as a result of interrupting large veins in the sylvian fissure.

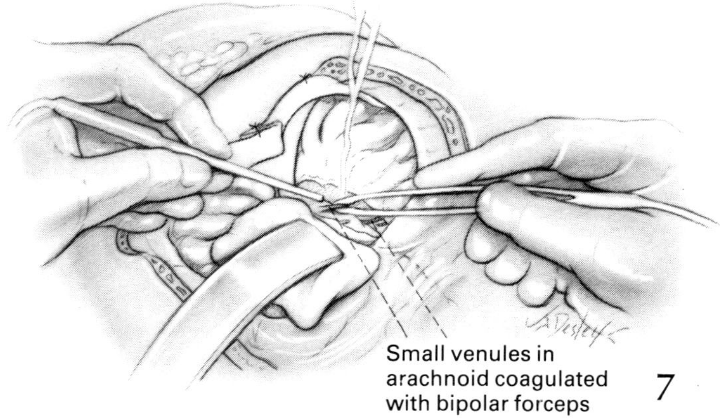


7

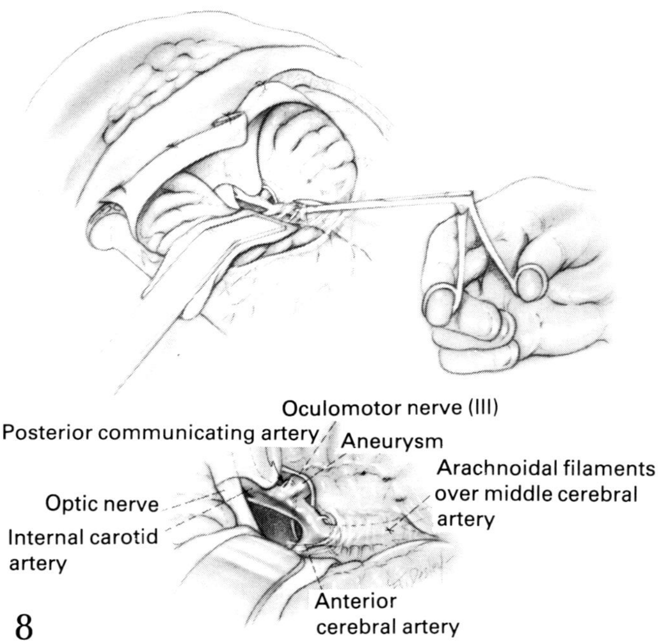


8

# 8

The arachnoidal incision is carried as far proximally as the area where the internal carotid artery divides. While it is not necessary to mobilize the middle cerebral artery, it is wise to leave some filaments of the arachnoid overlying it and not to 'skeletonize' the vessel. Preservation of these small arachnoidal filaments protects the vital perforating branches off the posterior aspect of the middle cerebral artery. Once the more superficial layers of the fissure have been divided, the single blade of the Yasargil retractor is placed gently on the frontal lobe and the traction adjusted by rotating the foot plate of the retractor blade. In most instances it is also necessary to release the arm at the base, as minor changes in the position of the fulcrum point are usually required to allow accurate placement of the blade.

After the arachnoid has been divided and the exposure carried as far medially as the area of the internal carotid bifurcation, the arachnoid overlying the optic nerve is incised with the tip of a No. 11 blade knife and the incision extended laterally, where the two arachnoidal incisions are joined. This permits good relaxation in the frontal lobe without disturbing vital structures in the area of the aneurysm itself.

The optic nerve is the anatomical landmark to which all other structures in this area can be related. Its early identification is essential.

## SACCULAR ANEURYSMS

Saccular aneurysms of the internal carotid artery commonly arise in one of four general locations, which will be considered in order of frequency: posterior communicating, ophthalmic, carotid bifurcation and anterior choroidal.

### *Aneurysms of the posterior communicating artery*

# 9a, b & c

In general, these aneurysms are best exposed by tracing the optic nerve proximally to its point of exit through the dural sheath in the optic canal and then working laterally from the optic nerve to the internal carotid artery on its dorsal medial surface. The aneurysm frequently projects laterally against the third nerve (*a*). In some cases, it is located so far proximally that it is necessary to resect the anterior clinoid process in order to obtain a good view of the anterior surface of the aneurysm. However, in general this is not necessary.

Although these aneurysms are perhaps the easiest of all aneurysms in the head to expose, they can be very difficult, particularly if bleeding develops before the entire sac has been identified. Very rarely in such instances one is presented with only a hole in the base of the internal carotid artery, and no sac to accept the clip. This will be dealt with in further detail below (*see Illustration 10*).

Almost invariably, these aneurysms project at an angle of 45° away from the direction of origin of the posterior communicating artery. It is essential to identify the origin of this artery and to preserve the vessel if at all possible since it carries vital perforating branches to the hypothalamus and in some instances serves as the primary source of blood supply to the posterior cerebral artery in patients with a fetal type circle of Willis. Using the microvascular dissector, the sac of the aneurysm is worked away from the origin of the posterior communicating artery and a plane of dissection created between these two structures (*b*). The aneurysm clip is then placed across the base of the aneurysm in a direction that preserves the origin of the posterior communicating artery (*c*). Once the aneurysm has been clipped, the posterior communicating artery should be inspected at its origin and traced distally under the internal carotid artery to ensure that it is free of the tips of the clip and has not been occluded where it is hidden from direct view by the internal carotid artery. It is wise to open the aneurysm after clipping to be certain that there is no bleeding.

It is seldom necessary to carry the dissection as far laterally as the third nerve. This merely inflicts more damage on the nerve in patients who already have a third nerve palsy as a result of the aneurysm.

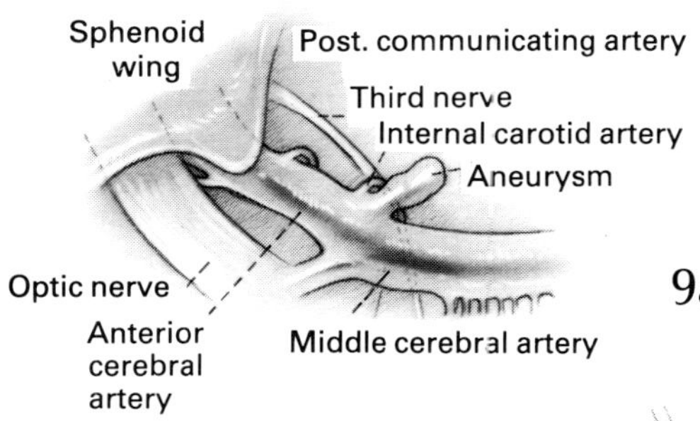


9a

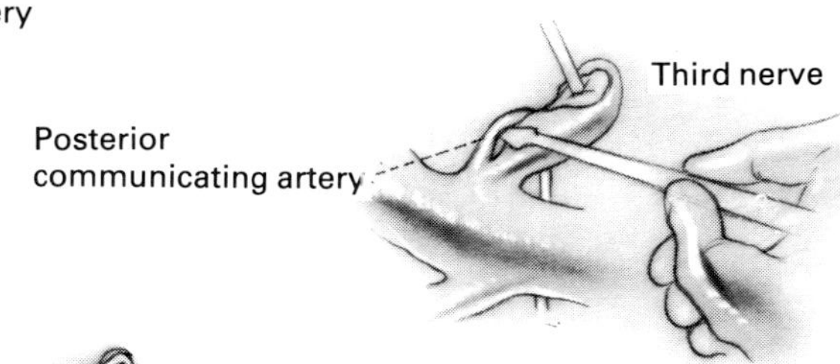


9b

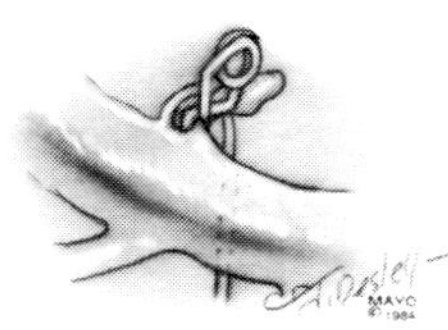

9c

# 10

Occasionally the sac of a posterior communicating artery aneurysm may be very friable and tear at its base, leaving nothing but a gaping hole in the wall of the internal carotid artery. In such cases, the artery is best repaired using a Sundt–Kees clip graft. This graft is available in diameters ranging from 2 mm to 4 mm and in lengths from 2.5 to 7 mm. For aneurysms of the internal carotid artery, a diameter of 3.5 mm is usually appropriate; the clip should be as short as possible to avoid encroachment on the origin of the anterior choroidal artery. Tears at the base of a very friable posterior communicating artery aneurysm usually involve the origin of the posterior communicating artery so that the vessel cannot be preserved. As noted earlier, a leash of perforating vessels to the hypothalamus arises from the posterior communicating artery, but fortunately in many patients there is sufficient retrograde flow from the posterior cerebral artery to supply these arterioles. Obviously, in these cases, preservation of the posterior communicating artery is of less importance than maintaining the integrity of the internal carotid artery. In the few patients in whom this type of repair has been necessary, there were no demonstrable ill-effects from occlusion of the posterior communicating artery.

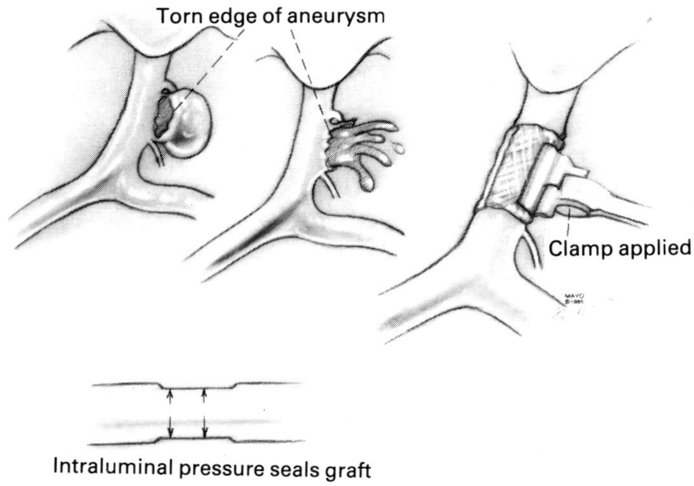


10

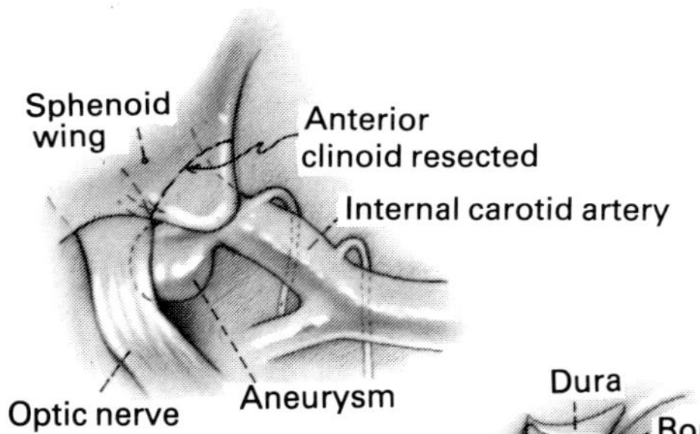


11a

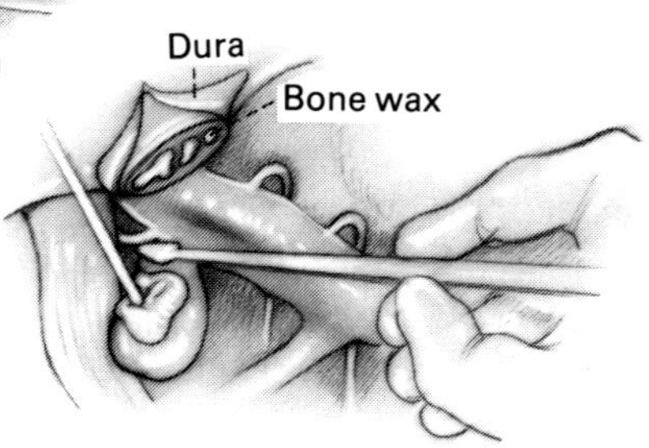


11b

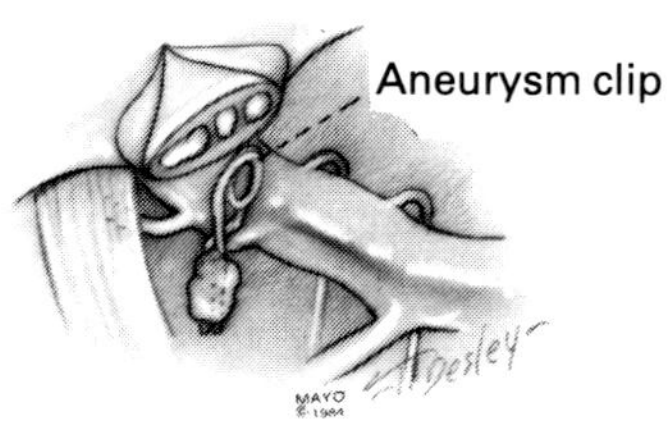


11c

# 11a, b & c

## *Ophthalmic aneurysms*

With most of these aneurysms it is necessary to resect the anterior clinoid process (*a*) to obtain a good view of the aneurysmal base. (For technique of resection *see* p. 189 and *Illustration 15*). Once the anterior clinoid has been resected, the internal carotid artery is traced proximally to the point of origin of the ophthalmic artery. A true ophthalmic artery aneurysm arises at an angle of about 90° to the long axis of the ophthalmic artery. However, many aneurysms in this area do not really arise at the origin of the ophthalmic artery but are displaced slightly in one direction or another.

Moderate hypotension is now induced. The base of the aneurysm is then dissected free from its fascial and arachnoidal attachments (*b*), and planes of cleavage are created anteriorly and posteriorly around the base of the aneurysm through which the aneurysm clip can be applied (*c*). In these patients under moderate hypotension, a small pledget held on the aneurysm sac with the suction unit can be used to manipulate the sac and isolate the base of the aneurysm. The aneurysm should be opened after it has been repaired.

# 12a–d

## *Aneurysms of the internal carotid artery bifurcation*

Aneurysms arising at the bifurcation of the internal carotid artery are particularly common in children. Although they arise at a point that is free of perforating vessels, the sac is invariably adjacent to perforating vessels, and in many cases these are adherent to the sac of the aneurysm. Standard microvascular techniques are used to prepare the aneurysm for clipping. These include: creation of appropriate cleavage planes in the tissue for passage of the aneurysm clip; compression of the aneurysmal sac with a small pledget held in place with a microsuction unit; and freeing of vital perforating vessels from the sac of the aneurysm. With these aneurysms it is not uncommon for the recurrent artery of Heubner to be intimately adherent to the undersurface of the aneurysm in a medial to lateral direction and for the anterior choroidal artery to be immediately subjacent to the inferior aspect of the aneurysm in an anterior to posterior direction (*a*). Small carotid perforating arteries can also be adherent to the base of the aneurysm. All of these vessels must be separated from the base of the lesion before it is clipped (*b*). After the aneurysm has been isolated, it is repaired with a standard aneurysm clip and then collapsed (*c*). This is particularly important with these aneurysms, not only to verify the adequacy of the clipping, but to confirm the patency of the small perforating vessels arising in and traversing the area of the aneurysm (*d*).

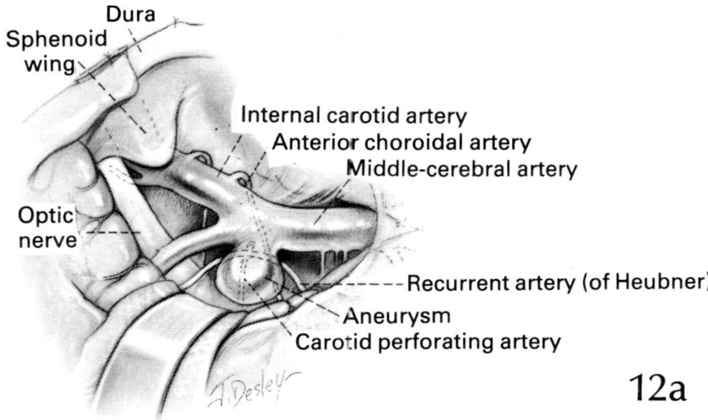


12a

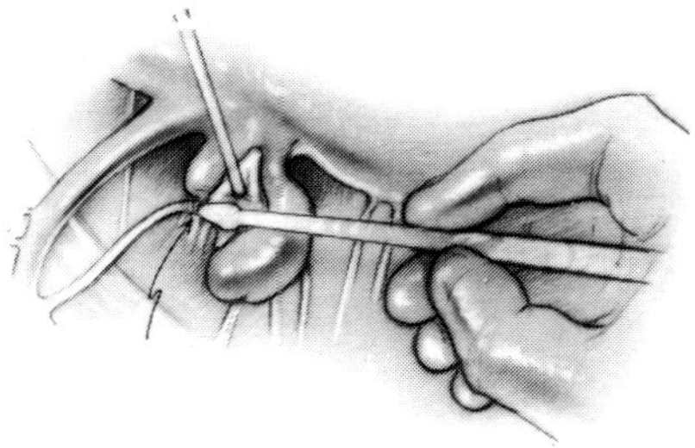

12b

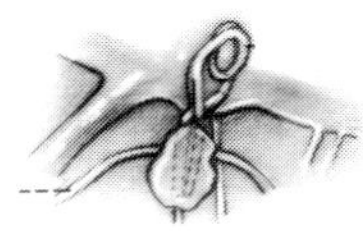

12c

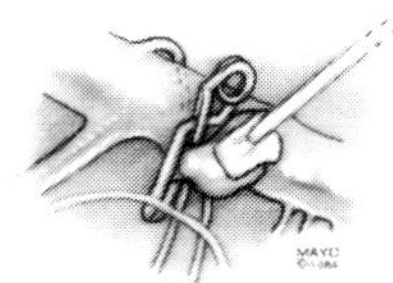

12d

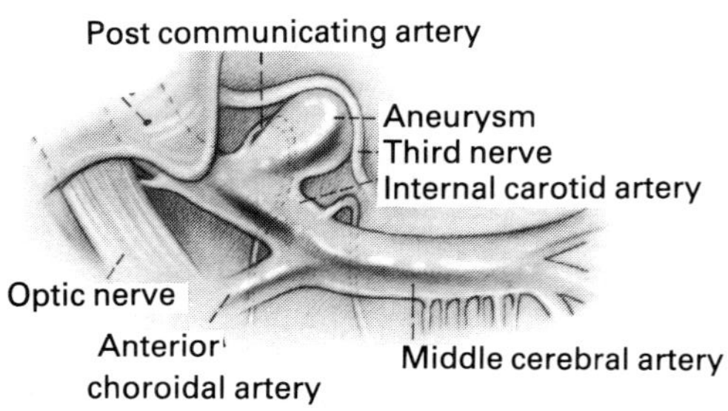


13a

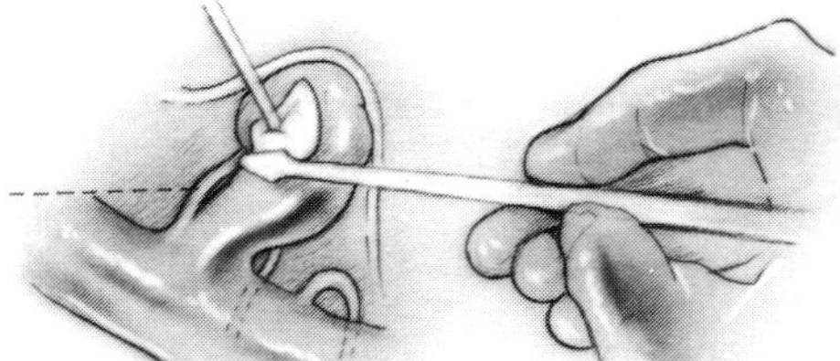

13b

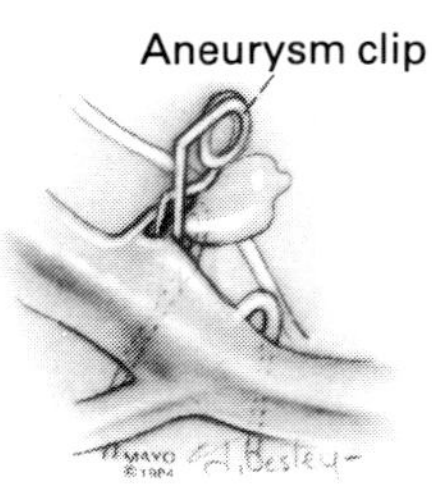


13c

# 13

## *Anterior choroidal artery aneurysms*

Aneurysms of the anterior choroidal artery are uncommon and can be very difficult to repair, as the integrity of the artery itself must be maintained under all circumstances. The anterior choroidal artery is a totally unforgiving vessel and, in the author's experience, occlusion will almost invariably result in a capsular infarct. Sometimes the anterior choroidal artery has two branches rather than one. In these cases, it is necessary to preserve both branches.

The techniques of dissection and repair are similar to those described for saccular aneurysms arising elsewhere along the internal carotid artery. The anterior choroidal artery runs slightly more laterally than the posterior communicating artery after it takes its origin, so that it is easier to trace its entire length after repair of the aneurysm than to trace the entire length of the posterior communicating artery after repair of an aneurysm arising near the origin of that vessel. The techniques for repair of these two aneurysms are similar.

## GLOBULAR AND GIANT ANEURYSMS ARISING FROM THE INTERNAL CAROTID ARTERY

# 14

The internal carotid artery is a preferred site for the origin of giant (more than 2.5 cm in diameter) and globular (1.5–2.5 cm in diameter) aneurysms. In our practice, globular and giant aneurysms accounted for 40 per cent of all aneurysms arising from the internal carotid artery. Thus, we have had a particular interest in the surgical approaches to these lesions.

Globular and giant aneurysms arising from the internal carotid artery can be divided into different categories according to the direction of their projection: superior, inferior, posterior, medial and lateral. The posteriorly projecting aneurysms usually involve the bifurcation of the internal carotid artery and are, in our experience, extremely difficult to repair directly.

We have used intraoperative cerebral blood flow measurements and continuous electroencephalographic monitoring to assess crossflow capabilities and thus the tolerance for temporary internal carotid artery occlusion in these patients, and have found excellent correlation between cerebral blood flow and electroencephalographic activity during temporary occlusion of the internal carotid artery.

The internal carotid artery is exposed through a transverse cervical incision. This incision is then temporarily closed, the electroencephalographic wires are removed, the head is prepared and draped in the usual manner, and the craniotomy is turned.

Normal cerebral blood flow under isoflurane (Forane) anaesthesia with normocapnia approximates 40 ml/100 g of brain tissue per minute. In most cases blood flow reductions to 15 ml/100 g of brain tissue per minute are tolerated quite well without electroencephalographic changes. Obviously, the length of time for which the internal carotid artery can be safely occluded is closely related to the adequacy of crossflow through the circle of Willis and over the surface of the brain in the leptomeningeal collateral vessels. If the blood flow falls below 10 ml/100 g per minute with internal carotid artery occlusion, both barbiturate protection and hypertension will be necessary during the period of temporary occlusion of the artery for the aneurysm repair.

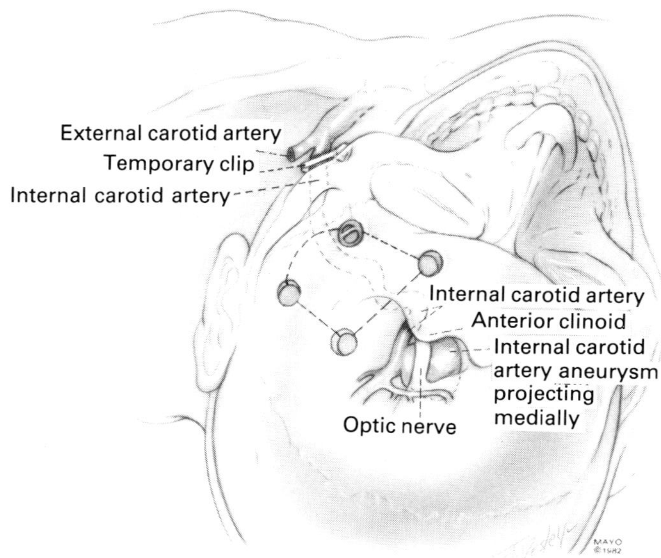


14

## *Aneurysms projecting superiorly and medially*

# 15

These aneurysms are exposed by a standard pterional approach in combination with a cervical exposure of the carotid bifurcation. Invariably, it is necessary to resect the anterior clinoid process. The dura overlying the anterior clinoid process is cut with the cautery unit and bone exposed for a distance of 4–5 mm (see *inset*). The bone is then resected using the high-speed air drill with a diamond bit. It is essential to remove all patties and loose particles of bone, etc. during drilling, as these could be sucked into the air drill with catastrophic consequences. Any patties which are left in the wound must be kept well away from the suction unit. Using the diamond bit allows the surgeon to resect the anterior clinoid process by 'feel'. The drill unit is held in one hand and a small suction unit in the other to clear the field of bone dust and blood from the bone itself and from openings into the cavernous sinus.

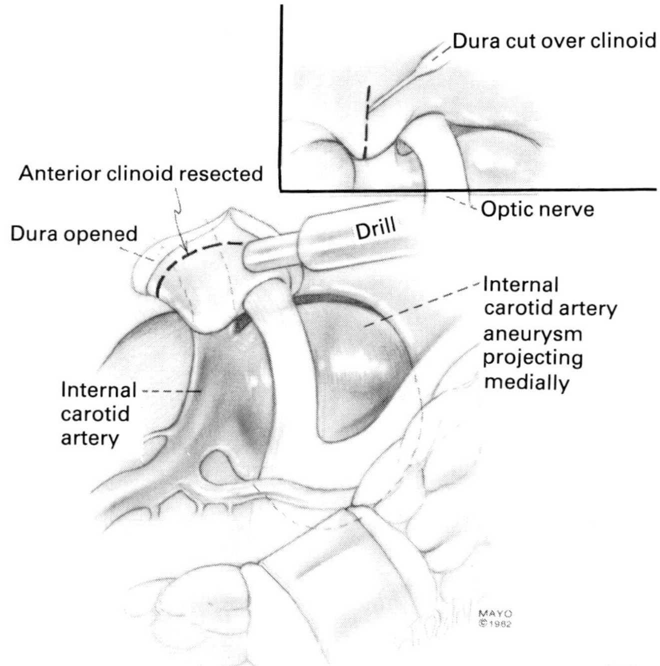


15

# 16

Once the anterior clinoid process has been removed, the anterior limit of the giant aneurysm can usually be seen. Appropriate planes of dissection are now created anteriorly and posteriorly around the base of the aneurysm using the aneurysm dissector. This should be done before applying the temporary clip to minimize the occlusion time. Occasionally, a giant aneurysm can be repaired directly, without being opened, but in the author's experience this is uncommon. In general, one must plan to occlude the internal carotid artery temporarily and to open the aneurysm.

The distal occluding clip should be placed proximal to the origin of the anterior choroidal artery if possible. The aneurysm is then opened with the tip of a No. 11 blade knife and a thrombectomy performed. This converts the base of the aneurysm to a pliable sac which will accept an aneurysm clip. It is not necessary to remove thrombus from the entire aneurysmal sac but only from the base of the aneurysm.

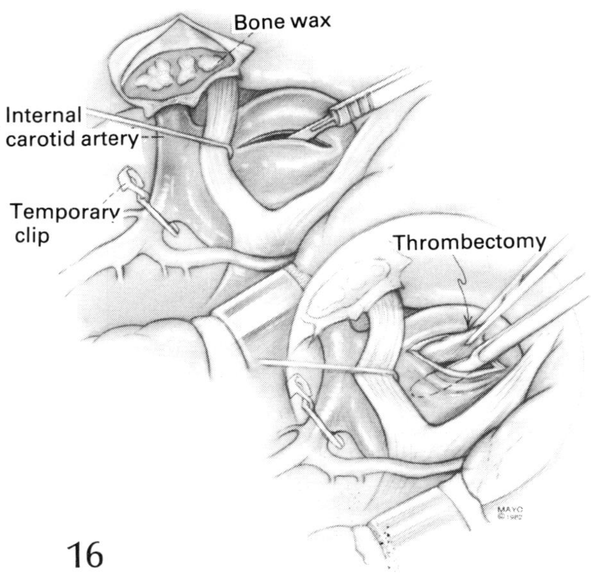


16

## 17

A conventional aneurysm clip is then positioned along the entire base of the aneurysm, leaving enough cuff of aneurysmal base so that there is no encroachment upon the lumen of the internal carotid artery.

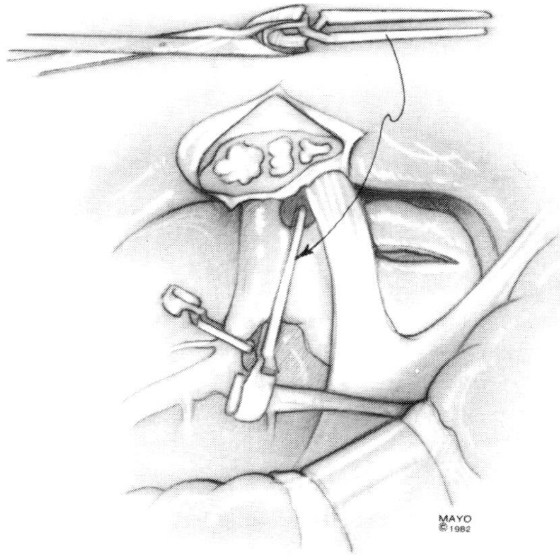


17

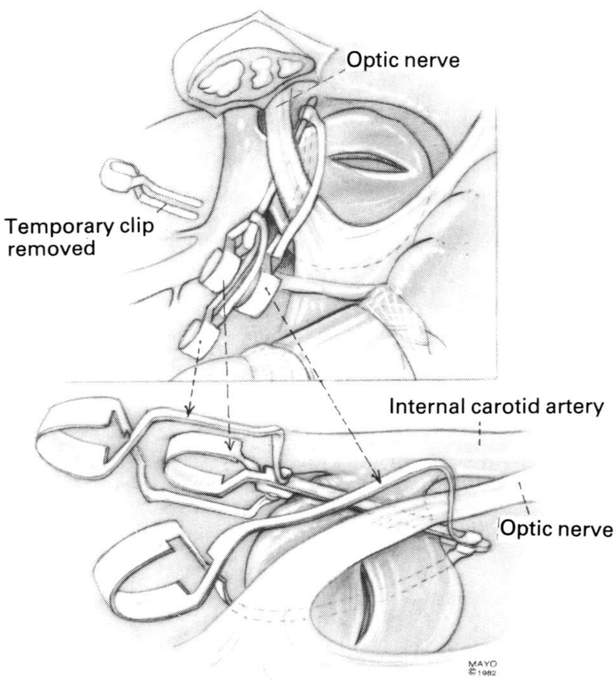


Enlarged view (medial aspect)

18

## 18

The extensile force in the base of these giant aneurysms is enormous and the author has found that conventional aneurysm clips lack the necessary tension to ensure permanent closure. For this reason, special booster clips have been developed with which to reinforce the aneurysm clip proximally and distally. After proper clipping of the aneurysm, the temporary occluding clips are removed to restore flow through the parent vessel.

# 19 & 20

## *Inferior projecting aneurysms*

Giant aneurysms projecting inferiorly are in general more difficult to repair than those projecting superiorly and medially, as it is more difficult to preserve the integrity of the anterior choroidal artery. Standard microdissection techniques are used to isolate the points of entry and exit of the internal carotid artery from the aneurysm. The vessel is then temporarily occluded in the cervical area distally. While the aneurysm is opened and decompressed the clips are appropriately positioned.

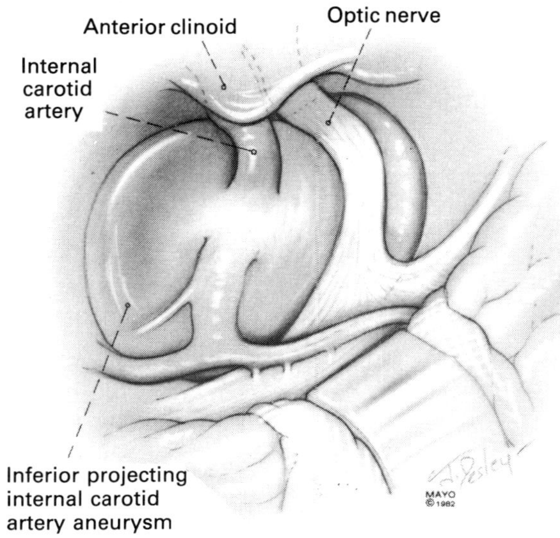


19

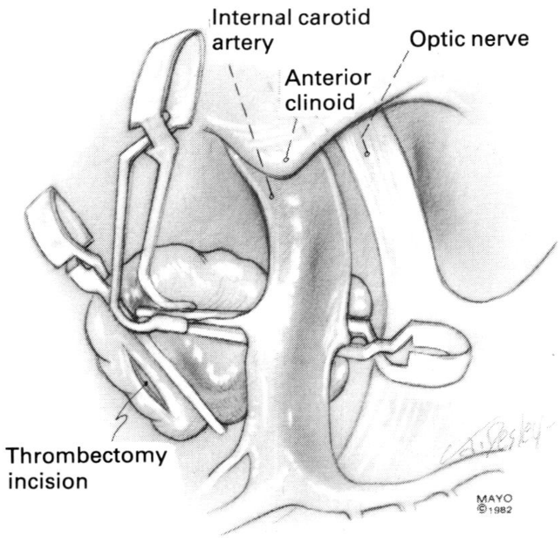


20

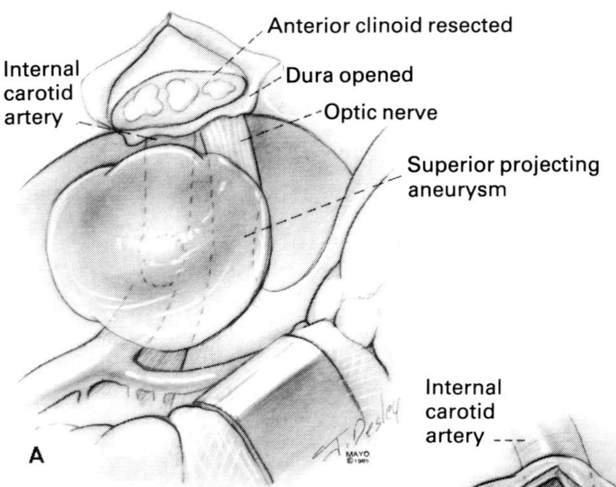


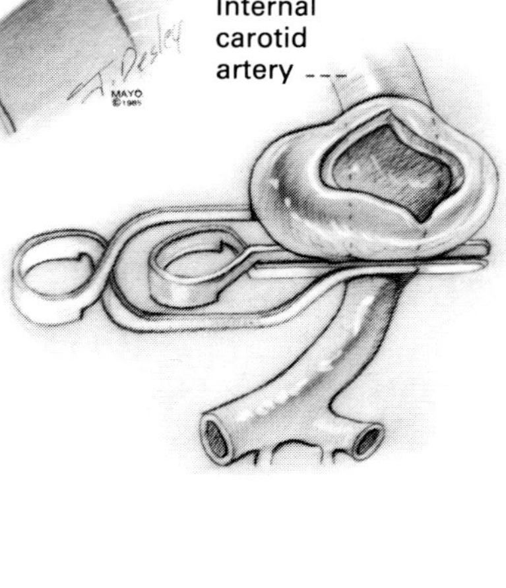


21

# 21

## *Lateral–superior projecting aneurysms*

Giant aneurysms projecting laterally pose major difficulties because both the perforating vessels and the parent artery are obscured from view by the lesion. In these cases it is particularly important to remove the anterior clinoid process and to isolate as much as possible of the internal carotid artery in the area of the siphon. Once the course of the internal carotid artery has been identified in the area of the cavernous sinus, the dissection is continued distally to uncover the important perforating vessels arising from this artery.

# 22

## *Bifurcation aneurysms*

Aneurysms arising at the bifurcation of the internal carotid artery are, in our experience, extremely difficult to approach directly. With growth, they have usually incorporated into their walls, at widely separated points, the origins of the anterior cerebral and middle cerebral arteries. Thus, it is virtually impossible to preserve the integrity of these vessels by direct repair of the aneurysm. It is recommended that these lesions be treated by a combination of internal carotid artery ligation and either interposition saphenous vein bypass grafting to one of the M-2 segments of the middle cerebral artery or a superficial temporal artery to a cortical branch bypass. The type of bypass selected will depend on the adequacy of collateral crossflow and the quality of the patient's superficial temporal artery. For high flows it is preferable to use an interposition saphenous vein graft.

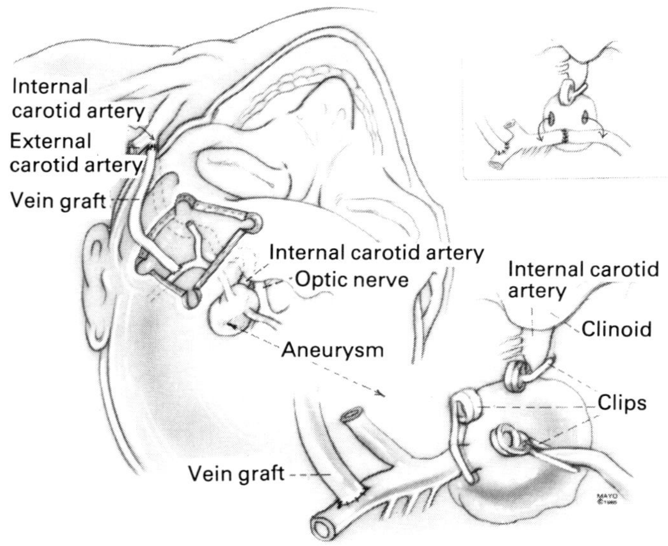


22

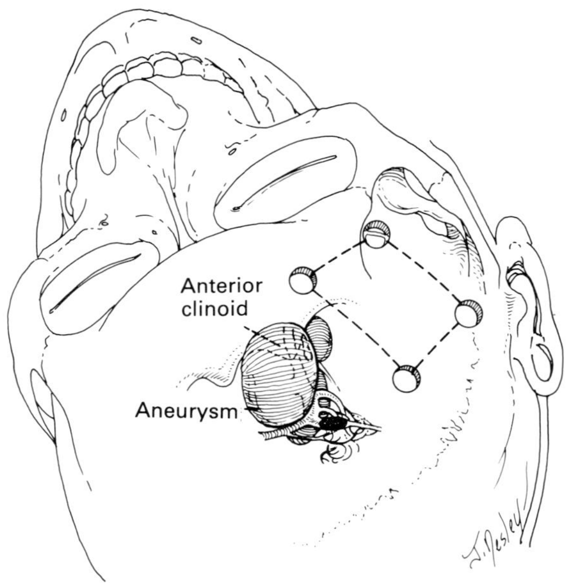


23

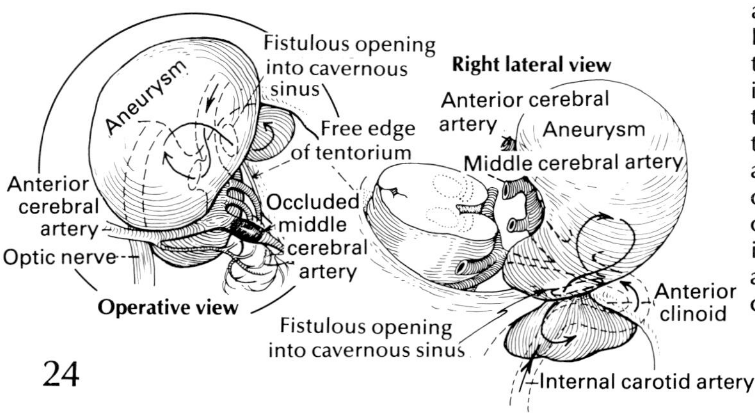


24

## FALSE ANEURYSMS

# 23 & 24

True aneurysms develop secondary to incomplete rupture or degeneration of the arterial wall whereas false aneurysms are the result of complete interruption of the arterial wall with formation of a perivascular haematoma which subsequently develops a fibrous wall by organization. In the perivascular area of the internal carotid artery, for example, a false aneurysm may develop in one of the arachnoidal compartments surrounding the artery if the membrane of that compartment has served to contain a haemorrhage from the primary vessel. In the case illustrated here, there was a coexistent fistula, but the approach to the false aneurysm would have been the same had there been no fistula. The internal carotid artery had already been ligated in the cervical area previously so it was not necessary to expose that vessel for temporary ligation.

The false aneurysm is exposed through a pterional approach using spinal drainage. The sylvian fissure is opened, and the right middle cerebral artery is identified and traced to its origin at the right internal carotid artery. In this case, the middle cerebral artery was patent up to the point of its origin just distal to the bifurcation of the internal carotid artery. A rete of small blood vessels from the artery of Heubner, the anterior choroidal artery and the posterior communicating artery had developed to anastomose with the striate arteries and anterior branches of the anterior temporal artery. Such small collaterals must obviously be preserved. The cross-filling from the left internal carotid artery was diverted entirely into the aneurysmal sac and fistula with no filling of the middle cerebral artery.

## 25

Under controlled hypotension to 70 mmHg, the thin-walled aneurysm is carefully dissected away from adjacent structures using the tip of a No. 11 blade knife and a cotton pledget. The right internal carotid artery is traced proximally, and the right anterior choroidal and posterior communicating arteries are identified. In this case, there was not sufficient room to apply an aneurysm clip without compromising the lumen of these perforating vessels. Hence, the segment of the right internal carotid artery feeding the aneurysm and fistula was doubly ligated with a 7/0 monofilament nylon suture. Both the right anterior choroidal artery and the right middle cerebral artery now appeared much larger and under better perfusion pressure than before ligation. There had obviously been a significant 'steal' into the aneurysmal sac and from there into the fistula.

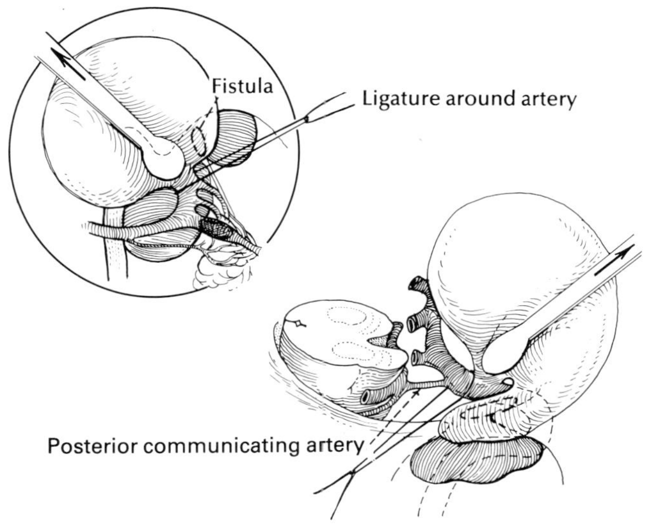


25

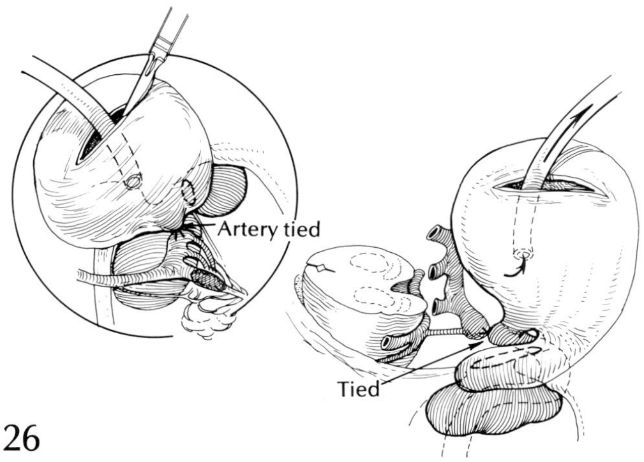


26

## 26 & 27

Opening the dome of the false aneurysm resulted in profuse bleeding from the cavernous sinus and ophthalmic veins. These venous bleeding points were identified and the bleeding controlled by packing with Surgicel (Ethicon, UK).

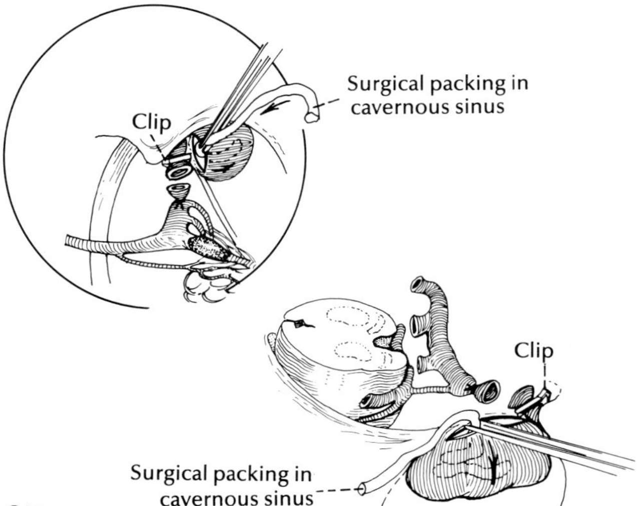


27

## *Further reading*

Drake, C. G., Vanderlinden, R. G. (1967) The late consequences of incomplete surgical treatment of cerebral aneurysms. Journal of Neurosurgery, 27, 226–238

Ferguson, G. G., Drake, C. G. (1980) Carotid-ophthalmic aneurysms: the surgical management of those cases presenting with compression of the optic nerves and chiasm alone. Clinical Neurosurgery, 27, 263–307

Hunt, W. E., Hess, R. M. (1968) Surgical risk as related to time of intervention in the repair of intracranial aneurysms. Journal of Neurosurgery, 28, 14–20

Lougheed, W. M. (1969) Selection, timing, and technique of aneurysm surgery of the anterior circle of Willis. Clinical Neurosurgery, 16, 95–113

Mullan, S., Hanlon, K., Brown, F. (1978) Management of 136 consecutive supratentorial berry aneurysms. Journal of Neurosurgery, 49, 794–804

Reddy, S. V., Sundt, T. M. Jr. (1981) Giant traumatic false aneurysm of the internal carotid artery associated with a carotid-cavernous fistula: case report. Journal of Neurosurgery, 55, 813–818

Rhoton, A. L. Jr., Saeki, N., Perlmutter, D., Zeal, A. (1979) Microsurgical anatomy of common aneurysm sites. Clinical Neurosurgery, 26, 248–306

Sugita, K., Kobayashi, S., Shintani, A. *et al.* (1979) Microneurosurgery for aneurysms of the basilar artery. Journal of Neurosurgery, 51, 615–620

Sundt, T. M. Jr., Whisnant, J. P. (1978) Subarachnoid hemorrhage from intracranial aneurysms: surgical management and natural history of disease. New England Journal of Medicine, 299, 116–122

Sundt, T. M. Jr., Piepgras, D. G. (1979) Surgical approach to giant intracranial aneurysms. Operative experience with 80 cases. Journal of Neurosurgery, 51, 731–742

Sundt, T. M. Jr., Sharbrough, F. W., Piepgras, D. G., Kearns, T. P. Messick, J. M., O'Fallon, W. M. (1981) Correlation of cerebral blood flow and electroencephalographic changes during carotid endarterectomy: with results of surgery and hemodynamics of cerebral ischemia. Mayo Clinic Proceedings, 56, 533–543

Sundt, T. M. Jr., Kobayashi, S., Fode, N. C., Whisnant, J. P. (1982) Results and complications of surgical management of 809 intracranial aneurysms in 722 cases. *Related and unrelated to grade of patient, type of aneurysm and timing of surgery. Journal of Neurosurgery, 56, 753–765

Sundt, T. M. Jr., Piepgras, D. G., Marsh, W. R. (1984) Booster clips for giant and thick-based aneurysms. Journal of Neurosurgery, 60, 751–762

Symon, L., Vajda, J. (1984) Surgical experiences with giant intracranial aneurysms. Journal of Neurosurgery, 61, 1009–1028

Weir, B., Aronyk, K. (1981) Management mortality and the timing of surgery for supratentorial aneurysm. Journal of Neurosurgery, 54, 146–150

Yasargil, M. G., Smith, R. D. (1977) Surgery on the carotid system in the treatment of hemorrhagic stroke. Advances in Neurology, 16, 181–209

Illustrations by D. Hutchinson

# Aneurysms of the posterior circulation

**Charles G. Drake** OC, MD, FRCS(C)
Professor and Chairman, Department of Surgery; Professor, Division of Neurosurgery, Department of Clinical Neurological Sciences, Faculty of Medicine, The University of Western Ontario, Canada

Isolated reports of surgical encounters with large posterior circulation aneurysms exposed under the impression that they were tumours have appeared in the literature since 1915. However, it was only in the late 1940s and 1950s that occasional deliberate surgical attack was described on ordinary ruptured aneurysms on this circulation. Initial results were gloomy for the most common aneurysms, at the basilar artery bifurcation, although it was evident that aneurysms along the trunk of the artery and those on the posterior cerebral and vertebral artery seemed more amenable to surgical obliteration. As experience expanded, improved results at the basilar bifurcation and continued good results with truncal aneurysms prompted description and illustration of the techniques used to deal with basilar aneurysms[1–3]. This chapter describes subsequent experience indicating that basilar and vertebral aneurysms have become as amenable to safe surgical treatment as those on the anterior circulation.

## Morbid anatomy

The incidence of aneurysms on the vertebral–basilar tree is estimated to be about 14 per cent (9 per cent basilar and 5 per cent vertebral artery)[4]. The commonest site for saccular aneurysms is at the basilar artery bifurcation (6 per cent of all aneurysms), followed by the vertebral artery at the posterior inferior cerebellar artery (PICA), the basilar–superior cerebellar artery and, with the fewest, the basilar–AICA (anterior inferior cerebellar artery) and the vertebrobasilar junction.

Hamby[5] described three varieties of aneurysm on the vertebral and basilar artery or their branches.

1. Large, tortuous, dilated, S-shaped atherosclerotic vertebral or basilar aneurysms.
2. Large, spherical vertebral or basilar aneurysms.
3. Smaller saccular aneurysms with subarachnoid haemorrhage.

Although Hamby considered the first two groups to present with signs of focal disturbance of brainstem or cranial nerve function, it is now clear that both may rupture spontaneously. Experience has shown that surgery has something to offer in the treatment of the large spherical aneurysms and even the occasional S-shaped aneurysms. The author has therefore modified Hamby's classification to correspond more specifically to the dimension of the aneurysm, recognizing that such classification omits important considerations in relation to the detailed anatomy of the neck of the aneurysm, the degree of atheroma and the extent of mural thrombosis in the sac. Aneurysms have therefore been classified as small (less than 12.5 mm), large (12.5–25 mm) and 'giant' (more than 25 mm). They will be described in this chapter under the anatomical relationships of the branching vessels from which they arise.

1. Basilar bifurcation
2. Posterior cerebral artery for first and second segments (P1 and P2)
3. Basilar–superior cerebellar artery (SCA)
4. Basilar–anterior inferior cerebellar artery (AICA)
5. Vertebrobasilar (VB) junction
6. Vertebral–posterior inferior cerebellar artery (PICA)

Less commonly, aneurysms arise at the sites of small unnamed vessels; these have been labelled according to the nearest named branch. A few aneurysms arise peripherally on the cerebellar arteries.

The critical size for rupture of posterior aneurysms (5–6 mm) appears to be similar to that in the anterior circulation, but intracerebral bleeding occurs only rarely with these lesions, and then into the third ventricle or temporal lobe from the top of the basilar artery.

## Natural history

The large fusiform S-shaped aneurysms probably arise on an atherosclerotic basis, but large bulbous and giant globular aneurysms almost certainly result from enlargement of small saccular aneurysms, and subarachnoid haemorrhage is not uncommon as a presenting feature or as a previous historical feature in their course. Numerous series of detailed follow-up studies of known vertebrobasilar aneurysms have indicated that their natural history is no more benign than that of their anterior counterparts.

## Clinical features

In general, small aneurysms present with subarachnoid haemorrhage (often under the influence of emotional and physical stresses), as do aneurysms of the anterior circulation. Initial minor warning leaks seem to be as common as vicious, recurrent bleeding.

There are few specific signs which would indicate a posterior fossa source of haemorrhage, although transient paresis of upward gaze has been seen after rupture of basilar bifurcation aneurysms. Third nerve palsy is commonly seen with laterally projecting basilar–SCA aneurysms, which should therefore be considered when carotid studies are negative in association with the IIIrd nerve palsy.

The VIth nerve is infrequently involved and the lower cranial nerves are rarely involved despite their proximity to ruptured vertebral or vertebrobasilar junction aneurysms.

The phenomena associated with vascular spasm are similar to those seen in the anterior circulation except that brainstem syndromes are more commonly featured. Arterial narrowing may occur remotely in the carotid circulation, where it may be associated with severe cerebral hemisphere oedema and ischaemia.

Enlarging posterior fossa aneurysms proclaim their localization through compression of neighbouring structures, producing various hindbrain syndromes. Tortuous atherosclerotic S-shaped aneurysms may compress neighbouring structures and may also produce recurrent brainstem ischaemic episodes due to partial thrombosis within them.

## Radiological diagnosis

The first neuroradiological investigation in patients with aneurysms of the posterior circulation, whether presenting with mass effect or haemorrhage, is usually a CT scan. In most cases, both non-contrast and contrast-enhanced scans of the head are appropriate to give the greatest information. Most substantially sized aneurysms will be shown on a contrast scan, as will the relationship of thrombosed portions of large aneurysms to portions that are still filling.

Angiography, however, remains the most important and definitive study for aneurysms, including vertebrobasilar lesions, in order to allow proper management decisions and operative care. The size and shape of the sac or sacs, the relationship of the neck to the parent and adjacent vessels, and any displacement of surrounding vessels, suggesting a larger mass effect, will be shown, as well as spasm in the post-haemorrhage cases. Overlying bone densities demand subtraction films in the majority of patients with posterior circulation aneurysms. Various oblique views and injection of both vertebral arteries when necessary provide sufficient information in most instances, although on occasion stereoscopy or angiotomography may be useful.

Routine views include a lateral and a Townes projection with a tilt of 30–35° to show the region of the foramen magnum more clearly. Oblique Townes views are sometimes needed but the head should usually be turned only 10–15° from the midline to avoid overlapping and distortion of the vessels. A true anteroposterior (Caldwell) view is often helpful to show an aneurysm and also to obtain a better view of the true relationships of the vessels to each other and to the aneurysmal sac. Basal views may also be necessary.

All studies should include demonstration of both carotid and both vertebral systems by selective injection so that the overlap of anterior and posterior circulations is avoided; transfemoral selective catheterization is the favoured route. Views with vertebral injection and compression of the carotid circulation will elucidate potential collateral supply to the posterior circulation through the posterior communicating artery. One should not be misled by streaming phenomena from a single vertebral injection which can be mistaken for spasm. Bilateral separate vertebral injections are usually sufficient to confirm the true size of the basilar artery.

Greater displacement of adjacent vessels than would be expected from the size of the opacified sac, and an irregular concave border to the aneurysm, may suggest that the sac is considerably larger than it appears. Correlation between angiographic and CT scan findings will allow understanding of the overall picture. If no source of bleeding has been shown following unequivocal haemorrhage, examination should be repeated in a week to 10 days' time. It is the author's practice to perform postoperative angiography in nearly all cases. There will still be occasions when the surgeon has an unpleasant surprise, although these are less frequent with magnification at surgery and routine aspiration of the sac following clipping. Cases of incompletely clipped aneurysms are more likely to have part of the neck remaining below a clip. Since the demonstration of remaining portions of a neck sometimes requires special views to avoid overlap with the clip itself, it is believed that intravenous digital angiography is insufficient to verify that all of the neck has been included in the aneurysm clip.

## Notes on technique and results

This review is based on surgical experience with over 1100 patients with aneurysms on the vertebrobasilar circulation. The overall results are given in Table 1, in three groups related to the size of the aneurysm. The particular results for small and large (bulbous) aneurysms are summarized in Tables 2–6 (which appear under the appropriate sections in the text). These have been divided into categories relating to site and projection, which are important at this stage in the evolution of the technical aspects of their surgical treatment. Giant aneurysms,

**Table 1 Vertebrobasilar aneurysms: results of surgical treatment***

| | *Number of cases* | *Excellent* | *Good* | *Poor* | *Dead* |
|---|---|---|---|---|---|
| Small aneurysms (<12.5 mm) | 715 | 560 | 79 | 48 | 28 |
| Large bulbous aneurysms (12.5–25 mm) | 195 | 125 | 36 | 25 | 9 |
| 'Giant' aneurysms (>25 mm) | 278 | 118 | 61 | 70 | 29 |
| | 1188 | 803 | 176 | 143 | 66 |

* Includes all grades and intervals from bleeding.

because of their special problems, are discussed separately.

Of most importance to the treatment of posterior as well as anterior aneurysms are the surgical adjuncts which have been developed to a fine degree in the last decade or so: brain relaxation, deep hypotension, magnification of vision and instrumentation.

A slack brain has always been important in providing room in which to work along the base of the skull. Now it can be provided almost routinely with the brain-shrinking agents mannitol and frusemide (furosemide; Lasix), and lumbar drainage of all the spinal fluid as the dura is opened. The significance of brain retractor pressure (BRP) is just being recognized, and it now appears that a BRP above 20 mmHg is associated with underlying ischaemia while a pressure near to 40 mmHg produces haemorrhagic infarction. Induced hypotension further aggravates the deficit in perfusion pressure. Soon, facilities for measuring BRP and local EEG will be incorporated into brain retractors so that the surgeon will be aware of the force he is using. It is probable that retractor injury has been much more significant than previously recognized.

The use of deep hypotension greatly reduces the stress on the aneurysm wall so that the aneurysm can be handled and dissected free of its connections with some boldness to reveal all the intimate connections at the neck for accurate occlusion without fear of massive rupture and its problems. A mean arterial pressure (MAP) of 40 mmHg is quite safe for an hour or more during the dissection and clipping of the aneurysm in otherwise healthy individuals who are not severely hypertensive.

Dissection of aneurysms has been facilitated particularly by the use of magnification of vision, first with loupes, now with the surgical microscope. With excellent coaxial illumination, even the finest details of the origin of the sac are revealed, allowing great accuracy in freeing the neck from branches (large and tiny), nerves and other adherences. In addition, now we have beautiful, fine, new instruments with which to perform these intricate dissections. Bipolar coagulation deserves special mention, for with it the neck of the aneurysm can be shrunk and rendered firm to reveal hidden connections and facilitate dissection and clipping. 'Baby' aneurysms, often no more than blisters and too small to be seen in an angiogram, are not infrequently discovered nearby and can be coagulated down to a thickened stump for packing.

In addition to these technical improvements, there has been a growing knowledge of the anatomy of an aneurysm. It is now known that most saccular aneurysms arise at the distal carina or 'crotch' of the branching of a major artery along the base of the brain. This means that in every site there are important vessels arising from or near the crotch which must be identified and preserved. They may be only the branches forming the crotch, but in most sites there are a few if not a host of tiny perforating vessels whose integrity is very important to the outcome.

The dissection must be carried to the very neck of the sac; under magnification and deep hypotension even sharp dissection can be used on the fragile wall to clear it from all these vital structures. The clip or ligature must be placed flush with the origin of the neck so that the arterial wall will heal firmly. Even a small portion of the neck remaining proximal to a clip has the potential of 'blowing out' to form another dangerous aneurysm. If the surgeon is not satisfied with the placement of a clip or if other structures are caught in the blades, it should be removed and replaced as many times as is necessary to obtain the ideal position. Admittedly, there are circumstances where a portion of the neck must be left to prevent kinking or to avoid injury to a dangerously adherent branch or hard atherosclerotic plaque. Then it should be packed with gauze or coated with plastic. If there is any doubt or if the sac has not been aspirated and collapsed to verify its obliteration, then postoperative angiography can help to assure the patient that the aneurysm is no longer a danger to him.

The extent and firmness of atheromatous involvement of the neck and parent branching are important. Ordinarily, 'soft' atheroma in the neck will conform to a clip or ligature, but 'hard' atheroma is dangerous because it may prevent the blades from staying in the ideal position and cause them to slide in on the artery or out on the waist of the sac. It is most dangerous if manipulation of the clip causes fracture of the atheroma and intima so that thrombosis may spread into the parent trunk.

Surgical ingenuity has known no bounds in the search for other methods of obliteration of aneurysms, such as plastic coating, or insertion of thrombogenic hair, wire or iron filings; however, the clip or ligature remains most effective for the majority of aneurysms. The other methods tended to be used if the dissection of an aneurysm had been left incomplete for fear of rupture or of obstructing branches arising from the sac. It is now known that the latter does not occur in saccular aneurysms except when they enlarge to the point that the parent branching becomes ectatic and forms the base of the aneurysm. Furthermore, it is now usually possible to clear the neck of the aneurysm safely for accurate and permanent occlusion.

## Choice of clips

Any good clip can be used for posterior aneurysms with a neck in clear view. The author tends to prefer the Sugita clip for most aneurysms: it is strong, has a reasonably narrow handle and clip applier, and exists in sufficient shapes and sizes and even with a bayonet design for clearer visualization of the blades during application in narrow confines. Not infrequently, a neck is shrunk down and firmed with coagulation so that a much smaller clip can be used very accurately. Because of the special problem of the larger bulbous basilar bifurcation aneurysms, a new clip was designed in 1969 with an aperture in its base to accommodate P1 (*see Illustration 11*). Because the blades used must be exactly the width of the compressed neck so that the opposite P1, perforators or IIIrd nerve are not caught in the tips, this clip is available in many lengths up to 24 mm for giant aneurysms. If the proper length is not available, a longer set of blades may be trimmed and filed for an exact fit. The fenestration at the clip base has been found to be very useful to enclose structures other than P1, such as nearby perforating vessels and (rarely) the IIIrd nerve. It has also been used for other aneurysms, and many other arteries – SCA, AICA, vertebral, basilar, carotid, M2 and A2 – have been accommodated in the opening. The long blades were reasonably satisfactory for very large-necked aneurysms and now the tandem principle, using one or more straight clips in tandem with a Drake clip, has solved the problem for most giant aneurysms with soft necks[6]. The Sugita modification of the Drake clip, with various angles and a larger aperture, has been most helpful. Since 1982, temporary clipping of the parent vessel, with clips specially designed for this gentle purpose (Klement-Kutz, Suzuki, Sugita), has been used more and more. A long Drake clip, whose handle has been sprung many times, is useful for deep-lying arteries.

## THE SUBTEMPORAL APPROACH

Aneurysms in the region of the basilar bifurcation, including those arising at the SCA, are exposed quite satisfactorily by an anterior subtemporal approach across the floor of the middle fossa and tentorial edge into the mouth of the incisura in front of the midbrain (*see Illustration 17*). Ordinarily, the right side is used unless the projection or complexity of the aneurysm, or a left oculomotor palsy or right hemiparesis demands an approach under the dominant temporal lobe.

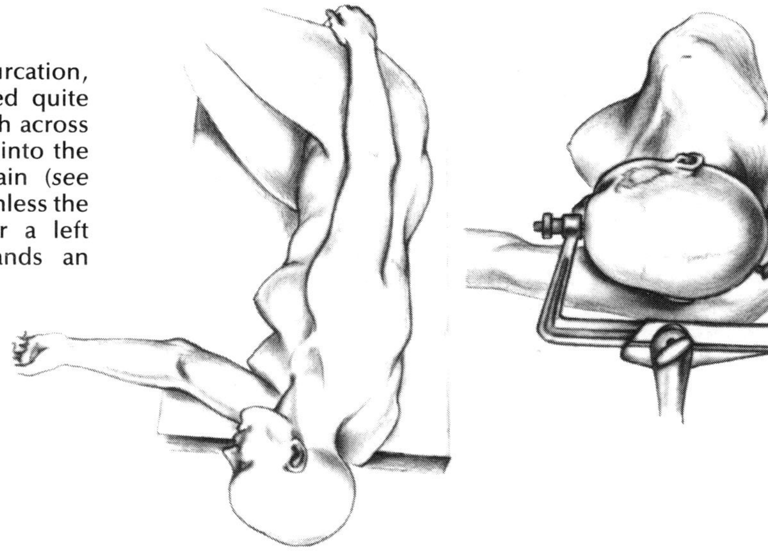

1

### Position of patient and incision

# 1–4

The patient is placed in the lateral decubitus position, with the head slightly flexed downward. A small subtemporal craniotomy through a linear incision as for the Frazier–Spiller operation for tic douloureux has been found quite sufficient and is now used routinely at University Hospital for most ordinary aneurysms in the region of the basilar bifurcation. It is important to remove the temporal squama down to and in front of the root of the zygoma in an inverted pear shape for better line of sight along the floor of the middle fossa. A temporal bone flap is now used only when it appears necessary to divide the inner third of the tentorium for a low-lying basilar bifurcation or superior cerebellar aneurysm, or to see and clear enough of the basilar artery for a temporary clip. Even so, the scalp should be prepared so that either a temporal flap may be turned posteriorly or a frontotemporal flap anteriorly if conversion to a pterional trans-sylvian exposure in combination seems necessary.

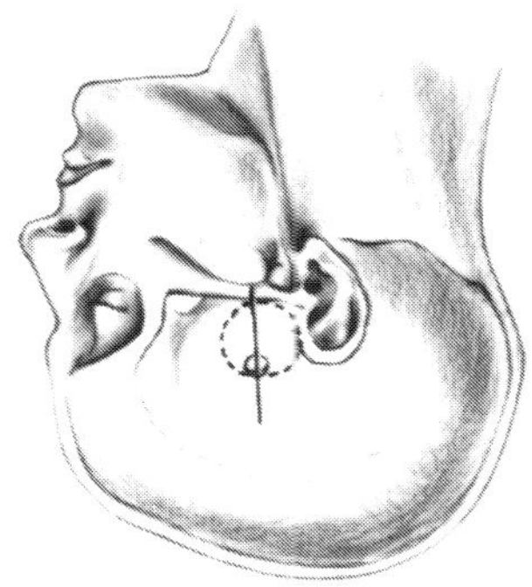

2

Normally, a week or more after bleeding, the brain will be very slack after mannitol, furosemide and lumbar drainage of all the spinal fluid as the dura is being opened so that very little brain retractor pressure will be needed to elevate the anterior temporal lobe out of the floor of the middle fossa. In the author's experience it has never been necessary to resect any portion of the temporal lobe. In recent years, it has been found that even during acute or early surgery a similar slackness can be obtained. Any large inferior temporal arteries should be protected and spared if possible. The vein of Labbé must be identified, protected with absorbable gelatin sponge, and spared. A sheet of compressed, moist gelatin sponge is used to cover the brain, for, if irrigated, it does not adhere to the brain even after several hours of retraction. The surgical microscope may now be moved into position. Most of the dissection can be done under ×10 or ×16 magnification but higher powers may be advisable for critical sharp dissection.

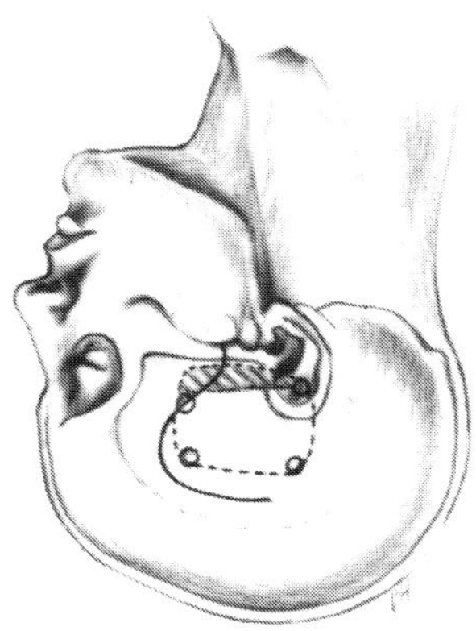

3

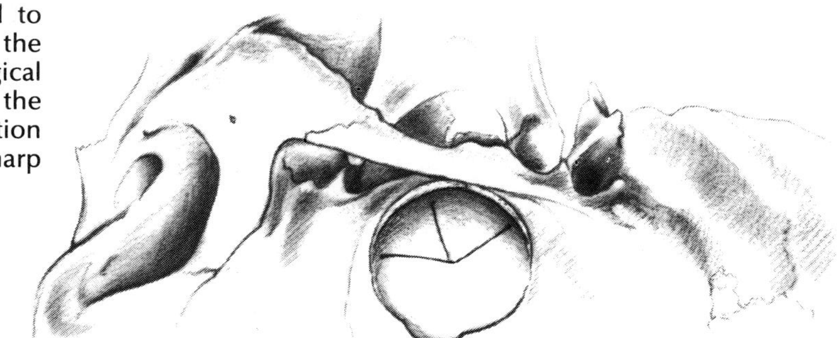

4

# 5

As the edge of the tentorium comes into view, the uncus will be seen disengaging from its position inside the edge of the tent. It marks the ideal position for the tip of the retractor as it lies just in front of the crus at the entrance to the interpeduncular cistern. The IIIrd nerve is almost always adherent to the tip of the uncus, so that, as the uncus is raised with the tip of the retractor, this nerve is elevated with it to spare it any unnecessary manipulation. It is usually possible to work underneath the nerve to clip the aneurysm except in the case of a high basilar bifurcation aneurysm or a giant sac, when it may be necessary to separate it from the uncus. The lessening of IIIrd nerve manipulation by this simple expedient has resulted in fewer postoperative IIIrd nerve palsies, and earlier and more complete recoveries in those that do occur.

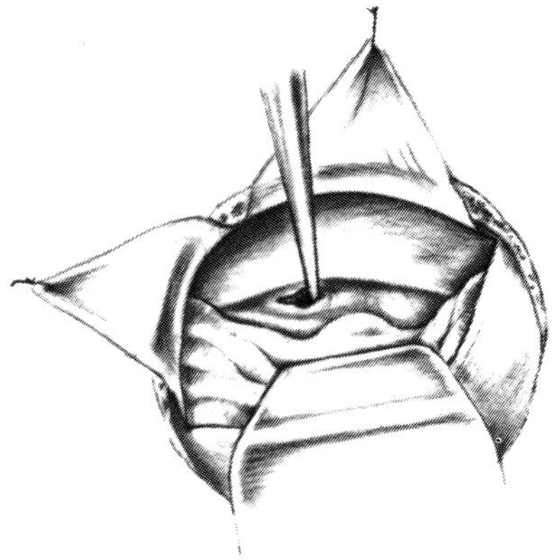

5

# 6

To increase the opening into the interpeduncular cistern substantially, a suture is placed in the edge of the tent just in front but free of the insertion of the IVth nerve. After passing it through the dura of the floor of the middle fossa, it can be tied tightly, thus tenting the edge of the tentorium downward, often for 1 cm or more. The IVth nerve can be tucked below the tentorial edge for safety. This simple but effective manoeuvre to open the entrance into the interpeduncular region obviates the need to divide the tentorium for aneurysms at the basilar bifurcation or as low as those at the superior cerebellar artery.

Opening the arachnoid in front of the crus and below the IIIrd nerve exposes the interpeduncular cistern. To avoid heavier retractor pressure to see the posterior cerebral artery, it is convenient to follow the superior cerebellar artery back to the basilar artery where it arises just below the origin of P1 as it curves upward.

In our experience, it has never been necessary to divide the posterior communicating artery. In fact, it should be carefully preserved in case some injury to P1 occurs or it becomes necessary (as it rarely does) to include P1 in the clip. Furthermore, this communicating artery gives rise to important diencephalic branches (anterior thalamo-perforating arteries) whose integrity would be compromised by its occlusion.

The blood pressure is now lowered to mean arterial values of 35–40 mmHg in otherwise healthy individuals. It is important to ensure that the intra-arterial pressure measurements are made with the transducer or manometer at head level if the patient is tilted so that mean *intracranial* arterial pressure is being recorded. Isoflurane has proved to be an excellent anaesthetic, as well as a most convenient way to induce easily controllable hypotension.

In recent years, the author has used one of the gentle temporary clips on the basilar artery below the superior cerebellar arteries but clear of perforators. This produces even more dramatic slackness of the sac, even after the anaesthetist has allowed the MAP to rise. These special temporary clips are used only when considered necessary, as in dissecting a partially hidden fragile sac, removing adherent perforators or clipping large bulbous awkward necks, and are not normally left in place for more than 2–3 minutes at a time as the dissection proceeds. They should only be used with mannitol 2 g/kg, which is thought to give some protection against cerebral ischaemia. In over 100 cases, each with postoperative angiography, there has been no evidence of arterial injury or occlusion, even though in a few critical situations the clip has been in place for more than 30 minutes. While significant arterial injury from temporary clipping seems not to occur, the safe length of occlusion time remains unknown; this depends greatly on the degree of collateral circulation involved.

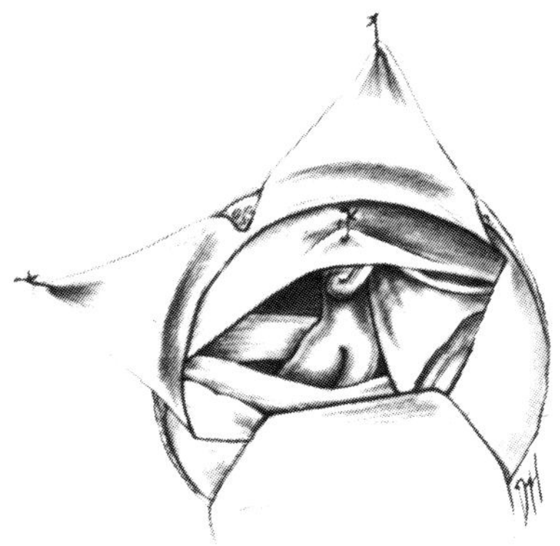

6

# SACCULAR ANEURYSMS ARISING AT THE BASILAR BIFURCATION

These arise in the crotch of the bifurcation and most commonly project *upward* in line with the curve of the basilar artery. The next most common projection is *posteriorly* into the interpeduncular space. Least common are those projecting *anteriorly*, with the dome above the dorsum sellae or adherent to its posterior surface. Rarely, they project laterally from a bifurcation that may be rotated nearly 90° in the coronal plane.

The host of perforating vessels seen in the angiogram in this region are often interpreted as arising from the aneurysm. This is fallacious since smaller saccular aneurysms cannot be the origin of perforators because of their origin as a 'blow-out' of unknown cause of the intimal lining through an opening in the media at the distal carina of the branching. These small vessels are named according to their distribution: interpeduncular, circumflex, mesencephalic, and posterior thalamoperforating arteries. They arise most often from the P1 segments at or very near their origins and are usually applied to the sides of the sac posterolaterally. A few interpeduncular vessels may arise from the back of the basilar bifurcation and be applied to the posterior aspects of the sac.

A characteristic feature of these aneurysms is the associated ballooning of the basilar bifurcation, which seems to become ectatic almost routinely as they enlarge, so that, when viewed from the side, the P1 segments seem to emerge from the sac itself. This ectasia, however, must have normal arterial wall; clipping above it can result in a 'blow-out' of a new aneurysm beneath the blades. The height of the basilar bifurcation is also very important, and varies considerably. Normally, the crotch is at or just above the dorsum sellae. However, it may be much higher, e.g. at the apex of the interpeduncular space behind the mammillary bodies, and even, if the basilar artery is elongated and tortuous with atheroma, so high as to indent the floor of the hypothalamus and third ventricle, although this is rare. The greater the height above the dorsum sellae, the more the retraction of the temporal lobe. As the neck of the sac reaches the apex of the interpeduncular space, it and the perforators are more effectively hidden by the mammillary bodies in front and the peduncles behind. However, only with one smaller aneurysm was it necessary to abandon clipping for gauze packing because of this obscuration by height. In our experience, gentle retraction of the mammillary bodies or crus has not produced any known serious deficit.

On the other hand, the bifurcation may be quite low, at the base of the dorsum sellae or even lower. This position of the neck is confining to the surgeon because the edge of the tent cannot be reflected inferiorly enough by the 'tenting' suture (*see Illustration 6*) and tends to hide the base of the sac and the upper basilar artery from a temporary clip, as they are wedged between the pontomesencephalic junction and clivus. However, dividing the inner third of the tentorium and working above and below the thin strand of the IVth nerve with retraction of the base of the crus will show enough of these low bifurcations for more accurate safe clipping. To gain a clear line of sight for this, it may be necessary to turn a temporal bone flap posteriorly (*see* under 'Basilar–AICA aneurysms', p. 211).

Another X-ray fallacy is the apparent position of the P1 segments clear of the neck in the Townes view. It must be remembered that P1 takes a compound curve forward and outward to cross above the IIIrd nerve before turning around the edge of the peduncle hidden over the hippocampal gyrus. The first curve and position of P1 are therefore not seen in the Townes view, so that it seems to come out straighter from the side of the neck. Furthermore, even when the neck seems to be clear for a few millimetres at its origin in the angiogram, P1 may well be adherent because of the unseen walls of the aneurysm and P1. Therefore, at operation, P1 will usually be applied to the side of the neck with its perforators. In larger, bulbous sacs it may seem to be arising from the base of the sac itself, although it really arises from the very common ectatic widening of the bifurcation.

## UPWARD PROJECTING ANEURYSMS

# 7 & 8

Following the superior cerebellar artery to its origin reveals the basilar artery and the origin of P1 immediately above, with the fibres of the IIIrd nerve crossing underneath. This nerve is elevated far enough up by the uncal adherence and its retraction to expose enough of the P1 origin and neck to complete the dissection and clipping underneath it. It is best to look at the front of the neck first, as there are no perforators, and it is usually simple to cross in front to identify the origin of the opposite P1 and even its perforators and obtain a view of the expanse of the neck, although the sac may have to be depressed a little with a dissector.

The difficulties with this aneurysm lie behind the sac. Rarely, it stands free in the interpeduncular space; more commonly, it is buried in the space hidden by the crus. Gentle retraction of the crus is well tolerated and exposes the posterolateral aspect and its perforators, which can be carefully separated at this stage with a tiny dissector. The pterional trans-sylvian approach may ease this problem, although the perforators behind cannot be as well seen.

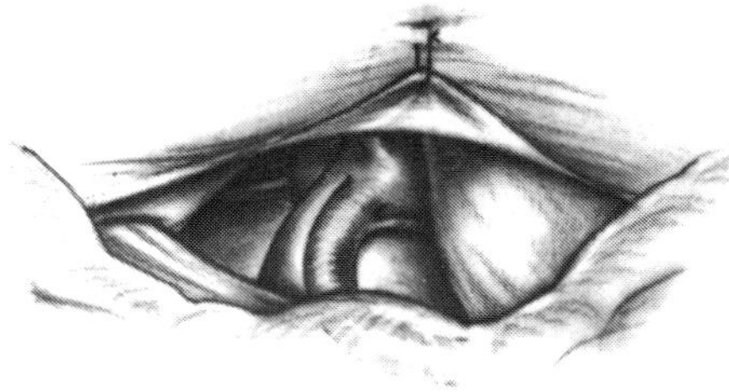

7

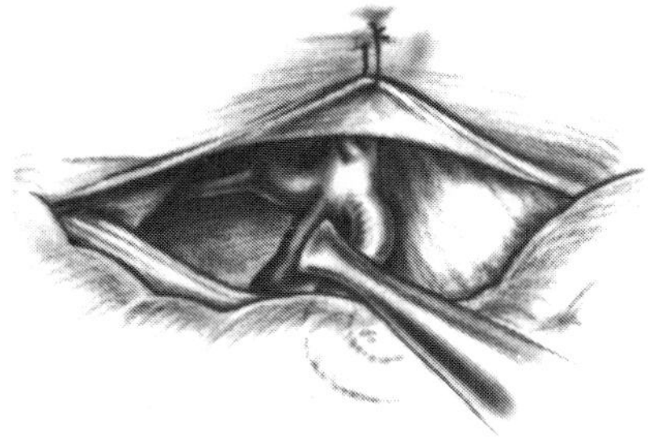

8

# 9

In order to expose the posterior aspect of the neck and waist it is usually necessary to indent and displace the waist of the sac anteriorly with the dissector or small sucker tip while slightly retracting the crus with the other instrument. This will reveal the whole of the interpeduncular space, the exit of the opposite IIIrd nerve, the origin of the opposite P1 and the perforators arising from it, and the basilar artery, which must be freed enough to allow a clip blade to slide underneath. A general widening or ballooning ectasia of the basilar bifurcation is common even with small aneurysms, and both are often patchily yellow with atheroma.

As noted earlier, P1 commonly arises nearly vertically from its origin beside the base of the sac, to which it gently adheres, before crossing laterally over the IIIrd nerve. To apply an ordinary spring clip in this circumference, P1 with its perforators must be freed carefully from this adherence so that one blade can be slipped underneath it, either from in front or from behind, to cross the neck. This is quite manageable where P1 ascends toward the front or back of the sac. However, when it is placed midway on the side of a more bulbous sac, it can be awkward and dangerous to try to free a firm adherence or slide one blade underneath P1 at nearly right angles to the surgeon. In this case the new clip with the aperture in its base for P1, designed for much larger sacs, is very satisfactory. It is not even necessary to separate P1, and perforators may safely be included in the aperture. Most important, however, with this clip is that blades can be selected or trimmed (with wire-cutting pliers) and filed to fall only across the neck so as not to impinge on P1 or perforators on *either* side.

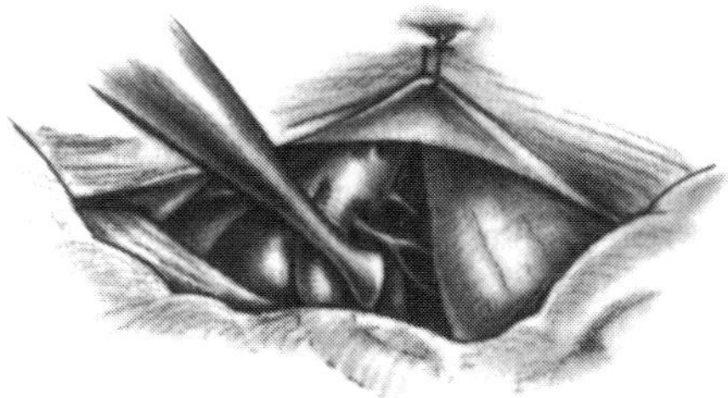

9

# 10

As the posterior blade of the clip is passed behind the neck, it must be kept inside the perforators. As the blades are allowed to close and narrow the neck, the opposite P1 will come into view so that a final alignment flush with the neck at the upper origins of P1 on each side can be made before closing the clip. The posterior blade must not be placed too far across, for the root of the opposite IIIrd nerve courses up behind the opposite P1 and can be brushed or even injured by this blade. As for any aneurysm, the position of the clip should be assessed immediately after the first placement by rotating it forward and backward to see the position of each blade. Not infrequently the blades will be found to be too high or too low on the opposite side and a perforator may be inadvertently caught, as shown in the illustration. A common error is to use blades that are longer than necessary and to place them up on the neck. In spite of apparent width, the neck is often narrower at its very origin, and much shorter blades can be used. The clip is removed, modified and replaced as many times as is necessary for perfect position. Usually this is no problem with deep hypotension. It may even be possible to take advantage of a malpositioned clip by quickly separating adherent perforators from the slack sac or P1, or if necessary the sac itself from higher reaches of the interpeduncular fossa.

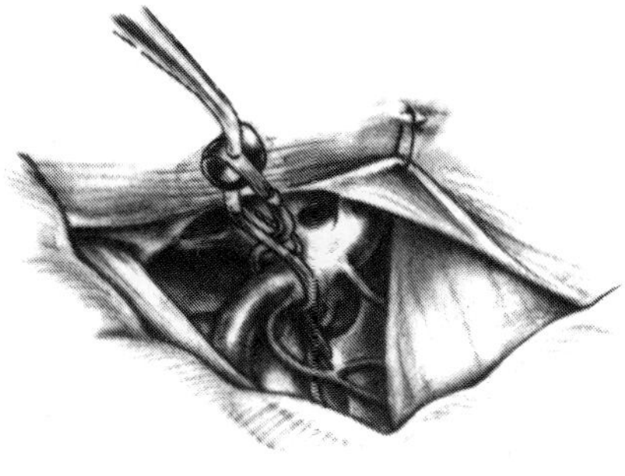

10

# 11

After final positioning, the aneurysm should be needled and collapsed. This will provide an even better view of the position of the clip. Should any final readjustment be required, the bleeding from a needle hole can always be stopped with a little pressure and waiting so that a dry field will be available for repositioning.

The slope to one side of the basilar bifurcation in the coronal plane, and hence the slope of the neck of the aneurysm, also deserves comment. The angle may be considerable, and, if down and away from the surgeon, make clip application awkward since not enough temporal retraction can be gained safely to achieve a line of sight along the angle of the neck. Even so, except in the rare circumstance of a laterally directed basilar bifurcation, this is not enough of a problem to warrant an approach under the dominant temporal lobe. It is usually possible to rotate the clip in its applier, or to retract P1 downward enough to level the neck for accurate placement.

Rarely, as the neck is closed by a clip, the dome of the sac is dragged inferiorly away from an attachment to the hypothalamic floor, and will bleed. If the clip has to be removed and replaced, the dome will usually stop bleeding as it re-expands and is tamponaded against its former adherence, if the rent is not too large.

When can a perforator be occluded? Ideally never, but in a few cases one or two tiny, very adherent ones on the back of a very thin neck have been included without evident deficit. Most can be dissected free with a tiny dissector, but a large adherent perforator may require special effort during temporary basilar clipping under high magnification. If still dangerously adherent posterolaterally, a Drake clip can be placed with the perforator in the aperture and a tandem clip added up to the perforator to complete the occlusion. Sometimes, thickening the wall of the sac with bipolar coagulation underneath a perforator will make it possible to dissect it free more safely without rupturing the aneurysm. With a lateral subtemporal approach, vertical aneurysms are perhaps the only ones on the basilar circulation whose neck cannot easily be shrunk and firmed up with coagulation since usually P1 is squarely in the way of closing forceps blades.

Frank rupture is handled as for any other aneurysms, primarily without panic and always keeping in mind that the dissection must be completed before the clip is applied. Frantic application of the clips leads only to disaster. Small rents will stop spontaneously with a little pressure. When bleeding from larger rents is directed into the sucker, the aneurysm tends to collapse, exposing its origin nicely for completion of the dissection. A rent at or near the neck may require meticulous placement of clip blades, but it is wise to take a P1 only if a generous posterior communicating artery is present.

In critical situations or when dealing with giant aneurysms, it may be possible to occlude P1 at its origin in certain circumstances. A good posterior communicating artery is a prerequisite for deliberate occlusion and no perforator should be included in the clip, which must be applied very accurately to leave the small vessels originating from the distal stump to be irrigated retrogradely by the communicating vessel. This action, however, should not be undertaken lightly, and only after careful consideration of the situation and the risk.

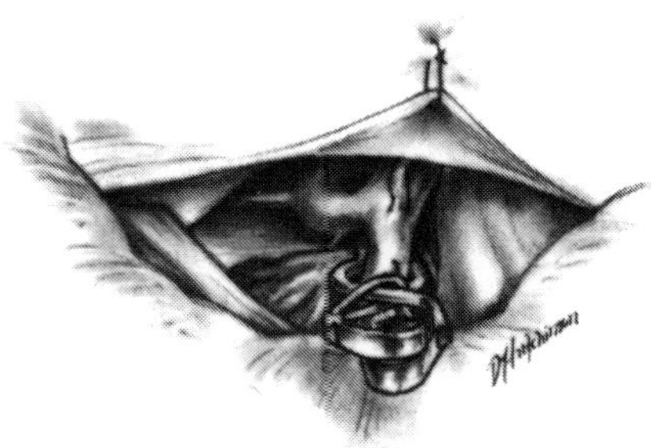

11

# 12

The common frontotemporal or pterional trans-sylvian approach to carotid and anterior communicating aneurysms has also been proposed for those in the region of the basilar artery bifurcation[7]. After splitting the inner two-thirds of the sylvian fissure, the approach is on the lateral side of the carotid artery, medial to the IIIrd nerve and its insertion. Only rarely is there sufficient space to see enough between the carotid and the chiasm. The author has used it from time to time over the years, especially when an anterior aneurysm is to be performed at the same sitting. For example, a left pointing superior cerebellar aneurysm can sometimes be done from a right approach to a carotid or anterior communicating aneurysm, whereas it is difficult to expose properly by a purely right subtemporal approach. However, this approach can be narrow and confining and its advocates advise division of the posterior communicating vessel for more space. It is most suitable for aneurysms with small necks lying in an ideal position, just above or below the dorsum sellae and pointing upward or forward. However, the height of the bifurcation varies greatly in relation to the dorsum, and backward-pointing sacs or those lying well below the dorsum are poorly seen.

Very high bifurcations may be exposed by a route above the carotid bifurcation, taking great care to spare the perforators here. This approach reduces the need for IIIrd nerve manipulation and provides a good face-on view of the basilar bifurcation and those P1 perforators that rise on the lateral sides of the sac. It may also allow the neck to be shrunk with coagulation although it must be certain that no hidden perforators posteriorly are caught in the tips of the forceps. Of more concern is that it does not allow nearly the same visualization behind the neck, especially on the opposite side, where perforators commonly hide, or below the neck when the sac projects posteriorly.

Division of the posterior communicating artery is often innocuous, but it may put its vital thalamoperforating vessels at risk and removes collateral flow to P2 when the origin of P1 has to be occluded with the neck, although this is rarely required. Also, the neck of the bifurcation aneurysm, as in the case of other broad bifurcation necks, is more completely obliterated if the clip is placed parallel to the bifurcation, and there is less risk of kinking. When placed at right angles, 'dog ears' may remain in front and behind as the sides of the neck are approximated and in a few cases these have been responsible for the development of new aneurysms at least on the carotid artery. Lateral placement of the clip obviates the necessity and hazard of dissecting free P1 segments which are commonly adherent to the neck and waist of the sac.

The disadvantages of the subtemporal route have been ascribed to the need for more temporal lobe retraction; the necessity to put some traction on the IIIrd nerve; and the relative difficulty in visualizing the origin of the opposite P1 and its laterally placed perforators. However, with modern techniques of brain relaxation, measured temporal lobe retraction is usually below 1.3 kPa (10 Torr) and with experience IIIrd nerve paresis is usually mild and transient. Temporary basilar clipping so softens the sac that its displacement with a small dissector or sucker tip usually affords an excellent view of the structures on the other side and, most importantly, behind.

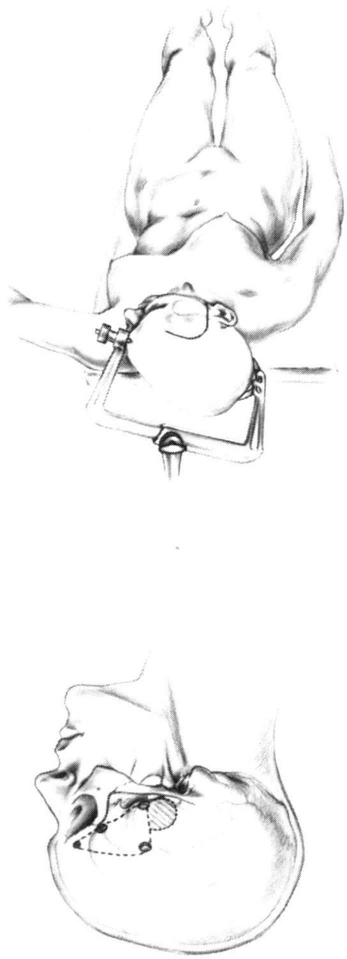

12

# 13a–e

The author, after many trials, prefers the subtemporal approach initially but with the option to go either trans-sylvian or more posteriorly temporal as needed. The advantages of each approach have frequently been used in complementary fashion, for the sylvian approach can be modified quickly to be subtemporal (*see Illustration 12*) by merely displacing posteriorly or elevating the temporal pole if the anterior temporal squama has been removed. Further, a 'half-and-half' combination of the two approaches is useful when the sylvian exposure does not allow visualization of the back of the neck of a larger aneurysm or when the neck has a more horizontal take-off posteriorly. The mobile temporal pole may be elevated or displaced backward enough to allow dissection on either side of the IIIrd nerve. Behind it, the posterior aspect of the neck can be seen and cleared of perforators, after which the clip is applied from in front of the nerve over the dorsum sellae, with all the vessels in view. Much of the merit of any exposure is a matter of continued use and familiarity with the anatomy. There have been three deaths among our patients in the last 5 years which were related to early rebleeding when clip blades were placed a little short of the far side of the neck. Now, when there is any doubt, we make quite certain that the blade of the Drake clip occludes the far side perfectly; if not, a tandem straight clip is added to any portion of the neck remaining open in the aperture on the near side containing P1.

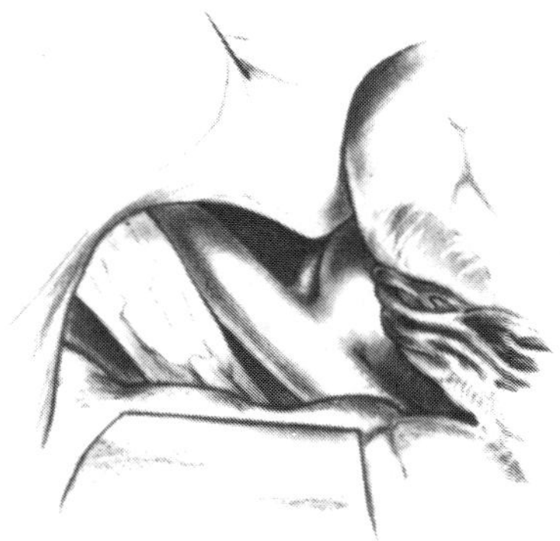

13a

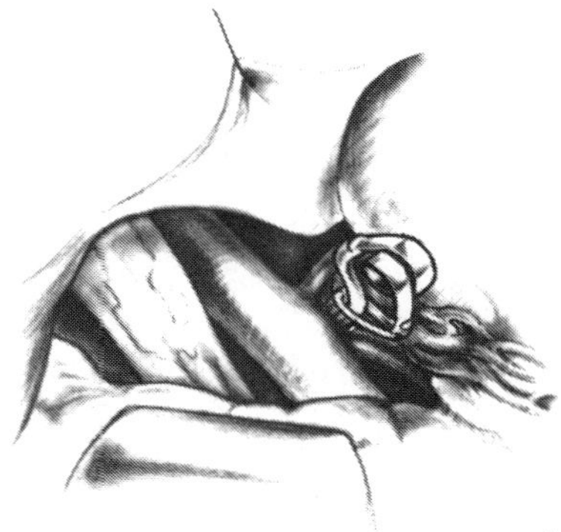

13b

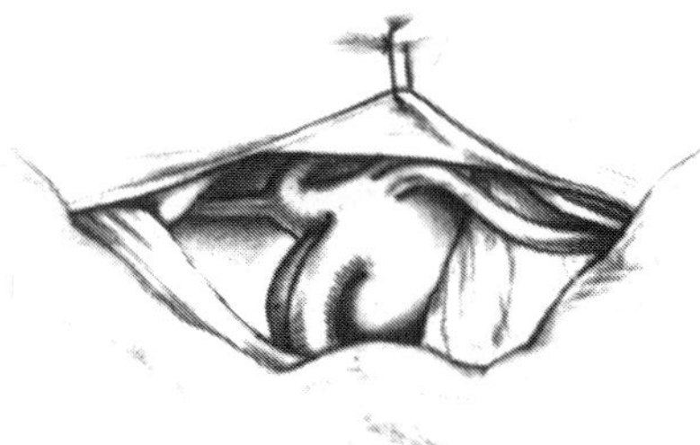

13c

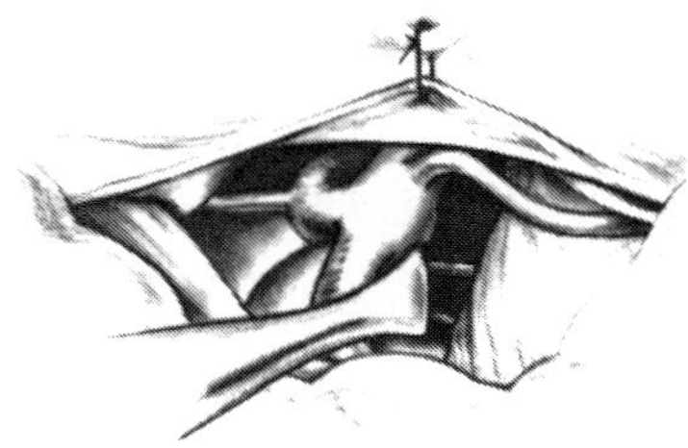

13d

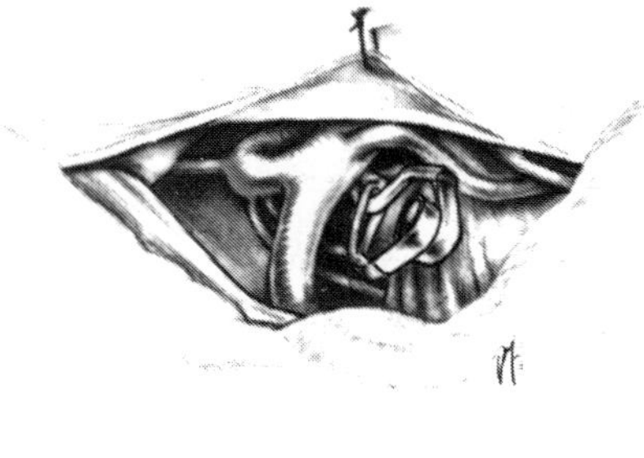

13e

*Treatment of two aneurysms, one carotid communicating and one at the basilar bifurcation; ruptured sac unknown. (a) Carotid communicating aneurysm exposed by usual subfrontal approach, and (b) aneurysm clipped, sparing the posterior communicating and anterior choroidal arteries. A paracarotid approach to the basilar bifurcation is too narrow and dangerous. (Carotid aneurysms can be clipped by pure subtemporal exposure.) (c) After additional squamous temporal craniectomy and subtemporal exposure the backward projecting basilar bifurcation aneurysm is seen. (d) Sac displaced to see and separate the perforators. (e) Clip free of perforators from opposite P1.*

## POSTERIOR PROJECTING ANEURYSMS

These aneurysms used to be considered difficult and dangerous to treat, but have proved to be a good group for surgical treatment. Once the neck is exposed, the perforators paradoxically seem to be either free or can easily be freed from the sac, although one or two may be above the neck as well as on both sides and below.

Again, the subtemporal approach is used, but the IIIrd nerve is more in the way because of its slope from above and behind P1 to cross down and below it, often across the neck. Only a glimpse of the neck is seen from in front although the opposite P1 is seen clearly. Because of the rise of P1 from its origin, it is necessary to work behind and below it and either above or below the IIIrd nerve, depending on its position and its easiest point of displacement. As the crus is retracted, the neck will come into view, although the dome, buried in the interpeduncular space, is usually not seen. Occasionally, there are perforators on top of the neck but the usual leash will be present on either side of and below the belly of the neck. They seem to separate as the crus is retracted or the neck is teased into view by gently pulling outwards on P1 with the sucker tip. As the blades of the spring clip are allowed to close slowly, the gradual narrowing of the neck will reveal its opposite side, the perforators there, and the opposite IIIrd nerve. The opposite P1 is usually not in the way of the blades, and as long as the blades close only across the far side of the neck it is unlikely that any unseen perforator will be caught. The author has even seen one or two small perforators free between the tips of the blades which were held just far enough apart by the bulk of the neck to accommodate them, but this is not a circumstance on which to rely. Aspiration and collapse of the sac will reveal clearly whether the clip has been placed accurately. It is essential to ensure that what appears to be a backward-projecting sac is not a right-angled saccule coming off posteriorly from what is really a neck with an initial upward projection, which should be treated as an upward projecting neck. This mistake cost the life of one patient when 3 years later the base of the vertical portion of the neck, left inadvertently proximal to the horizontally placed clip, blew out.

## ANTERIOR PROJECTING ANEURYSMS

It is unfortunate that these are the rarest, for they are the most straightforward to treat. They project forward and upward from the line of the basilar artery, usually above the dorsum sellae, and are free in the interpeduncular space. They are free of perforators since none arise from the anterior aspect of the basilar artery. In low basilar bifurcations, caution is needed, for the dome is often adherent to the dorsum or clivus and may be torn loose. It is also important to ensure that the clip blades do not encroach on the opposite P1 although remaining flush with the origin of the neck.

## BILOCULAR ANEURYSMS

Bilocular aneurysms are not uncommon at the basilar bifurcation. They may be difficult to clip because of the width of the angle forming the neck of the sac, which may approach 180°. However, if the neck (which may only be broad in the sagittal plane) is not large, it can be 'gathered' with the clip as the blades are forced gently upward from their original position at the top of the basilar artery. If the saccules are too large, each can be clipped separately since the first clip narrows the other sac conveniently for the second clip.

## LARGE (OR BULBOUS) BASILAR BIFURCATION ANEURYSMS

Most of these project vertically and have bulbous necks whose size is directly proportional to the difficulties of exposure and clipping. The problem is that the basilar bifurcation is almost always ballooned with ectasia and seemingly a part of the neck. Consequently, the P1 segment also seems to originate from the side of the neck, rising vertically with its perforators in close application to it. However, enough experience has been gained to suggest that this ectatic bifurcation is composed of reasonably normal arterial wall and has not 'blown out' to form another aneurysm over the years, below a clip that has been properly placed between the medial portions of the P1 origins. The sheer bulk of the neck makes it more difficult to see either in front of or behind across to the other side. The origin and neck of this aneurysm are more likely to be yellow and firm with atheroma.

Once exposed, the waist of the sac should be indented anteriorly, using firm pressure, to allow a glimpse of the origin of the opposite P1 and perhaps its perforators. It is most important to identify the opposite P1 accurately and not to mistake the superior cerebellar artery for it, for if the blades of the clip rest just above the latter artery, the basilar apex and the opposite P1 will be occluded. This mistake was the cause of death in one of our patients. The opposite P1 may be identified by confirming either that the opposite IIIrd nerve (usually clearly seen) courses beneath it or that the opposite posterior communicating artery can be seen entering it. Behind, these large aneurysms tend to bulge far back into the interpeduncular space, and fairly firm retraction of the peduncle is necessary even to expose part of the back of the neck. One can often get a 'feel' of the curve and extent of the neck by blindly but gently working a small curved dissector backwards beside the neck inside the medial aspect of the peduncle. It is remarkable how much retraction the peduncle will take without producing any deficit. Finally, it is necessary to work either the sucker tip or a dissector gradually behind the neck at the appropriate angle, displacing the waist forward as the instrument is advanced and separating perforators until the apex of the curve is reached, when more bold forward displacement will tilt the waist of the sac forward to disclose the contents of the interpeduncular fossa, the opposite perforators and usually the opposite P1. As this is done, the top of the origin of the opposite P1 should be noted to obtain a line on the angle for the clip blades.

The new clip designed specially for this aneurysm should be used unless P1 has an unusual course upwards on the anterior or posterior portion of the neck, when an ordinary spring clip blade can be worked underneath it. During the foregoing inspection, an estimate should be made of the width of the neck between the P1 origins. This cannot be exact, for, as the neck is closed by the blades, it widens somewhat. However, the final length of blades used must be exactly the width of the closed neck.

If the neck is not too broad, the blades can gradually be worked across with a rocking motion, inside the perforators on the moistened neck, and slowly allowed to close. Because of the breadth of the neck, it will probably be necessary to use the sucker tip to indent again the waist of the sac from behind in order to expose the base of the neck and the perforators in the interpeduncular fossa for initiating clip application. In its present form, this clip is slightly awkward to apply, as the handle and tips of the applier hide the aperture so that it is sometimes difficult to be sure that P1 is free in the opening. Narrowing of the handle or off-setting or angling the blades would solve this problem.

If there are no significant perforators behind, the blades can be started low on either side of the basilar bifurcation and then gently worked up on the neck by rocking and sliding just high enough to clear each P1 before closing. As the blades close, the opposite P1 will be seen so that adjustments of their angle can be made. The opposite IIIrd nerve is in more jeopardy during application of the clip, for it is thinned and flattened on the far side and apt to be brushed or even torn by the widely opened posterior blade.

A significant difficulty with these aneurysms is the yellow atherosclerotic firmness of their base which causes the blades, although initially placed open in good position, to slide down and occlude the bifurcation as they close. Sometimes the anterior blade can be held up on the far side of the neck with the sucker tip as the blades are allowed to close. Repeated trials seem to 'soften up' the neck so that blades will hold, but often drastic narrowing of the waist of the sac is required, using forceps or the sucker tip, to produce a slope on which they will close and remain. It may even be necessary to place the blades up on the waist deliberately and then try to place another set of blades across below them or, failing that, to pack the remaining base in gauze. (A 'hobnailed' clip blade might be a solution to this dilemma.) If there is a good posterior communicating artery, then the ipsilateral P1 can be cautiously taken in the clip, provided there is no alternative and no perforators are included. The bulk of these necks is often such that the tips of the blades will not fully close on the other side, still allowing blood into the aneurysm, which will bleed on needling. If the blades are in a good position, they should be left, for a strong clip will finally occlude the neck. Sometimes, rotation of the clip about its long axis will complete the occlusion; this can be maintained, if necessary, by suturing the rotated handle to nearby dura.

Another abnormality seen occasionally with bulbous sacs, and which results from the ectasia of the bifurcation, is that the P1 segments emerge vertically *downward* from the base of the sac. Here, it is almost impossible to prevent the blades of a clip from stenosing each P1 orifice, and consideration must be given to basilar artery occlusion just below, using the tourniquet after the patient wakes from the anaesthesia.

**Table 2 Basilar bifurcation aneurysms: results of surgical treatment**

| | *Number of cases* | *Excellent* | *Good* | *Poor* | *Dead* |
|---|---|---|---|---|---|
| Small (<12.5 mm) | | | | | |
| Upward projecting | 258 | 189 | 35 | 25 | 9 |
| Posteriorly projecting | 50 | 35 | 9 | 3 | 3 |
| Anteriorly projecting | 39 | 30 | 4 | 4 | 1 |
| | 347 | 254 | 48 | 32 | 13 |
| Large bulbous (12.5–25 mm) | 155 | 99 | 28 | 21 | 7 |

## Results

The overall results with 347 small aneurysms (less than 12.5 mm) at the basilar bifurcation operated on at our Unit since 1958 are shown in Table 2. The overall mortality and morbidity of 3.7 and 9.2 per cent respectively was almost halved in the 141 cases operated on in the last 5 years, to 2 and 5.6 per cent respectively. This is no doubt due to the experience accumulated, but particularly to the determination to preserve the perforating vessels, recently with the help of temporary basilar clipping. A persisting morbidity has been due to operation on poor-grade patients, a rare perforator occlusion, and rebleeding in three patients in whom the clip blades did not completely occlude the neck.

The consistently poorer results with the large bulbous aneurysms sitting more deeply in the interpeduncular fossa in good-risk patients are mostly due to inadvertent perforator or P1 occlusion. The overall mortality for these aneurysms was 4.5 per cent, and 13.5 per cent had a poor result. Here too, temporary basilar occlusion is proving very useful for more accurate clip placement or tandem clipping, and recent results are most encouraging.

# POSTERIOR CEREBRAL ANEURYSMS

These arise principally in two places: at the junction with the posterior communicating artery, and at the first major branching on the side of the midbrain. However, a few appear to arise at the origin of large perforating branches from P1 and (more rarely) peripherally on the occipital lobe.

Those arising from P1 are approached in the same fashion as those at the basilar bifurcation and may have much the same intimate involvement with perforating vessels.

The posterior cerebral artery is hidden under the hippocampal gyrus as it winds around the side of the midbrain, and this gyrus must be elevated with the tip of the retractor to expose aneurysms arising at its first major branching. It may even be necessary to remove a small amount of the overlying hippocampal gyrus to expose a high-placed or complex aneurysm where it lies on the midbrain in the choroidal fissure. The same care is needed in the dissection of the neck to preserve the branching, although usually perforators are not a problem here. For aneurysms lying more posteriorly, the posterior cerebral artery may be followed to the midline behind the midbrain by the subtemporal approach. Beyond this, an occipital flap should be used so that the mobile occipital pole can be retracted laterally and upward from the dural surface of the falx–tentorial junction.

Experience in the treatment of giant posterior cerebral artery aneurysms has shown that this vessel has a remarkable collateral circulation from many leptomeningeal vessels from the middle and anterior cerebral arteries. In our experience of 15 P1 clip occlusions, including four trappings, there were no field defects from occipital infarction. In most of these cases, no filling of P2 could be seen from posterior communicating vessels, which were probably occluded with the thrombosis of the aneurysm. P2 was occluded on four occasions with only one pre-existing field defect, but of five trappings of giant P2 aneurysms, three developed field defects.

**Table 3 Posterior cerebral aneurysms (<12.5 mm): results of surgical treatment**

| *Grade* | *Number of cases* | *Excellent* | *Good* | *Poor* | *Dead* |
|---|---|---|---|---|---|
| 0 | 8 | 7 | 1 | 0 | 0 |
| 1 | 25 | 22 | 3 | 0 | 0 |
| 2 | 1 | 1 | 0 | 0 | 0 |
| 3 | 6 | 2 | 0 | 1 | 3 |
| 5 | 1 | 0 | 0 | 0 | 1 |
| | 41 | 32 | 4 | 1 | 4 |

## Results

Posterior cerebral aneurysms included only small and giant sizes. Results with the small aneurysms (*see Table 3*) have been good, presumably because of their easier exposure, although perforating vessels are a concern with those arising on the P1 segment. One death resulted from massive pulmonary embolism and the poor result was in a patient already severely hemiparetic who failed to improve.

# BASILAR-SCA ANEURYSMS

## 14

These arise at the distal crotch of origin of the SCA; as they enlarge, the neck comes to involve most or all of the lateral portion of the basilar artery between the SCA and P1. They usually project laterally, rarely forward, lying in a shallow bed in the peduncle. There is always an intimate relation to the IIIrd nerve, which will course either over or under the sac or be flattened by the dome. Rarely, this aneurysm arises inferiorly to the SCA.

The subtemporal approach is used on the side of the projection of the aneurysm. Although this aneurysm can be treated from the opposite side, it is awkward to work across in front of the basilar artery in the narrow confines behind the clivus. Furthermore, it may be necessary to dissect underneath the basilar artery to free perforators which not infrequently arise here and cannot be seen as well from this side as from the ipsilateral side. These disadvantages are greater than those of an approach on the dome of the aneurysm, i.e. some increase in the risk of rupture and, in those projecting to the left, retraction of the dominant temporal lobe, although this is less than for bifurcation aneurysms.

The suture tying down the edge of the tentorium usually suffices for exposure without necessitating division of the tentorium, except for very large aneurysms. However, if there is any doubt about the adequacy of exposure, the inner third of the tent can easily be divided through the subtemporal craniectomy, as for the low basilar bifurcation. Preparation for a posterior temporal flap should be in place in case it is necessary to see much farther down behind the clivus. The thin strand of the IVth nerve must be constantly watched to guard against tearing it (as occurred in three of our early cases). The fragile dome with its adherent clot can be avoided by working down the sides of the aneurysm, starting in front. If necessary, the sac can be depressed against the peduncle to reveal the neck emerging from the basilar artery and the superior cerebellar artery below it. P1 may be readily visible too, depending on its course, but if the sac is of any size it is often hidden above and behind.

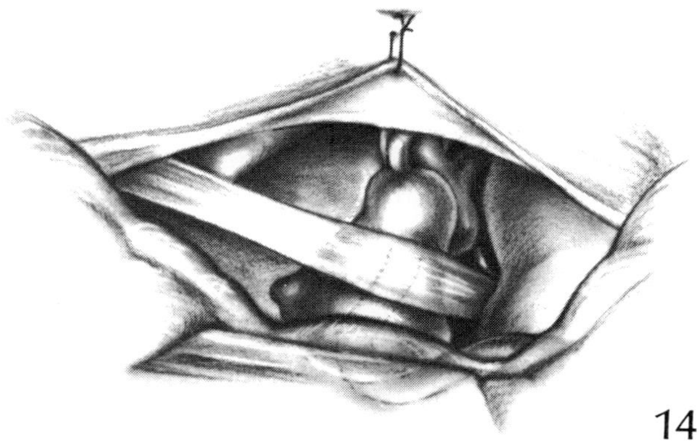

14

## 15

Then, working behind, the aneurysm is gently dissected and teased out of its bed in the peduncle, using a fine spatula to lift it to show the plane of cleavage. The waist and neck are freed from P1 and the SCA in the same way, although the latter is usually not as adherent. With the aneurysm freed and displaced forward, the neck with any nearby perforators is seen clearly. During these manipulations, great care must be taken not to injure the IIIrd nerve, which may wind around the neck itself. If the nerve makes application of the clip awkward, then a ligature can be slipped gently around inside it and tied firmly, or the neck can be shrunk with coagulation. The tiny bifurcation sac is coated in gauze before clip placement.

Occasionally, the SCA emerges from the side of the neck below, so care must be taken not to kink it with a clip.

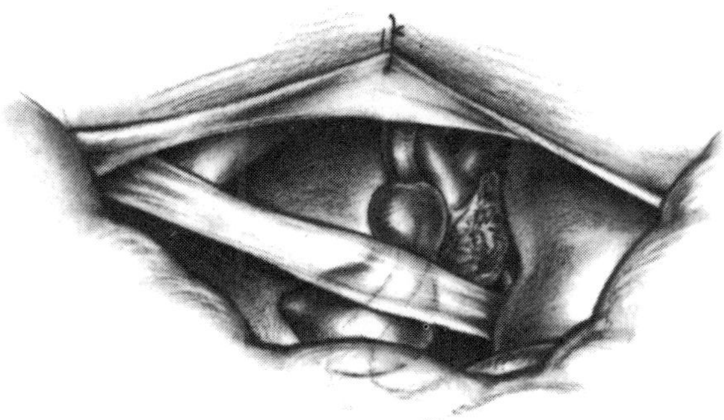

15

# 16

A curved clip in the long axis of the basilar artery often fits well across the curve of a larger neck created by the slopes of origin of P1 and the SCA.

Aspiration and collapse of these aneurysms is important to relieve any IIIrd nerve compression if present.

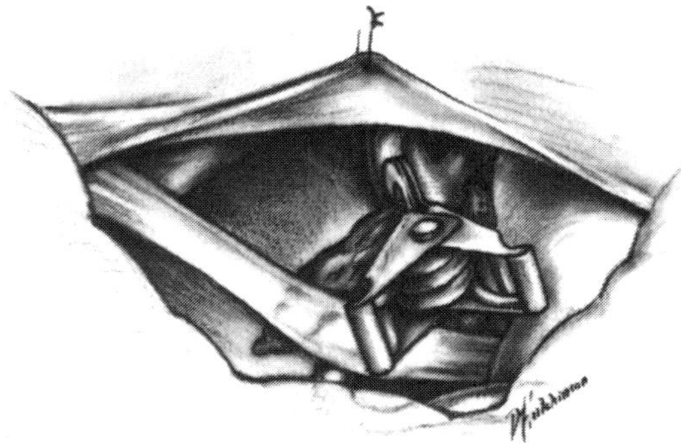

16

These aneurysms can also be treated by the sylvian approach on the side to which they project (or the opposite side if necessary).

Rarely, they project forward toward the dorsum sellae or are adherent to it. Obliteration is then quite straightforward, for there are no perforators involved. Care must be taken not to injure the opposite IIIrd nerve as the clip is applied and closed.

The bulk of *large bulbous aneurysms* obscures the field more, but they too should be approached on the dome and dissected free in the same way to expose the neck, although more forceful retraction of the sac will be necessary to free it from its bed to see the neck behind. Often, P1 is very adherent above and may have to be dissected free with a knife. Coagulation of a thin neck will not only shrink it but firm it up for freeing a very adherent vessel. The IIIrd nerve is always displaced and flattened by these large sacs and is more prone to injury.

Aneurysms lying distally on the SCA on the upper surface of the cerebellum are rare. They may be approached subtemporally through the tentorium but the more distal ones are easily seen by a suboccipital–subtentorial exposure in the sitting position.

## Results

In our experience, obliteration of ordinary basilar–SCA aneurysms has been very satisfactory, with only one death (due to a postoperative extradural clot) and six poor results, four of whom had been in poor condition (*see Table 4*). The morbidity was high in the large bulbous sacs, and was due to rupture at the neck in two cases, and basilar spasm and midbrain ischaemia in the others.

**Table 4 Basilar trunk aneurysms at the SCA: results of surgical treatment**

| | *Grade* | *Number of cases* | *Excellent* | *Good* | *Poor* | *Dead* |
|---|---|---|---|---|---|---|
| Superior cerebellar | 0 | 21 | 21 | 0 | 0 | 0 |
| | 1 | 73 | 71 | 1 | 0 | 1 |
| | 2 | 26 | 16 | 8 | 2 | 0 |
| | 3 | 9 | 2 | 3 | 4 | 0 |
| | | 129 | 110 | 12 | 6 | 1 |
| Large bulbous (12.5–25 mm) | 0 | 3 | 2 | 1 | 0 | 0 |
| | 1 | 14 | 6 | 3 | 3 | 2 |
| | 2 | 2 | 1 | 1 | 0 | 0 |
| | | 19 | 9 | 5 | 3 | 2 |

# BASILAR-AICA ANEURYSMS

These aneurysms arise in the crotch of origin of the AICA over the middle third of the clivus, usually nearer its junction with the lower third. They tend to project laterally but sometimes project forward against the clivus or even posteriorly into the pons. There is always a near or intimate relation to the VIth nerve.

## 17

### Choice of approach

These aneurysms may be exposed in one of two ways. The whole of the basilar artery and even the upper vertebral arteries may be visualized through the subtemporal–transtentorial approach (*b*). However, from behind and below through the standard lateral suboccipital exposure, the whole of the vertebral artery and the basilar, at least as far as the AICA, can also be exposed (*c*). The choice of approach depends on the height of the aneurysm on the clivus, its size and projection, and certain other disadvantages of each approach.

1. An approach from above could result in injury to the Vth, VIth, VIIth or VIIIth cranial nerve and the necessity of approaching under a dominant temporal lobe.
2. An approach from below could cause injury to the Xth or XIth nerve.

Ordinarily, the author prefers to go through the tent because the final exposure in front of the pons is a little larger, and unilateral deafness or a temporary facial or VIth nerve paresis is far less distressing and dangerous than a vagal palsy. Even so, with experience, it is possible to work at the vertebral artery junction and above through the posterior fossa underneath the medulla between the pharyngeal filaments of the XIth nerve and the vagal fibres with no or minimal injury. The size and projection of the aneurysm also determine which route is most likely to expose the neck and AICA while avoiding the dome. Generally those over the lower third of the clivus are approached from below and those above through the tentorium. The transoral–transclival approach has been abandoned for aneurysms because it is confining, dangerous and now unnecessary.

A combined subtemporal–transtentorial and suboccipital-transmastoid approach, which avoids the dangerous division of the lateral sinus, can be very useful for certain awkwardly placed or large aneurysms. After turning a posterior temporal flap in continuity with a lateral suboccipital craniectomy to expose the lateral sinus, enough of the mastoid is removed to uncover the whole of the upper half or more of the sigmoid sinus and enough dura in front of it for a watertight closure. The mastoid emissary vein must be anticipated and occluded with a pin suture if necessary. After dividing the tentorium to the junction of the lateral and sigmoid sinuses, the dura in front of the sigmoid over the cerebellum is divided up to the same point. This trifoliate dural confluence contains the superior petrosal sinus, which can be divided just medial to the lateral sigmoid sinus confluence. The lateral and sigmoid sinuses are then untethered and retracted posteriorly with the superolateral corner of the cerebellum to give a much wider view through the cerebello-pontine angle to the whole of the basilar and upper vertebral arteries, which can be approached above or below the VIIth and VIIIth nerves.

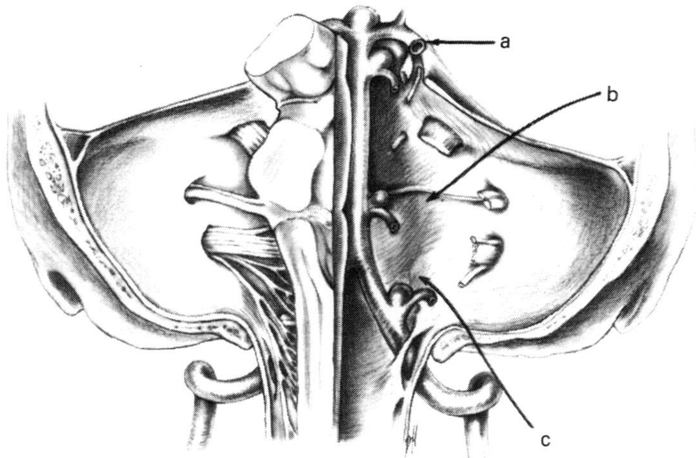


17

# 18

The subtemporal–transtentorial approach requires a temporal bone flap placed more posteriorly, as otherwise the posterior edge of the bony opening will prevent the retractor from angling far enough backward for a line of sight down the posterior slope of the petrous bone. It is most important to preserve the integrity of the vein of Labbé during temporal lobe retraction; in one case tearing resulted in a fatal venous infarction postoperatively. The midtemporal lobe is elevated to display the edge of the tentorium beside the crus cerebri. This edge is picked up 1–2 cm *behind* the insertion of the IVth nerve, clipped and/or coagulated and divided, and the tentorium is then incised 1–2 cm behind the petrous ridge far laterally to near the lateral sinus.

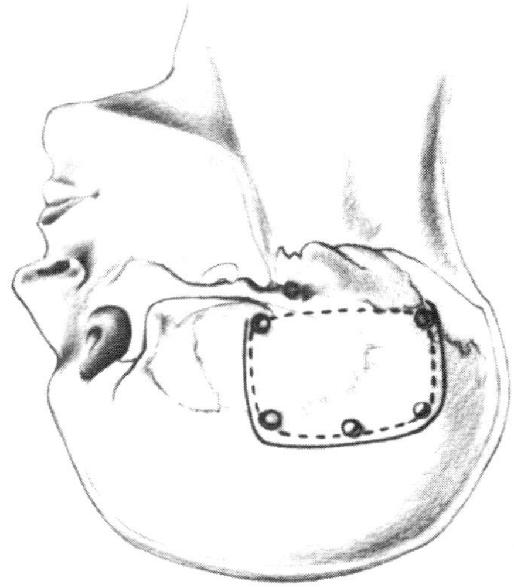

18

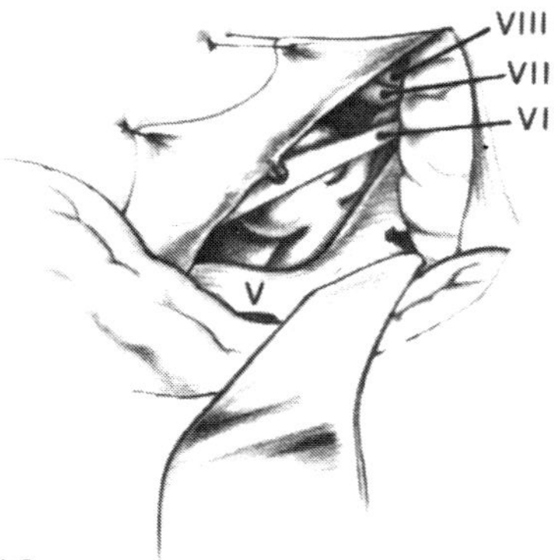


19

# 19

The anterior leaflet is then folded forward on its attachment to the ridge and tied firmly to the floor of the middle fossa, usually with three sutures. This exposes the IVth and Vth nerves medially under the arachnoid and petrosal vein(s) midway, bridging the petrosal sinus and anterior cerebellum. The vein or veins are divided after careful coagulation, the arachnoid is opened, and cerebrospinal fluid is evacuated.

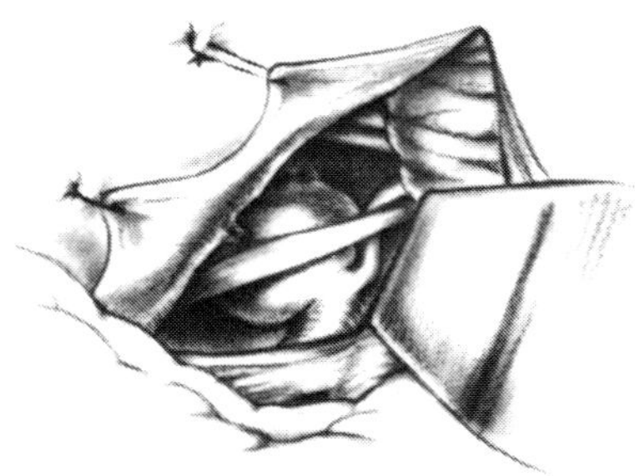

20

# 20

With a slack brain, very little retraction of the temporal lobe is required as the tip of the same retractor is worked down along the anterior edge of the cerebellum just lateral to the Vth nerve. As the tip gently retracts the pons from the petrous bone and clivus, the bundle of the VIIth and VIIIth nerves will come into view laterally. The final exposure will be in the opening between the Vth nerve medially and the VIIth and VIIIth nerves laterally. At first, the space may seem too confined, but with suction and further gentle retraction it opens up considerably to reveal first the VIth nerve, then the basilar artery above the aneurysm. The arachnoid sheet in front of this space may be a nuisance in the sucker and have to be divided. If there is much old clot in the cistern, it is best to suck it away in a direction away from the presumed position of the dome of the aneurysm.

The VIth nerve is slack enough to be placed up against the clivus or held gently with the retractor tip on the pons. Often, it has to be separated from an adherence to the aneurysm. Handled gently, the VIth nerve, like the IIIrd nerve, has a remarkable propensity for complete recovery of function.

# 21

The aneurysm may be disclosed by following the AICA back to the midline or following the basilar artery down from above, depending on its projection and size. Forward projecting sacs are commonly adherent to the clivus and those projecting laterally or posteriorly are embedded shallowly in the pons. Occasionally, the neck will stand out clearly, with the AICA below, but usually it is necessary to dissect the neck free and to separate the vital AICA from any adherence, using blunt or even sharp dissection. The fundus can often be held forward against the clivus to facilitate this dissection.

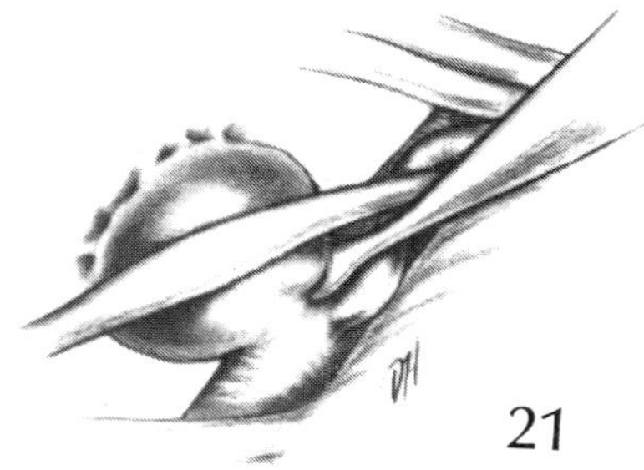

21

With a backward projecting sac it is quite possible to work *behind* the basilar artery to free the neck and perforators. Rupture of the sac is a frustrating possibility because of the narrow confines but is handled no differently. Clip application can be awkward in this region, mainly because the tips of the appliers and the handles are so large as to be difficult to work in the right direction, out of line of sight, in between the nerves. It may even be necessary to guide the applier in laterally to the VIIth and VIIIth nerves.

We have encountered a few aneurysms whose origin from the trunk of the basilar artery is clearly midway between that of the AICA and SCA, probably at the site of an unnamed vessel or possibly at the origin of the primitive trigeminal artery. This can be an awkward segment of the basilar artery to see even though the tent is widely divided, for the broad Vth nerve crosses the field and it is necessary to work above and below it. However, it has not been necessary to divide either it or the IVth nerve.

Three of the aneurysms arising from the basilar artery at the AICA were *bilateral* ('butterfly' aneurysms). In each case, it was possible to clip both aneurysms, although in two it meant working beneath the basilar artery to expose the neck of the posteriorly projecting sac. Both AICAs have to be cleared before clipping. It is wise to place the first clip so that the blades or the handle do not interfere with placement of the second clip.

Most *large bulbous* aneurysms at the AICA were approached through the tentorium. Coming down on a large upward projecting aneurysm may be precarious because the dome will obscure the neck or may be torn. Because of this, in two cases the necks were approached through a tentorial opening on the opposite side to dissect across the midline either over or underneath the basilar artery. While this was feasible in both cases, visualization of the neck was not as good; more recently, therefore, such cases have been approached on the same side as the projection of the aneurysm. It is a matter of working down the sides of the sac and displacing the waist of the aneurysm with a spatula or narrow retractor to visualize and clear its connections at the base for clipping. The AICA may be difficult to see below the neck of a large sac and this may have to be considerably displaced to be sure that the vital AICA is freed.

The results of surgery on basilar trunk aneurysms at the AICA are summarized in Table 5.

**Table 5 Basilar trunk aneurysms at the AICA: results of surgical treatment**

| | *Grade* | *Number of cases* | *Excellent* | *Good* | *Poor* | *Dead* |
|---|---|---|---|---|---|---|
| <12.5 mm | 0 | 4 | 3(1) | 1 | 0 | 0 |
| | 1 | 34 | 26(5) | 2 | 5(1) | 1 |
| | 2 | 6 | 4(4) | 1 | 0 | 1 |
| | 3 | 4 | 1(1) | 1 | 2 | 0 |
| | | 48 | 34(11) | 5 | 7(1) | 2 |
| Region of union of vertebral arteries | 0 | 1 | 0 | 0 | 1 | 0 |
| | 1 | 32 | 30(6) | 2(1) | 0 | 0 |
| | 2 | 9 | 5(1) | 3(2) | 0 | 1 |
| | 4 | 1 | 0 | 1 | 0 | 0 |
| | | 43 | 35(7) | 6(3) | 1 | 1 |

The numbers in parentheses refer to large bulbous aneurysms (12.5–25 mm).

# VERTEBROBASILAR JUNCTION ANEURYSMS

Because saccular aneurysms always seem to arise at the *distal* carina of a bifurcation on which the axial flow impinges, it would seem unlikely that the crotch of union of the vertebral arteries could be the site of aneurysm formation. However, the author is reasonably convinced that he has seen aneurysms arising at least in the neighbourhood of this junction. Three have occurred in cases where the opposite vertebral artery ended in the PICA and did not join its fellow, giving rise to the aneurysm.

The vertebral artery union usually overlies the junction of the lower and middle thirds of the clivus. This region can be approached from above or below, as in the case of basilar–AICA aneurysms, and the same considerations prevail. However, since it has been learned that in most cases the unilateral posterior fossa approach is quite satisfactory for visualization of the vertebral arteries up to and including the VB junction, this approach has been used routinely for these aneurysms. When difficulties arise with this exposure, especially if there is scarring from a previous operation, the combined transtentorial–suboccipital–transmastoid will be more revealing and helpful.

The results of surgery are summarized in Table 6. There were only two large aneurysms, each with an excellent result. The morbidity was related to rupture of an associated arteriovenous malformation or other aneurysm, arterial spasm, extradural clot, poor preoperative condition and probable pontine retractor injury (in two early cases).

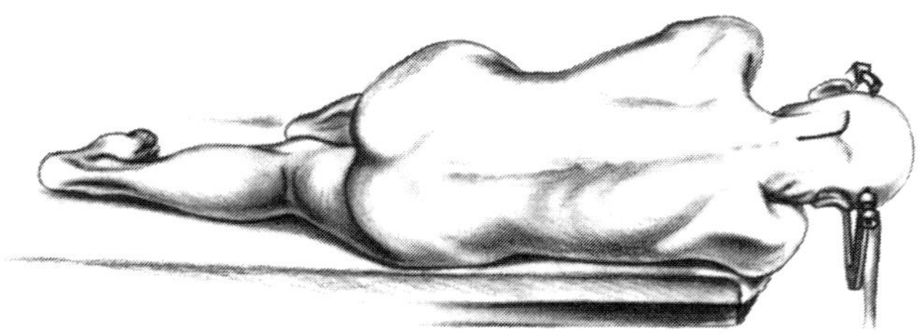

22a

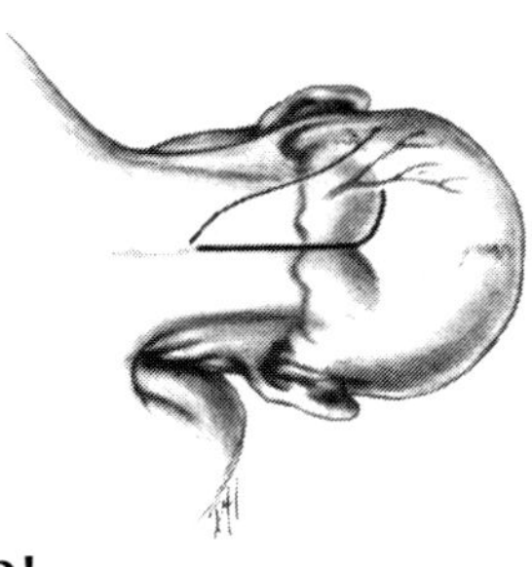

22b

# VERTEBRAL ANEURYSMS

Although their principal origin is at the distal crotch of the origin of the PICA, because of the notorious tortuosity and wandering of the vertebral artery and the varying level of origin of the PICA, these aneurysms have been found from near the intracranial entry of the vertebral artery under the first dentate ligament to near the vertebrobasilar junction, and from the lip of the foramen magnum to the middle third of the clivus. A right vertebral aneurysm has been seen lying to the left of the midline. Most project upward, lying shallowly in the medulla, either on its side or in front. A few project posteriorly into the medulla, or forward with the dome adherent to the clivus. Most common in this aneurysm is the tendency for the PICA to arise from the side of the neck. A few arise distinct from the PICA, probably at the site of origin of the anterior spinal artery or possibly at the origin of small unnamed branches. Most have an intimate relation to the hypoglossal nerve, which usually lies on the upper side of the neck but may be split by the aneurysm or lie in a groove between loculi.

**Table 6 Vertebral artery aneurysms: results of surgical treatment**

| *Grade* | *Number of cases* | *Excellent* | *Good* | *Poor* | *Dead* |
|---|---|---|---|---|---|
| 0 | 8* | 8* | 0 | 0 | 0 |
| 1 | 97* | 88* | 5 | 0 | 4 |
| 2 | 16 | 14 | 2 | 0 | 0 |
| 3 | 6 | 2 | 1 | 1 | 2 |
| 4 | 2 | 0 | 0 | 1 | 1 |
| | 129 | 112 | 8 | 2 | 7 |

* Including one large bulbous aneurysm (12.5–25 mm).

# 22a & b

The 'park bench' position (*a*) is very useful for vertebral and lower trunk aneurysms, allowing the surgeon to sit while providing a good angle for dissection up the side of and under the brainstem. It eliminates most of the risk of air embolism and allows a combined subtemporal–transtentorial exposure if necessary. A midline L-shaped incision is used, with the horizontal limb (4 cm or 1½ inches long) stopped just short of the occipital nerves (*b*) to preserve sensation in the scalp above. The patient's face is tilted a few degrees to the floor for comfortable access to premedullary and pontine regions.

The cerebellum is slackened off by opening a cistern, and then elevated off the medulla with the retractor at the base of the tonsil to expose the XIth nerve with its medullary pharyngeal filaments, the Xth and IXth nerves, the caudal loop of the PICA, and the vertebral artery as it emerges from under the first dentate ligament. Lower aneurysms will be seen immediately at this stage, as will those unusual ones lying up on the side of the medulla above the IXth and Xth nerves.

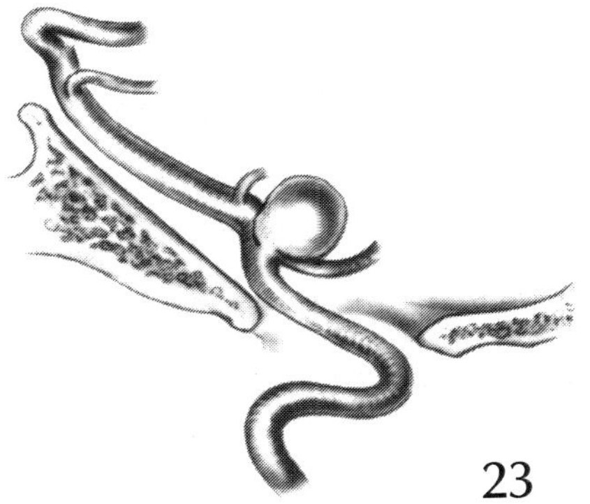

23

## 23 & 24

It is usually necessary to follow the vertebral artery upward toward the assumed site of the neck. Fortunately in this regard, the origin of the PICA is just proximal to the neck so that it will be seen first as a landmark to denote the presence of the neck just beyond, even though it may be under the midline of the medulla.

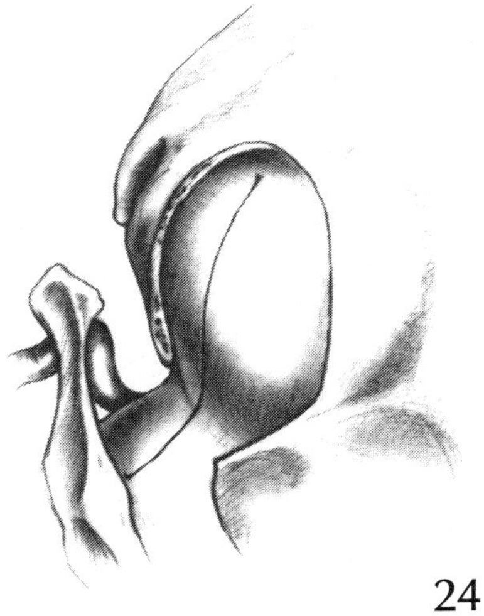

24

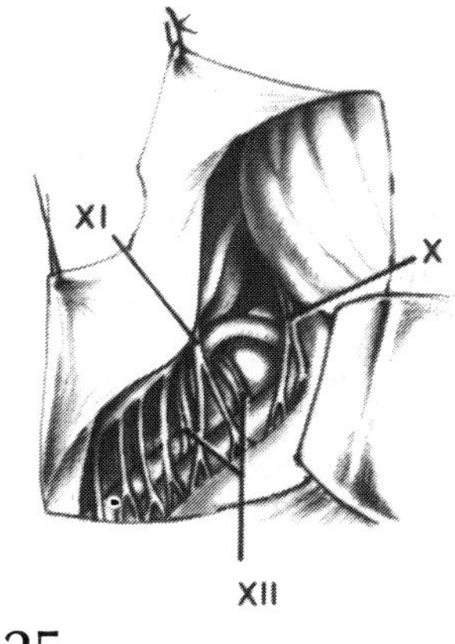


25

## 25

In most cases the route is below the lower filaments of the vagus but between the fragile pharyngeal filaments of the XIth nerve. Great care must be taken, for these filaments appear to be the principal innervation of the pharynx and larynx. (Dysphagia and hoarseness are not only distressing but dangerous consequences.) The hypoglossal nerve may be divided into two bundles by the aneurysm.

As the vertebral artery runs under the medulla, the latter must be gently retracted to follow it. Spontaneous breathing is used as a guide to retractor pressure. At first, as in the case of pontine retraction from above, it will seem that there is not enough room, but further gentle retraction and suction increase the exposure sufficiently to allow visualization of midline aneurysms over the lower middle third of the clivus. (A left vertebral aneurysm was once treated inadvertently from the right side when the opening was made on the wrong side.)

# 26

As the neck of the aneurysm is glimpsed, it may be best to work on either side of the PICA up the sides of the vertebral artery to the neck and then underneath the vertebral artery to follow it beyond the neck.

This portion of the artery and its direction must be seen to prevent its inadvertent occlusion during clip alignment. If it is difficult to obtain a good view of this segment, it can be visualized by holding the aneurysm closed with forceps or allowing the blades of the clip to close slowly to collapse the neck; the blades can then be realigned and positioned correctly just before final closure. The XIIth nerve will usually be seen on the far side of the neck and is gently freed so that the clip will not injure it.

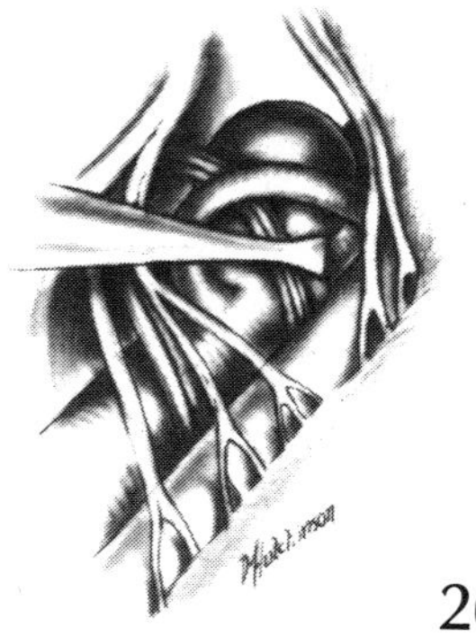

26

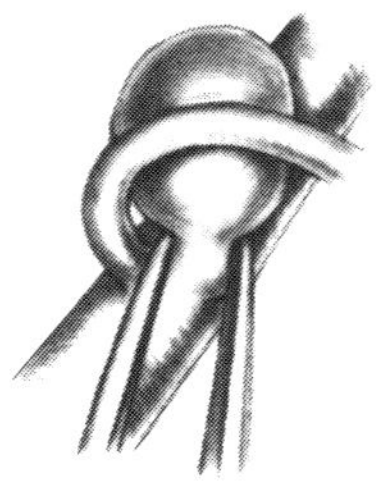

27

# 27

The fact that the PICA emerges from the near side of the neck often makes clipping awkward, for the angle of the neck will be oblique to the exposure and the clip tends to slip down to occlude the PICA. Coagulation to shrink the neck just above the PICA will result in narrowing for clip application. The illustration shows the neck held with forceps for coagulation or for determining the ideal position of the clip. Aspiration of the sac after clipping is routine.

# SURGERY OF GIANT VERTEBROBASILAR ANEURYSMS

Giant aneurysms (over 25 mm in diameter) usually arise from enlargement of smaller saccular aneurysms, but occasionally they are elongated fusiform serpentine dilatations of the vertebral and basilar arteries arising from atherosclerotic weakening of the wall. Surgical management of the latter is currently virtually impossible. However, our Unit has had experience with over 500 giant aneurysms, of which 278 have been on the posterior circulation. Although they have proved more difficult than those on the anterior circulation, most are surgically treatable, and about two-thirds of such patients have a satisfactory result.

As the natural history of giant aneurysms is bleak, surgical treatment should be considered in most cases. In our Unit, the therapeutic options have been reduced to neck clipping or Hunterian ligation of the parent artery, sometimes with trapping if opening and evacuation of the sac is essential to relieve brainstem compression. Other methods to obliterate the sac by promoting intraluminal thrombosis, such as injection of thrombogenic wire, have been found wanting since the neck of the sac usually remains open and subject to the pounding axial stream, and dilates to produce another dangerous aneurysm beneath.

## NECK OCCLUSION

It is surprising how often the neck of a giant aneurysm is small enough or can be made so for a strong spring clip to be applied. Neck clipping in this series was accomplished in 93 of 249 cases. Great care must be taken when applying the clip, as severe stenosis or occlusion of the parent artery, a major branch or a vital perforating vessel may result from a sliding clip or crimping of the neck tissue. Temporary occlusion of the parent artery or even trapping during the dissection around the neck and clip application is helpful. In our experience, the use of modern, gentle, temporary clips has never produced arterial injury sufficient to promote occlusive thrombosis in well over 100 cases, all of which have had postoperative angiography. Temporary clipping is only undertaken with mannitol 2 g/kg in the circulation as some protection against cerebral ischaemia. Ordinarily, the occlusion time is only 2 or 3 minutes, during which much dissection can be accomplished. For neck occlusion the Drake clip is commonly used so that an adherent vessel may be accommodated in the aperture at its base. This clip, as modified by Sugita in various angles, may be used in tandem with a straight clip which occludes that portion of a large neck remaining in the aperture while its blades are occluding the far side. Once the orifice is closed, the aneurysm may be aspirated or opened to evacuate its contents and relieve mass effect. Of the 93 patients with giant aneurysms that could be clipped, 63 per cent had a good result but 11 per cent died and 26 per cent had a poor result. However, when only patients in good condition are considered, 76 per cent had good results. The greatest morbidity occurred when attempting to clip giant aneurysms in the region of the basilar artery bifurcation. It is hoped that CT scanning for fleeting or vague neurological syndromes will allow earlier recognition of a larger number of patients in whom the neck may be occluded more safely.

Unfortunately, the necks of the majority of giant aneurysms are impossible or dangerous to clip because either too much of the parent artery is incorporated into the neck, or the bulbous steep slope of a firm neck allows the closed blades of the clip to slide in and thus occlude the parent artery or major branch; this is particularly problematic when the neck is stiffened with atheroma or mural thrombosis. Occasionally, with temporary occlusion of the parent artery, an aneurysm may be opened and thrombus evacuated to make the neck clippable. In a few pliable broad-necked aneurysms, the tandem clip principle, using multiple Drake clips in tandem or in parallel, can be used to reconstruct the arterial lumen, a procedure that has been so successful for giant carotid aneurysms.

## PROXIMAL PARENT ARTERY OCCLUSION

For unclippable necks, currently the best option is occlusion of the parent vessel as near to the aneurysm as is feasible to stop the high pounding axial flow into the sac. The stagnation in the sac thus isolated usually promotes intraluminal thrombosis which obliterates all or most of the aneurysm. Of course, this manoeuvre requires adequate circulation into the territory of the obliterated artery by communicating arteries or leptomeningeal collateral flow. Unfortunately, in contrast to the carotid circulation, there is no safely reliable extracranial–intracranial bypass to the basilar artery via the posterior cerebral or superior cerebellar arteries. However, when posterior communicating arteries (even of modest dimensions) exist, occlusion of the upper basilar artery is usually possible for aneurysms in the region of the basilar bifurcation. Even the lower basilar or both vertebral arteries have been occluded successfully.

The presence and calibre of the posterior communicating arteries may not be known from routine carotid and vertebral studies. However, these vessels can be opacified routinely by Allcock's method, using first right, then left carotid compression during vertebral angiography. Clip occlusion of the basilar or both vertebral arteries may be used when one or both communicating vessels are obviously sufficient to carry the basilar circulation above the point of occlusion. Clip occlusion of the basilar artery in 33 patients produced good results in 70 per cent, while 9 per cent died and 21 per cent had poor results. Again, if only patients in good condition are considered, the results were very much better.

If the circulation is marginal, a special tourniquet, designed to test the adequacy of the collateral flow when the patient is conscious, can be used. If it is impossible to clip the aneurysm during surgery, a snare is made by placing a plastic suture around the basilar or vertebral artery and bringing the ends out of the head in small polyethylene tubing through a stab wound. When the patient is awake, the tourniquet can be closed by hand during angiography and the closure maintained by small artery forceps while the patient is carefully monitored for any ischaemic deficit. If none appears after 30 minutes or so, then the stem of the tourniquet may be clipped to hold the occlusion and the patient kept under close observation. The snare can be quickly opened with clip-removing forceps if ischaemia develops. After 24 hours, the stab wound is enlarged under local anaesthesia. The tourniquet can be reclipped as deeply in the wound as possible to maintain the occlusion, and the ends cut off and buried subcutaneously. Tourniquet occlusion of the basilar artery in 32 patients with presumed marginal collateral circulation produced good results in 16. Once again, patients in good condition fared much better. Remarkably, there was little correlation between the number and size of the posterior communicating arteries and subsequent ischaemia, as tiny vessels were sometimes able to maintain the upper basilar circulation.

Giant aneurysms on the trunk of the basilar artery may be trapped to allow evacuation of the aneurysm if this is considered essential to relieve critical brainstem compression. In six such cases, there were four excellent results, one poor result and one death. In four cases, the anterior inferior cerebellar arteries and some perforators were undoubtedly included in the trapped segment, and in two of these there was sufficient collateral circulation to the territory of these vessels bilaterally. In three of the trappings, the tourniquet was used to test the collateral flow in the conscious patient.

For giant unclippable aneurysms arising at the VB junction or the vertebral artery, occlusion of one or both vertebral arteries is necessary. One vertebral artery may be occluded beyond the PICA almost routinely as long as the other exists and fills the basilar artery. Occlusion proximal to the PICA risks medullary infarction, although it is remarkable how often the PICA fills retrogradely through a channel underneath the thrombosed aneurysm or by collateral flow from the AICA. Complete thrombosis of an aneurysm restricted to one vertebral artery is usual.

Similarly, where one vertebral artery is atretic or ends in the PICA, giant lower basilar trunk aneurysms can be treated by occlusion proximally of the only vertebral artery filling them, but this requires sufficient posterior communicating collateral flow, which may have to be tested with the tourniquet. Detached balloon occlusion of an intracranial vertebral segment is undoubtedly dangerous because the ostia of perforating branches may also be occluded. Unilateral vertebral occlusions for giant vertebral aneurysms produced good results and complete obliterative thrombosis in all seven patients so treated. Unilateral occlusion for giant basilar trunk and VB aneurysms was very satisfactory in 10 of 14 patients, but two were made worse and two died largely from brainstem ischaemia.

For most giant VB junction aneurysms, bilateral vertebral occlusion will be necessary, but this requires sufficient posterior communicating collateral flow. Clip occlusion of one vertebral artery with placement of the tourniquet on the other during the initial exploratory craniotomy has merit in marginal situations.

Huge VB junction aneurysms which involve a considerable segment of the basilar artery with its branches (especially AICAs) are particularly dangerous since bilateral vertebral occlusion is very efficient in promoting complete thrombosis in the sac, which may result in severe brainstem infarction. Recently, a Drake clip has been used to produce severe stenosis of the second vertebral artery and thus promote the development of collateral supply over a period of months. Bilateral vertebral artery occlusion has been used in 16 patients, with good results in nine. The four poor results and three deaths were mostly related to brainstem infarction after branch occlusion from massive thrombosis within the aneurysm.

Only a few giant posterior cerebral aneurysms are clippable, whether they arise on the first (one of four on P1) or second (one of three on P2) segments. Many tend to be fusiform. However, the results with P1 and P2 occlusion have been excellent in promoting complete obliterative thrombosis but without occipital infarction. This complication did not occur after any of the 15 P1 occlusions and in only three of nine P2 occlusions, in five of which the aneurysm was trapped for evacuation. While the posterior communicating artery may confer some protection for P1 occlusion, this is seldom the case with these aneurysms since the communicating artery tends to be occluded by aneurysmal thrombosis. In those cases where no field defect occurred, leptomeningeal collateral flow from A2 and M2 branches has been spectacular, even filling P2 retrogradely to or near to the aneurysm. The results in all 15 P2 aneurysms were good, whether neck occlusion (six), proximal clipping (four) or trapping (five) was used. P1 occlusion (10) or trapping (seven) was used in 17 of 22 patients with giant P1 aneurysms, with only two poor results (from midbrain ischaemia because of perforator isolation). Another patient died when the proximal P1 trapping was improperly placed or slipped, and the previously intact aneurysm burst.

While surgical treatment of giant aneurysms on the anterior carotid circulation is successful in 85 per cent of cases, and posterior cerebral and vertebral giant aneurysms have a surgical success rate of 85 and 90 per cent respectively, only about 66 per cent of patients with giant aneurysms arising on the basilar artery fare well.

## *Acknowledgement*

The author is indebted to Dr A. J. Fox, Director of Neuroradiology at The University of Western Ontario, who has carried out the majority of studies in this series.

## *References*

1. Drake, C. G. (1965) Surgical treatment of ruptured aneurysms of the basilar artery. Experience with 14 cases. Journal of Neurosurgery, 23, 457–473
2. Drake, C. G. (1968) Further experience with surgical treatment of aneurysm of the basilar artery. Journal of Neurosurgery, 29, 372–392
3. Drake, C. G. (1979) The treatment of aneurysms of the posterior circulation. Clinical Neurosurgery, 26, 96–144
4. Fox, J. L. (1983) Intracranial Aneurysms, p. 22. Heidelberg: Springer–Verlag
5. Hamby, W. B. (1952) Intracranial Aneurysms. Springfield: Charles C. Thomas
6. Drake, C. G. (1979) The treatment of aneurysms of the posterior circulation. Clinical Neurosurgery, 26, 96–144
7. Yaşargil, M. G., Antic, J., Laciga, R., Jain, K. K., Hodosh, R. M., Smith, R. D. (1976) Microsurgical pterional approach to aneurysms of the basilar bifurcation. Surgical Neurology, 6, 83–91

Illustrations by Robert Lane after S. Badell

# Surgery of intracranial arteriovenous malformation

**H. Hunt Batjer** MD
Assistant Professor, Division of Neurological Surgery, University of Texas Southwestern Medical Center, Dallas, Texas, USA

**Duke S. Samson** MD
Professor and Chairman, Division of Neurological Surgery, University of Texas Southwestern Medical Center, Dallas, Texas, USA

## Patient selection

Following the initial pioneering attempts at surgical treatment of intracranial arteriovenous malformations by Krause[1], Dandy[2], and Cushing and Bailey[3], diagnosis and therapeutic strategies were revolutionized by the introduction of cerebral angiography[4]. Despite modern microsurgical and neuroanaesthetic advances, however, selection of patients for whom operative intervention should be offered remains controversial even among arteriovenous malformation surgeons. While natural history data suggest that the long-term risk of death or disability from haemorrhage, ischaemia or seizures approaches 50 per cent[5,6], the short-term risk of rebleeding is considerably lower than that present with aneurysmal rebleeding and is approximately 6 per cent during the first year and 3 per cent per year thereafter[7,8]. As accurate non-invasive neuroimaging techniques have become increasingly available in small as well as large communities, neurosurgeons are confronted with an expanding group of patients with asymptomatic or minimally symptomatic arteriovenous malformations. To make matters more complicated, more and more elderly patients are being similarly diagnosed.

The decision whether to offer surgical therapy to a given patient must be highly individualized and must take into consideration a number of variables in the heterogeneous population. Important elements in our decision-making process are discussed below.

### The patient

The general medical condition of the patient presenting with a major intracranial haemorrhage or progressive disability from ischaemic symptoms influences anaesthetic decisions such as the potential use of hypotension or high-dose barbiturates and perioperative cardiopulmonary care, but usually does not influence our decision to offer a surgical procedure. Notable exceptions to this general rule include patients with end-stage heart, renal, pulmonary or hepatic disease or those who have only a slight chance of survival owing to an unassociated malignancy. The medical status assumes paramount importance in the patient with an asymptomatic or minimally symptomatic arteriovenous malformation. In general, we require that these patients could reasonably expect to live 15–20 years if their neurological threat were eliminated before surgical treatment can potentially favourably compete with their natural history.

### Life-threatening haemorrhage

We recommend operative resection to all but a very select group of patients who present with a new intracranial haemorrhage or a documented prior history of bleeding. While the previously quoted natural history data are somewhat reassuring in terms of a low risk of early recurrent bleeding, our experience suggests that there may be subgroups of patients who, once symptomatic, will continue to bleed repetitively. Patients with small periventricular arteriovenous malformations with solitary drainage may be particularly susceptible to early rebleeding due to venous compromise by the clot or increased intracranial pressure. For patients evaluated following intracranial haemorrhage from extremely large or eloquently located arteriovenous malformations, careful scrutiny of computerized tomography (CT) and magnetic resonance imaging (MRI) studies not infrequently reveals that the haematoma has actually dissected portions of the neurologically most dangerous planes. This makes it more likely that a well planned procedure can be carried out with only a small risk of increasing the neurological deficit. For patients who survive intraventricular or intracerebral haemorrhage from thalamic, bithalamic or brainstem arteriovenous malformations we require occasionally that the patient must have sustained multiple bleeds, proving their malignant natural history, before recommending surgical treatment or stereotactically directed radiotherapy.

## Progressive neurological deficit

In our experience, patients presenting with ischaemic symptoms from typically large, high-flow lesions will become progressively disabled fairly quickly if not treated aggressively. Unfortunately, many patients in this group are elderly and have other medical problems increasing their operative morbidity. Owing to their poor outlook if untreated, however, we usually recommend surgery.

## Intractable and disabling seizures

Despite literature to the contrary, our experience is that patients with seizures are usually medically controllable after arteriovenous malformation resection. We are quite aggressive in recommending surgery to patients with arteriovenous malformations located in relatively non-eloquent brain tissue when the use of intraoperative electrocorticography and subsequent resection of additional tissue would offer substantial hope of seizure control. We are also aggressive in offering resection to patients with temporal lobe arteriovenous malformations in whom electrophysiological evidence suggests ipsilateral origins of the seizure disorder. In these patients, resection of the hippocampus and the mesial temporal structures follows routine microsurgical removal of the malformation.

## Characteristics of the arteriovenous malformation

While we do not routinely grade arteriovenous malformations by the published grading scales, we include a number of radiographic and cerebral blood flow (single-photon emission computed tomography or xenon-enhanced computed tomography) parameters in our initial evaluation. Location of the arteriovenous malformation in relationship to the Rolandic fissure, motor and sensory speech (using the Wada test), thalamus and brainstem are major concerns, particularly in patients who have not suffered life-threatening complications. Extremely large arteriovenous malformations (greater than 6 cm) carry a higher risk regardless of their location owing to the volume of shunted blood which must be redistributed acutely at the time of excision, and the risk of loss of control intraoperatively increasing morbidity and mortality. While our experience of evaluating non-angiographic aspects of haemodynamics using cerebral blood flow techniques is limited, it is likely that lesions with extremely high flow and the presence of large volumes of ischaemic and dysautoregulated tissue carry higher surgical risk. The presence of wide cortical representation is a favourable parameter which lessens the amount of retraction necessary on adjacent healthy brain tissue during operation. In our experience, the incorporation of lenticulostriate or thalamoperforating vessels into the feeding system increases the risk of surgical morbidity[9]. This may simply relate to the fact that substantial filling of the arteriovenous malformation will remain during the deep dissection near the internal capsule or basal ganglia, producing a bloodier operative field and decreasing the likelihood of a perfect microsurgical removal. In the presence of associated aneurysms in the arteriovenous malformation feeding system, frequently we recommend at least clipping of these lesions even if arteriovenous malformation resection is not contemplated. Patients with these aneurysms may be at higher risk of rupture owing to the high flow in the parent vessels than patients with asymptomatic aneurysms without an arteriovenous malformation[10].

## Surgical team

It is not possible to offer these patients an optimal chance of a favourable surgical outcome without a carefully organized team of professionals. Valuable components of this team include the surgeon, neuroanaesthetist, neuroradiological support, neurosurgical intensive care and operating room nurses.

*Surgeons(s)* Perhaps no other neurosurgical patient is as dependent on a highly skilled and experienced microsurgeon as the patient with an arteriovenous malformation.

*Neuroanaesthetist* Many resections require protracted anaesthesia which can be complicated by major blood loss and cerebral haemodynamic crises.

*Neuroradiological support* Skilled neuroradiologists with interventional capabilities are required for state-of-the-art diagnostic and therapeutic embolization procedures, as well as their availability for intraoperative angiography.

*Neurosurgical intensive care* Skilled nurses trained in the management of haemodynamically unstable patients as well as in the subtleties of neurosurgical postoperative surveillance are vital in early detection of postoperative complications.

*Operating room nurses* A qualified and vigilant nursing staff is critical during these procedures which can quickly deteriorate into life-threatening emergencies.

### Realistic expectations

In this surgery, the team is critically dependent on the realistic understanding of the patient and his family and their support in the face of a protracted acute recovery phase and extended rehabilitation.

### Non-microsurgical therapy

Intravascular embolization or surgical ligation of feeding vessels is not recommended if resection is not planned. Leaving the low-resistance shunt *in situ* sets the stage for the well-described complications of recruitment of myriads of dural, tentorial and leptomeningeal feeding vessels over time which can convert the removal of a relatively straightforward arteriovenous malformation into a procedure that is exceedingly difficult and dangerous to the patient. However, we feel that occasional patients may benefit, at least temporarily, from this approach. The elderly patient with progressive neurological disability from a large or eloquently located lesion, and who would not be a surgical candidate owing to poor cardiopulmonary status and limited life expectancy, may be neurologically improved if flow through the malformation can be decreased. Additionally, patients suffering intracranial haemorrhage from inoperable thalamic or brainstem arteriovenous malformations may be protected from early rebleeding during the period which is required for stereotactic radiotherapy to potentially eliminate the lesion.

### Intangibles

Occasionally, well-informed asymptomatic patients simply cannot enjoy a normal life knowing that they harbour an unpredictable and potentially lethal disease, and request treatment regardless of risk. After consideration of this and other variables, it is likely that the most sensitive predictor of selection of the patient who will have a poor future if left untreated and a successful outcome if operated upon is the gestalt of an experienced surgeon as he evaluates the patient and radiological studies. This general impression frequently influences our decision-making.

## Timing of surgery

As a general rule we make every attempt to manage patients with fresh intracerebral or subarachnoid haemorrhage from an intracranial arteriovenous malformation medically with steroids, intermittent diuresis, intracranial pressure monitoring and ventricular drainage (when necessary) to avoid craniotomy for decompression. As long as intracranial pressure can be controlled and patients remain neurologically stable, we continue with a non-operative course. If this protocol is successful, it is often surprising how much neurological recovery can occur over the first 2 or 3 post-haemorrhage months. We recommend early definitive angiography shortly after admission so that the vascular architecture is known and an appropriate bone flap can be constructed in the event of acute deterioration, allowing control of the afferent and efferent vessels. In the event of failure of medical management, we recommend a generous craniotomy and an initial attempt at simple haematoma decompression, avoiding injury to the malformation itself. We ligate a few of the arterial feeding vessels found in the subarachnoid space prior to closure routinely in this setting. If medical management is successful, the patient is followed closely by CT scanning for signs of haematoma resolution and improvement in mass effect. We do not recommend therapeutic embolization in the first 1–2 weeks after haemorrhage because any resultant oedema or infarction may precipitate intracranial decompensation from mass effect. The timing of definitive craniotomy is individualized and determined by the rate of neurological recovery, clinical and radiographic evidence of normalization of intracranial pressure and the rate of haematoma resorption. A compromise must be made between avoiding attempting resection while the brain is swollen or hydrocephalic, and operating prior to complete obliteration and gliosis in the haematoma cavity. The plane dissected by the haematoma can be used to significant advantage during microsurgical resection. In general, we tend to operate between 3 and 6 weeks post-haemorrhage. We strongly recommend repeat angiography immediately before the planned procedure because the haematoma may have compressed portions of the lesion, resulting in non-visualization on the acute angiogram.

The patient who is rendered comatose from the initial haemorrhage or who is deteriorating rapidly during evaluation presents a difficult problem to the neurosurgeon. If at all possible, we recommend angiography before craniotomy to avoid an inappropriate bony exposure. Barbiturate coma may offer some advantage in providing brain protection for the additional hour of preoperative evaluation required during angiography. If immediate angiography is not available, CT scanning with and without contrast, or MRI, can both yield useful anatomical information before emergency craniotomy to help the surgeon avoid entering the nidus of the malformation. Our goal in this type of procedure is to decompress the haematoma and ligate available feeding vessels. This is often not possible and if malformation bleeding is not controllable the lesion should be resected. We usually perform a non-microsurgical removal in this setting and have had optimal results in performing a modified lobectomy where appropriate and avoiding dissection on the bleeding nidus itself. The use of high-dose barbiturates has been a useful surgical adjunct in these difficult situations and seems to reduce brain volume, control systemic blood pressure, and, if continued for 12–24 hours postoperatively, prevent wide swings in systolic pressure during the acute recovery phase.

# Important preoperative considerations

## Embolization

1

Many cerebral hemisphere and posterior fossa arteriovenous malformations can be successfully removed with minimal morbidity or mortality without preoperative diminution of their arterial supply by interventional radiological techniques, such as liquid, particulate or balloon embolization. However, the experience of most surgeons involved in this surgery would suggest that not only does the liberal use of these innovative techniques markedly reduce the risks and potential complications associated with the removal of large and difficult lesions, but also that their routine application facilitates the uncomplicated surgical excision of many if not most arteriovenous malformations of modest (2.5–4.0 cm) diameter. While an in-depth discussion of the variety of techniques currently availabe is beyond the scope of this chapter, our own experience with intraoperative and preoperative embolization using isobutyl 2-cyanoacrylate, preoperative embolization with flow-directed Silastic (Dow Corning, UK) and polyvinyl alcohol particles, and preoperative embolization using selective intracranial catheterization with polyvinyl alcohol slurry would support the concept that small-particle embolization close to the malformation itself is the most satisfactory current alternative in terms of efficiency and risk. The goal of embolization is twofold: (*1*) to embolize the nidus of the malformation itself; and (*2*) to provide a decrease in proximal arterial flow by the occlusion of major arterial channels at the margin of the lesion. These goals are best accomplished by transfemoral catheterization under local anaesthesia followed by superselective cannulation of the major feeding arteries of the malformation with repetitive injection of small-fragment emboli into the body of the lesion. Neurological status should be monitored closely throughout the embolization procedure, which should be terminated with the appearance of any neurological deficit, or with dramatic angiographic reduction in vascularity.

While preoperative embolization is not without potential morbidity, the efficacy and safety of therapeutic embolization will depend greatly on the skill and experience of the neuroradiologist involved. For this reason, it is imperative that the interventional neuroradiologist functions as an essential member of the surgical team involved with the overall preoperative planning of the therapeutic approach to each individual malformation. As a general rule, definitive surgical excision of a malformation should be carried out 7–14 days following embolization. This time period allows for maximal effect of the embolization procedure on both the arteriovenous malformation and the haemodynamics of the surrounding brain, and is brief enough to minimize the enlargement of collateral sources.

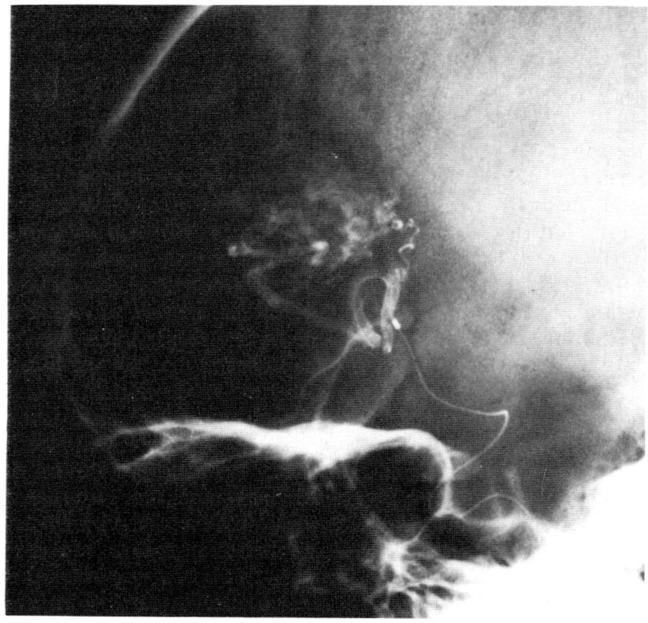

1

## Cosurgeons and arteriovenous malformation excision

Many small arteriovenous malformations can be removed with relative ease without the benefit of preoperative embolization. Many such surgical excisions do not require great technical skill, nor protracted periods of operative time. Unfortunately, larger and more complicated malformations frequently necessitate and demand the protracted concentration and manual dexterity of an accomplished microvascular surgeon over an extended operative period. Not infrequently the most delicate, difficult and potentially dangerous aspect of removal comes in the latter stages of the surgical procedure when the surgeon is completing the periventricular portion of the dissection. In cases of large lesions particularly, this portion of the procedure occurs late in the dissection, often many hours after the skin incision; therefore, the presence of two experienced and accomplished surgeons alternating with relative frequency throughout the day can both speed the completion of the procedure and avoid potential complications due to fatigue, tremor or inattention during the final stages of resection. The routine use of cosurgeons or two surgical teams in procedures directed at the removal of malformations larger than 3 cm in diameter, or those located in either the brainstem or cerebellopontine angle, will be rewarded by an enhanced level of surgical care for the patient[11].

### Early postoperative angiography

The use of microsurgical techniques, which enables the neurosurgeon to work on the very margin of the lesion, carries with it the risk of inadvertent isolation of irregular portions of the lesion, which protrude into normal brain parenchyma. Even under microscopic visualization these small segments are difficult to identify and form a significant risk of postoperative haemorrhage and associated morbidity if unrecognized and untreated. Furthermore, postoperative complications including cerebral oedema and 'normal perfusion pressure breakthrough' bleeding[12] are impossible to distinguish from haemorrhage due to retained arteriovenous malformation fragments, a distinction with very important therapeutic implications. For these reasons, intraoperative or early postoperative angiographic evaluation of the results of resection have proved to be of great benefit in our own series of over 250 such surgical procedures. Despite this experience, we continue to find residual malformation requiring reoperation in one of every eight to ten patients. In each case the patient is returned immediately to the operating room for completion of the resection. This rather surprising incidence is matched by a low incidence of normal perfusion pressure breakthrough bleeding (approximately 3 per cent), suggesting that haemorrhage from undetected retained arteriovenous malformation may not infrequently be misdiagnosed as the occurrence of breakthrough bleeding.

### Normal perfusion pressure breakthrough bleeding

This clinical phenomenon was initially recognized and subsequently described by Spetzler *et al.* and has subsequently been the subject of a large amount of both clinical and experimental consideration[12]. It represents the delayed appearance of cerebral oedema and/or confluent haemorrhage in the brain parenchyma surrounding the site of a recently resected arteriovenous malformation. This complication occurs most frequently following a single-stage removal of a large and highly vascular malformation and is believed to represent the sequelae of redistribution of large volumes of blood into chronically underperfused brain parenchyma. It occurs most commonly within 48 hours following surgical excision and is clinically manifested by neurological deterioration and the appearance of focal neurological deficit. The CT picture is most frequently one of a combination of haemorrhage and low-density oedema that may involve extensive areas of previously normal cortex. Essentially, the diagnosis of the phenomenon involves exclusion of the possibility of haemorrhage from retained malformation. Once this has been done, mass effect considerations may necessitate the resection of a portion of the involved brain parenchyma and/or evacuation of intracerebral clot. However, the most effective management of this complication is the protracted use of barbiturate coma with global reduction in cerebral blood flow[13]. More importantly, several measures are available to decrease the probability of this feared and morbid complication. Sequential preoperative reduction in arterial flow to the malformation with concomitant restoration of normal flow to the surrounding brain parenchyma before excision of the malformation is perhaps the most important of these, and has been documented to occur by cerebral blood flow studies in several patients[14]. While theoretically this can be accomplished by surgical ligation of arterial feeders intraoperatively, certainly the most effective and least invasive method of such flow reduction is by selective preoperative catheterization and embolization of these feeding vessels. This procedure, used in association with sequential cerebral blood flow evaluations, provides the best preoperative insurance against the changes in cerebral haemodynamics implicated in the production of normal perfusion pressure breakthrough bleeding. Furthermore, in cases in which this complication would seem to be a reasonably likely occurrence or in which some brain engorgement occurs late in the procedure, the elective use of postoperative barbiturate coma for a period of 48 to 72 hours may offer additional security.

## Technical considerations in arteriovenous malformation surgery

There are certain principles which deserve the surgeon's close attention in the planning and execution of every surgical procedure which has as its goal the removal of an arteriovenous malformation. While the location, size, vascular anatomy and status of the brain parenchyma, as well as the patient's overall condition and age, will influence and modify the application of these tenets in each individual case, an appreciation and observation of these principles will consistently result in the best possible operative outcome.

### Anaesthetic considerations

Excellent neuroanaesthetic support is an absolute requirement for the performance of this surgery and can prove a serious challenge to even the most accomplished and experienced anaesthetist. These operative procedures are often protracted and necessitate the early establishment and close maintenance of an adequate, but not excessive, level of anaesthesia/analgesia coupled with judicious ventilator and fluid management, both to maximize brain tissue relaxation and often to ensure the preservation of optimal haemodynamic function in the event of significant volume depletion owing to serious intraoperative blood loss. These considerations mandate close preoperative consultation between the anaesthetist and surgeon followed by close intraoperative surveillance of all available parameters, including electrocortical activity, somatosensory evoked responses, arterial blood pressure, central venous pressure, pulmonary capillary wedge pressure and systemic vascular resistance.

### Operative exposure

The cortical projection of all arteriovenous malformations should be easily localized before the surgical procedure using imaging techniques currently available in the preoperative period (especially MRI in the sagittal and coronal planes). In almost all superficially located malformations and some deeply located lesions (such as in the cerebellar vermis or cerebellopontine angle), the degree of superficial exposure should be extensive. Large craniotomy flaps with wide stellate dural openings permit inspection of an extensive area of cortex surrounding the suspected site of the arteriovenous malformation and identification of important feeding and draining vessels at some distance from the lesion, from which points they can be tracked in the subarachnoid space and/or sulci to the margins of the lesion itself (*see Illustration 2*). Furthermore, this degree of exposure is often necessary if the use of intraoperative electrical cortical stimulation is anticipated, or if postoperative electrocorticography is planned. Similarly, access to deep lesions, such as those in the cerebellopontine angle or involving the corpus callosum, is facilitated and brain retraction is minimized with extensive exposure of the entire length of the lateral and sigmoid sinuses or of the cortical aspect of the interhemispheric fissure.

## Early access to the arterial supply

Proximal control and sequential ligation of the arterial input remains the keystone to successful removal of these vascular lesions. The surgical approach to each lesion should be planned in such a fashion as to provide the surgeon with the greatest degree of early proximal control over the maximum amount of arterial feeding. While many of these lesions receive a significant amount of arterial input which traverses the brain parenchyma, most arterial supply enters the lesion almost directly from large conducting vessels in the subarachnoid space. These arteries are found beneath the arachnoid in cortical sulci or in the subarachnoid cisterns and should be identified and isolated before making the initial cortical incision. If these points of isolation lie at some distance from the suspected margin of the malformation, the arterial feeders should not be ligated at this time, but rather should be stripped of their arachnoid covering and prepared for temporary clip placement later in the procedure. The vessels can be marked by small cotton patties so that the surgeon can easily return to them quickly should their ligation become necessary during the dissection. The use of proximal occlusion, both by preoperative embolization and by clip ligation in the initial stages of the procedure, serves two roles; the first is to reduce the vascularity and potential for haemorrhage from the malformation itself, the second is to decrease the distension of the malformation by arterial blood, thus facilitating the compression and dissection of the malformation from the surrounding brain and therefore minimizing the degree of brain tissue retraction.

## Preservation of venous drainage

Despite reports to the contrary, it is the authors' belief that preservation of all venous drainage until obliteration of all arterial input has occurred is an extremely important principle in the resection of these lesions. While the nature and location of the principal draining veins should be fixed in the surgeon's mind prior to the procedure, there is no way to estimate the reserve capacity of the drainage in the face of early sacrifice of important venous channels. It is true that the superficial venous drainage of a malformation may appear to limit access to the margins of the lesion, but this limitation is more apparent than real as careful microscopic dissection of the draining vessels themselves will permit their elevation from the underlying cortex and preservation of their integrity, facilitating circumferential dissection of the margins. This dissection of a venous pedicle is important, as not infrequently bound tightly to the veins are important entering arterial feeders to the malformation whose identification can only be made by extensive mobilization of the venous structures. As with early control of the arterial inflow, preservation of the venous drainage will both prevent undue haemorrhage from the malformation during the time of dissection and also serve to provide maximum decompression of the malformation, permitting its mobilization and retraction during exposure.

## Circumferential dissection

When maximum access has been gained to the feeding arteries of the malformation, and the venous pedicles have been identified, freed from the surrounding cortex, and carefully preserved, the surgeon turns his attention to the actual resection of the malformation. This dissection will first pass through the pia–arachnoid, the superficial cortical layers and then extend deeply into the white matter and ultimately into the periventricular tissue, the ependyma and finally into the ventricular system itself. This exposure should be planned so that a relatively constant depth of dissection throughout the entire circumference of the malformation is maintained, avoiding extending the exposure deeply in any one site until the entire periphery of the malformation is freed from the surrounding brain parenchyma. This technique involves frequent movement of the microscope as the malformation is repetitively circumnavigated, and provides for relatively brief periods of retraction on any one portion of the lesion and the adjacent brain. As exposure is shifted from place to place, the depth of dissection should be marked with a non-adherent strip of Instat (Johnson & Johnson, New Brunswick, New Jersey, USA) or Mericel (American Corporation, Mystic, Connecticut, USA) so that the surgeon can return to the appropriate depth with ease in a later portion of the procedure. Careful attention to the concept of circumferential dissection maximizes the mobility of the malformation at any given level in the dissection process, prevents protracted retraction on either malformation or brain tissue, and decreases the possibility of encountering difficult bleeding in a deep and narrow exposure. In this way, the surgeon will move throughout the three sequential stages of dissection (arachnoid/cortical, white matter and periependymal/ventricular) around the periphery of the malformation rather than having very superficial exposure on one margin and deep and perhaps threatening exposure on another.

## Maintenance of haemostasis

Preservation of a dry field of dissection is often difficult and may tax even the most experienced microvascular surgeon. The two mechanisms which the authors have found most beneficial in their practice have been the use of bipolar cautery forceps and the use of numerous small aneurysm clips.

While bipolar cauterization plays a large part in all microvascular surgical technique, the fragile primitive vessels require special care if cautery is to be both effective and reliable. Vessels to be cauterized should be moist with irrigation fluid and cautery should be maintained on the lowest setting consistent with vascular sealing. Short bursts of cautery delivered while the tips of the forceps compress the vessel are preferred to longer bursts delivered while the vessel is clamped forcefully and sealed by the forceps; the gentler approach prevents charring of the vessel, adherence to the forceps and subsequent avulsion of the vessel. Additionally, we prefer to use forceps with intermediate size tips rather than the very fine tipped forceps most commonly used in subarachnoid dissection, as the latter have a tendency to burn through the very fragile small arterioles. Unfortunately, many vessels are not amenable to closure with bipolar cautery, particularly the dilated arterioles in the periventricular area which often rupture and then retract into the white matter when attacked with even the most gentle bipolar technique. For that reason, we have found it beneficial to use small Yaşargil aneurysm clips on these distended vessels, a technique which both speeds the procedure and provides a reliable and repetitive degree of haemostasis for vascular structures which are otherwise most difficult to close. The smallest clips possible should be employed to facilitate further dissection in the area and after placement can be covered with a thin cottonoid or Mericel patty. Subsequently, a retractor can be placed directly on the clips to permit continued exposure of the periphery of the malformation. Microaneurysm clips are preferred to any type of haemoclip because of the ease of application, precise closing pressure and capacity for removal and reapplication.

## Wide ventricular exposure

As almost all arteriovenous malformations abut on to and involve a significant portion of the ependymal lining of the ventricle, and often receive important arterial feeding through the ventricle and periependymal tissue, it is important to extend the exposure and dissection well into the ventricular cavity. Additionally, haemostasis, which is often awkward to obtain in the periventricular white matter, becomes much simpler when the ventricle is opened and the malformation can be mobilized away from the ventricular wall. Ventricular exposure should be extensive to ensure that no residual malformation is left in the periependymal tissue and early in the dissection the floor of the ventricle should be identified with a cottonoid or Mericel strip both to facilitate rapid identification when returning to the area and also to prevent haemorrhage into the ventricular system. Once the ventricle has been identified and opened, most commonly the ependymal portion of the malformation can be quickly separated from the surrounding healthy tissue using bipolar dissection, and the malformation can be raised on its venous pedicles and then removed. Following removal of the lesion, the ventricle should always be closely inspected and all ventricular clot evacuated. The choroid plexus is infrequently involved with the malformation itself, but its close proximity and the emergence of vessels of an uncertain type from the choroid plexus often demands at least a partial resection of the plexus to ensure complete removal and this should be done without trepidation.

## Postoperative induced hypertension

The use of microtechniques, permitting a surgeon to work on the margin of an arteriovenous malformation sparing brain tissue, may on occasion induce him to transgress the margin of the malformation inadvertently, leaving a finger of residual arteriovenous malformation in the normal brain parenchyma. This area of retained malformation can ultimately produce catastrophic bleeding in the postoperative period and may necessitate a repeat surgical procedure for the patient if it goes unnoticed following the removal of the bulk of a malformation. Furthermore, the presence of dysautoregulated vessels in the brain adjacent to the malformation bed may on some occasions lead to postoperative parenchymal haemorrhage, significant brain oedema, and other complications which have been described under the title of 'normal perfusion pressure breakthrough'. In order to ensure that no malformation remains and also to evaluate the brain parenchyma around the arteriovenous malformation bed for the complications of dysautoregulation, we prefer to raise the systolic blood pressure 15–20 mmHg and to maintain it there for a period of 10 to 15 minutes while the raw brain margins are inspected. If no haemorrhage or overt oedema is identified, the blood pressure is returned to normal after this period of time and the brain edges are coated with Surgicel (Ethicon, UK) prior to closure. On several occasions, especially when dealing with large or ill-defined malformations, this technique has enabled us to identify a small area of retained malformation or to detect a propensity for brain swelling which has subsequently influenced us to maintain the patient in barbiturate coma in the postoperative period for a protracted time. While this technique would seem to have the greatest utility with large malformations, it is also beneficial in the small or irregularly shaped arteriovenous malformation in which the presence of residual malformation may be unexpected.

# Stages of arteriovenous malformation resection

The operative procedure for resection of an arteriovenous malformation can somewhat arbitrarily be divided into three sequential stages during each of which the focus, goals and techniques of the surgeon in addition to the complications which may occur are unique. A preoperative appreciation and continued intraoperative awareness of these concerns can prevent less experienced surgeons from becoming confused and conceptually disorientated during a protracted operation.

## Superficial cortical/subarachnoid dissection

2

The initial technical segment of the removal deals with dissection in the subarachnoid space and the establishment of the dissection plane through the pia and into the superficial layers of the cortex. Depending on the size of the malformation and the degree of cortical representation of the lesion, this portion of the procedure can be either extremely extensive or quite limited in scope; however, regardless of the size of the malformation, this portion of the dissection encompasses three distinct steps, each with its particular technical concerns.

### *Establishment of proximal arterial control*

This important manoeuvre is the keystone of all arteriovenous malformation surgery. It represents the most important prerequisite in beginning to develop the dissection plane around the malformation itself. Ideally, the major arterial feeders to the malformation should first be localized using the preoperative arteriogram and then identified in the subarachnoid space at the margin of the malformation, where they can be ligated with either permanent or temporary aneurysm clips. Quite commonly one or more of these principal feeding arteries cannot be identified within the subarachnoid space adjacent to the lesion, but can and should be isolated at some distance from it. Temporary clips placed on the vessels here will provide adequate arterial control and can be exchanged for permanent clips placed in greater proximity later in the procedure. In most large malformations, some of the entering arterial supply will only be identified once the cortical incision is made and deepened to expose the contents of the deep sulci, but a diligent effort should be made to identify all principal arterial supplies to the lesion before beginning its exposure.

### *Preservation of cortical venous drainage*

As mentioned previously, the preservation of patency of venous drainage until late in the dissection process is an established and important maxim in the successful operative removal of such lesions. However, because the

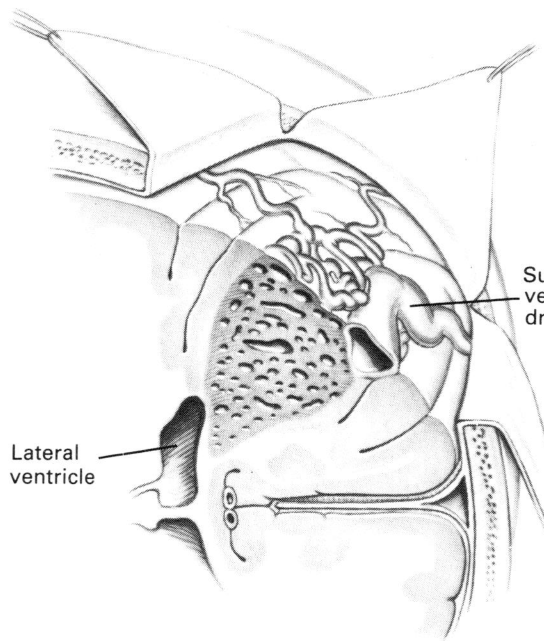


2

cortical venous drainage of these lesions often obscures the margins of the malformation and impedes access to delineation of the periphery of the lesion, it is important to isolate each venous pedicle carefully with meticulous sharp dissection early in the initial phase of exposure. This manoeuvre will often uncover significant arterial channels either bound tightly to the venous pedicle by arachnoid adhesions or hidden from view deep to overlying venous structures. Furthermore, isolation of the cerebral venous pedicles will provide access to the entire peripheral margin of the malformation and facilitate rather than impair its ultimate mobilization. Haemorrhage from these draining veins produced by good sharp dissection technique can be quickly closed with bipolar cautery forceps without compromise of the venous patency and should never be a cause of either alarm, or premature abandonment of pedicle dissection.

### *Identification of cortical arteriovenous malformation margin*

Actual dissection of the lesion begins when the subarachnoid space is abandoned and is extended through the pia–arachnoid into the superficial layers of the cortex at the margin of the malformation. In certain arteriovenous malformations this step is straightforward and uncomplicated, but in many malformations identification of the actual margin of the arteriovenous malformation can be more difficult. Often the cortical representation of the lesion will be quite distinct in one area of the malformation, providing the surgeon with an excellent starting point from which the cortical incision can be extended in circumferential fashion to uncover the hidden boundary of the malformation which frequently lies beneath an extremely thin shelf of unremarkable overlying cortex. Additionally, previous dissection done in order to identify the principal arterial input to the lesion and to dissect the cortical venous drainage completely will delineate margins of the malformation which can then be developed and extended into other less well demarcated areas. Occasionally, even when dealing with a malformation which by radiographic evaluation appears to have significant cortical representation, no true malformation margin can be perceived on the cortical surface of the brain. Most commonly in these situations, the cortical representation of the margin is to be found within one or more sulcus, but the simplest and most expeditious way to identify this margin is to carry the dissection of the venous pedicles into the substance of the brain itself. By gently opening the pia at its point of contact with the enlarged draining vein, the vein can be dissected for several millimetres into the brain tissue to encounter the malformation. This margin can then be identified and dissected in a circumferential manner. It may be necessary in some cases to develop this plane of dissection along each of the major cortical venous drainage channels and then to connect the individual sites of dissection to each other as they reach the margin. This technique will avoid random incisions and associated damage to overlying brain parenchyma which may be both normal and functional.

As soon as the margin of the malformation is encountered and dissection is begun along its periphery, it is important for the surgeon to focus retraction on the malformation itself and to spare the adjacent brain tissue from all possible retractor pressure. Similarly, access to the deeper portions of the malformation is facilitated if the lesion is dissected throughout its circumference through the superficial cortical layers before extending the exposure into the deep white matter. This attention to circumferential exposure will maximize the mobility of the malformation and thus facilitate the maintenance of haemostasis and enable the surgeon to remain in a gliotic plane at the very margin of the lesion without transgressing normal brain parenchyma. The initial phase of dissection ends as the entire circumference of the malformation is exposed to a depth greater than that of the surrounding sulci.

## Intermediate white matter planes

# 3

At this point the surgical procedure enters its second stage, that of the deep white matter dissection. This phase is technically the simplest and easiest portion of the procedure, as the nidus of the malformation dissects quickly and cleanly from the adjacent white matter. As there are few significant entering or exiting vessels which transgress this portion of the brain, dissection can be relatively rapidly deepened again in a circumferential fashion with continued retraction on the lesion itself to identify and develop this normally avascular dissection plane. Gentle strokes of a small suction tip delivered in parallel and adjacent to the margin of the malformation, coupled with a stroking closing motion of the bipolar forceps, are very useful in elaboration of this plane; care should be taken to work on the very periphery, maintaining its coils and knuckles in view at all times. As the dissection moves circumferentially around the malformation it is wise to mark the depth of dissection at each area using a thin Mericel strip which will facilitate the surgeon's return to the exact limits of his prior dissection as the malformation is continually mobilized.

The major dangers during the white matter stage of dissection are excessive retraction on the brain and overaggressive pursuit of the margin of the malformation into the periependymal tissue. The first of these is avoided by a continual conscious attempt to maintain retraction on the malformation, rather than on the brain tissue. The second and potentially more dangerous complication can be avoided by continued awareness of the depth of exposure as dissection proceeds through the white matter and by recognition of the change in the consistency and vascularity of the tissue as one enters the periependymal zone. If this area is entered and bleeding is encountered, the lack of circumferential exposure makes haemostasis difficult to obtain. In general, unless the bleeding is profuse, it is better to pack this area and return to complete the white matter portion of this section throughout the circumference of the malformation before attempting to deepen the dissection into the ventricular system in order to control the area of haemorrhage.

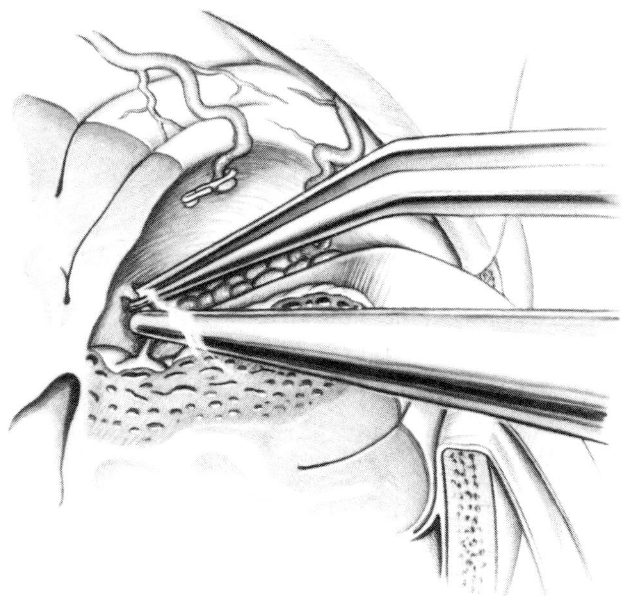

3

## The periependymal/ventricular stage

# 4

The final stage of removal involves the dissection adjacent to the ventricular system. By the nature of their development almost all arteriovenous malformations have some representation on the ventricular wall; in this region the lesion receives its deep arterial input and admits the deep aspect of its venous drainage. The microvasculature in the area adjacent to the ventricle consists of very small, fragile, dilated arterioles and venules which are not part of the proper malformation itself but represent one of the most difficult and challenging problems of neurosurgical haemostasis. By this stage, the malformation has been disconnected from its major cortical arterial supply but maintains its cortical venous drainage and, in the case of most larger lesions, remains distended by the considerable arterial input which enters through the deep periependymal tissue. This continued engorgement of the malformation often makes visualization deep to the malformation difficult and the degree of retraction necessary to gain exposure can carry a significant risk of haemorrhage from the malformation itself.

In the ideal situation, the periependymal dissection is carried out in the same fashion as in the previous two stages; that is, in a circumferential fashion with dissection being deepened through the ependyma into the ventricular system. This plane is then followed around the margins of the malformation with final sacrifice of the deep venous drainage as the last stage in the deep dissection. The malformation is then disconnected from its cortical venous pedicles and removed intact. Care must be taken when the ventricle is initially opened to mark the floor of the ventricular system and simultaneously to block the accumulation of blood in the dependent aspect to prevent the intraoperative development of obstructive hydrocephalus, a cause of significant cerebral distension in the latter phases of removal. Once the ventricle has been opened, increased attention should be paid to close control of all bleeding points and as the dissection is carried around the margin of the malformation, the numerous small distended vessels should be carefully cauterized at relatively low voltage settings and then cut sharply to avoid avulsion. Unfortunately many of these vessels will rupture during cauterization, and it is with these fragile periependymal vessels that we have found

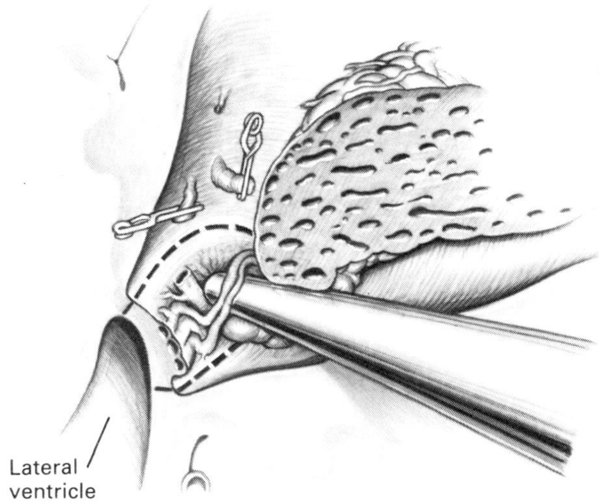


4

the use of numerous small aneurysm clips to be of most benefit. The gentle closing force of the clip approximates the margin of the distended vessel and allows for subsequent sectioning of the vessel on the malformation side of the clip without attendant haemorrhage. The surgeon should avoid repetitive futile attempts at control of this myriad of small vessels with cautery; if, as is so often the case, they prove refractory to cauterization, the willing use of multiple aneurysm clips can both speed the procedure and increase the surgeon's effectiveness as the deep margin is further developed.

All deep venous drainage should be carefully inspected to ensure that the vessels being sacrificed do in fact represent the venous outflow from the malformation rather than the important intraventricular components of the deep venous drainage of the brain. Before permanently occluding any major deep drainage, the vessel should be temporarily occluded with a small temporary aneurysm clip and the malformation carefully observed for a period of minutes to ensure that the lesion does not engorge owing to premature sacrifice of a major venous outflow channel. At the time of permanent occlusion, all deep draining veins should be secured with permanent aneurysm clips before being sectioned.

5

Almost inevitably the choroid plexus will be found to be in some spatial relationship with the malformation and its arterial/venous supply. While the malformation may not in fact involve the adjacent choroid plexus, it is often necessary and advisable to remove a portion of the plexus in association with the malformation to ensure complete resection, and this can be done with impunity as long as the vascular components of the plexus are secured prior to its amputation. Once the margin of the resection has been deepened into the ventricular surface throughout the periphery of the malformation, and the deep venous drainage and choroid plexus component of the malformation successfully dealt with, the lesion can be elevated from its bed and its cortical drainage cross-clipped and cut. With the bulk of the lesion now out of the way, the periependymal area along the margins of the bed can be carefully inspected for any residual vessels and any clot carefully evacuated from the chamber of the ventricle. The bed of the malformation should be covered with a thin coating of haemostatic material such as Surgicel and the systolic blood pressure raised 15–20 mmHg for a period of 15 minutes prior to dural closure.

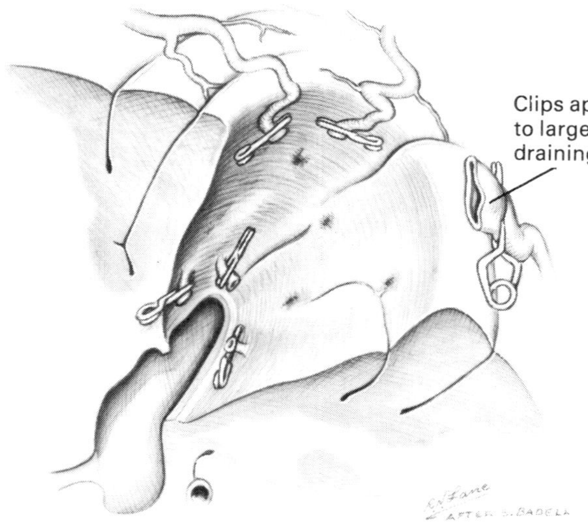


5

## Conclusion

Once the decision has been made to treat a patient with a large arteriovenous malformation radically, the conceptual problems associated with the development of a well-thought-out radiological and surgical strategy and the technical problems encountered in excising the lesion can challenge even the most experienced and skilled surgeon. We believe that consideration of these preoperative, intraoperative and postoperative principles modified to meet the subtleties of each individual case offer the surgeon a reliable framework that will consistently ensure excellent chances of a patient's favourable recovery. While the goal of any therapeutic strategy in dealing with arteriovenous malformations is to minimize the risk of uncontrolled haemorrhage, this potentially lethal complication must be anticipated in every case. There is perhaps no surgical situation more taxing to the surgeon and more dangerous to the patient than protracted and poorly controlled bleeding, which, despite efforts to clear the field, simply obscures the source of the haemorrhage. It is vital for the surgeon to be constantly aware of the likely remaining sites of arterial supply throughout the dissection so that they can be aggressively pursued in a bloody field if necessary. It is equally vital for the surgeon to be aware of the three-dimensional aspects so that the lesion can be quickly delivered or resected with adjacent parenchyma if necessary as a life-saving manoeuvre. Refusal to cease the procedure and clear-headed consideration of surgical options in extremely stressful circumstances can be rewarded by awakening a surprisingly well patient.

## References

1. Pia, H. W. (1975) The indications and contraindications for treatment or assessment in cerebral angiomas. In: Pia, H. W., Glieve, J. R. W. eds. Advances in Diagnosis and Therapy, pp. 1–7. Berlin: Springer–Verlag

2. Dandy, W. E. (1928) Arteriovenous aneurysm of the brain. Archives of Surgery, 17, 190–243

3. Cushing, H., Bailey, P. (1928) Tumours Arising from the Blood Vessels of the Brain. Angiomatous Malformations and Hemangioblastoma. Springfield: Charles C. Thomas

4. Egas Moniz, A. C. de A. F. (1934) L'Angiographie Cerebrale: ses applications et resultats en anatomie, physiologie et clinique. Paris: Masson et Cie

5. Crawford, P. M., West, C. R., Chadwick, D. W., Shaw, M. D. (1986) Arteriovenous malformations of the brain: natural history in unoperated patients. Journal of Neurology, Neurosurgery and Psychiatry, 49, 1–10

6. Stein, B. M., Wolpert, S. M. (1980) Arteriovenous malformations of the brain. II. Current concepts and treatment. Archives of Neurology, 37, 69–75

7. Graf, C. J., Perret, G. E., Torner, J. C. (1983) Bleeding from cerebral arteriovenous malformations as part of their natural history. Journal of Neurosurgery, 58, 331–337

8. Jane, J. A., Kassell, N. F., Torner, J. C., Winn, H. R. (1985) The natural history of aneurysms and arteriovenous malformations. Journal of Neurosurgery, 62, 321–323

9. Batjer, H. H., Devous, M. D., Seibert, G. B. *et al.* (1988) Intracranial arteriovenous malformation: relationship between clinical and radiographic factors and ipsilateral steal severity. Neurosurgery, 23, 322–328

10. Batjer, H., Suss, R. A., Samson, D. S. (1986) Intracranial arteriovenous malformations associated with aneurysms. Neurosurgery, 18, 29–35

11. Batjer, H., Samson, D. (1986) Arteriovenous malformations of the posterior fossa: clinical presentation, diagnostic evaluation and surgical treatment. Journal of Neurosurgery, 64, 849–856

12. Spetzler, R. F., Wilson, C. B., Weinstein, P., Mehdorn, M., Townsend, J., Telles, D. (1978) Normal perfusion pressure breakthrough theory. Clinical Neurosurgery, 25, 651–672

13. Day, A., Friedman, W., Sypert, G. W., Mickle, J. P. (1982) Successful treatment of the normal perfusion pressure breakthrough syndrome. Neurosurgery, 11, 625–630

14. Batjer, H. H., Devous, M. D., Meyer, Y. J., Purdy, P. D., Samson, D. S. (1988) Cerebrovascular hemodynamics in arteriovenous malformation complicated by normal perfusion pressure breakthrough. Neurosurgery, 22, 503–509

Illustrations by Barbara Hyams

# Surgery of gliomas

**J. J. Maccabe** MB ChB, FRCS (Ed)
Consultant Neurosurgeon, King's College Hospital and Maudsley Hospital, London, UK

## Introduction

The gliomas (astrocytoma, oligodendroglioma and ependymoma) constitute about half of all intracranial tumours. They are all, to a greater or lesser degree, malignant. About 55 per cent are malignant astrocytoma or glioblastoma multiforme, both terms signifying a rapidly growing tumour with a short clinical course. Without treatment the average survival time from diagnosis is 2–3 months. Gliomas spread by infiltration, making their boundaries impossible to define. The forepart of the brain is most often involved, the frontal and temporal lobes being equally affected. The occipital lobe is a rare site. Central areas of the brain are frequently infiltrated by the time of diagnosis, with the tumour extending into the basal ganglia, or across to the opposite hemisphere through the corpus callosum. Cure by surgical excision is therefore impossible. Areas of necrosis and cystic degeneration are common. Extensive oedema in the surrounding brain accompanies rapid tumour growth, aggravating the symptoms and signs of hemisphere disturbance.

In the majority of patients the onset of symptoms is gradual. At first there may be only complaint of headache or lethargy. Epilepsy occurs in over one-third of patients as the initial symptom. The rapid growth of the tumour and the pathological changes which accompany it soon produce focal symptoms and signs, indicating the principal part of the brain involved. By the time of admission motor weakness is present in at least half the patients and about a quarter are suffering from impaired consciousness. These signs may represent infiltration and destruction by tumour, but they can also have their origin in reversible local or general pressure effects.

Opinions vary as to the place of surgery in the management of the malignant astrocytoma. A few regard surgery as totally unwarranted beyond the need to establish a tissue diagnosis by biopsy. A more general view is that where appropriate, formal excision of tumour, although always incomplete, will help to lengthen survival time by reducing the total tumour burden and by relieving intracranial pressure and brain displacement.

Internal decompression may certainly result in dramatic improvement in the condition of the patient. Relief will be short-lived, however, unless additional treatment follows to delay residual tumour growth. This is usually a course of radiation therapy.

In selecting patients for excisional surgery there are two major considerations. First, the tumour removal should be as complete as possible, consistent with maintaining function. Limited resections are of no value. The mass must be accessible so that the resection can be carried out from within the tumour while disturbing surrounding brain as little as possible. If the tumour is in a non-vital area such as the right frontal or temporal lobe, adjacent brain tissue may also be excised to supplement the decompression, without adding to the patient's disability. In the parietal lobes and in the dominant temporal lobe there are obvious limitations, and heroic measures in these areas are usually better avoided. Tumours in the basal ganglia, thalamus and corpus callosum are not suitable for excision. There are therefore serious limitations to the number of patients suitable for major surgery.

A second consideration must be the quality of survival expected. There is no kindness in lengthening survival when the neurological deficit is profound and irreversible from destructive tumour growth. On the other hand, drowsiness and moderate motor deficit may be due to brain oedema and displacement, and may be dramatically reversed by a timely resection. Preoperative steroid preparation, by reducing brain swelling, will usually indicate the likely improvement in neurological function.

For malignant astrocytoma there are few other points to guide patient selection. Frontal lobe tumours are more often associated with a worthwhile recovery, although only a small percentage of patients return to their former employment. Patients presenting before 40 years of age may have a more favourable outlook. The nature of the pathology determines the outcome and is the reason why survival beyond 18 months is unusual even with energetic treatment.

Of the other gliomas, some 30 per cent are more slow growing astrocytomas. They have a more firm, uniform structure and are ill-defined. They are associated with better survival rates after excisional surgery alone. Patients under 20 years of age or with a long preoperative symptomatology and without major neurological deficit appear to do best, a reflection of the slower rate of growth of these lesions. Oligodendrogliomas form some 5 per cent of gliomas. These are also widely infiltrative and many are heavily calcified. Five-year postoperative survival rates are similar to those of the low-grade astrocytomas. Excisional surgery is usually supplemented by radiation treatment.

## Special investigations

# 1, 2 & 3

A high index of suspicion is the prime requirement for the early diagnosis of an intracranial glioma. If the history suggests the possibility, and even if a detailed neurological examination reveals little or nothing abnormal, more definitive investigation should be undertaken.

Computerized tomography (CT) is the basic radiological investigation. This rapid, non-invasive technique, carrying minimal risk, has completely altered the approach to investigation for intracranial tumour. Two abnormalities may be revealed on the films. First, an alteration in brain tissue density from the normal range; second, displacement or distortion of normal anatomical patterns, particularly the ventricular system. Malignant tumours may be represented by areas of low density or decreased attenuation, although mixed pictures are also frequent. Areas of necrosis and cystic degeneration can be identified. Contrast enhancement, reflecting damage to the blood–brain barrier, delineates the tumour more accurately, and displays surrounding oedema clearly. A correct diagnosis of glioma can be made in over 90 per cent of cases.

The most malignant lesions are usually of mixed attenuation, with obvious mass effect and surrounding oedema. Contrast enhancement is almost universal. Lower grade astrocytomas are usually of low attenuation, but they may be isodense with brain. Oligodendrogliomas are also low attenuation tumours, usually showing calcification on CT and enhancing irregularly with contrast. The details of tumour location and spread, of brain swelling and ventricular displacement, provide nearly all the information required for biopsy or more major surgery.

Angiography can also prove diagnostic, outlining not only vessel displacements but occasionally displaying characteristic vascular features. The tumour may appear as a highly vascular localized mass, superficially resembling an arteriovenous malformation, with numerous feeding vessels and arteriovenous shunts. About 50 per cent of gliomas are largely avascular, although an early filling vein may provide a clue to the diagnosis. The principal value of angiography is in alerting the surgeon to possible problems associated with an unusually vascular tumour.

Radioisotope scanning is useful when CT scanning is not available. An abnormal uptake of isotope occurs in the majority of malignant astrocytomas, but the more slowly growing tumours are not regularly demonstrated. The method is in general much less reliable than CT.

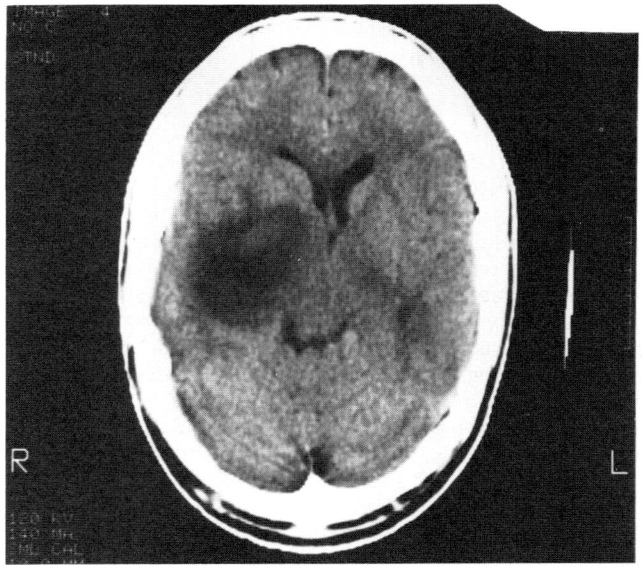


*Figure 2. Low grade astrocytoma. A large low density mass in the right temporal lobe, with mass effect. No contrast enhancement.*

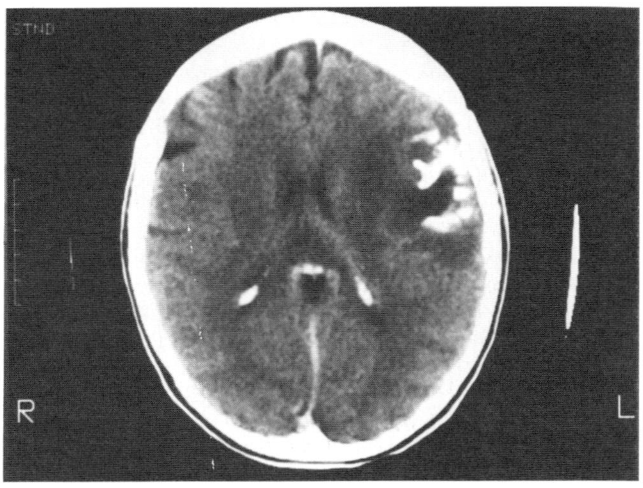


*Figure 1. Malignant astrocytoma. Mixed attenuation lesion, with irregular wall enhancement. A large solid component with cystic charge arteriosity oedema in surrounding brain with mass effect.*

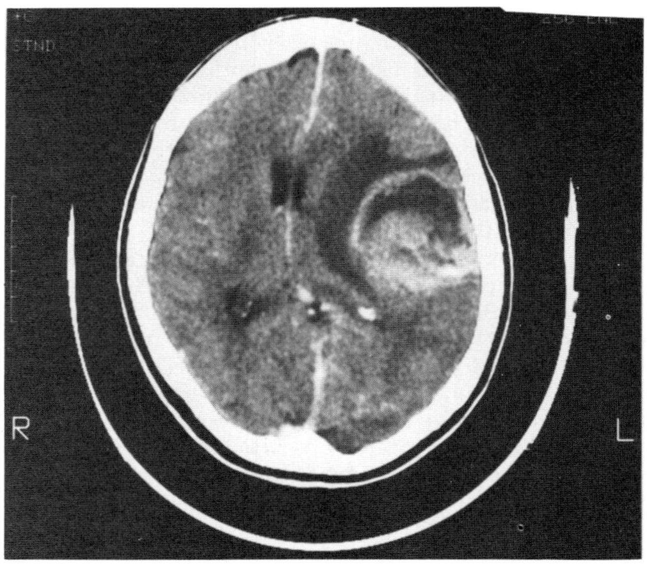


*Figure 3. Oligodendroglioma. A large low density lesion with characteristic calcification, causing mass effect.*

# The operations

A diagnosis based solely on clinical and radiological criteria carries the risk of at least occasional error. A tissue diagnosis should be established wherever possible, whether or not treatment is to follow. Where craniotomy and tumour resection are inappropriate, needle biopsy through a burr hole provides a suitable method for obtaining tissue.

Reduction of raised intracranial pressure by steroid therapy is an essential preliminary to all surgery on patients with glioma. Such preparation reduces mortality and morbidity from burr hole biopsy, and accelerates a smoother recovery after major resection. Steroids alone can benefit patients with malignant astrocytoma, improving their state of alertness and degree of mobility. They may also be used to sustain the patient during a course of radiation.

## BURR HOLE BIOPSY

In experienced hands, tumour biopsy via a burr hole is a very safe procedure in patients who are properly prepared. Free hand and stereotactic methods are available. It is appropriate for patients unsuitable for craniotomy owing to the location of their tumour, or those with established severe neurological deficit. A large tumour cyst may be drained through a burr hole with benefit. Haemorrhage is the main hazard of the procedure, and may result in increased disability and occasionally mortality. Care and experience are required to obtain a representative tissue specimen, for gliomas vary greatly from one area to another. A reliable opinion can be given quickly on smears of tumour and the technique has an accuracy rate of 95 per cent, judged by comparison with subsequent paraffin sections.

The procedure can be carried out under local analgesia, with sedation, but if there is any doubt as to the patient's airway then general anaesthesia is safer. The position of the patient will depend on the location of the burr hole. The tumour is approached by the shortest route from the surface, if possible avoiding passage through eloquent areas. CT films of the tumour, preferably in at least axial and sagittal views, will locate the lesion in relation to the patient's head and its various surface markings. For most lesions, an approach from the top or posterior aspect of the skull, parallel to the midline, is simplest. The anteroposterior location of the burr hole can be decided with reference to the coronal or lambdoid sutures, which can be felt through the scalp. The inclination of the cannula forwards or backwards can be guided further by reference to other identifiable points, notably the external auditory meatus. For lesions in the temporal lobe a lateral approach is employed. The zygomatic arch indicates the floor of the middle fossa. After opening the dura and incising the pia, a blunt side-holed brain cannula with an external diameter of 2 mm is introduced until a change of resistance is felt. Some estimate of the likely distance to be traversed should be made beforehand so that too deep and perhaps damaging penetration does not result.

The stylet is removed and the cannula gently rotated, while suction is applied with a 5 ml syringe. The right hand is used to operate the syringe while the left hand, resting on the head, controls movement of the cannula. Soft tumour will emerge without difficulty, as will softened brain. The material obtained is used to make smears and to provide specimens in formol saline. For tumours located more deeply in the brain, in the thalamus, basal ganglia or vicinity of the third ventricle, a stereotactic method for biopsy is essential.

## CRANIOTOMY

Good surgical conditions are ensured by preoperative steroid administration, careful anaesthetic management and dehydration of the brain. Controlled respiration is always employed with nitrous oxide–oxygen anaesthesia and relaxants, with or without volatile supplements. Monitoring is carried out by ECG recording and by an arterial line and pulse oximeter. Five hundred millilitres of 20 per cent mannitol is rapidly administered after induction and an in-dwelling catheter provides for the subsequent diuresis.

According to the position of the tumour and the craniotomy opening, the patient will usually be placed either supine or in the full lateral position. To avoid venous obstruction, the neck must not be unduly rotated. A modest head-up tilt is helpful. A pin-fixation head rest stabilizes the operation site. The skull opening is placed to allow tumour exposure by transcortical incision where it comes nearest to the surface. Axial, coronal and sagittal views of the lesion provided by the CT scan are translated to the patient's head using surface landmarks. The most favourable tumour locations for craniotomy are in the frontal and temporal lobes on the non-dominant side, where formal lobectomy can be combined with tumour reduction. A relaxed brain facilitates all procedures. Incision of the cortex is safer and haemostasis easier and quicker. When the dura is opened, the gyri will be broad and flat as a result of oedema. A brain cannula may be used to locate the main tumour which can then be exposed by a short cortical incision, gradually widened. Tumour is removed by suction or by an ultrasonic aspirator where it is soft and necrotic, and where it can be clearly identified. This process continues until more firm or normal areas are reached where the brain architecture is preserved and where it is best to stop. It is essential to remain strictly within the tumour area unless a formal lobectomy is intended. The brain should never be subjected to undue traction. At the end of the operation the dura is repaired as completely as possible and the bone flap always replaced.

Patients are returned to an intensive care area for some 48 hours after surgery. A suction drain left in the subgaleal space is removed after 24 hours. Stitches are removed after 5 days. Steroid therapy is gradually reduced to a maintenance level over 7 days and continued during subsequent radiation therapy.

## FRONTAL LOBECTOMY

# 4 & 5

The patient is placed supine with the head turned to the opposite side. The ipsilateral shoulder may be elevated on a wedge to prevent undue rotation of neck structures. The scalp incision begins in the midline about 3 cm above the nasion. It turns downwards behind the coronal suture to reach the zygoma within the hairline. The frontal branch of the facial nerve should be avoided.

The temporalis muscle is incised anteriorly and posteriorly with cautery to expose the anterior end of the temporal line and the squamous temporal bone. The first burr hole is placed on the temporal line to enter the lateral part of the anterior cranial fossa. Care is required to avoid the orbital cavity. The second and third holes are centred almost on the midline with care to avoid the superior sagittal sinus. The anterior burr hole is placed above the frontal sinus and the posterior one at the coronal suture. The fifth burr hole is behind the pterion. The osteoplastic flap is reflected on the temporalis muscle, the bone across the base being first reduced by rongeurs. The dura is opened as a U-shaped flap based on the medial margin of the opening and the sagittal sinus.

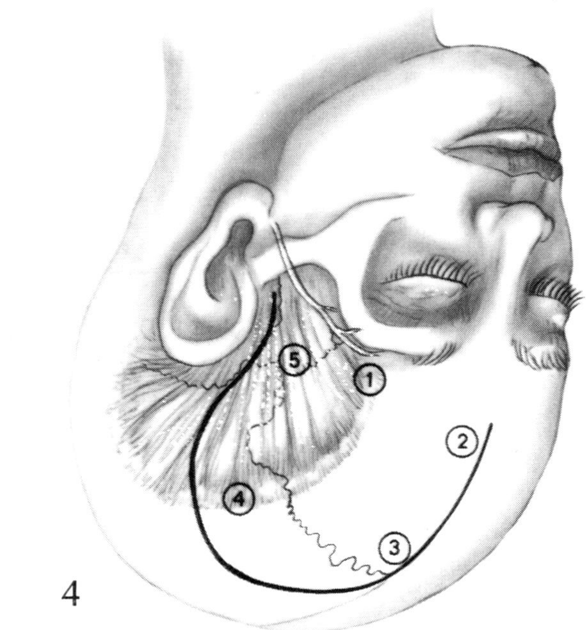


4

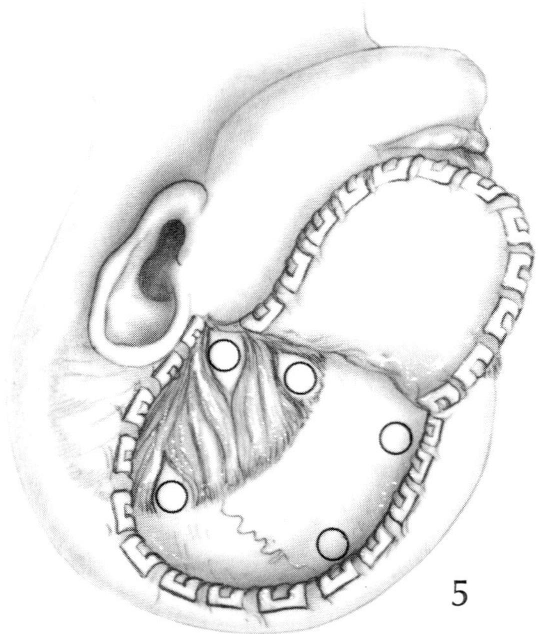

5

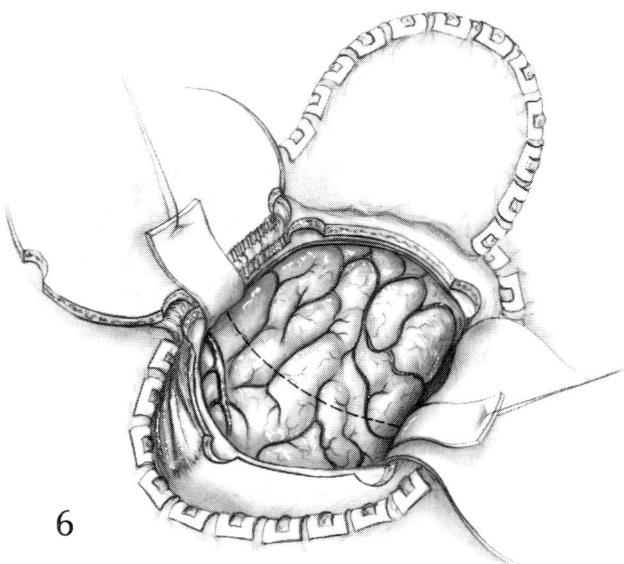

6

# 6

The line of the cortical incision extends from a point some 8 cm from the frontal pole on the medial margin of the hemisphere to the lesser wing of the sphenoid inferiorly. Both points are marked with cottonoid strips. On the dominant hemisphere the posterior half of the inferior frontal gyrus must be preserved to avoid speech disturbance.

# 7, 8 & 9

The pia arachnoid covering the brain surface is coagulated along the line of the incision and divided with scissors. Larger vessels are isolated and coagulated separately before division. The white matter is cut using a small metal sucker or an ultrasonic aspirator, the part to be removed being held forward by a hand retractor. As the incision is deepened, care is taken to incline the plane of section anteriorly. The cut surface of the hemisphere and the exposed brain are generally kept moist and protected by cottonoid strips. If the anterior horn of the lateral ventricle is opened it should also be covered with cottonoid to prevent blood collecting within the ventricular system. At its medial end the white matter incision is inclined forwards so that the pia is divided where the two hemispheres are clearly separate, anterior to the corpus callosum, to avoid damage to the anterior cerebral vessels. The ipsilateral frontopolar artery is divided near the orbital surface. When the amputated portion of the frontal lobe is withdrawn the olfactory tract and bulb should be preserved if possible. The residual cavity is filled with wet cotton wool packs which are left in place for some minutes. Thereafter gentle irrigation with warm saline allows the recognition of any persisting oozing points. Finally, the dura is closed as completely as possible and the bone flap securely replaced.

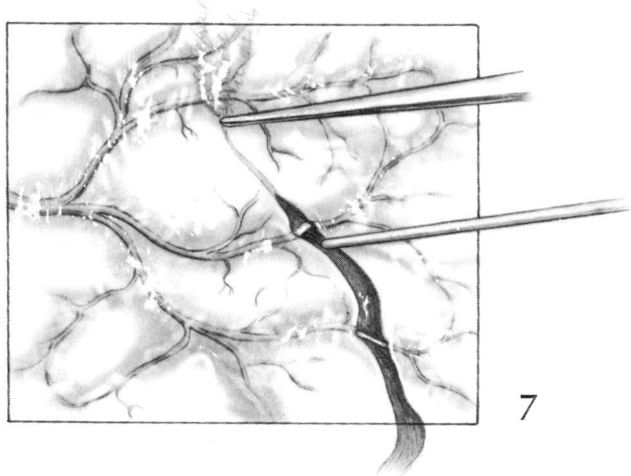

7

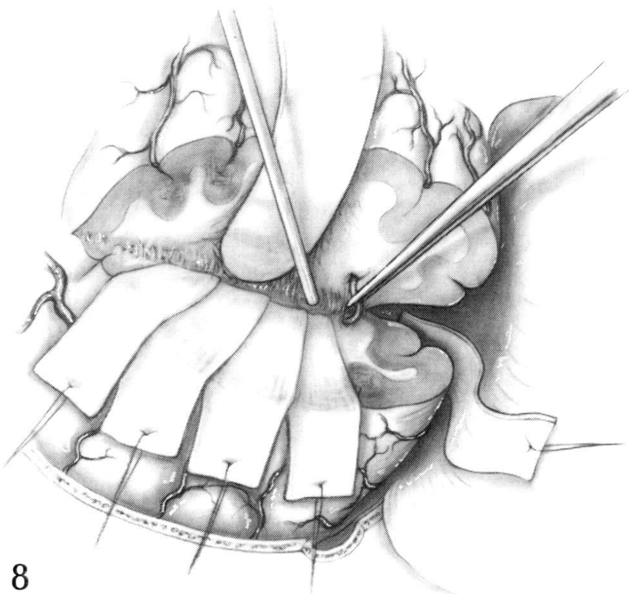

8

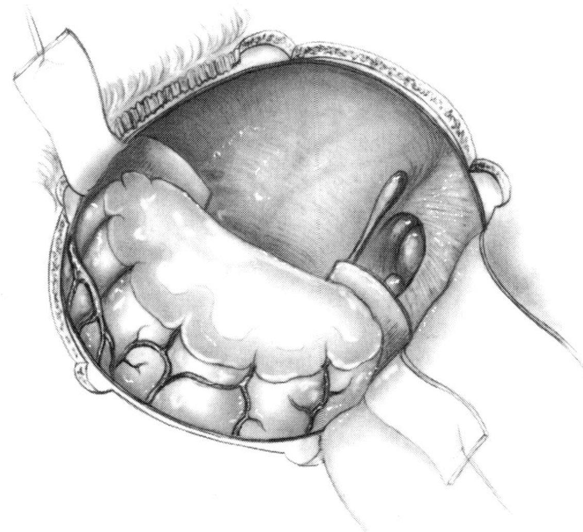

9

## TEMPORAL LOBECTOMY

# 10

For temporal lobectomy the patient is best placed in the full lateral position. The brachial plexus in the underarm must be carefully guarded. The scalp incision begins closely in front of the ear and passes backwards above it. It then curves forwards above the temporal line.

The first burr hole is beneath the temporalis muscle just below the temporal line and just behind the external angular process of the frontal bone. The fifth burr hole is also under the muscle, just above the root of the zygoma, almost level with the floor of the middle fossa. The other burr holes are outside the attachment of the temporalis muscle. After reflection of the bone flap, additional bone is removed by rongeurs towards the floor of the middle fossa. The dura is opened as a U-shaped flap based superiorly. The inferior dural edge is stitched to the temporalis muscle to assist with haemostasis.

On the dominant hemisphere it is preferable to spare the superior temporal gyrus to avoid speech disturbance. On the non-dominant side, a thin layer of superior gyrus should always be preserved to protect the middle cerebral vessels.

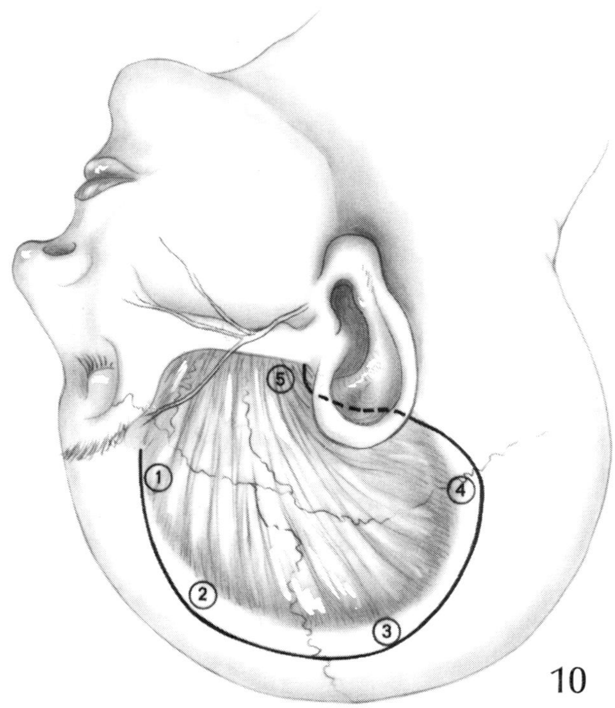


10

# 11, 12 & 13

The cortical incision extends backwards to a point level with the Rolandic fissure where it turns inferiorly towards the middle fossa floor. The white matter is divided first in this posterior portion to enter the temporal horn, then turning downwards and medially to the floor of the middle fossa. The middle temporal gyrus is then retracted downwards, and dissection by sucker or aspirator continued until the medial part of the under surface is reached at the fusiform gyrus.

The medial part of the temporal lobe should be removed by subpial suction to avoid injury to the cerebral peduncle, the posterior cerebral artery and the third cranial nerve. The uncus may be extensively herniated through the tentorial hiatus, and the use of the operating microscope may facilitate dissection at this point. Excision of an uncal herniation greatly reduces complications from postoperative swelling.

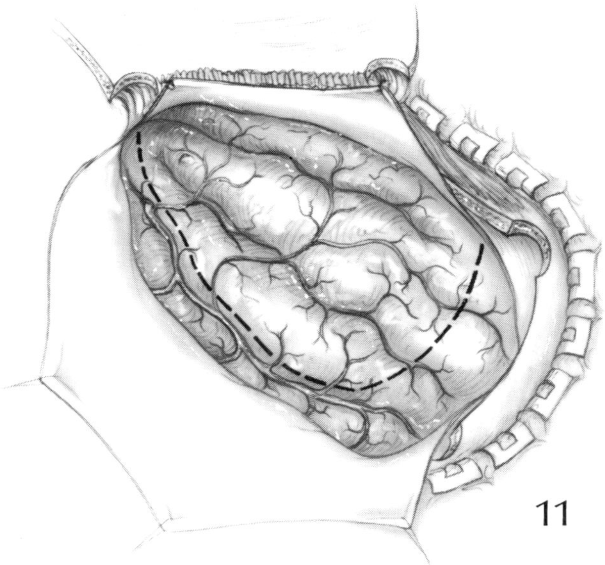

11

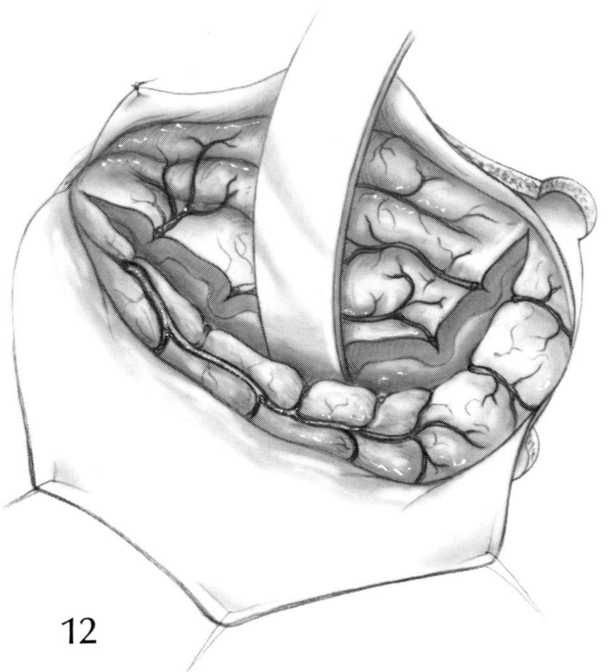

12

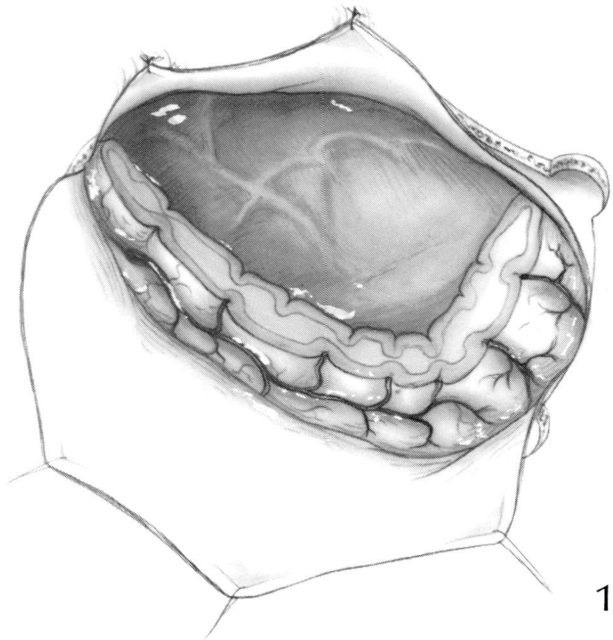

13

## OCCIPITAL LOBECTOMY

# 14

The patient is placed in the lateral position with the head slightly rotated to bring the occipital region uppermost. The scalp incision begins in the midline near the superior nuchal line, and ends above and behind the ear. The scalp flap is reflected posteriorly, preserving occipital vessels and nerves.

The first two burr holes are placed 2 cm from the midline, and the fifth just above the transverse sinus. The bone flap may be reflected forwards based on the temporalis muscle. The dura is opened as two flaps based on the adjacent venous sinuses.

# 15 & 16

On the non-dominant side the cortical incision will begin some 7 cm from the occipital pole on the superior margin of the hemisphere. On the dominant side only 3.5 cm is permissible to avoid the angular gyrus. The posterior cerebral artery is coagulated and divided in the calcarine fissure; finally, division of the veins at the torcula will allow the lobe to be removed. A complete homonymous hemianopia will always follow.

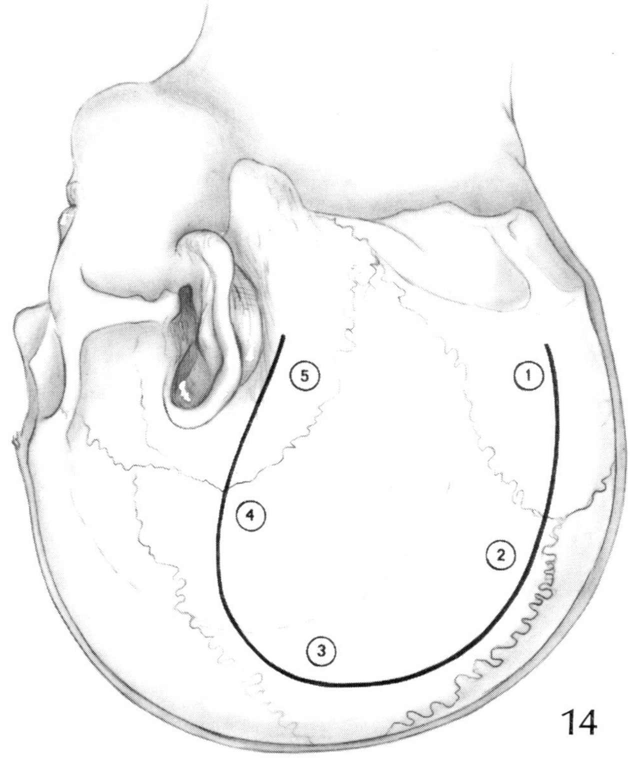

14

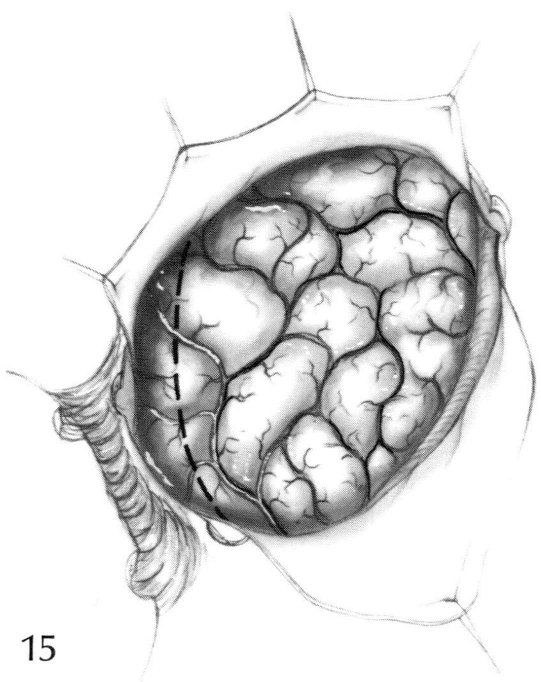
15

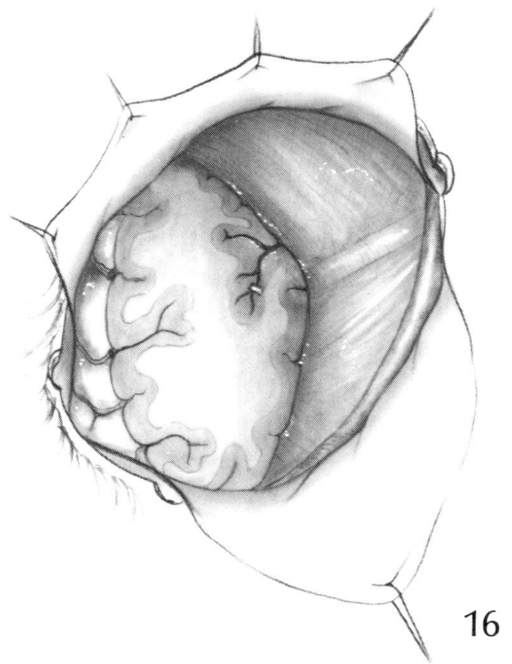
16

## *Further reading*

Jelsma, R., Bucy, P. C. (1967) The treatment of glioblastoma multiforme of the brain. Journal of Neurosurgery, 27, 388–400

Laws, E. R. Jr., Taylor, W. F., Clifton, M. B., Okazaki, H. (1984) Neurosurgical management of low-grade astrocytoma of the cerebral hemispheres. Journal of Neurosurgery, 61, 665–673

Marshall, L. F., Jennett, B., Langfitt, T. W. (1974) Needle biopsy for the diagnosis of malignant glioma. Journal of the American Medical Association, 228, 1417–1418

Salcman, M. (1980) Survival in glioblastoma: historical perspectives. Neurosurgery, 7, 435–439

Steinhoff, H., Lanksch, W., Kazner, E. *et al.* (1977) Computed tomography in the diagnosis and differential diagnosis of glioblastomas: a qualitative study of 295 cases. Neuroradiology, 14, 193–200

Van Buren, J., Fedio, P., Frederick G. C. (1978) Mechanisms and localization of speech in the parietotemporal cortex. Neurosurgery, 2, 233–239

Weir, B. (1973) The relative signif cance of factors affecting post-operative survival in astrocytomas, grades 3 and 4. Journal of Neurosurgery, 38, 448–452

Illustrations by A. Besterman and Angela Christie

# Surgery of meningiomas

**Valentine Logue** FRCS, FRCP
Emeritus Professor of Neurosurgery, Institute of Neurology, London, UK

**Lindsay Symon** TD, FRCS
Professor of Neurosurgery, Gough-Cooper Department of Neurological Surgery, Institute of Neurology, National Hospitals for Nervous Diseases, London, UK

## Introduction

Meningiomas constitute between 13 and 16 per cent of all primary intracranial tumours. They were amongst the first tumours to be recognized as benign and their detailed description by Bailey and Cushing constituted one of the landmarks of neurosurgical development.

The principles of removal have been well established for many years although a number of technical adjuncts such as bipolar diathermy, ultrasonic dissection apparatus, and the availability of lasers have been developed in recent years, and these have undoubtedly increased the neurosurgical armamentarium in the handling of these masses.

Perhaps more important, however, is the development of detailed arteriography, an excellent imaging technique which has made the planning of surgical approaches progressively easier. The large flaps of previous years, imposed upon the surgeon by the inability to distinguish accurately between the mass itself and surrounding oedema, have been replaced by smaller flaps with lesser exposure of normal brain, intracranial pressure being progressively more easily controlled by steroids and dehydrating agents.

The use of induced hypotension and ventilation to control venous pressure by lowering the arterial $P\text{CO}_2$, and, if necessary, preoperative embolization of major external blood supplies, have all contributed to a more radical removal of difficult tumours and a steady reduction in morbidity.

## Meningioma sites

| | | |
|---|---|---|
| Convexity | | 30% |
| Parasagittal and falx | | 28% |
| Basal | | |
| Sphenoidal ridge | 18% | 31% |
| Suprasellar and parasellar | 5% | |
| Other sites (olfactory groove, subtemporal, tentorial, peritorcular) | 8% | |
| Posterior fossa | | 9% |
| Intraventricular | | 2% |
| | | 100% |

Convexity meningiomas are defined as arising from the dura over the cerebral hemispheres free of attachment to the superior sagittal sinus or to the base of the skull.

A parasagittal meningioma is a tumour which covers or has extended onto the wall of the sagittal sinus.

The falx tumour arises entirely or mainly on the falx when its edges may often involve the lower margin of the sagittal sinus.

Occasionally a tumour may spread widely over the falx, sagittal sinus wall and convexity dura.

With extensive tumours it may be quite difficult to decide exactly under which heading to classify them, an example being the extensive apical petrous tumour. This extends onto the clivus, often across the midline widely in the cerebellopontine angle, and extends above the petrous ridge into the middle fossa, sometimes as far forward as the chiasm. The usual practice is to take a guess at the origin of the tumour and classify it accordingly.

## Radiological diagnosis

The plain X-ray is helpful in about 55 per cent of cases in suggesting the diagnosis of a meningioma by the demonstration of one or more of the following features: tumour calcification; an enostosis or exostosis; an area of bone sclerosis, decalcification or bone erosion; or hypertrophied meningeal channels with an enlarged foramen spinosum.

### *Computerized tomography and magnetic resonance scanning*

# 1 & 2a, b & c

These two techniques of imaging have vastly improved the accuracy of diagnosis and the localization of the tumour. Of the two, in general, computerized tomography is undoubtedly the more useful in routine meningiomas. It has the advantage of enabling contrast enhancement to be given; the majority of meningiomas take up contrast avidly and the comparison between a mass of brain density or slightly above unenhanced, and a mass which is brightly enhanced after contrast renders the differential diagnosis relatively straightforward. It is particularly useful in tracing the development of recurrences or following the size of residual tumour in inoperable sites, and it will also pick out the multiple lesions of central neurofibromatosis.

Gamma scintigraphy used to be of considerable use but has now been largely superseded. However, in the absence of computerized tomography it remains a useful adjunct. The computerized tomogram will now reconstruct in parasagittal and coronal cuts, and the last possible advantage of scintigraphy, its capacity to produce anteroposterior and posteroanterior views, has disappeared.

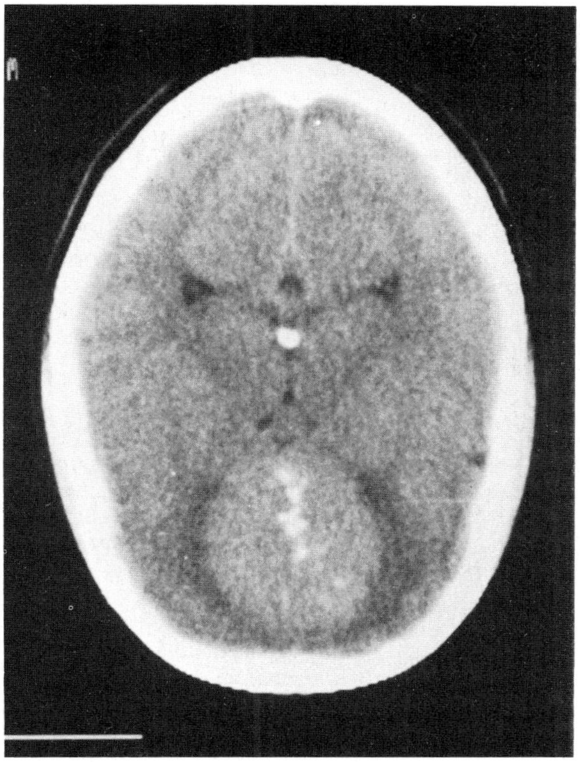

1

*Figure 1. Typical scan appearances of a convexity meningioma. The lesion is of slightly increased density compared with brain on the unenhanced scan and on contrast enhancement lights up strongly.*

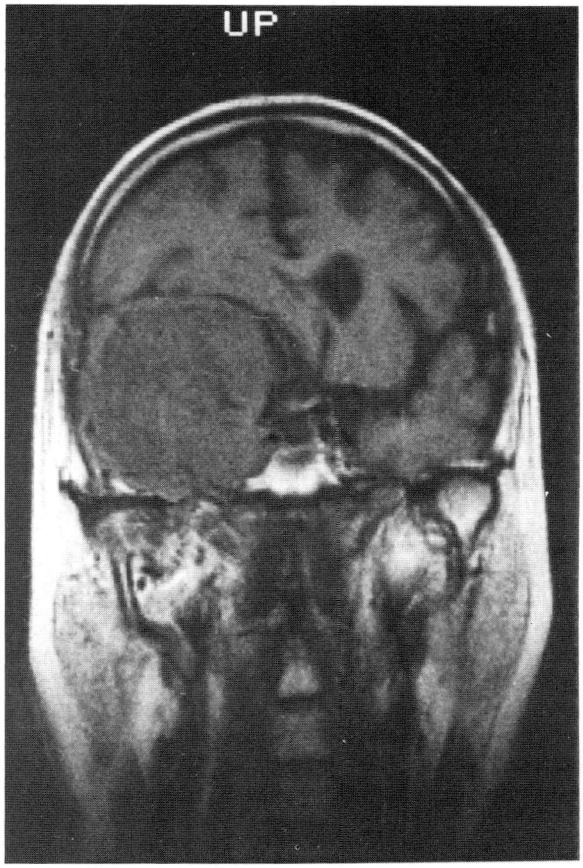


2b

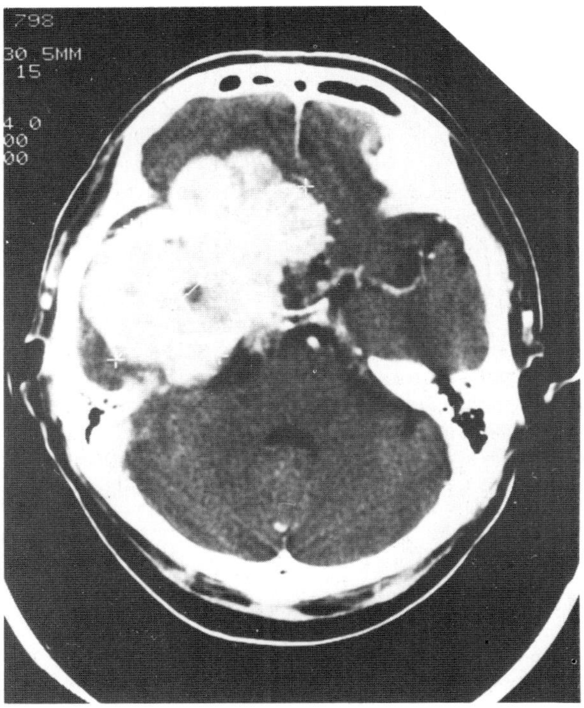


2a

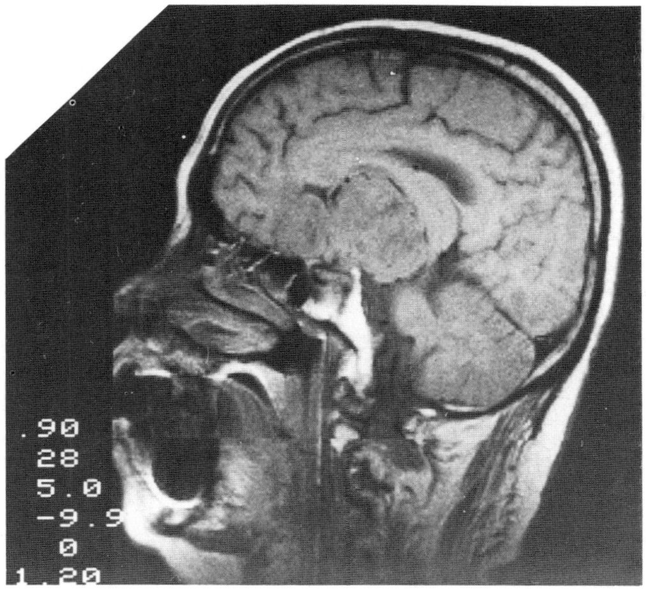


2c

*Figure 2. CT (a) and magnetic resonance imaging (b & c) of a huge middle and anterior fossa meningioma. Details of its relations with cerebrospinal fluid spaces are particularly well shown on the magnetic resonance image.*

# 3

Magnetic resonance scanning is of particular use in masses close to the midline where the delineation of central structures on the sagittal cuts of the scan can produce a picture virtually identical to an anatomical textbook.

*Angiography*

In planning the resection of a meningioma knowledge of its blood supply is of cardinal importance. In supratentorial tumours, carotid arteriography, generally performed by the femoral route, enables selective injection of the internal and external circulations. Meningiomas are supplied by dural blood vessels as a rule and internal carotid injection alone may very well miss the characteristic blush of a meningioma. On the other hand, subfrontal and olfactory groove tumours are predominantly supplied by branches of the internal carotid artery, either direct or through the ophthalmic artery, and careful internal carotid arteriography with subtraction may be necessary to delineate this fine blood supply.

In the posterior fossa, vertebrobasilar arteriography may indicate the displacement of blood vessels and supply from the dural branches of the vertebral artery. However, it is important to remember that most tumours arising from the area of the clivus and the medial aspect of the posterior fossa receive their blood supply from the meningohypophyseal branches of the internal carotid artery, or in more lateral tumours from the external carotid artery through its dural or occipital branches. A petrous apex or lateral petrous meningioma may show no pathological circulation on vertebrobasilar injections, and yet show profuse circulation from meningohypophyseal or external carotid supply.

Arteriography draws the following information to the surgeon's attention.

The vascularity of the tumour. If this is thought to be overwhelming, selective external carotid embolization may be employed about a week preoperatively (not more) to reduce the dangers of surgery.

The relationship of both the supplying vessels and the major arterial branches to the capsule. This is of particular importance in preserving the integrity and function of surrounding brain.

The degree of encroachment on any related venous sinus.

The proximity of a large draining vein to the parasagittal, pterional and tentorial tumours.

Air encephalography was commonly employed in the past for the diagnosis of midline or parasellar tumours. It has been almost totally replaced by magnetic resonance scanning or fourth-generation CT scanning. Ventriculography is no longer employed.

## Principles of surgery

The dominating principle in the removal of a meningioma is the avoidance of damage to the surrounding brain, either directly by traction and distortion or indirectly by interference with arterial trunks or major veins.

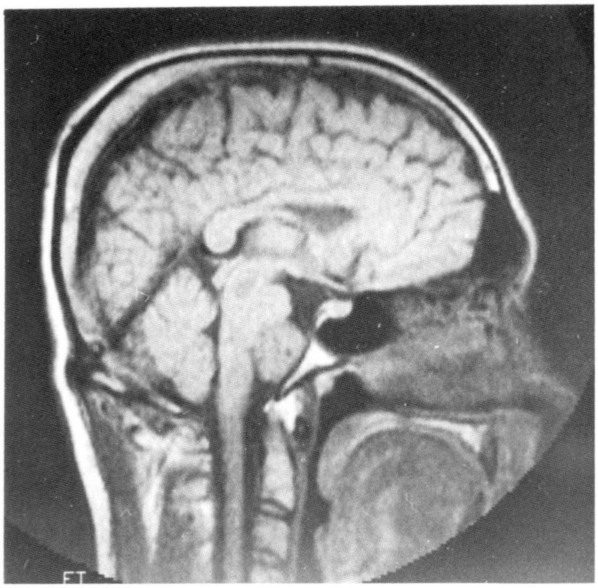

3

*Figure 3. Magnetic resonance image of a midclival meningioma. A frequent posterior fossa artefact in CT scans makes magnetic resonance imaging in the posterior fossa of immense value.*

It is not only that trauma produces or increases neurological signs, for example speech disturbance, hemiparesis, hemihypoaesthesiae or visual impairment, but it tends also to exacerbate oedema. Oedema follows virtually every meningioma removal, even the smallest (despite the use of steroid medication). It can be recognized from the CT scan and is also confirmed by the bulging of the scalp flap postoperatively when the bone flap has been removed. This oedema may persist from a matter of days to several weeks. Excessive oedema stretches and distorts the cortex and white matter, thus increasing the extent of the residual scar and adding to the risks of perpetuating or producing epilepsy, which remains too often as a permanent and disastrous aftermath to an otherwise satisfactory tumour removal.

To achieve the optimum conditions for avoiding trauma to the brain it is essential that every effort is made to reduce raised intracranial tension, preferably to a level just above atmospheric pressure at the time of working on the tumour. If the pressure is not properly controlled once the dura is incised, cerebral herniation along with protrusion of the tumour occurs, resulting in stresses and small-vessel damage in the surrounding brain which exacerbate the oedema at an early stage in the operation. In addition, excessive tension will make separation of the capsule from the brain-bed more difficult and more traumatic.

### Reduction of intracranial tension

Principles of management of intracranial tension are outlined in the chapter on 'Control of intracranial tension', pp. 1–11. The main measures to be undertaken are as follows.

*Preoperatively*

It has become clear that a generous period of fairly heavy steroid administration vastly enhances the ease of removal of meningiomas. It is now the authors' practice to administer dexamethasone in doses of 16 mg a day for at least a week prior to surgery unless surgery has presented as an urgent necessity because of the rapid deterioration of the patient. With the increased availability of scanning this is becoming less frequent. Dehydrating agents such as frusemide (Lasix) may be added but are as a rule best avoided in the preoperative period. They may become necessary to control reactive swelling in the postoperative period, but once again with the availablility of high steroid administration for 5 or 6 days postoperatively this is becoming less frequent.

*During operation*

*Positioning* The head of the table is raised to reduce brain and cerebrospinal fluid pressure (particularly important when operating on, or near, the larger venous sinuses) and to potentiate arterial hypotensive techniques.

*The use of controlled respiration* For many years the authors preferred to maintain spontaneous respiration during the resection of basal or posterior fossa tumours. Considerable experience in respiratory pattern disturbances proved a valuable monitor, but this has largely been replaced by continuous electrocardiographic monitoring, supplemented if necessary by monitoring of brainstem and somatosensory evoked responses. The vast improvement in operating conditions available, with controlled respiration lowering the arterial $P\text{CO}_2$ to the region of 25–30 mmHg, has made its use invariable in clinics throughout the world.

*Induced hypotension* The vessels of a meningioma do not autoregulate. Reduction in arterial blood pressure, therefore, results in a fall in arterial perfusion in the tumour. This, accompanying the reduction in venous pressure induced by artificial ventilation, considerably reduces the blood loss which could attend removal of these often highly vascular tumours. The level of hypotension should be considered carefully in relation to the patient's preoperative blood pressure. Thus, an elderly hypotensive patient will have a higher autoregulatory threshold in normal brain than a fit and healthy young patient with a normal blood pressure. What might be safe hypotension for the latter might constitute unsafe induced ischaemia in the former.

*Dehydrating agents* The most popular is mannitol which is best given before the induction of hypotension so the renal perfusion remains adequate to eliminate fluid and so that its hypervolaemic effect on capillary bleeding has largely subsided when the exposure is being made. The optimum dose is 1 g/kg. Excessive dosage adds little to the reduction of the tumour-brain-bed tension and increases extradural bleeding. Use of these agents, almost universally popular 10 years ago, has steadily declined in recent years, probably owing to the generally earlier diagnosis of tumours, the acceptance of increased steroid dosage for a longer period preoperatively, and better anaesthesia.

## Reduction of local tension between tumour capsule and brain-bed

This is achieved by the invariable practice of exenterating the interior of the tumour to produce a thin and pliable capsule which can be retracted away from the brain with minimal trauma to reveal the course of vessels running from the brain onto the tumour.

The brain itself should never be retracted. An overhanging lip of tissue such as occurs with the basal 'submerged' tumours may be held up, but no retraction is put upon it. In particular, no patties should ever be pushed down between the tumour (exenterated or not) and the adjacent brain. This procedure contuses the brain, tears blood vessels and so adds to local oedema long before the tumour is ready for removal.

## Monitoring

The electrocardiogram is used throughout the operation and blood pressure is monitored continuously, usually by radial artery catheterization. Estimation of the blood gases is carried out at appropriate intervals in a prolonged operation. More sophisticated monitoring techniques such as evoked response monitoring for localization of the motor and sensory cortex or evoked response monitoring of cranial nerves may be indicated in special situations.

## Magnification

The use of the loupe previously and now the operating microscope has particular value in dissecting the tumour capsule away from the walls of large venous sinuses, from the optic nerves and chiasm, and from arterial trunks such as the internal carotid and its anterior choroidal and posterior communicating branches. It is also useful in defining the following smaller vessels supplying the tumour, particularly from the anterior communicating/anterior cerebral complex and also from the middle cerebral artery.

In the surgery of basal meningiomas, the microscope is essential. Dissection of cranial nerves in the tentorial hiatus and branches of the basilar and cerebellar arteries is impossible without the use of the microscope. It is also of great help in the dissection of arteries and veins which actually run through tumour tissue, a situation that may be encountered in parasagittal and pterional lesions.

## Bipolar coagulation

This is particularly helpful when working near the optic nerve and chiasm and in the posterior fossa when dealing with vessels on and about the brain stem.

## Mechanical retractors

A retractor such as that developed by Yaşargil is of help in holding up overhanging brain when dealing with a 'submerged' basal or posterior fossa tumour. It should be adjustable so that actual retraction is avoided and should be relaxed at intervals during the operation.

# SUPRATENTORIAL TUMOURS

## The operation

### EXCISION OF A CONVEXITY MENINGIOMA

The removal of a meningioma with a bony exostosis in the frontoparietal zone will be described. This illustrates the basic surgical principles employed.

# 4 & 5

### The incision

The incision is planned so that the tumour lies in the centre of the exposure and there is generous access on all sides. The scalp is then incised, haemostasis is achieved in the usual fashion and the flap is separated from the pericranium.

The bone flap is cut either by the conventional method of burr hole and saw incision or by employing an air-driven cutting drill utilizing two burr holes at the base of the flap. This latter method is expeditious and helpful with heavily vascularized bone, but with a flap that is hyperostotic or with an irregular inner surface it may cause difficulty, resulting in tearing of the dura and, if the tension is high, extrusion and damage to the veins which may be of serious import in the parasagittal zone.

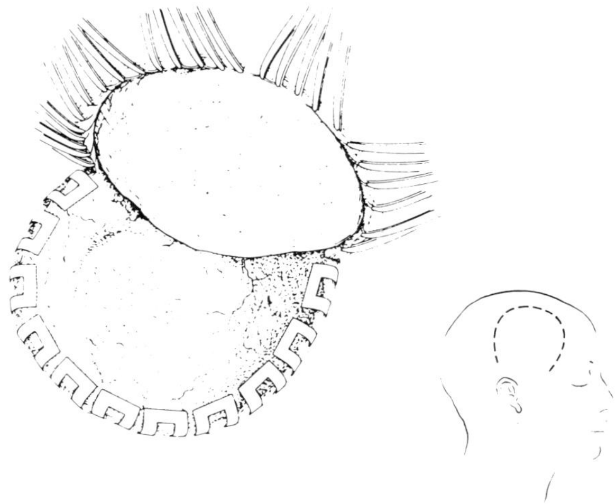

4

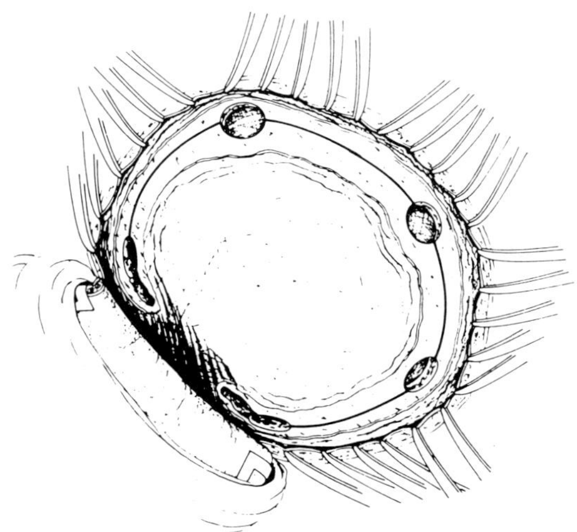

5

# 6 & 7

## Elevation of bone flap

Tumour which is attached to or is infiltrating the inner table of the bone flap is freed by lifting with one elevator just sufficiently to enable a second elevator to be inserted with its curve reversed to conform with that of the inner table. The blunt point of the second elevator is used to dissect gently and separate the tumour and dura completely from the bone.

This elevator is now discarded for a fresh one and the bone flap is fully elevated. This method avoids any tendency to pull the tumour out of its bed prematurely, so distorting the brain and possibly tearing vessels.

Elevation of the bony flap may be associated with profuse blood loss from the tumour surface and dural vessels and has to be carried out expeditiously. The bleeding can be quickly controlled by the application of two layers of cottonoid held gently but firmly in place covering the dura.

With large convexity tumours where appreciable brain swelling may be expected it may be sound practice to remove the bone flap completely. This may be done at this stage by cutting through the muscle and pericranial attachment, or may be postponed until the tumour has been removed and the dura excised. The bone flap is frozen in an antibiotic mixture and stored for replacement at a later date, usually some 3 months after the initial procedure. With the use of several days preoperative steroid and the general diagnosis of meningioma before the intracranial pressure is appreciably raised, removal of the bone flap is less necessary now than in previous days.

At this stage the dural tension should be assessed by palpation and optimally it should be just above atmospheric pressure, bulging slightly. If it is felt to be too high a further dose of mannitol may be given.

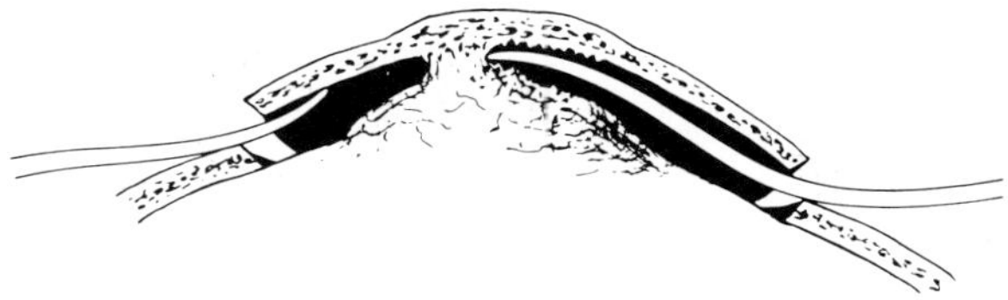

6

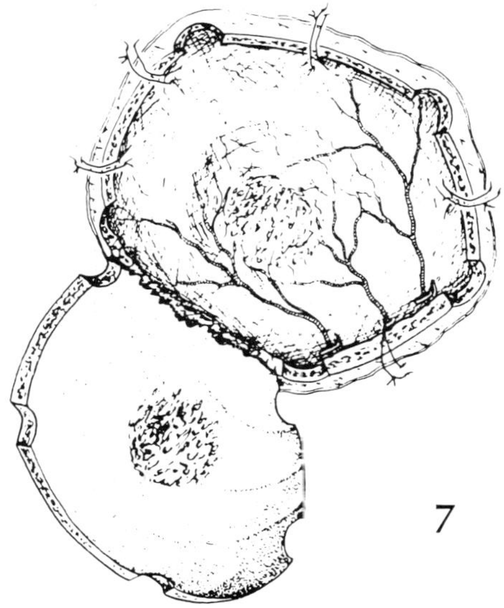

7

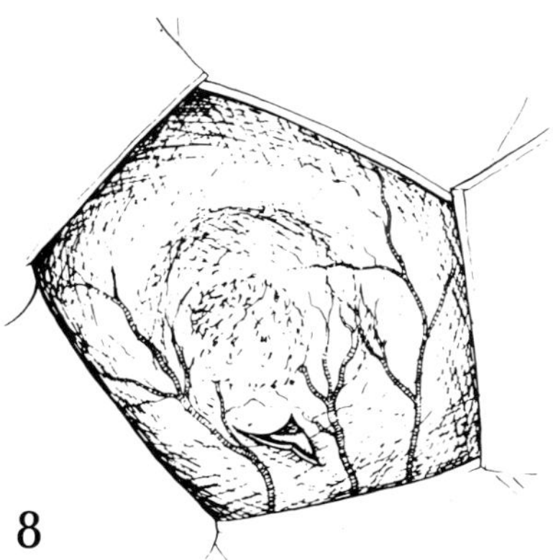

8

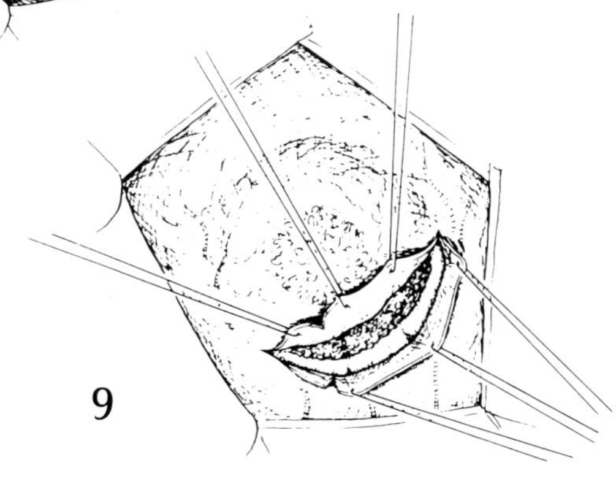

9

## Treatment of dura and meningeal vessels

Venous channels in the bone are occluded with wax; the dura is then hitched up to the bone with duroperiosteal sutures about 3 cm apart. When used for underpinning meningeal vessels the ligature should be tied firmly around the vessel before the ends are passed through the pericranium so that if the stitch should cut out from the latter it will not leave a blood vessel unoccluded. The larger arterial channels are best closed with a tantalum clip inserted through a slit made in the dura alongside them.

# 8 & 9

## Incision of dura

The edge of the tumour is palpated through the dura and a radial incision is made and continued medially until the fringe or edge of the neoplasm is exposed. The incision is then continued circumferentially, keeping no more than 3 mm peripheral to the tumour fringe, thus avoiding the production of a large opening between tumour and dura through which brain herniation could occur. The dural vessels are clipped or coagulated. Any irregularities of the contour are followed closely with the incision. Every 1.5 cm a stitch is put through the dural edge on each side. The stitches on the convexity dura are weighted with clips to evert the dura mater and so prevent any indentation of the brain. Those in the dural attachment of the tumour are tied with a single knot and used for retraction later. When the dural incision is completed and if control of intracranial tension is correct, the tumour should protrude a few millimetres out of the head at most and there should be no brain herniation.

# 10 & 11

## Exenteration of tumour

A circular opening 2 cm in diameter is made through the dural base or presenting tumour. Subsequent removal depends largely on the consistency of the neoplasm.

If the tumour is very soft the centre may be sucked out, often in a few minutes. The remaining thickness of tumour capsule can be assessed by palpation at intervals with blunt forceps (*see Illustration 12*) to avoid undue thinning and possible penetration or inversion by the sucker, resulting in tearing of blood vessels on the subjacent brain surface. Bleeding vessels within the cavity are caught up in the mouth of the sucker and clipped or coagulated together.

The ultrasonic dissection apparatus (Cavitron) is of some use in the excision of meningiomas. However, the fibrous septa which commonly traverse even soft tumours may very well defeat the ultrasonic dissector; the second author of this chapter has found the combined use of an ultrasonic dissector and a large sucker commonly of more value in the rapid exenteration of tumours than the use of either alone. The ultrasonic dissector is generally inadequate to deal with very hard tumours even at maximum power. In relation to delicate basal nerves or vessels some authorities recommend the use of lasers, and in the treatment of the base of the tumour the neodymium-YAG laser may be of value, with its increased penetration through tissue enabling the bone to be heat-sterilized to the depth of a few millimetres.

If blood loss is excessive, removal of the centre of the tumour can be done in stages with control of the bleeding achieved with cotton wool tampons at each step.

If the tumour is of firmer consistency and will not suck away it is exenterated with a diathermy loop of appropriate size. Bleeding points are coagulated after every slice.

In some cases the meningioma may be hard but may contain extremely friable thin-walled blood vessels which do not coagulate easily and may need repeated application of diathermy. This makes removal a very slow process, but it is essential in these cases to complete the haemostasis at each step before proceeding to the next loop incision. Unless this is done considerable blood loss may occur and if the cavity is not kept dry assessment of the thickness of the capsule may be hindered.

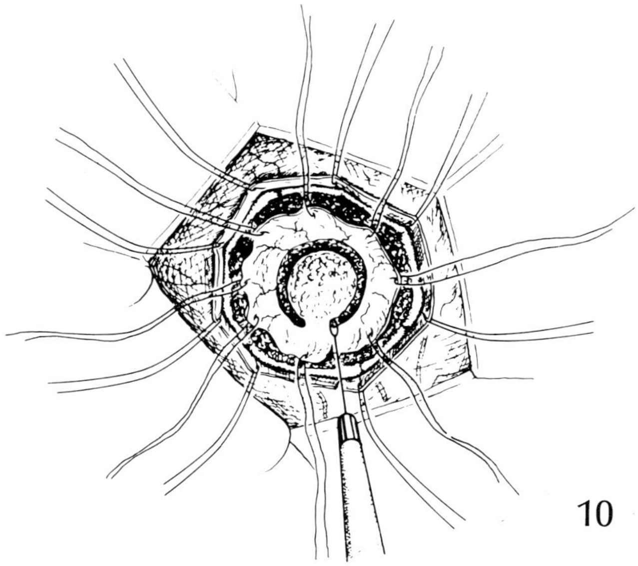

10

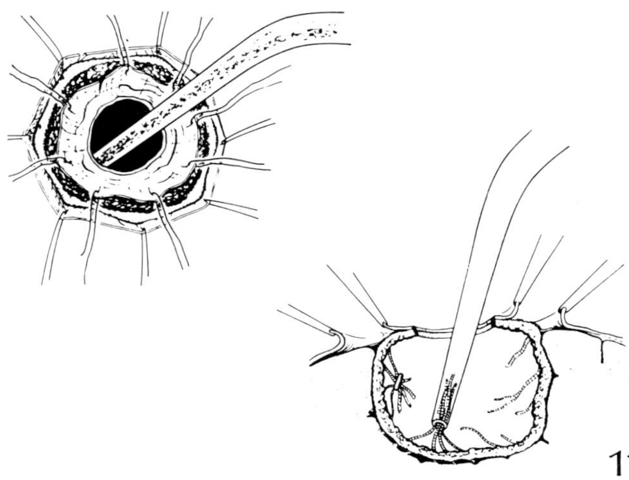

11

# 12

## Assessment of completeness of exenteration

A blunt pair of forceps or a narrow brain retractor is gently pressed against the inside of the tumour capsule and if sufficient has been removed to leave a shell about 3–5 mm in thickness (more for the softer tumour, less for the harder), a characteristic springiness and displaceability will be perceived. If the wall is rigid and unyielding, more shavings with the loop will be required until the correct degree of laxity is obtained. If the capsule is knobbly and bears protuberances, it must be borne in mind that the adjacent major arteries may run in the crevices of the surface of the tumour. The location of the vessels will have been shown by the arteriogram and in their vicinity the capsule should not be excessively thinned.

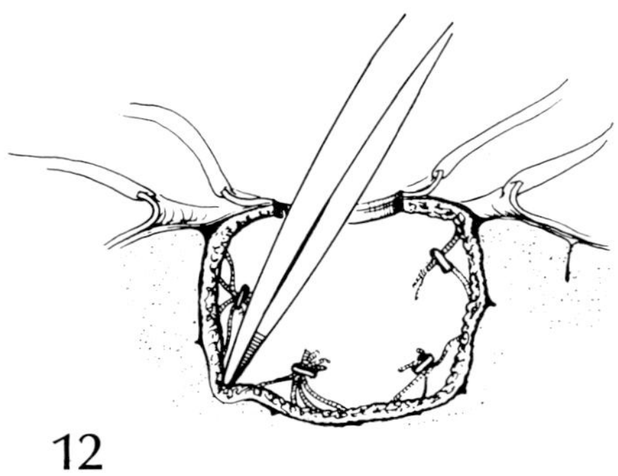

12

# 13

## Tumour excision

When the correct amount of tumour has been removed the capsule will be lax and the local tumour–brain-bed tension will be reduced. Sufficient room for manoeuvre has now been achieved and the tumour can be peeled away from the brain without any disturbance of the latter, or any need for its retraction, and without any tendency towards displacement or rocking of the tumour as a whole.

The sutures through the dural edge attached to the tumour are now gently retracted over a short segment to stretch the arachnoid which is now opened to expose the blood vessels running from adjacent brain to the meningioma. The use of the microscope and bipolar coagulation is particularly helpful in the division of tiny branches passing from vessels in the pia–arachnoid into the tumour.

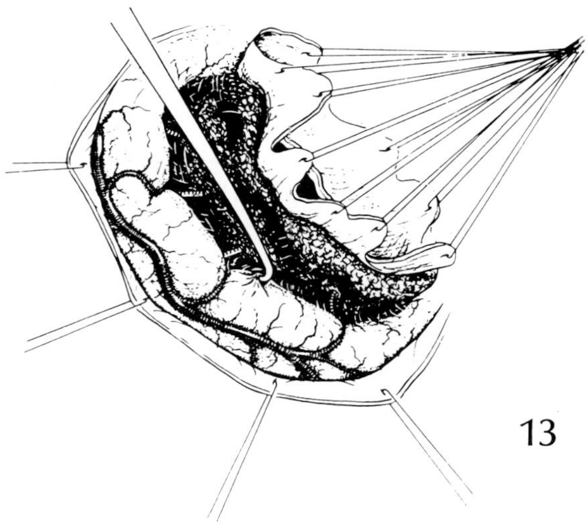

13

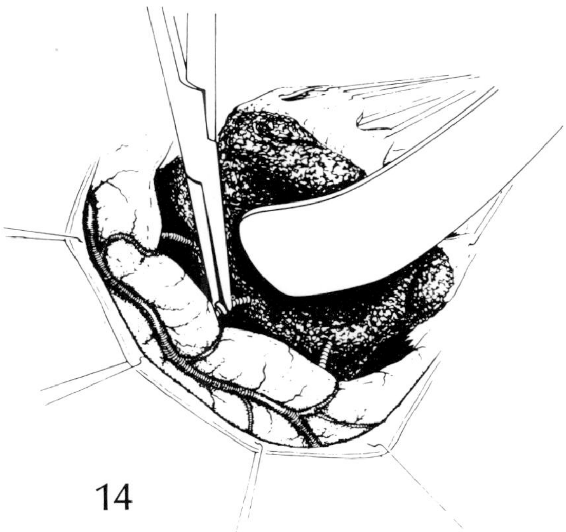

14

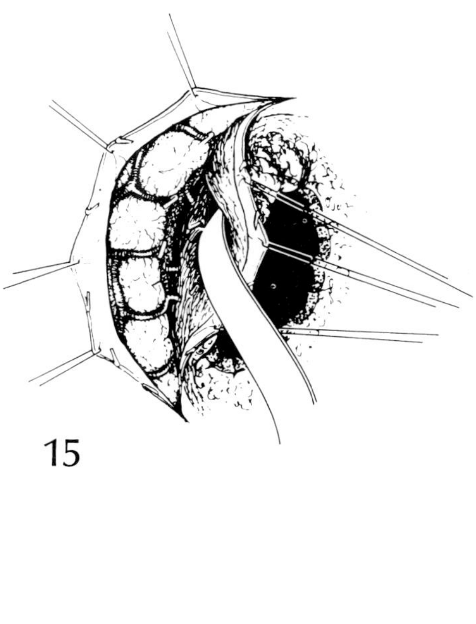

15

# 14 & 15

## Occlusion of blood vessels

When it has been confirmed that the distribution of a blood vessel is confined to the tumour it can be clipped or coagulated. With more room available a brain spatula is now applied to the tumour to separate the capsule deeper in. If in doubt whether a vessel is concerned solely with the supply of the neoplasm it is best to delay occluding it until more of the capsule has been exposed so that a longer length of the vessel's course may be revealed. This is of particular importance in the pterional and parasagittal/falx zones.

# 16 & 17

## Completion of dissection

This dissection is continued the entire way around the periphery of the meningioma, so that only its deep surface in contact with the white matter remains to be cleared. If the tumour is very large it may overhang the spatula in redundant folds, preventing visualization of the fundus. This is dealt with by excising a wedge of the wall and then retracting the adjacent segments of the tumour inwards to give access to the deep surface.

Further wedges are excised until the fundus is clearly exposed. It is then gently retracted away from the white matter, the few vessels being defined, clipped or coagulated.

It is essential that any blood vessels coming through the white matter are occluded cleanly and not broken off, as they may retract into the white matter and excessive fibre tract damage may be caused in pursuing them to arrest haemorrhage.

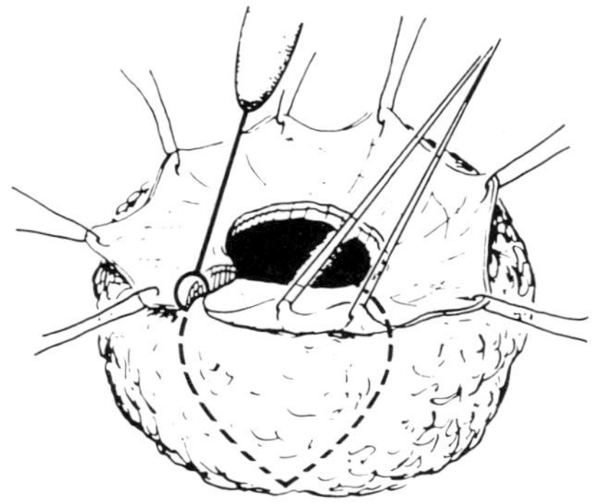

16

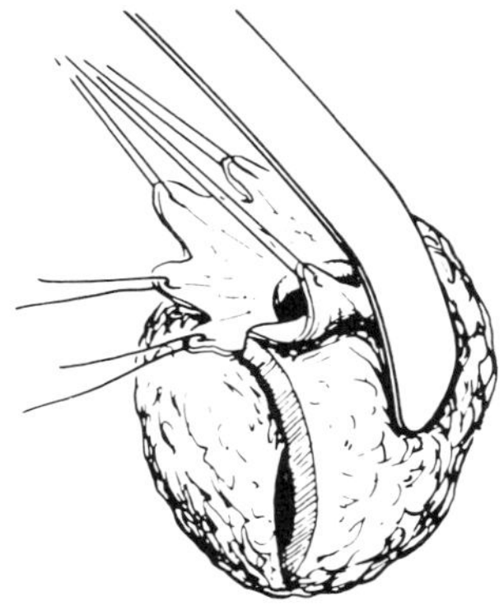

17

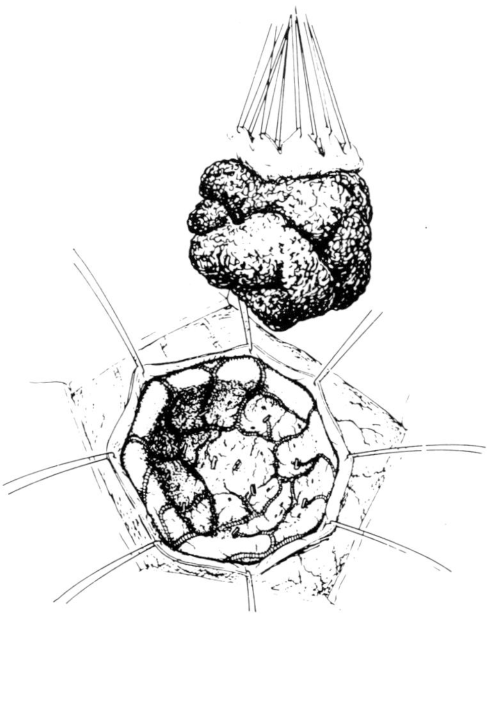

18

# 18

## Removal of tumour

The tumour can now be lifted out completely. Inspection of the bed should show no bruising or laceration of the cortex or white matter. The cavity at this stage is usually contracting down due to surrounding oedema. This may occur quickly.

# 19 & 20

## Removal of dura

It is the author's practice to excise all the dura in the exposed area (this does not apply to 'submerged' tumours), its vessels being clipped or coagulated. An edge of 3–4 mm is left projecting beyond the bone to retain the duroperiosteal sutures previously inserted and is then coagulated to shrink it up to the bone margin.

The reasons for complete dural excision are as follows.

1. To ensure total microscopic removal of the tumour because a thin fringe or a layer of cells may extend subdurally for a considerable distance from the edge of the main neoplastic mass to remain as one source of recurrent growth at a later date.
2. If a central dural defect is left following tumour removal any extradural bleeding will tend to run over the margins into the tumour site to produce a cavity clot.
3. Any significant rise of tension, as when the brain has been traumatized, will produce a brain hernia which, with the ring constriction of its 'neck', will result in venous obstruction, so increasing the herniation.
4. Complete dural excision provides a much larger area of decompression, allowing the brain to bulge, and even with a considerable rise in tension there is little risk of any obstruction to its veins. The decompressive effect results, in the author's experience, in a less disturbed postoperative neurological course.

With the increased use of preoperative steroids and earlier diagnosis it is more frequently possible than hitherto to reconstitute the dura safely. It must be remembered, of course, that reconstituted dura will prevent brain swelling and may embarrass the blood supply of the superficial cortex if it proves impossible to control such swelling by other means. The materials which have been used to reconstitute dura are legion; the safest is undoubtedly fascia lata although this requires another incision. Occasionally adequate pericranium may be available and a variety of artificial membranes have been produced commercially. Lyophilized dura, which used to be of extreme value and was used by the authors for a number of years, has recently come under some suspicion as possibly harbouring the virus of Jakob–Creutzfeldt disease; in at least one case the transmission of this deadly illness was probably attributable to such dura. Its use at the present time, therefore, cannot be recommended.

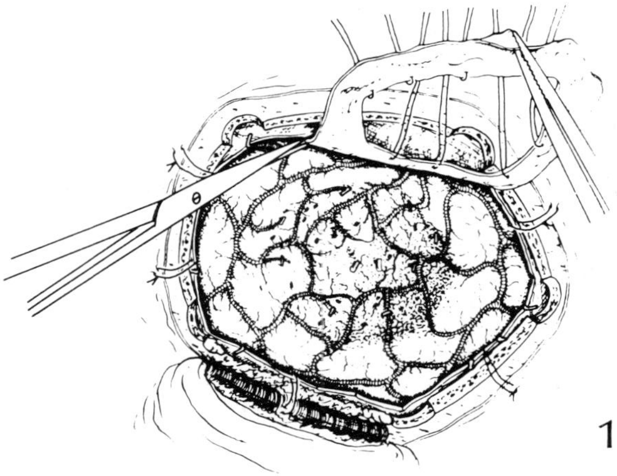

19

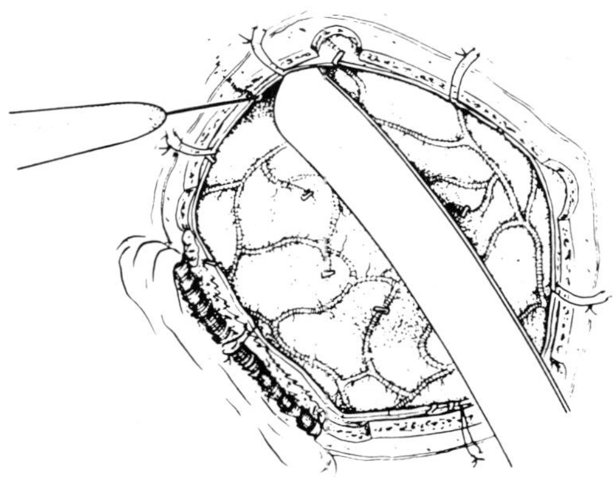

20

# 21 & 22

## Removal of bone flap

*Closure of the craniotomy*

In the course of closure, controlled respiration will have been reversed and the blood pressure encouraged to rise. Any unoccluded vessels in the dura or in the bed of the tumour will be clipped or coagulated and particular attention paid to cut temporal muscle in the deep aspect of the scalp flap if the bone has been removed.

If it has been decided that the bone flap should be removed, this may already have been done; if not, it may now be done by cutting through its remaining attachment of temporal muscle and pericranium, these being left attached to the flap for its subsequent replacement. If, on the other hand, it has been decided that the bone flap may be replaced, the dura will have been reconstituted and attention must be turned to possible invasion of the flap by the meningioma. Any involved area of the flap should be drilled away with an instrument such as the Hall Air Drill and the bone flap then replaced, usually with a single central perforating stitch tied over an opened clip anchoring the bone firmly to the dural substitute used. The pericranium and muscle may then be closed with interrupted stitches. It has never been the author's practice to wire down these flaps.

If it has been decided to remove bone, the exposed brain should be covered with a layer of Gelfilm to minimize adhesions to the scalp flap. It also tends to minimize leakage of blood from the scalp into the cavity left by removal of the tumour. With care, as described, damage to the arachnoid around the tumour site will be minimal and the tendency to adhesion formation reduced. It is remarkable how within about 3 months a complete layer of neodura will have formed.

The scalp is now closed in the usual two layers to prevent any tendency to a cerebrospinal fluid leak. No drainage is used if the bone has been removed, but if the bone has been replaced a standard subgaleal suction drain may be employed.

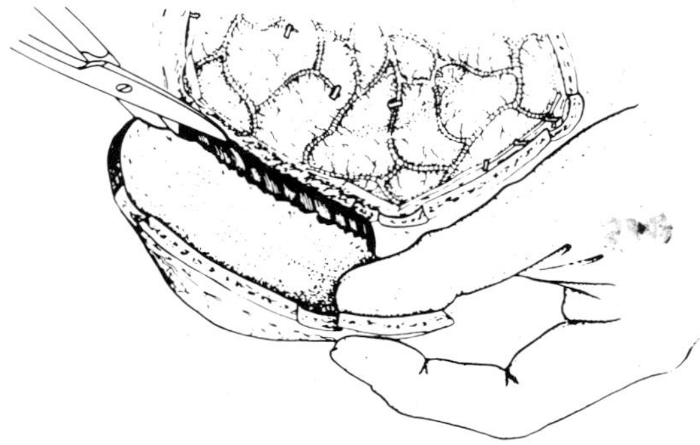

21

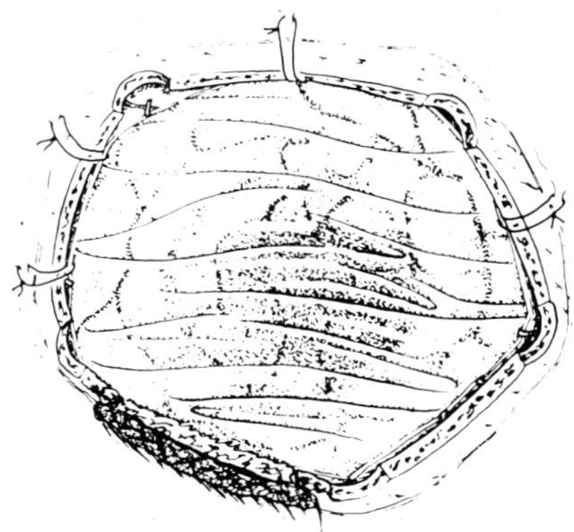

22

# Postoperative care

With the bone flap in place, the subgaleal suction drain should be removed in 48 hours and the stitches may be removed on the third postoperative day.

If the bone flap has been removed it will generally be found that the flap bulges during the first few days owing partly to brain swelling and partly to the collection of blood-stained cerebrospinal fluid. It is generally wise to aspirate this daily by introducing a blunt brain needle cautiously for a short distance only through the sutured incision, as far away from evocative cortex as possible. Sometimes for many days after such an excision of meningioma, dura and bone flap, there is a tendency for quite large quantities of fluid to collect and this may require control by repeated spinal taps supplemented by the use of the carbonic anhydrase inhibitor acetazolamide (Diamox), which tends to inhibit the choroid plexus production of cerebrospinal fluid. The use of mild dehydrating agents such as frusemide may also be necessary.

Stitches are removed at around the third day unless the tension in the flap is seriously raised, when it may be wiser to retain them for 5 or 7 days. Anticonvulsants such as phenytoin in a dose of 200–300 mg/day are given routinely postoperatively. Different units have differing anticonvulsant routines, but it has been the author's practice to administer anticonvulsants for a year postoperatively to all convexity meningiomas, and for longer should fits occur in the postoperative phase.

Where recurrent epilepsy supervenes soon after operation it is important that it be rapidly controlled as frequent uncontrolled fits may result in gross deterioration of neurological deficit and perhaps the production of quite a long-lasting hemiparesis. The author's preference is for the use of intravenous chlormethiazole (Heminevrin) which only rarely fails to stop such recurrent seizures. It should be given by intravenous drip in quantities sufficient to control the fits, and withdrawn gradually over a period of 24 hours thereafter. Only rarely in resistant status epilepticus is it necessary to consider the use of powerful anaesthetic drugs such as thiopentone. Diazepam, formerly liberally used in such epilepsy control, can no longer be recommended. It is accompanied by troublesome hypotension and is not very effective as an anti-epileptic drug.

# Treatment of bone flap

Where there is any concern about postoperative brain swelling the bone flap is likely to have been removed. However, many convexity tumours show little tendency to herniation these days and the dural defect can easily be reconstituted. In the case of submerged tumours which do not present at the brain surface, then the dural flap is completely closed and the bone flap replaced.

In cases where the flap has been removed it is replaced at a later date when the intracranial tension has returned to normal as shown by the craniotomy defect sinking in when the patient is upright. This may occur fairly rapidly, but it is usually wise to wait about 3 months for a firm neodura to form, and where troublesome brain swelling persists it may take much longer.

Replacement is mandatory in the parietal area because very occasionally a patient who has a large postoperative defect in this zone may, over a period varying from months to years, develop a parietal decompression syndrome which comprises headache, dizziness and a hemiparesis possibly with hemihypoaesthesia, predominating on the contralateral side. This appears to be the result of changes in the cortex and white matter caused by the oscillation of the brain in and out of the defect with alteration in posture such as standing and lying or by coughing and straining. The symptoms are reversed by replacement of the flap.

After removal, the bone flap is placed in a sterile metal container with penicillin and streptomycin in saline solution, covering it completely. It is frozen at a temperature of −10°C and preserved in this fashion until the time comes for replacement.

If the bone is seen to be invaded by tumour, with or without an enostosis or exostosis, a burr hole is made to one side of the involved area at the time of replacement, and this is cut away with rongeurs until normal bone is exposed all round. The resulting aperture can be filled with a small disc of acrylic, tantalum or titanium.

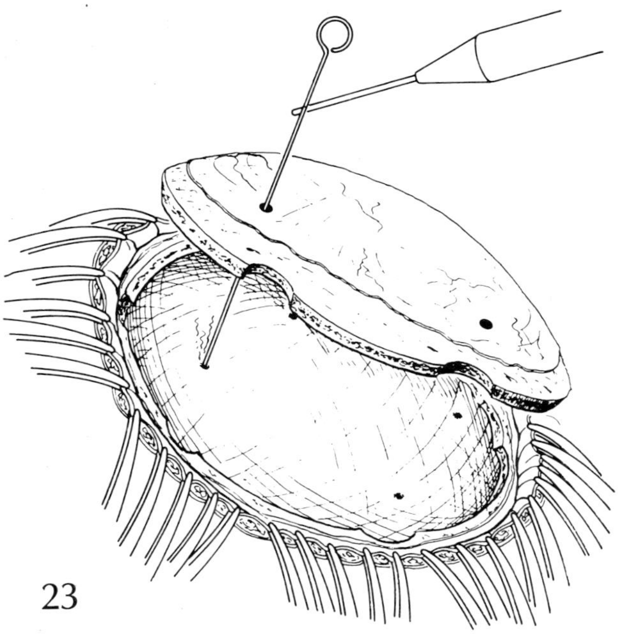

23

# 23

## Replacement of bone flap

With the induction of anaesthesia the craniotomy defect usually bulges so that controlled respiration is necessary, and although this is usually adequate to reduce the tension, mannitol may be required. It may be helpful to control tension further by the use of spinal drainage during the operation.

The scalp is reflected, leaving the newly formed dura intact. A good line of cleavage can be found in nearly all cases. Rather than dissecting the dura away from the bone edges to insert perforating stitches, which occasions a good deal of venous bleeding extradurally, the bone flap can be anchored directly onto the dura.

This is done by making four small-calibre drill holes 2–3 cm in from the periphery of the flap, the stilette of a brain needle being introduced through each hole onto the dura and coagulated briefly so as to mark the site for the stitch.

# 24 & 25

## Insertion of stitches

Stitches are then passed via the holes in the bone through the dura and tied in succession over opened-out tantalum clips. Pericranium previously left attached to the flap is sutured. The method produces a flap that is slightly mobile and which can adjust to intracranial pressure variations during the first few postoperative days.

If headaches develop, lumbar spinal taps may be necessary for 2 or 3 days postoperatively. Aspiration of the flap may be required for the first 2–4 days or, alternatively, continuous subgaleal aspiration through a vacuum bottle may be used for 24 hours.

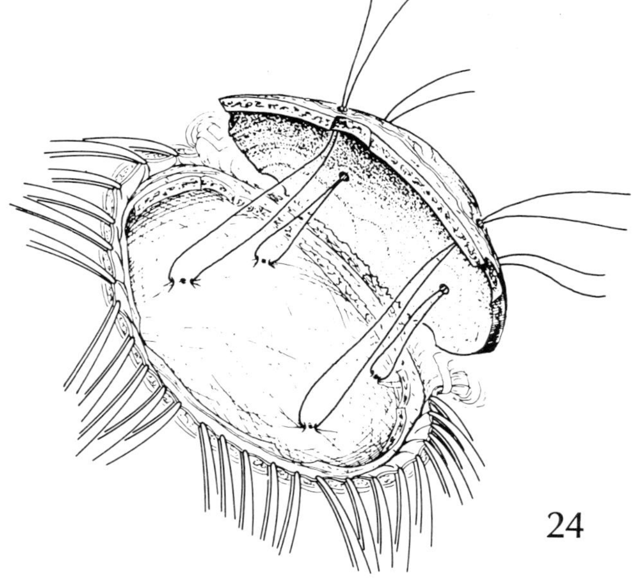

24

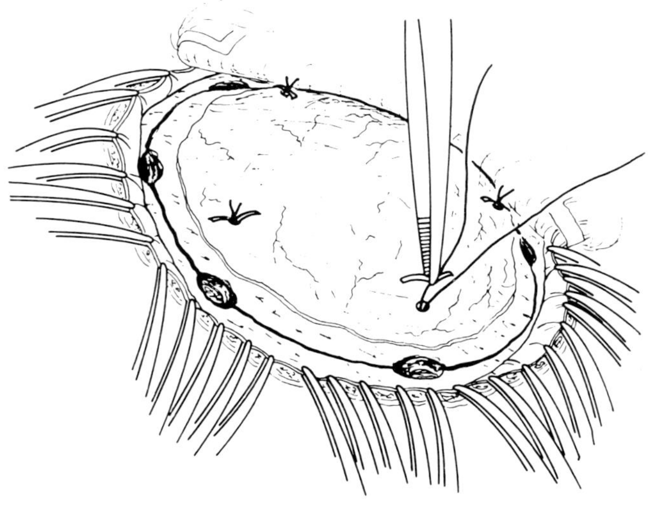

25

# SUPRATENTORIAL MENINGIOMAS IN SPECIAL SITES

In the following tumour situations greater control of tension, both general and local, in the brain-bed area is required than for convexity tumours.

1. Parasagittal and falx
2. Basal
   a. Sphenoidal ridge: middle and inner third, pterional, including bone sclerosing tumours
   b. Suprasellar and parasellar
   c. Olfactory groove, unilateral or bilateral
   d. Temporal fossa
   e. Tentorial
   f. Peritorcular

## Parasagittal and falx

### Investigations

Investigations are aimed at revealing the following essential features.

1. The precise site of the tumour in the anteroposterior plane. This may be obtained most conveniently by sagittal and coronal cuts on magnetic resonance scan, sagittal reconstruction of fourth-generation CT scan, or reference to scan planes in the scout film of a normal CT scan, usually with enhancement.
2. Whether the tumour is strictly unilateral or has extended through the falx and/or the sagittal sinus on the opposite side. In the latter case, the chances of complete excision are significantly reduced and the risks of residual neurological disability enhanced. One must, therefore, plan the approach to the opposite side with great care.
3. The degree of sinus involvement. With careful subtraction films of the venous phase of the arteriogram and the use of suitable oblique films the risk can now usually be determined without the necessity for the older method of open sagittal phlebography. In the posterior parts of the sinus some information may be obtained by retrograde phlebography from the jugular veins, but with modern digital methods of subtraction this is now unnecessary.
4. The situation and size of the sagittal veins on both hemispheres and the extent of any anastomoses between draining radicals over the surface of both hemispheres.
5. The relationship of the major anterior cerebral arterial branches to the tumour, as parasagittal and falx neoplasms are pre-eminent in providing vascular hazards during removal.

All the foregoing information is essential in order to assess the difficulties so that one can judge beforehand how radical and prolonged the operation should be. For instance, the surgical management in an elderly and frail patient with a history of tumour growth of about 6 or 7 years would be different from that in a patient aged 35 years with a history of a year or less.

It is conventional to divide the sagittal sinus with its related tumours into three roughly equal parts because their symptoms, the methods of dealing with the sinus, and the function of the adjacent brain with its neurological manifestations, differ in each site.

The anterior third extends from the crista galli to the level of the corona, the middle third from this point back to the lambda and the posterior third from the lambda to the torcula herophili. There is often overlap by a tumour from one zone to the next.

## The incision

# 26 & 27

*Anterior third*

A unilateral flap is adequate in most cases, but in the frontal region, if access to the opposite side is required, a slightly curved incision just behind the hair-line will permit a second small flap to be turned.

Alternatively, a cosmetic bifrontal flap may be marked from the outset permitting the formation of a unilateral or a bilateral bone flap as proves to be necessary. Using such a bilateral incision it may be difficult with the towels in position and the scalp turned down to find the midline of the forehead where the burr hole should be sunk for the best cosmetic effect. If during towel application a midline towel clip is placed over the glabella it is usually possible to palpate this through the turned down flap, or alternatively, a needle may be inserted directly in the midline using the nose as a guide after the towels have been placed, but before the scalp is turned back. This needle can be used to make a vertical scratch in the pericranium which may than be recognizable once the scalp has been turned down. In order to reduce the risk of damage to the sagittal sinus when making the burr holes, the margin of the burr is brought just up to the midline and does not transgress it.

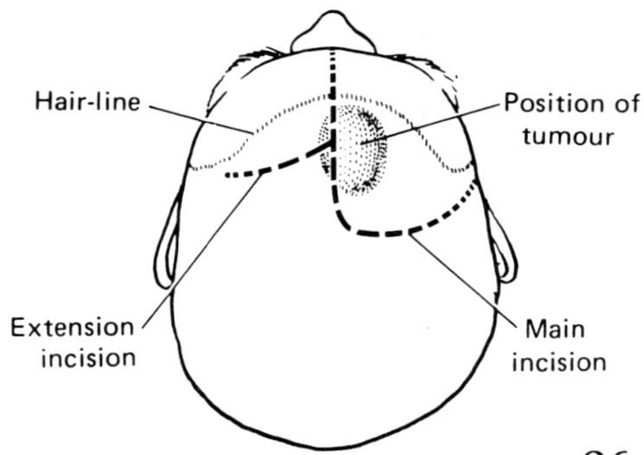


26

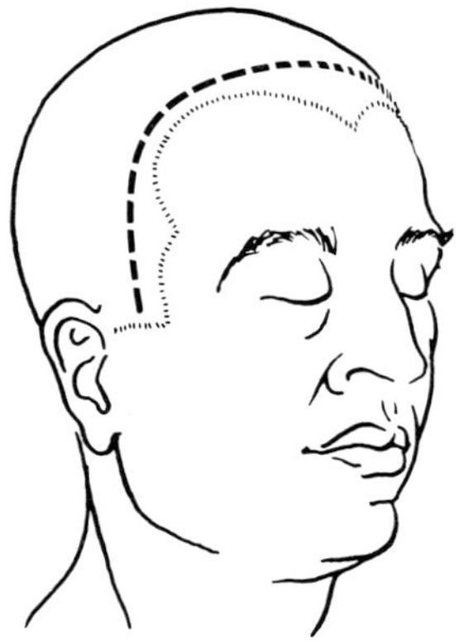

27

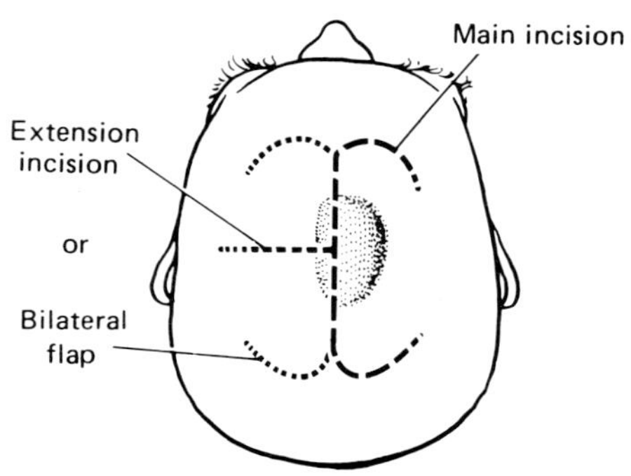


28

# 28

*Middle third*

If the tumour is known not to transgress the sinus, a horseshoe-shaped flap extending up to the midline is adequate. However, if the tumour has extended across the midline, either a contralateral transverse incision at the level of the tumour is made or, if the extension is considerable, then a further horseshoe-shaped flap will allow the necessary access. It is best to turn two bone flaps, one on each side, rather than to cut a flap right across the sinus because if the sinus is damaged by the saw or when the flap is being separated, considerable blood loss may occur before the bone is completely reflected and the bleeding controlled. Such troublesome blood loss is best controlled by the rapid adoption of fairly steep foot-down tilt controlling the venous pressure. It is important under these circumstances to avoid excessive negative phase on the respirator lest air embolism occurs.

# 29

*Posterior third*

This is best done with the patient in the semirecumbent position with the head flexed. A flap similar to that made in the frontal region can be fashioned, again with a horizontal extension to the opposite side depending on the size of any contralateral tumour. The principles of removal of meningioma in the parasagittal and falx region are exemplified in a description of the excision of a bilateral parietal falx and parasagittal tumour which has occluded the sinus (confirmed by arteriography) and infiltrated the bone.

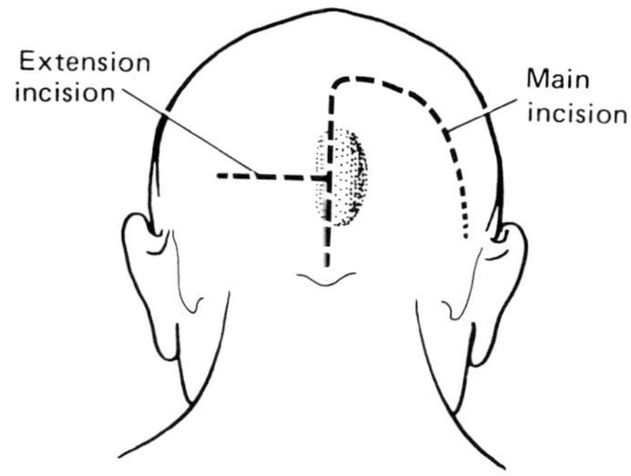


29

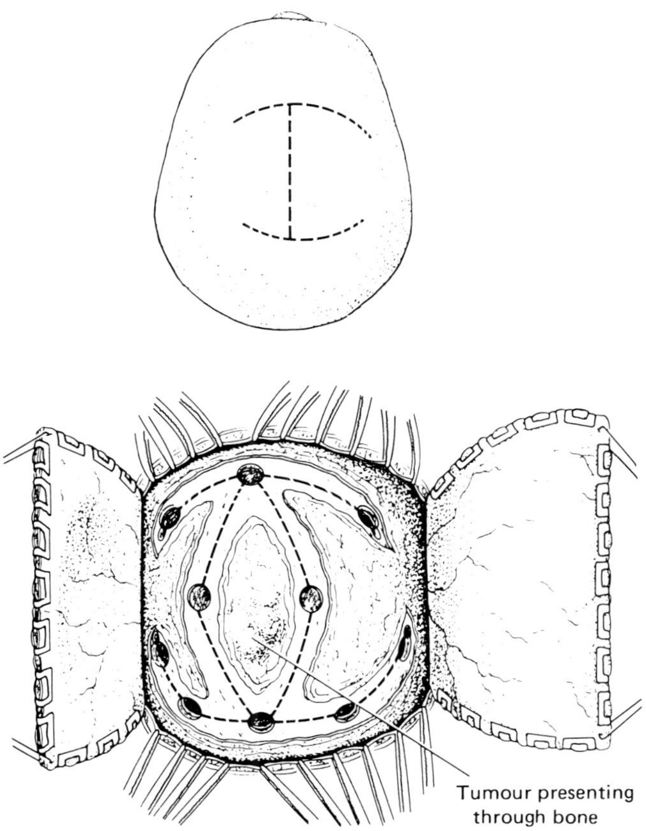


30

# 30

## Incision and exposure

It is better to make a bilateral exposure using two scalp flaps and two bone flaps so that the latter may be raised individually.

The scalp flaps are reflected and the burr holes sited to surround the exostosis or the area of the skull infiltrated with tumour, producing a lozenge-shaped island of bone. The lateral two bone flaps are then fashioned by dividing the pericranium; further burr holes are made so that the right and left flaps can be turned back individually.

# 31

## Separation of the bone from the tumour

With the lateral bone flaps turned, the central infiltrated zone of skull is separated rapidly from the bulk of the tumour presenting extradurally. Bleeding, which is often profuse at this stage, may be controlled by gentle pressure with cottonoid and then the individual bleeding points coagulated.

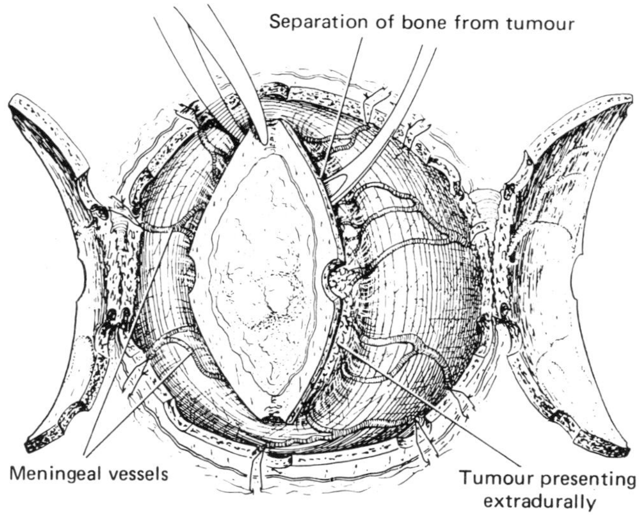


31

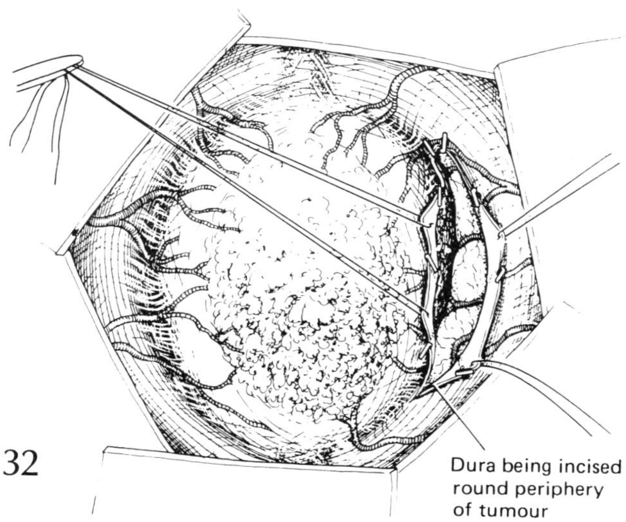


32

# 32

## Incision of dura

The edge of the meningioma may be recognized by palpation of the dura with blunt forceps. The usual peripheral incision is made, with care being taken to avoid any interference with the sagittal veins. The incision is carried up to the sinus both in front of and behind the tumour and the usual stitches are inserted into the cut edges of the dura on each side. A similar procedure is then carried out on the other side.

# 33

An opening is made in the dural attachment of the neoplasm and a thorough exenteration is carried out by suction or diathermy loop until room for manoeuvre is obtained, as described in the section dealing with removal of convexity meningiomas.

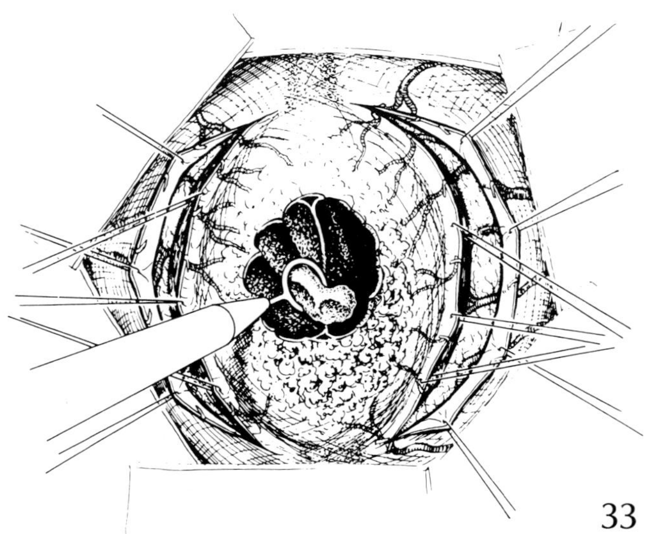

33

# 34

Traction is now made on the sutures through the dural attachment of the tumour to put the arachnoid on the stretch. The arachnoid is then opened and the lax tumour capsule retracted from the brain to identify the blood vessels which supply the neoplasm itself. These are clipped or coagulated and the dissection continued deeply from front to back, first on one side and then on the other until the falx is visualized.

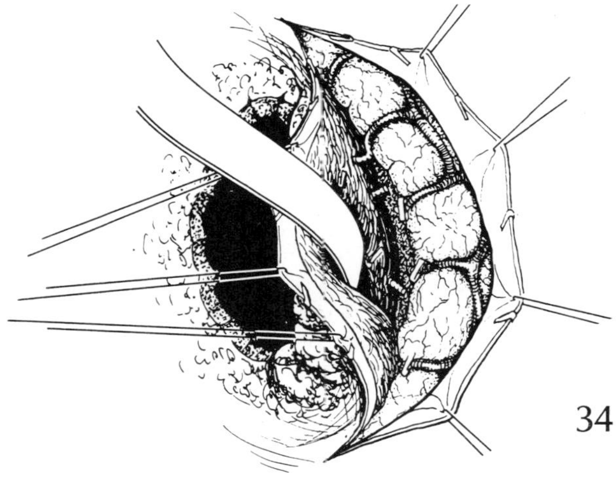

34

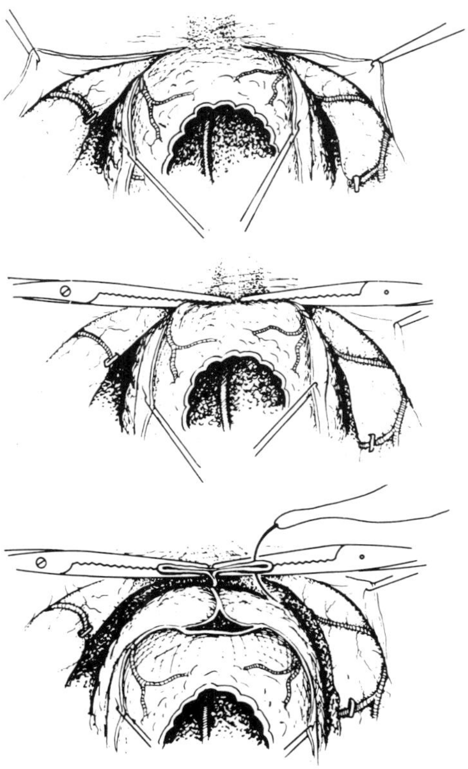

35

# 35

## Treatment of sinus

The junction of the occluded and non-occluded portions of the sinus anteriorly can be recognized by palpation with forceps or by aspiration with a hollow needle. Clamps are then applied from each side of this junction point to occlude the sinus completely, which is then cut through on the tumour side of the clamps. The edges of the patent sinus are now closed with a continuous suture from each side and the clamps removed. A similar procedure is carried out on the sinus at the posterior aspect of the tumour.

# 36

## Treatment of falx

As a result of sinus block an extensive collateral venous circulation may develop through the scalp veins, the sagittal veins over the hemispheres on both the medial and lateral surfaces, the convexity dura on each side in the vicinity of the block and, more importantly, the falx down to the inferior sagittal sinus. Therefore, an unnecessarily wide excision of the falx should be avoided, and an incision not more than 3 mm away from the edge of the tumour attachment is made from front to back. The neoplasm can now be lifted out of the head. The efficacy of the occlusion of the sinus is confirmed by the anaesthetist raising the pressure in the anaesthetic circuit.

The exposed brain, dura and bone flaps are dealt with in the manner previously described for the convexity tumour.

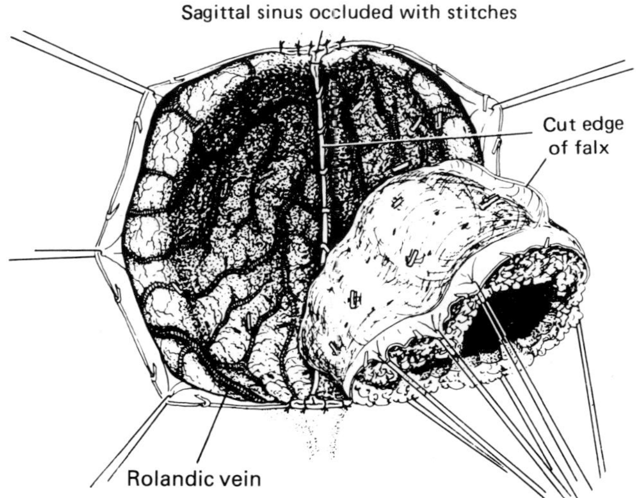


36

## UNILATERAL PARASAGITTAL MENINGIOMA

Every effort should be made preoperatively to determine the following.

1. To confirm from the CT scan and the arteriogram that the tumour does not extend across the midline
2. To ascertain whether the sinus is blocked, again from the arteriogram or, if doubt remains, by direct phlebography
3. To determine the relationship of the parasagittal veins to the tumour mass from the venous phase on the arteriogram. The degree of sinus involvement both of its wall and of its lumen will of course vary from case to case and the operator must be prepared to open the sinus if the need arises.

The same principles are employed as with the bilateral parasagittal tumour, with insistence on the need to reduce the intracranial tension and the venous pressure by controlled respiration, hypotension, posture and dehydrants. It is wise, before embarking on surgery, to arrange that the head of the table can be elevated over a good range if sinus bleeding should become a major feature, and that adequate quantities of blood are available for transfusion.

The early operative steps are the same as those for the bilateral parasagittal tumour.

# 37

The usual peripheral incision is made, with care being taken to avoid any interference with the sagittal veins. The incision is carried up to the sinus both in front and behind.

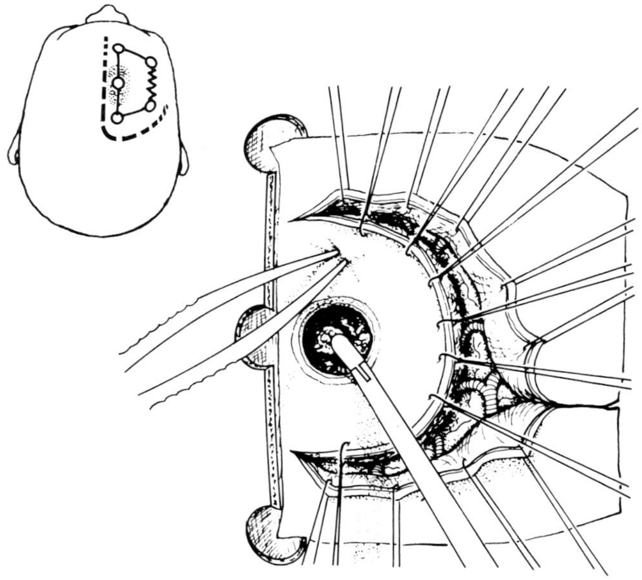

37

# 38

Exenteration of the tumour is now carried out. Owing to its fixation to the sinus the neoplasm will not rotate fully out of the head.

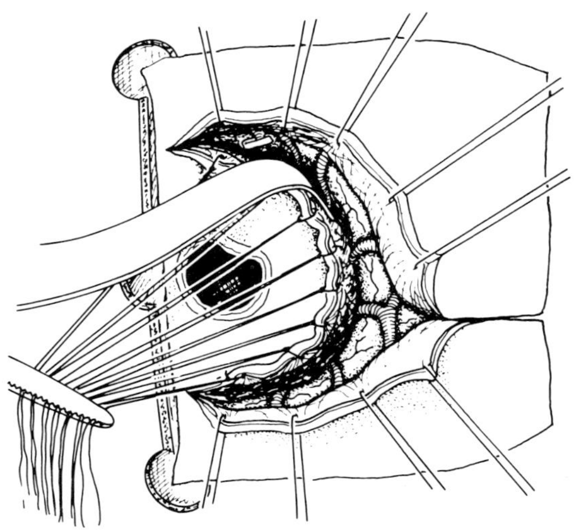

38

# 39

The capsule therefore has to be cut away in segments in order to narrow down its sinus attachment.

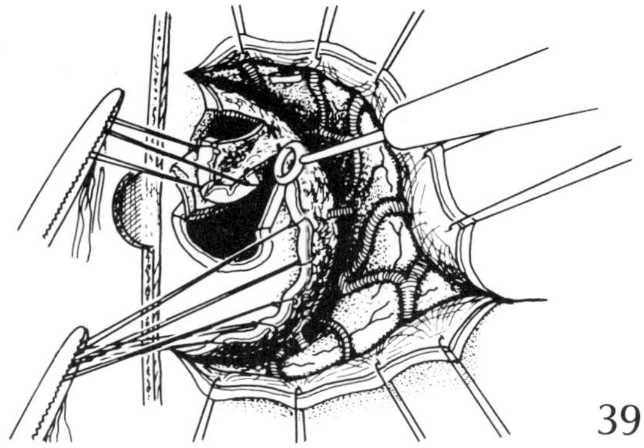

39

# 40

At this stage the falx is incised just peripheral to the tumour base so that by inspection one can confirm that there has been no extension through it to the opposite side.

With the bulk of tumour removed, room for manoeuvre will have been obtained to permit dealing with the sinus attachment.

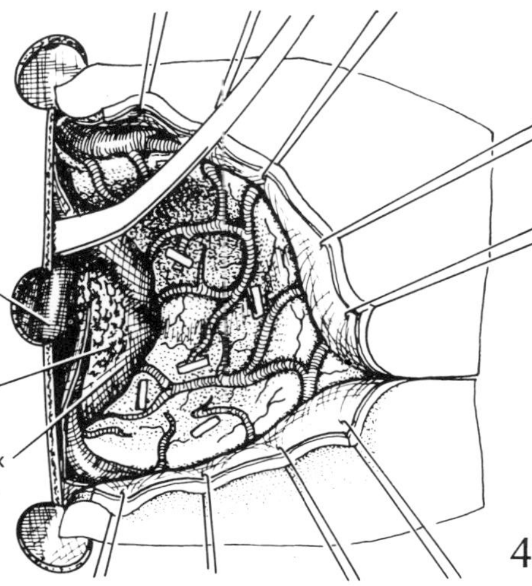


40

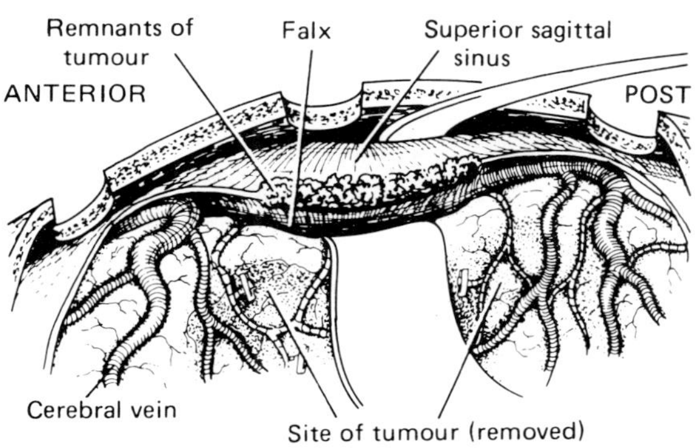


41

## Treatment of sinus attachment

In a number of cases the tumour may at first appear to have a wide attachment to the convexity dura and falx as well as to the sinus wall, but a good deal of this may merely be adhesive and can be stripped off with a blunt dissector. The area is subsequently lightly coagulated. This may leave only a small area of true infiltration of the sinus wall.

The sinus involvement may be confined to the lateral angle, which is excised in step-to-step fashion as follows.

# 41

The sinus is first separated and depressed from the overlying bone. It is now possible to apply forceps blades to the roof and the lateral wall medial to the tumour and squeeze them together with firm pressure.

# 42 & 43

An incision is made between the tumour margin and the forceps blades and a continuous suture inserted, drawn tight and tied to arrest any leakage of blood. The incision is now extended for another 2 mm and the next stitch insertion made. The procedure continues in successive steps until the whole area of involvement has been excised. There will tend to be some narrowing of the lumen of the sinus following this procedure, but it is unlikely to interfere significantly with the venous flow.

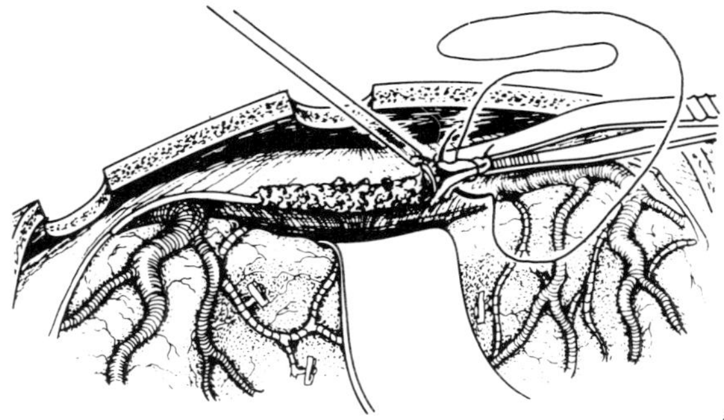

42

*Infiltration of the wall* This may or may not be associated with an intraluminal extension which will have been demonstrated in the venous phase of the arteriogram. The extent of involvement of the sinus wall will be demonstrated by thickening, both visible and palpable, of the dura for a varying distance around the tumour attachment. A small area of attachment less than 2 cm in diameter can be treated in an elderly patient simply by thorough coagulation, but in younger patients it is safer for the whole area to be excised and the gap replaced with a graft. This is best done by utilizing pericranium from the bone flap. This is immediately accessible, pliable and easily sutured, whereas fascia lata, lyophilized dura and synthetic materials tend to be too rigid and too difficult to suture in such a small space to provide a blood-tight anastomosis.

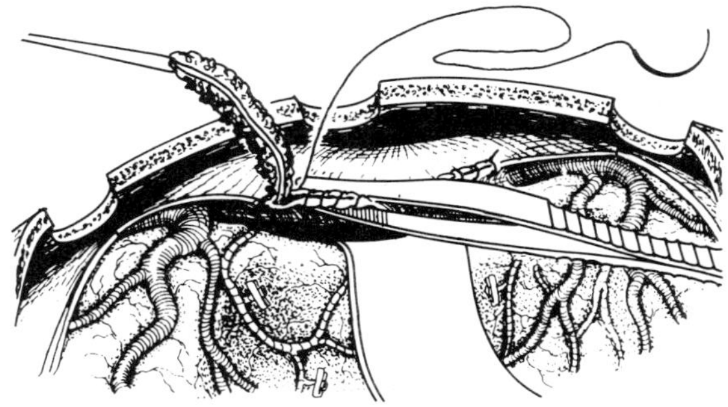

43

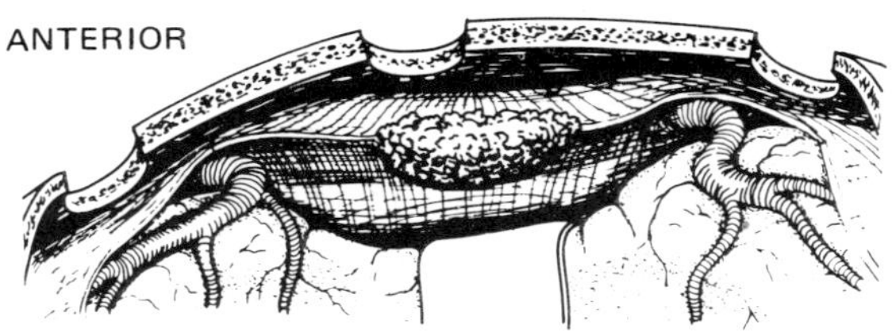


44

# 44

The sinus is separated and displaced downwards away from the overlying bone.

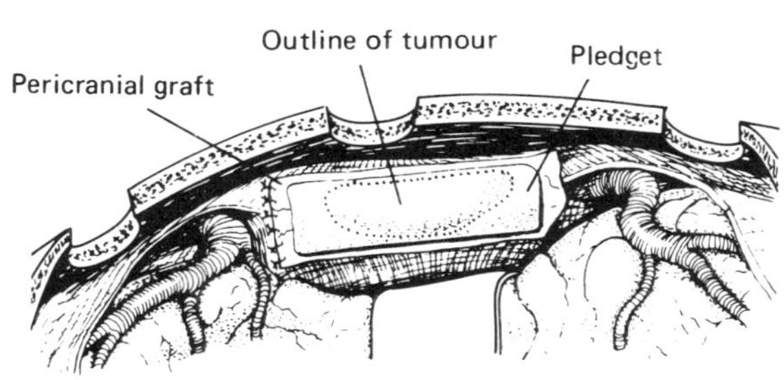


45

# 45

The affected portion of the sinus wall is overlaid with a graft which is trimmed to overlap the area by 2–3 mm.

The graft is covered by a cottonoid patty 2 mm narrower to expose the graft edge for suturing.

# 46, 47 & 48

The anterior end of the graft is sutured onto the sinus wall and the cottonoid and graft are turned back on themselves to expose the tumour. An incision is then made 2 mm away from the anterior edge of the tumour. A suture is inserted through the sinus wall on each side and the graft propelled forward by the finger or forceps to occlude the opening.

A further 2 mm incision is made above and below the neoplasm and the graft is again pushed forward and sutured at each edge. This is continued step by step until the area is completely excised. Any excess graft is trimmed off.

If bleeding should become excessive, occlusion of the sinus anteriorly with the finger which is holding the graft in position will usually control it, at least temporarily.

The integrity of the anastomosis is tested by the anaesthetist by raising the pressure in the respiratory circuit: any leakage of blood warrants another stitch.

An alternative method for small areas is the following: after the tumour has been excised a portion of fascia lata or pericranium is stuck on the surrounding sinus wall using plastic glue. This is supported with a stitch at each corner.

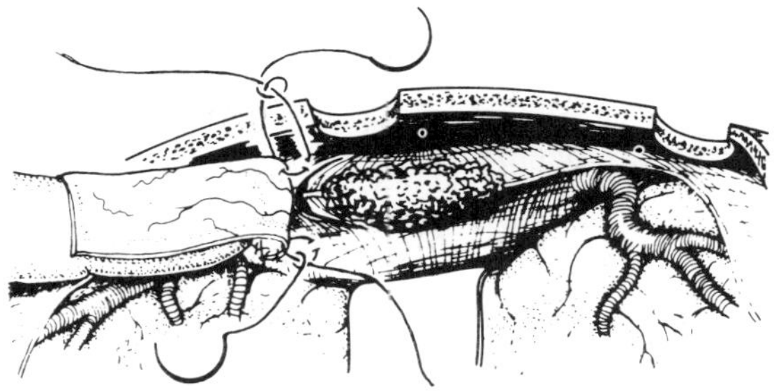

46

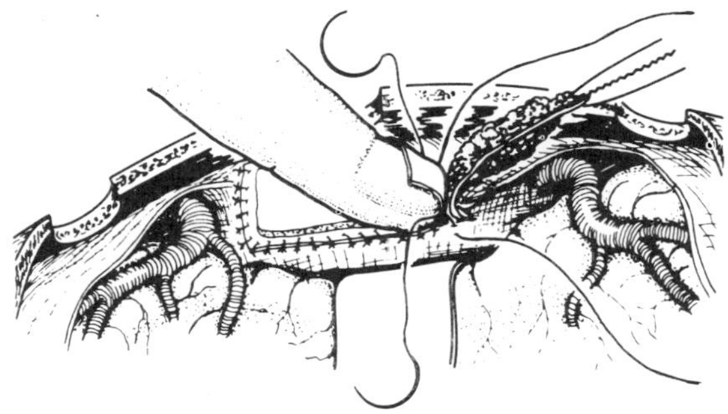

47

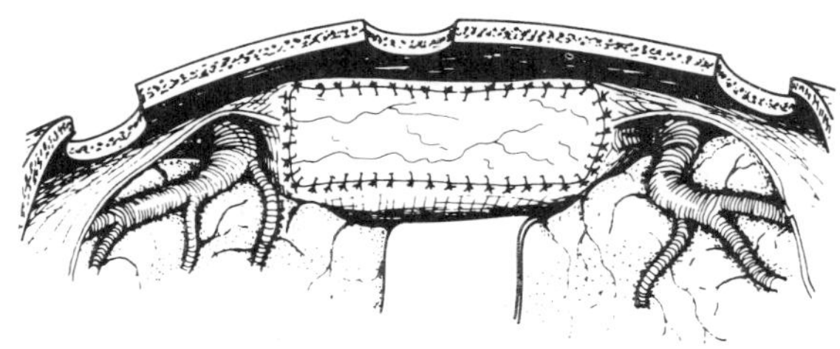

48

## Tumour recurrence

It must be accepted that if tumour is left behind in the sinus wall recurrent growth will occur at some time and possibly involve the sinus more extensively. It has been shown that even when, in the surgeon's assessment, a convexity tumour has been completely excised renewed growth appears in 9 per cent of cases; when tumour has been seen to be left behind the figure rises to 39 per cent.

However, recurrence may take a very long time to appear and as many of these patients are in their sixties a significant proportion will die of intercurrent disease rather than the meningioma. The decision to embark on a long procedure potentially associated with significant mortality and morbidity, rather than merely to rely on coagulation, will be influenced by the age and frailty of the patient, the speed of growth of the neoplasm, the extent of blood loss that has already occurred during the excision and the duration of the operation.

With regard to tumours in the anterior third of the sagittal sinus it may be thought easier and quicker to cut out the whole segment of an involved but still patent sinus rather than to excise and repair it as described above. However, the obvious fact that one interferes with the venous drainage of both hemispheres when excision is proposed should be borne in mind. Therefore it is essential to know beforehand that there is no anomaly in the anatomy of the veins on the opposite side, whereby a large amount of that hemisphere drainage runs into the sinus segment that it is proposed to excise.

## MENINGIOMAS OF THE MIDDLE THIRD OF THE SINUS

Tumours in this site provide a great challenge to neurosurgical judgement and skill and also carry a risk of serious morbidity.

The principle is to approach the tumour through non-evocative brain as far as possible, without traumatizing the motor and sensory zones. At the same time damage to the major veins, including the Rolandic, must be avoided. The difficulty of access is influenced by the site of the tumour in relation to the vertical plane, that is to say, whether it is superficial or deep.

When part of the tumour presents on the convexity surface the operation follows the previously described pattern. The tumour may be entered directly with little disturbance of brain, its centre excised and subsequently the capsule may be cut away to expose the sinus attachment (often by working between major sagittal veins) which may be dealt with as described elsewhere in this chapter.

It is when the tumour is submerged and extends laterally to undermine the motor and sensory projection fibres that difficulties are more obtrusive. Rather than retract evocative brain the approach is made to it obliquely from in front, or behind, depending on the relationship of the tumour to the motor and sensory zones.

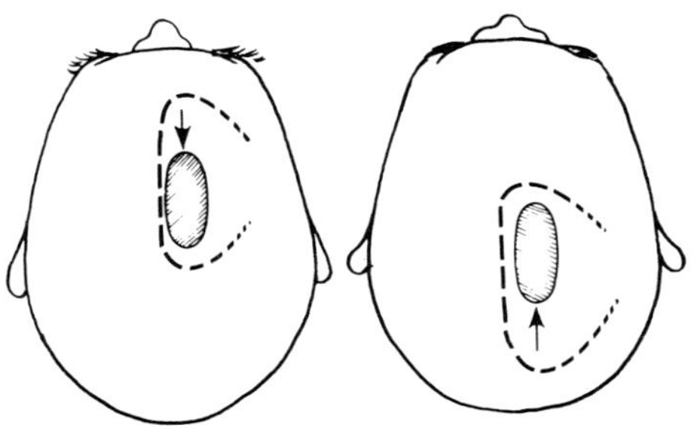

Arrows indicate direction of approach

49

# 49

If situated mainly under the motor strip the flap is positioned with its centre anterior to the tumour; if mainly under the sensory area the flap is sited with its centre posteriorly.

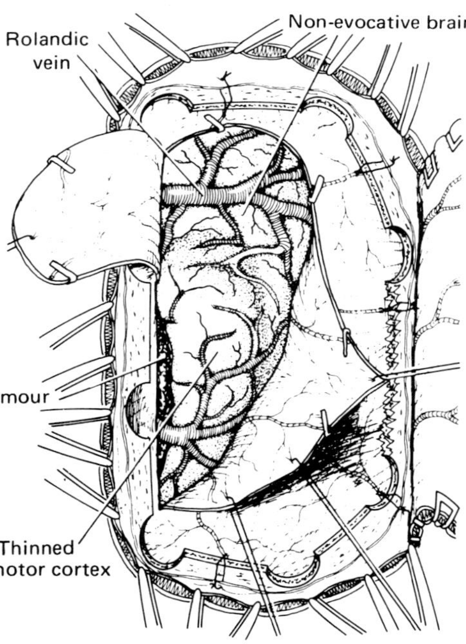


50

# 50

A semicircle of non-evocative brain is resected either in front of or behind the tumour to approach the anterior or posterior aspect of the capsule, respectively.

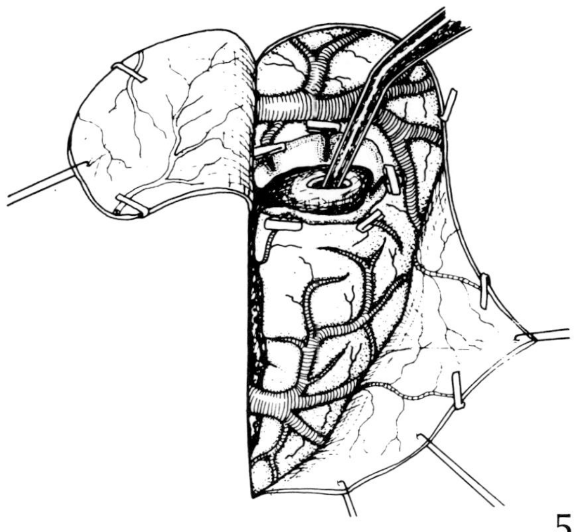

51

## 51 & 52

The tumour is eviscerated in the usual fashion and with the reduction in local tension the capsule can be excised and the brain will then tend to move sideways and down into the cavity. This exposes the tumour attachment which can be cut away and any necessary sinus repair carried out.

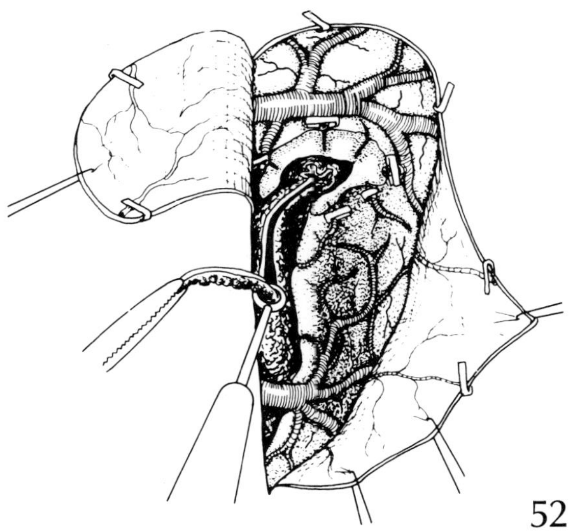

52

## TUMOUR OF THE POSTERIOR THIRD OF THE SINUS

# 53

In this situation access and the control of venous tension may be extremely difficult. The patient may be placed face down with considerable neck flexion and foot-down tilt, the knees being flexed on the foot rest in what the author has called the 'praying mantis' position, also known as the 'concorde' position by Japanese authors. Alternatively, the lateral or 'park bench' type position (*see* chapter on 'Control of intracranial tension', pp. 1–11) with the head rotated nose towards the floor may enable the area to be adequately exposed. The aim should always be to place the site of the tumour and the flap at the highest available point and as far as possible to convert everything into a simple frontal type craniotomy.

Fortunately, the venous drainage into the sinus from the posterior parietal/occipital zones is relatively sparse, and wider access is more easily obtained between the veins to the tumour.

The exposure and exenteration are carried out as described for the anterior third tumour.

The involvement of the sinus is now assessed. Mere adhesion is stripped off and the sinus is coagulated. If the wall is infiltrated there is a significant risk in trying to excise a segment. The sinus in this situation cannot often be obliterated with finger pressure because of the resulting engorgement of veins with brain swelling. One should, therefore, only excise an area of the wall in the fashion previously described if it can be confirmed that the intrasinus tension is at, or only just above, atmospheric pressure; otherwise treatment must depend on coagulation.

Very occasionally, a segment of the sinus known to be blocked completely can be excised as described elsewhere in this chapter.

When the tumour involves the torcula herophili the treatment of its attachment is limited to coagulation.

## FALX TUMOUR

Removal follows the same steps as for the parasagittal tumour except that, being more submerged, even greater reduction of intracranial tension is required by the methods previously described.

1. For tumours situated on the anterior or posterior third of the falx a semicircle of non-evocative brain with its base alongside the falx can be excised to give access to the capsule (*see Illustration 51*), should tension prohibit exposure without excessive retraction.
2. The centre of the tumour is eviscerated.
3. An incision is made in the falx round the periphery of the tumour between tantalum clips and the tumour is removed.

For those tumours on the middle third of the falx and thus lying below the middle third of the sagittal sinus the approach will be as for the similarly sited parasagittal tumour. Depending on the tumour's relationship to the motor and sensory zones, this will be either from in front or behind by excising a semicircle of 'silent' brain to avoid retraction.

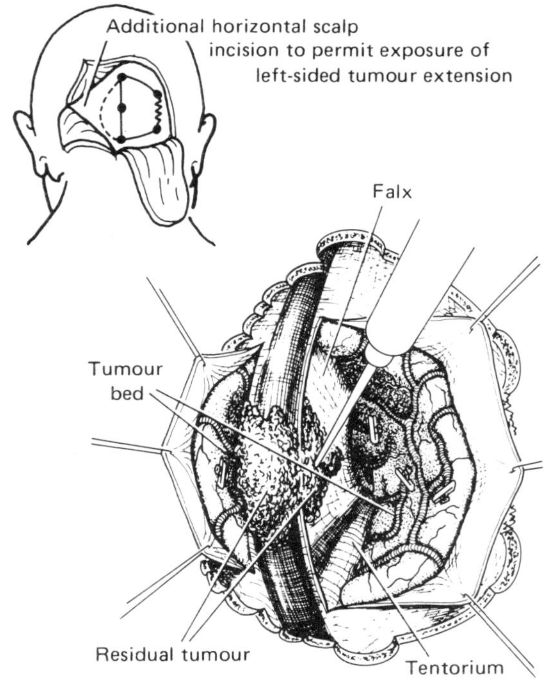


53

The falx tumour will not rotate at all out of the head and its attachment can be dealt with only by excising segments of the capsule, once the tumour has been eviscerated, in order to expose its base on the falx. This attachment is excised by making an incision in the falx 3 mm from its periphery and then continuing it around the tumour, in stages, between tantalum clips.

Sometimes the inferior angle of the sagittal sinus is involved. In this case the incision can be continued through the angle, a suture being put through the two lateral walls of the sinus at each 2 mm step to close the opening, as described when the lateral angle of the sinus is involved (*see Illustration 42*).

## Additional hazards

The callosomarginal and pericallosal arteries may run in grooves on the deep, inferior surface of these falx neoplasms, particularly when knobbly, and care must be taken during removal of their centres not to thin the capsule too radically.

A search is made for the arteries after evisceration has been completed and adequate room for manoeuvre has been achieved so that, starting anteriorly, the main trunk may be isolated and then gradually dissected off the neoplasm, small entering vessels being recognized, isolated, clipped and divided.

## Hydrocephalus

An excessive excision of the sinus and adjacent dura may reduce the cerebrospinal fluid absorbing area; particularly in elderly patients. Communicating hydrocephalus may result, sometimes requiring a shunt procedure to relieve it.

# BASAL TUMOURS

## Sphenoidal ridge meningiomas (pterional, globular and sclerosing)

The major hazard of tumours in this site relates to the basal blood vessels, the internal carotid in medially placed lesions and the middle cerebral artery and its branches in more peripheral lesions. Further hazards in medially placed lesions involve the optic nerve and the nerves to the superior orbital fissure in the cavernous sinus, and more laterally sylvian veins entering the sphenoparietal sinus may constitute a hazard. Rarely a large sylvian vein with little or no superior (Trolard) or inferior (Labbé) anastomosis may been seen. In such cases great efforts should be made to preserve such a vein which may be the sole drainage area for the inferior parietal zone. Its sacrifice tends to produce venous infarction manifested by focal fits and hemiparesis.

The middle cerebral artery and its branches vary in relationship to the tumour; where the meningioma has a rough and knobbly surface, vessels tend to run in grooves between the knobs and extreme care is necessary as the central tumour is evacuated. It is essential to look carefully round the capsule from time to time to ensure that the major vessels are identified as soon as it is practicable.

The situation of the internal carotid artery is dealt with subsequently.

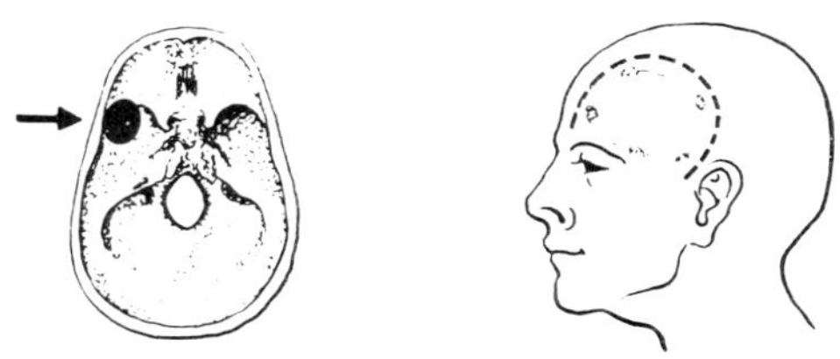

Arrow indicates direction of approach

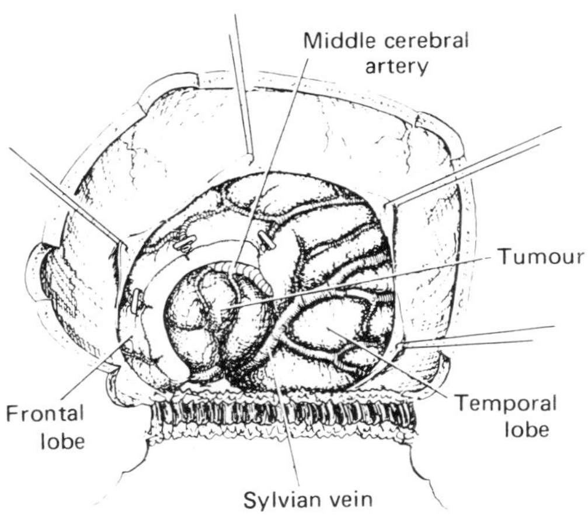


54

## 54

It may be necessary to use a large bone flap depending on the size of the tumour, and this may be sited more frontally or temporally depending on the exact situation of the mass. It is essential, however, that the flap be so designed to enable access to the medial surface of the tumour so that the relationship to the commencement of the often stretched middle cerebral artery may be early exposed.

The tumour may present against the dura without the interposition of brain substance, in which case a dural flap is reflected upwards and the tumour exenterated in the usual fashion.

In others, a layer of brain tissue is interposed between the tumour surface and the dura, i.e. the neoplasm is truly 'submerged'. In this instance a clean resection of a semicircle of the posterior portion of the inferior frontal convolution will give access to the capsule without the need for retraction.

The surface of the tumour is coagulated and the centre removed with suction or with a diathermy loop.

When adequate room for manoeuvre has been made, gentle traction on the capsule to draw it away from the sylvian fissure will expose the middle cerebral artery and its branches, which can be dissected off its surface. Vessels actually supplying the tumour can be clearly defined and clipped or coagulated.

With a large meningioma, wedge-shaped segments of the capsule may need to be excised.

The attachment of the tumour to the greater sphenoidal wing may be removed with its attached dura. Often the neoplasm has a very close relationship to the entry of the sylvian vein into the sphenoparietal sinus and this vein may need to be sacrificed. However, if the vein is shown by arteriography to be an important one on the dominant hemisphere, it may well be best to leave a small nub of tumour surrounding its entry point to preserve it.

At the conclusion the dural flap is sutured back into position, the bone flap is replaced and the dura held up to it with a perforating suture. The scalp is closed in the usual fashion with suction drainage.

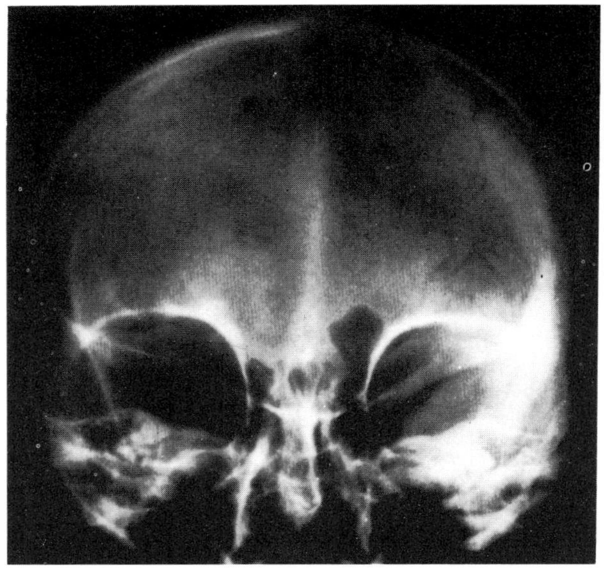

55

## Sclerosing pterional meningiomas

# 55 & 56

These tumours, common in middle-aged women, cause thickening of the greater sphenoidal wing, the roof and lateral wall of the orbit and encroach on its capacity, causing proptosis with, later on, diplopia. They are usually very slow growing and the main indication for their removal is for cosmetic reasons for proptosis.

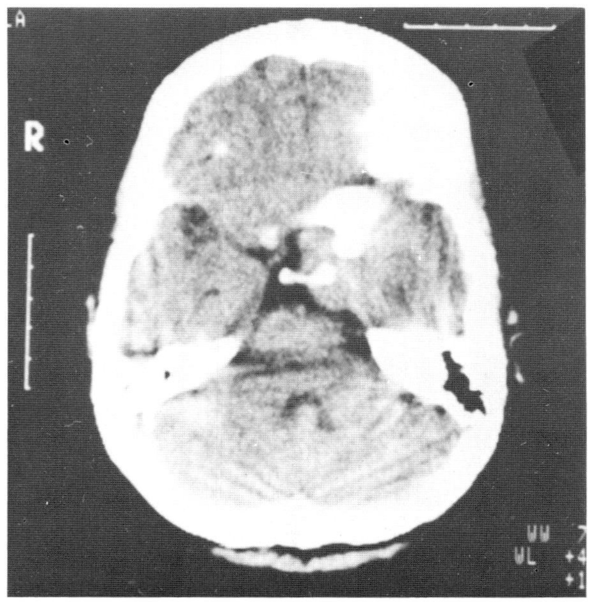


56

*Figure 56. Axial tomography (unenhanced) of a hyperostosing sphenoidal wing meningioma involving the anterior clinoid process.*

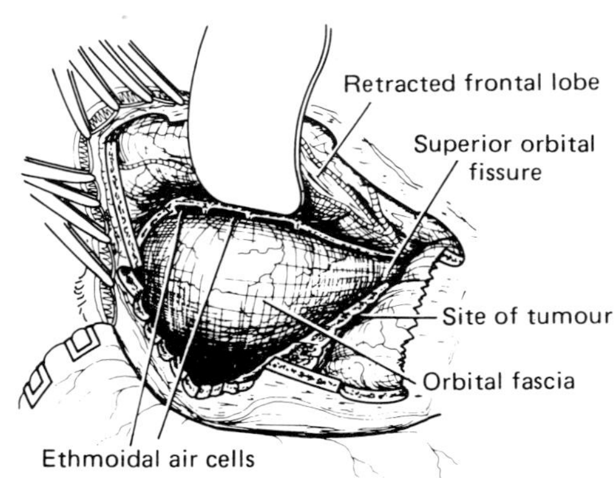


57

# 57

A large frontotemporal flap is marked out. This extends medially anteriorly to the midline so that access to the anterior aspect of the orbital roof in addition to the front of the temporal fossa can be achieved.

The bone flap hinged on the temporal muscle is turned backwards and downwards. The frontal dura is now dissected medially off the roof of the orbit, up to the olfactory groove, and held gently with a mechanical retractor.

An opening is made cautiously through the thickened and usually dense bone of the orbit with an air drill to expose the orbital fascia. This is preserved intact at this stage to prevent orbital fat, which is under tension, from herniating and hampering further removal of bone.

# 58

The orbital roof is now excised. This is done by enlarging the original opening with rongeurs and then painstakingly removing the orbital plate from the frontal sinus anteriorly to the clinoid ridge posteriorly and extending up to the ethmoidal cells medially.

The lateral wall of the orbit is now removed down to its floor, the bone removal reaching forwards to within 5 mm of the orbital rim and posteriorly to include the greater sphenoidal wing up to the lateral margin of the sphenoidal fissure. The lesser wing is not usually involved so that there is rarely a need to remove the roof of the optic foramen. To achieve adequate decompression, the floor and posterior wall of a large frontal sinus may need to be partly removed, as may a lateral extension of the ethmoidal cells. These openings in the sinuses are covered with Gelfoam strips and, later on, flaps of orbital fascia are turned upwards to help seal them.

The orbital fascia is now divided with several radiating incisions. This is the essential step in obtaining maximum reduction of the proptosis. When necessary, the flaps are fashioned to turn up and cover an open sinus or exposed air cells.

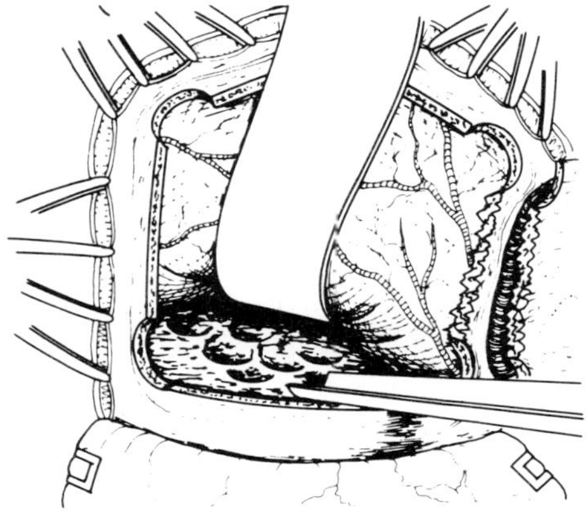

58

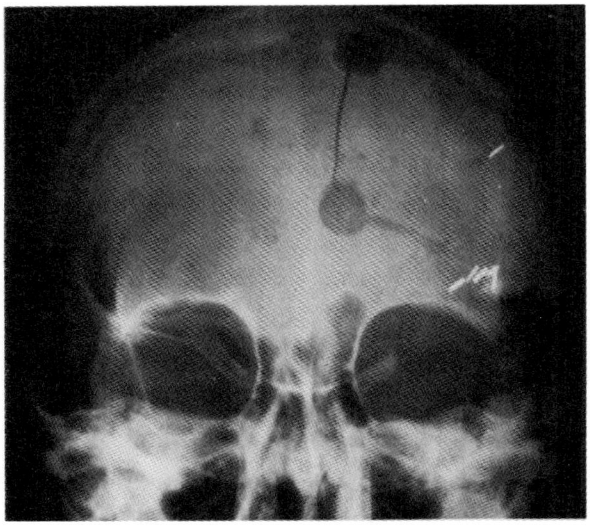

59

# 59

Finally the parent tumour is sought out. This is usually on the anterior wall of the temporal fossa, is small, often only 1–2 cm in diameter, and can usually be excised *in toto* with its dural attachment.

Sometimes it may be more extensive, extending medially to attach itself to the lateral wall of the cavernous sinus in which case this area has to be left *in situ* and coagulated.

Radiotherapy can be used later if any tumour is left behind as these seem to be one of that small group of meningiomas which are relatively sensitive to deep X-ray treatment.

The bone flap is replaced and the dura held up with a perforating stitch. The scalp is closed in the usual manner. At the conclusion a bandage is applied gently but firmly over a marine sponge placed on the closed eyelids to prevent excessive protrusion of the globe occurring in the subsequent 48 hours. The sponge is kept moistened.

# Middle and inner third sphenoidal ridge meningiomas

With these tumours the optic nerve, the internal carotid artery and the proximal parts of the anterior cerebral and middle cerebral vessels are the important hazardous points.

Not infrequently the internal carotid artery may run in a groove or even through the tumour, which will be demonstrated by the narrowing and irregularity of its wall shown on the arteriogram.

The bone flap needs to be large to reach to the midline anteriorly to give access to the medial margin of the tumour and the carotid artery and also to expose the pterion laterally.

It is essential to ensure that the intracranial tension is reduced to a low level with controlled respiration, dehydrating and hypotensive agents, provided, when using the latter, that the internal carotid is known not to be excessively narrowed and stretched.

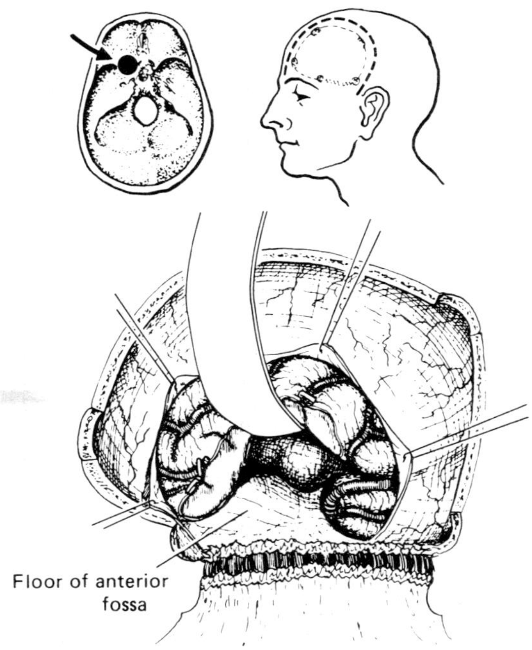


60

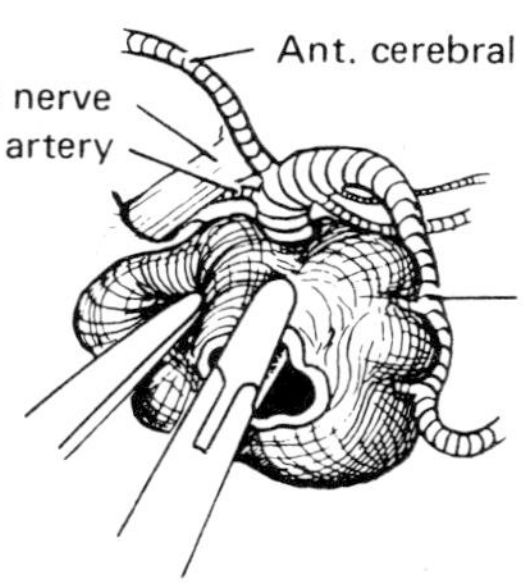


61

## 60

The initial approach to the tumour should be subfrontal rather than along the sphenoidal ridge to enable early identification of the optic nerve and carotid artery. It is seldom necessary to carry out even restricted resection of brain, but with the application of self-retaining retraction in the subfrontal zone, the olfactory tract should first be identified and followed back towards the sphenoidal ridge. Invariably it crosses the sphenoidal ridge at the point of emergence of the optic nerve and, even should tumour interpose, the olfactory tract points like an arrow back to the direction where one may expect to find the optic nerve and internal carotid. When these structures have been identified the tumour should be removed by gentle morcellment with either rongeurs, the ultrasonic dissector or suction coagulation. It is important to maintain control of the capsule with blunt forceps so that it is not rocked as tumour tissue is broken away, especially when the tumour is in contact with the optic nerve and internal carotid artery. The use of the microscope is essential.

At the completion the dura is incised round the attachment and the latter is freed from the bone with a periosteal elevator.

## 61

With a large tumour the centre is exenterated, again by breaking up the neoplasm with a blunt hook, the ultrasonic dissector or pituitary rongeurs, avoiding its basal attachment in the vicinity of the optic nerve. Once the capsule is pliable it can be retracted laterally to expose the nerve.

Segments of capsule are then cut away to reveal the dural attachment. This sometimes straddles the ridge to involve the anterior wall of the temporal fossa.

If this is so a lateral approach along the sphenoidal ridge with gentle retraction of the temporal pole backwards will give access to this area, which can then be removed, but if the mass in the temporal fossa is very large it may be wise to perform a limited 2.5 cm resection of the anterior temporal lobe to provide free access and minimize brain retraction.

In cases where the internal carotid artery and/or the middle cerebral vessel run in a groove in the tumour substance, it is often possible to dissect the vessel out under magnification using a blunt hook to break up the tumour attached to its wall.

However, when the artery runs through the neoplasm, although in some instances it is possible to dissect it free, it may be more prudent to leave the local cuff of tumour undisturbed in the hope that radiotherapy may influence it later. If dissection of the main trunk is in fact carried out, the course of the ophthalmic, the anterior choroidal and possibly the posterior communicating arteries needs to be borne in mind.

## Suprasellar and parasellar meningiomas

# 62a & b & 63

In the management of these tumours the CT scan with sagittal and coronal reconstructions and, more recently, magnetic resonance imaging have proved of great use. Nevertheless, angiography is still indicated to demonstrate both the blood supply of the tumour and its relation to the great vessels. Encephalography has now been completely superseded by magnetic resonance scanning which will give images of great clarity in such lesions in close relation to cerebrospinal spaces.

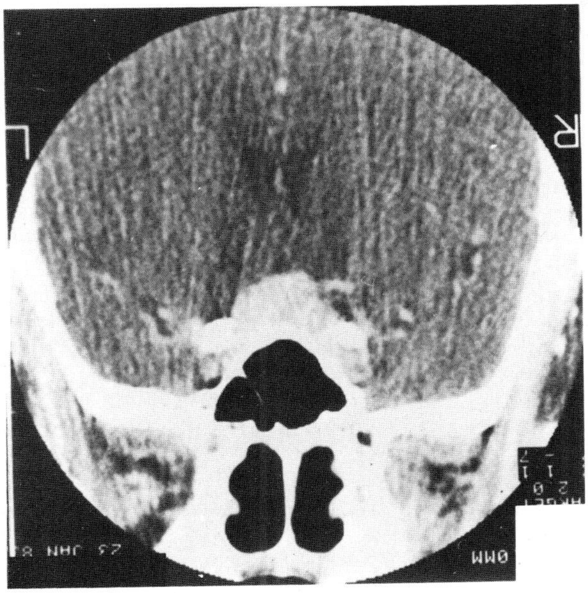

62a

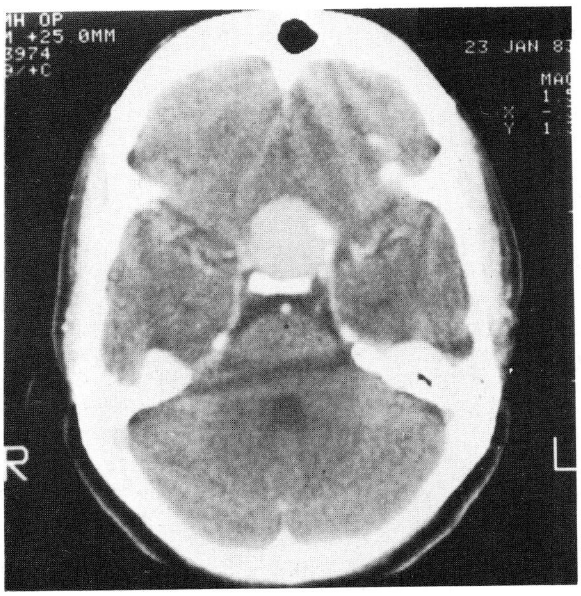

62b

*Figure 62. Axial (enhanced and unenhanced) and coronal (enhanced) sections of CT scan of a suprasellar meningioma. The relationship of the air sinus to the base of the meningioma is particularly well shown in the coronal cut.*

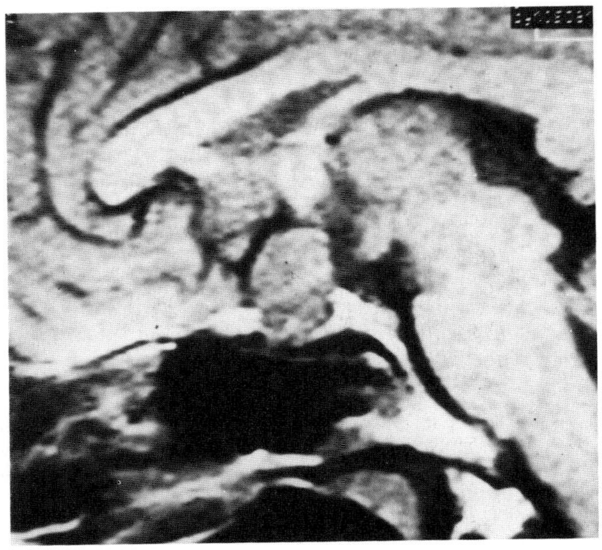

63

# 64

Access is usually adequate through a unilateral flap on the right, but an alternative is the use of a bilateral cosmetic scalp incision. With adequate relaxation and early opening of cerebrospinal fluid spaces in the inner third of the sylvian fissure, it is now usually possible to avoid the wedge excisions of the inferomesial part of the frontal pole which used to be popular. Self-retaining retraction in the subfrontal zone is usually sufficient.

The relationship of the tumour to the optic nerve and chiasm may vary, but identification of the right optic nerve is the first step in excision of the tumour and a guide to the situation of this nerve lies in the invariable relationship of the olfactory tract to the nerve as the two approach the inner end of the sphenoidal wing. The chiasm and optic nerves may straddle the tumour, giving it an hour-glass shape, or one or the other may be displaced downwards and lie beneath it. Quite frequently one nerve may lie below and the other run over the top of the opposite pole with rotation of the chiasm. The situation of the nerves may be predicted from careful examination of good quality magnetic resonance scans.

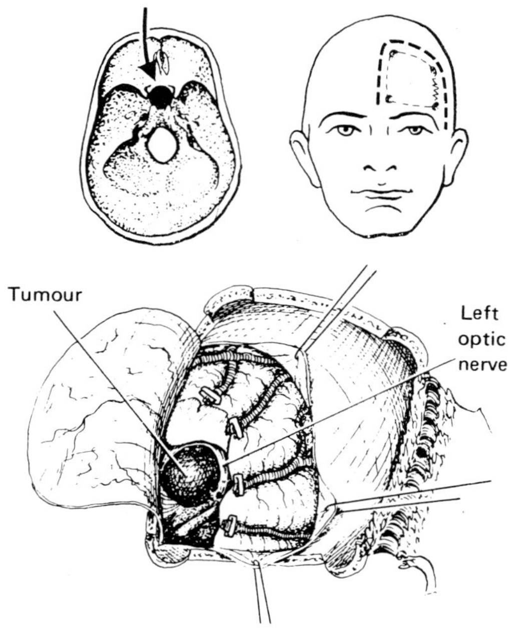


64

# 65

After the right optic nerve has been identified, the tumour should be gradually gutted, initially staying close to the jugum sphenoidale. It is important to remember that the sphenoidal air sinus may bulge up into the base of such meningiomas and if entered at this stage it will be necessary to repair it with pericranium to avoid a cerebrospinal fluid leak at the close of the procedure. Staying close to the jugum sphenoidale at this stage will enable the afferent blood supply of the tumour, which arises from perforating branches from the ophthalmic and posterior ethmoidal arteries, to be occluded. The tumour is then gradually exenterated and drawn down from contact with the nerves. If the neoplasm is hard it will require excision with a small loop diathermy or breaking up with a small pituitary rongeur and blunt hooks. The ultrasonic dissector (CUSA) may occasionally be of value. Soft tumours may be removed entirely by suction.

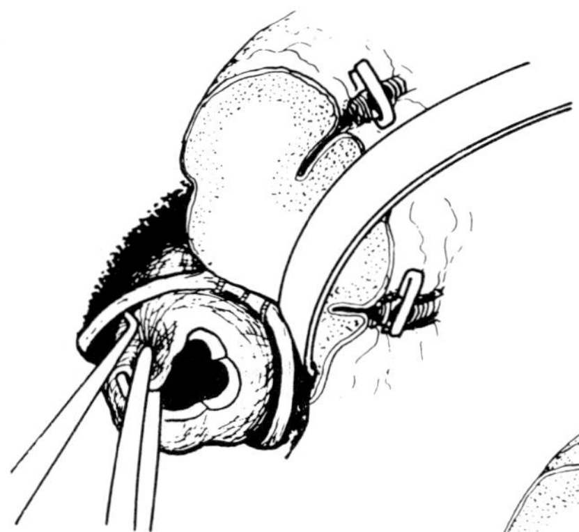

65

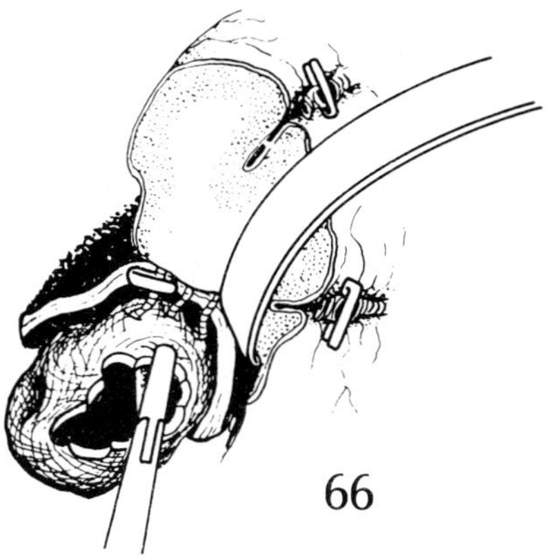

66

# 66

In large tumours the capsule may need to be thinned appreciably before sufficient mobility is obtained for even the ipsilateral optic nerve to be identified.

With the optic nerve in view the capsule can be freed from it and gently retracted down from under the chiasm. Small branches from the anterior communicating and anterior cerebral arteries supplying the tumour will often be present and will need to be clipped and divided.

The anterior cerebral artery complex may in fact actually be incorporated in the dome of the neoplasm and may require blunt dissection, utilizing the microscope, to free it. Occasionally involvement is so intimate that a small portion of the tumour surrounding the vessels may need to be detached from the main mass and left *in situ*.

Further back the tumour may involve one or both internal carotid arterial trunks and again careful dissection under magnification may free them, due note being taken of the relationship of the ophthalmic, anterior choroidal and posterior communicating arteries to the capsule.

In some cases the tumour sends a cuff around one or both optic nerves far into the optic foramina and a complete macroscopic removal may not be possible.

# Olfactory groove meningiomas

## UNILATERAL

## 67a, b & c & 68

These tumours have an origin which straddles the olfactory groove and may extend from the crista galli in front to the jugum sphenoidale behind and laterally out onto the orbital roof.

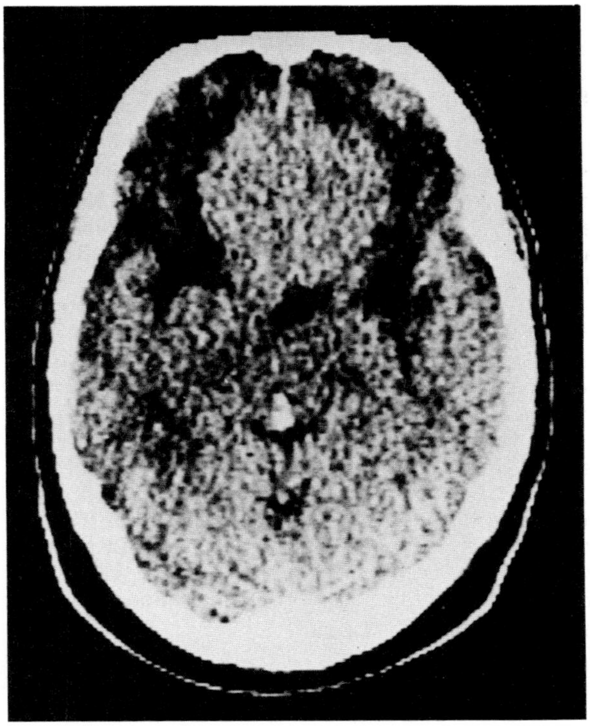

67a

*Figure 67. Plain and enhanced scans of an olfactory groove meningioma.*

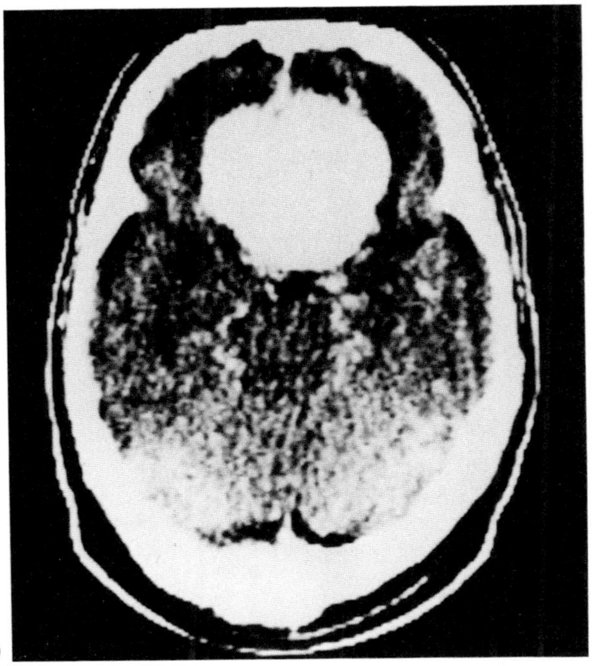

67b

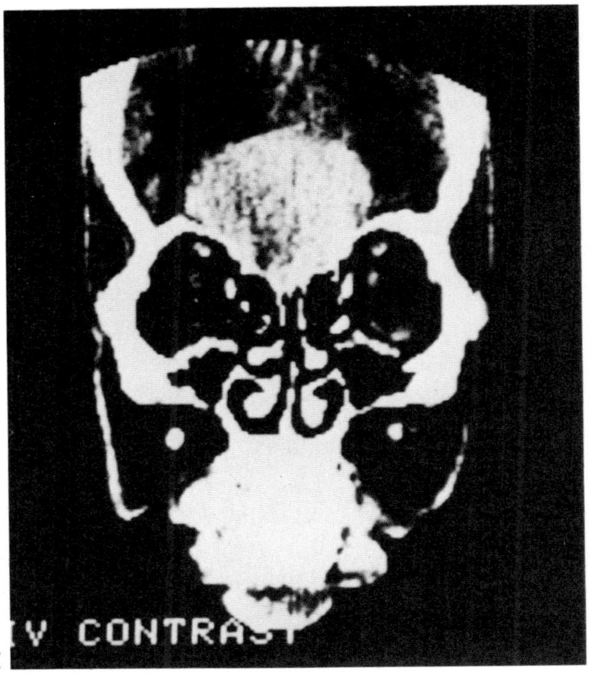


67c

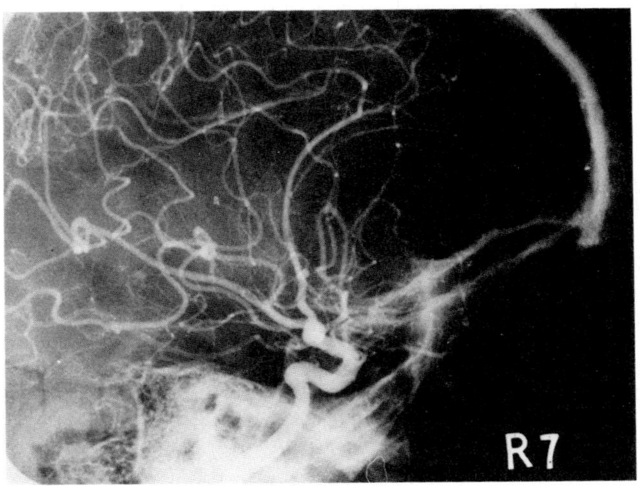


68

# 69

The approach to these tumours may be either through a unilateral frontal flap with the vertical limb strictly in the midline or a bifrontal curved cosmetic incision as described elsewhere in this chapter with a unilateral or bilateral bone flap.

The dural flap is turned medially and a brain needle introduced to determine how far from the brain surface the tumour lies. It is then wise to carry out a wedge resection of the medial frontal pole to deal with the tumour without significant brain retraction. If the intracranial pressure is appreciably raised despite mannitol, then the dural opening should be restricted to its posterior limb. Dissection through cortex should then be performed before the dura is widely opened to enable a rapid exenteration of the chosen portion of frontal lobe and avoid prolapse of the brain, rupture of the pia and troublesome bleeding.

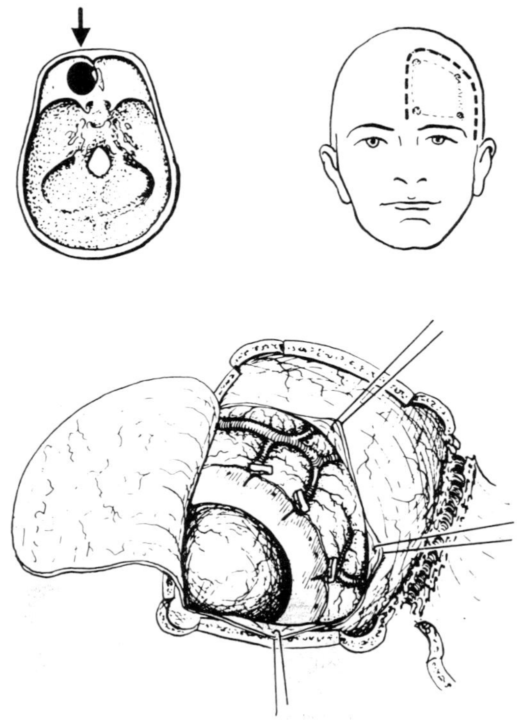

69

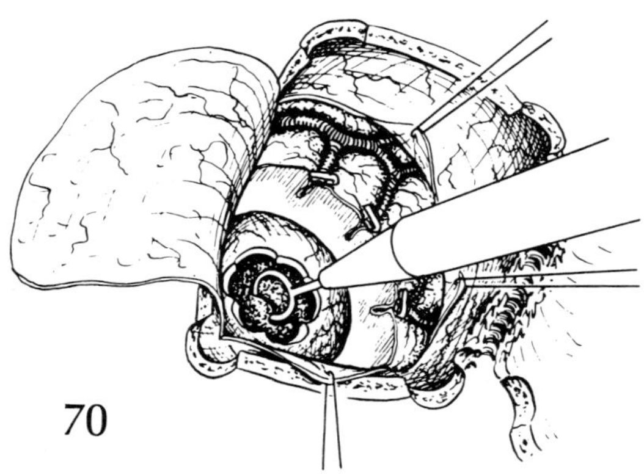

70

# 70

Subsequent treatment of the tumour is as for a convexity meningioma; an opening is made in its surface and then with a sucker or diathermy loop, depending on its consistency, the centre of the tumour is exenterated with careful arrest of haemorrhage at each stage.

# 71

When the capsule has been thinned sufficiently it can be displaced away from the brain-bed and the vessels of supply identified and coagulated or clipped. In posteriorly extending tumours search along the lesser wing will reveal the optic nerve which is usually displaced downwards. Occasionally a nub of tumour extends back under the chiasm, lifting it up and stretching the nerve, in which case appropriate care will be required. When the neoplasm extends across the midline it is usually possible to deal with it through the same unilateral right frontal exposure as used for the main tumour. If more than two-thirds of the tumour lies on the left side of the head it may be wise to perform the operation unilaterally from the left side. Only very rarely is a bilateral frontal flap required for truly massive tumours. Bilateral subfrontal retraction is often associated with appreciable intellectual impairment and is best avoided. It is astonishing how large portions of the tumour lying on the contralateral side may be removed following the removal of the greater part of the first side. It is the author's preference to perform these operations predominantly from the right side. When the centre of the tumour extension to the opposite side has been removed the capsule can be rotated over into the cavity previously created by the removal of the main tumour and subsequently excised. Occasionally access may need to be extended by incising the falx from its free edge up to the lower margin of the sagittal sinus and retracting the resulting triangular flaps with stitches.

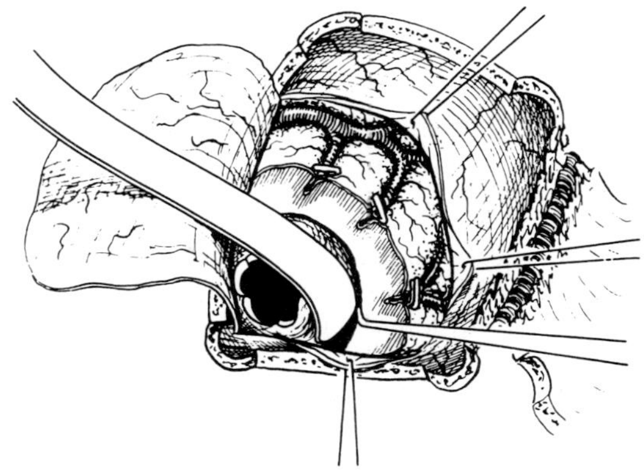

71

## Hazards

The anterior cerebral arteries may run in a groove in the posterior and superior aspects of the tumour surface, sending in branches which may, owing to their short course, be difficult to clip. Bipolar coagulation is usually capable of dealing with these.

## Dural attachment

When the bulk of the tumour has been removed an incision is made 3 mm away from the edge of the meningioma base down onto the bone, and the involved dura is then removed with a rugine. Care must be taken to detach all the tumour growing from the crista galli with its related dura mater.

If the bone, particularly over the lamina cribrosa, is excessively thinned by the tumour a pericranial or fascia lata patch may be laid over the whole raw area. This extends beyond its edge by 5 mm all round and is held in place with interrupted sutures or, more easily, is clipped onto the surrounding dura with tantalum clips inserted through small slits in the latter. The recent availability of fibrin glue has appreciably simplified the fixation of such grafts.

If there is no bone erosion, a layer of Gelfoam applied to the raw area of bone may minimize adhesions.

The dural flap is sutured back into position and held up to the bone by a single perforating stitch. The scalp is then closed with subgaleal suction drainage.

A number of these tumours pass through the ethmoidal plate into the roof of the nose. It is essential to recognize this on preoperative studies so that, perhaps with the collaboration of an ear, nose and throat colleague, a resection of the central portion of the ethmoidal plate may be performed and the floor of the frontal fossa reconstituted, usually with a graft of fascia lata superiorly and split-skin grafting to its lower surface on the nasal aspect. If such radical resection is not performed, these tumours invariably recur.

# Subtemporal tumours

In the dominant hemisphere particular care must be taken to see that there is no disturbance of the inferior parietal zone.

## 72

A low temporal flap extending right down to the floor of the temporal fossa is used. The standard exposure is that described by Penfield which, with retraction of the muscle, scalp and bone by sprung stitches, gives adequate access to the anterior temporal fossa. An alternative skin incision opening posteriorly was often used in the past, having the advantage that there is not a large bulk of muscle anteriorly. The cosmetic appearance of this flap was less satisfactory and it is not now commonly employed.

The cutting of the bone flap in these tumours may require considerable skill, particularly if there is extensive hyperostosis in the lateral part of the temporal fossa. It is frequently wise to use an instrument such as a Hall drill to cut the lower part of the flap and under these circumstances the temporal muscle may be entirely detached from the bone and a good deal of this will subsequently have to be excised if heavily involved by meningioma.

The situation of the tumour is confirmed by needling and then a semicircle resection confined to the middle and inferior temporal gyri is carried out to expose the capsule. If the tumour is sited further back, extending onto the tentorium, then this lateral–posterior temporal zone may be evocative with regard to speech, and brain resection should be avoided.

Any elevation of the temporal lobe must be extremely gentle. In addition, if Labbé's vein is the sole draining vessel of the parietal area, strenuous attempts should be made to spare it. Sacrifice of this vessel is likely to produce venous infarction, which in the dominant post-temporal zone may have disastrous effects on speech function.

The capsule, when exposed, is opened and eviscerated in the usual fashion. The dural attachment to the floor of the fossa may be dealt with as for olfactory groove tumours. If it should extend medially onto the lateral surface of the cavernous sinus, light coagulation is all that is necessary.

As mentioned earlier, recurrence of these basal tumours is much less frequent than with the parasagittal and falx meningiomas.

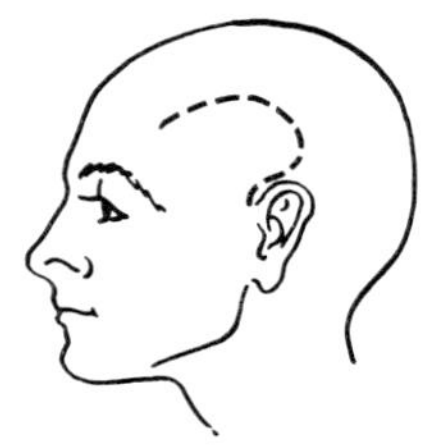

'PENFIELD' incision

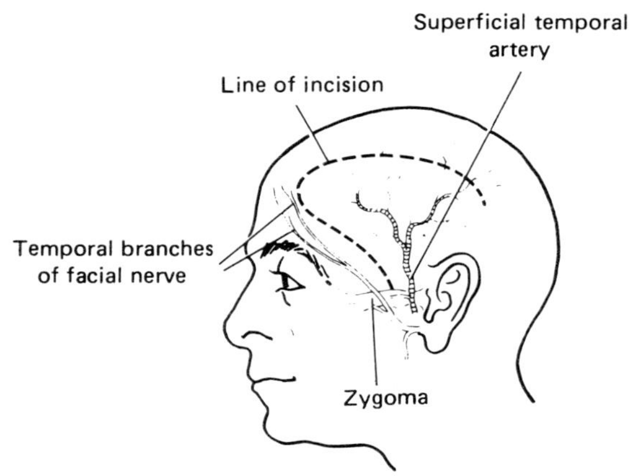


'LOGUE' incision

72

# Tentorial tumours

The tentorium forms a large proportion of the floor of the supratentorial compartment so that potential tumour sites may be widely separated. Those laterally situated may extend onto the base of the petrous bone, straddle the superior petrosal sinus and involve the lateral sinus; those posteriorly sited may involve the straight sinus and also the torcula herophili and lateral sinus.

## LATERAL TENTORIAL TUMOURS

# 73

On the side of the non-dominant hemisphere, if the tumour does not actually present against the convexity dura after the reflection of the dural flap, a semicircle brain resection with a base of perhaps 4 cm can be made which will give access to the capsule. On the dominant side any resection should be very restricted but may well be necessary with a large tumour in order to avoid excessive brain retraction which will cause more damage over a wider area. The other hazard is a dominant Labbé's vein which is draining most of the hemisphere with little blood entering the sylvian veins. The situation of this vein may very well determine the direction in which the tumour is approached. If the bulk of the tumour is anterior to the insertion of Labbé's vein, then on either side a small temporal resection may aid access, with the patient in the true lateral position recumbent. If the tumour is predominantly behind Labbé's vein a more true 'park bench' position with the head rotated towards the floor and access through a small resection of the inferior post-temporal region may be best. With the aid of dehydrating agents such as mannitol and continuous lumbar drainage the necessity for brain resection is fortunately confined to large tumours.

Tumour excision follows the usual pattern with removal of the centre of the tumour and excision of the capsule in segments. The attachment may prove difficult as it often straddles the superior petrosal sinus and may involve venous radicals running from the deep aspect of the occipital lobe. With an elderly patient, coagulation of the attachment may be all that is required, bearing in mind the relatively low recurrence rate. For a younger person an attempt should be made to excise it and an incision is made round the attachment in the usual fashion, extending forwards to the back of the petrous bone and the superior petrosal sinus. The lateral part of the petrosal sinus is now divided between clamps and its lateral opening closed with a continuous suture. It is then dissected medially out of its groove in the bone, the posterior fossa dura being divided below its inferior margin and cleared up to a point just above and lateral to the trigeminal nerve. A curved clamp is applied here to the sinus, which is cut through, and the medial end is closed with clips.

The closure of the convexity dura, bone flap and scalp is carried out in the usual manner.

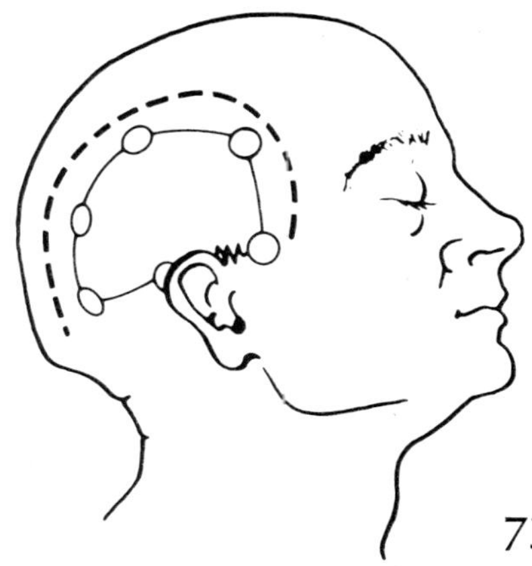

73

## MENINGIOMAS OF THE TENTORIAL HIATUS

With tumours attached to or overlapping the free edge of the tentorium the particular hazards are the proximity of the mesencephalon, the posterior cerebral and superior cerebellar arteries, the fourth nerve and sometimes the anterior portion of the straight sinus and entry of the great vein of Galen.

The 'park bench' position is probably the best for tumours of the tentorial hiatus. The difficulty of resection depends a good deal on how much of the tumour lies above and how much below the tentorium. Access will be determined by the situation of Labbé's vein which must be preserved. In large tumours extending both above and below the tentorium an approach dividing the lateral sinus and the tentorium down to the level of the tumour anterior to Labbé's vein may prove best. This approach is described in relation to meningiomas of the petrous apex.

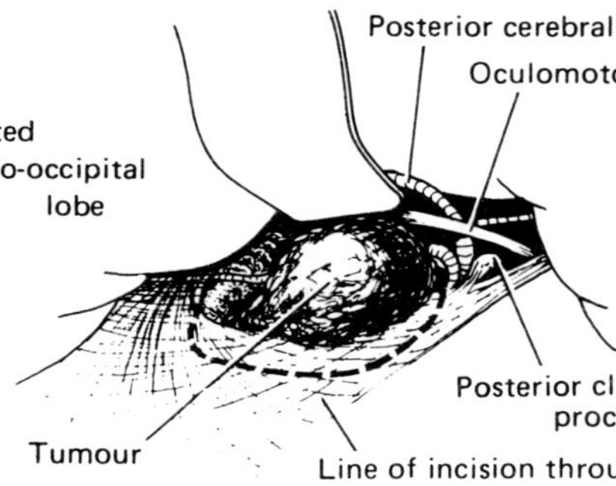


74

## 74

The interior of the tumour is excised thoroughly so that the collapse of the lax capsule will expose the brain stem and the related arterial trunks clearly and, higher up and medially, the vein of Galen entering the straight sinus.

The tentorium is incised laterally and posteriorly to the tumour attachment, and the incision, between tantalum clips, is continued in front of the neoplasm up to the hiatus medially. The small sinus in the edge of the free margin of the tentorium is clipped, avoiding and protecting the fourth nerve.

Posteriorly the incision skirts alongside the straight sinus to enter the hiatus just lateral to the Galenic–straight sinus junction.

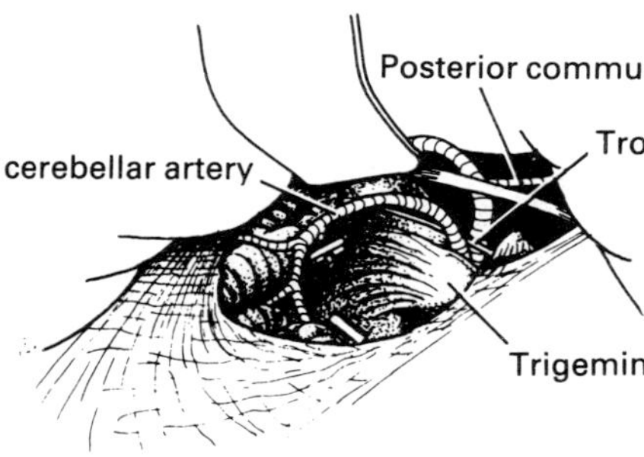


75

## 75

The collapsed capsule can now be rotated backwards to expose the indented mesencephalon. It is separated from the posterior cerebral and superior cerebellar arteries, and any vessels of supply to the tumour are clipped. It is important not to disturb the mesencephalic branch of the superior cerebellar vessel.

The capsule is rotated laterally and downwards onto the cerebellum to permit its separation from the vein of Galen on its posteromedial aspect; it is then lifted out.

Although there have been some reports of cases in which the vein of Galen has been divided without ill-effect it is wise to set out with the intention of preserving it.

After haemostasis the convexity dura is closed and held up to the bone with a perforating stitch. The scalp is closed with subgaleal suction drainage for 24 hours.

## POSTERIOR TENTORIAL MENINGIOMAS

These tumours tend to present with field defects and the hazards are mainly related to the visual pathways and to the straight and lateral sinuses and the torcula herophili.

Although these regions may be approached with a semirecumbent position with the head flexed and precautions against air embolism employed as usual, most surgeons now prefer to operate on such patients either in an exaggerated 'park bench' position with considerable rotation of the head towards the floor or in the prone position with extreme foot-down tilt and neck flexion, the so-called 'concorde' or 'praying mantis' position.

Fortunately the occipital pole and its lateral surface usually have little venous drainage running posteriorly. Veins from the undersurface drain forwards, towards the superior petrosal and adjacent zone of the lateral sinus, and the veins on the falx surface run upwards and forwards some distance to enter the sagittal sinus, so that the occipital pole can usually be moved out of the way without much disturbance of its veins.

With the tumour sited directly posteriorly the occipital pole tends to be displaced upwards and forwards by it, giving access directly to the capsule which is incised and the tumour eviscerated in the usual fashion.

Any attachment to the straight sinus, lateral sinus and torcula herophili are more safely dealt with by coagulation.

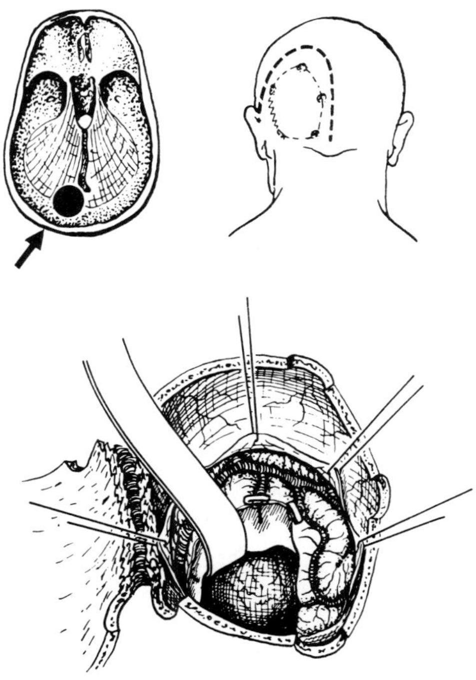

76

## 76

With large tumours extending further laterally, usually with dense field defects (in which usually there occurs relatively little recovery postoperatively), a semicircular excision of the inferior occipital zone posterolaterally will give access to the capsule, which can be treated in the usual fashion.

Particular care is needed in avoiding the calcarine artery and its branches and the medial occipital cortex.

A table derived from a personal series of the first author extending over many years is appended below (Table 1). It has not been surpassed.

**Table 1 Surgical results for supratentorial tumours**

| *Tumour* | *Cases* | *Deaths* | *Mortality (per cent)* |
|---|---|---|---|
| Parasagittal | 91 | 4 | 4.4 |
| Falx | 42 | 1 | 2.4 |
| Convexity | 83 | 2 | 2.4 |
| Total | 216 | 7 | 3.2 |
| Basal | 134 | 9 | 6.7 |
| Total | 350 | 16 | 4.57 |

# POSTERIOR FOSSA MENINGIOMAS

There are numerous classifications of the sites of these tumours. The following is a simplified classification which includes the important situations.

| | |
|---|---|
| Cerebellopontine angle | 43 per cent |
| Deep aspect of tentorium including the free margin | 22 per cent |
| Lateral and posterior walls of the cerebellar fossa (embedded in the cerebellar hemispheres) | 14 per cent |
| Clivus and basi-occiput | 8 per cent |
| Foramen magnum | 6 per cent |
| Others (including intraventricular, cerebellar hemisphere without dural attachment, torcula herophili with extensive dural attachment involving several areas) | 7 per cent |

The principles of surgery in the posterior fossa are identical to those used for supratentorial tumours, namely reduction of general intracranial pressure and then reduction of tumour–brain-bed tension so that a sufficient area of the capsule may be clearly visualized for adequate excision.

The approach to these lesions demands careful control of intracranial pressure and thoughtful positioning of the patient.

Cerebellar convexity tumours and tumours posteriorly placed in the region of the foramen magnum are probably best approached with the patient seated in the semi-recumbent position and with careful precaution against air embolism. This position may also be employed for tumours arising from the lower aspect of the tentorium since, in the lateral or prone positions the steep upward slope of the tentorium may make it extremely difficult to deal with these if they are near the midline. However, for the great majority of extracerebellar lesions in the posterior fossa the 'park bench' position is best. For the particular problems of apical petrosal and clivus lesions modification of this position with slightly less rotation of the head is preferable, the combined supratentorial and infratentorial approach being easier with the head almost completely laterally placed. Where the tumour is large and has produced raised intracranial pressure, preliminary ventricular drainage by catheter will often aid access and, where hydrocephalus and raised pressure are not a problem in the preoperative period, considerable additional help may be obtained by continuous lumbar drainage. Mannitol and other dehydrating agents are of relatively little value in the posterior fossa presumably because of the relatively small bulk of normal tissue to dehydrate. With such measures combined with the use of preoperative steroids for a few days, the extensive resection of cerebellum which used to be mandatory to avoid excessive cerebellar retraction is now thankfully less frequently required. Thus, in the past 10 years even in dealing with apical petrosal and clivus tumours it has not been found necessary to resect cerebellum in a series of over 50 cases.

## Cerebellopontine angle

Tumours in the cerebellopontine angle present problems similar to those of the acoustic tumour except that on the one hand they tend to be more vascular, whereas on the other hand the cranial nerves involved with such tumours (which may range from the fifth to the eleventh), tend to retain their discrete bundle formation and may prove easier to dissect off the tumour and to preserve than, for instance, the flattened and sheet-like seventh nerve often associated with an acoustic neuroma.

### Position

In general the best position for approach to the cerebellopontine angle remains the 'park bench' position. The additional aid of induced hypotension which is possible in this position is of considerable benefit in a vascular tumour.

### Procedure

The best access to the cerebellopontine angle is provided by a slightly S-shaped incision starting above the asterion and running down the posterior face of the mastoid, sloping towards the foramen magnum. The incision should normally reach to just above the spine of C2 near the midline. The incision is deepened through skin, muscles and fasciae to clear the lateral two-thirds of the occipital plate, the lateral half of the arch of the atlas and the area of bone above the lateral sinus. The craniectomy should be carried from the posterior face of the mastoid two-thirds of the way to the midline and should open the foramen magnum, but should not necessarily involve removal of the arch of the atlas unless the tumour is very low down. Superiorly, the craniectomy should be carried right up to the lateral sinus to permit access to the high angle, and it may well be advisable to remove bone above the lateral sinus if self-retaining retraction based on a skull-fixed base plate is used. Control of the intracranial tension will have been achieved either by spinal drainage or continuous ventricular drainage, but may be further aided by opening the foramen magnum at an early stage. The dura is commonly opened in a long-stemmed 'Y' with the upper limbs based anteriorly on the corner of the lateral and sagittal sinus and posteriorly extending up to the lateral sinus. The incision should pass down into the foramen magnum. The edges of the dura are sutured back to the muscle with silk sutures, and dissection pursued down the posterior face of the petrous bone. With correct positioning, the posterior face of the petrous will be almost vertical, and little retraction of the cerebellum will be necessary to detect the origin of the tumour. With self-retaining retraction it is now usually possible to dissect the cerebellum from the surface of the tumour under the microscope to a sufficient extent to enable preliminary identification of neighbouring nerves. The position of the posterior group (ninth, tenth and eleventh nerves) should be identified early as far as possible, since damage to these nerves during resection is a major cause of morbidity from difficulty in swallowing. Attempts should also be made to identify the relationship of the tumour to the seventh and eighth nerves, although from preliminary studies it may be clear that the bulk of the tumour lies behind them in which case they will be invisible. Superiorly, the fifth nerve may also be identifiable at an early stage. Important branches of the posterior inferior cerebellar artery are likely to have been defined by preoperative arteriography, and while the hemispheral branches of the posterior inferior cerebellar and anterior inferior cerebellar arteries may be sacrificed, the brain stem branches of both these vessels are of extreme importance and damage to the brain stem supply will result in a lateral medullary syndrome. It is, therefore, important to divide only branches of these vessels which directly supply the tumour, although if the hemispheral distribution of either vessel has a long course on the capsule, it may be divided for access if necessary.

A portion of the capsule should then be coagulated over an appropriate area and the tumour progressively exenterated. The ease of this manoeuvre depends entirely on the consistency of the tumour, as in the supratentorial compartment. Diathermy loop excision tends to be dangerous close to cranial nerves or the brain stem and must be employed with extreme caution in the posterior fossa. It is best to rely on breaking up the neoplasm with a blunt hook and rongeurs or the ultrasonic dissector, removing the small fragments by suction.

When the capsule is sufficiently lax, the upper pole is rotated laterally and gently dissected off the pons. It will usually be found that the fifth nerve runs over the upper pole of the tumour or around its medial surface.

Attention is now directed to the lower pole where dissection is continued upwards, separating it from the posterior inferior cerebellar artery (in the case of a large tumour, also from the vertebral artery). Any fine vessels running into the neoplasm are coagulated with bipolar diathermy.

Continuing cranially, the capsule is separated from the sixth nerve and then at a higher level from the seventh and eighth nerves, which are usually related to its medial surface, but may run around its inferior pole or laterally on its outer surface. The remaining tumour capsule is carefully dissected free from the anterior inferior cerebellar artery and removed.

The attachment is excised where this can be done without damage to the cranial nerves; otherwise it is treated by light coagulation.

Recurrence is very uncommon.

# MENINGIOMAS ON THE POSTERIOR AND LATERAL WALLS OF THE CEREBELLAR FOSSA

Tumours arising from these sites present no special features in surgical removal except that they may be extremely vascular and the subjacent bone may have a profuse blood supply from the branches of the external carotid, particularly the occipital arteries.

When the bony decompression has been carried out, the attachment of the tumour often presents and the usual encircling incision is made, followed by the circular opening in its basal attachment, and the meningioma is eviscerated. The capsule can usually be dissected easily from the surrounding cerebellar hemisphere and can then be removed complete with its dural attachment.

## TENTORIAL MENINGIOMA

There are three situations to be considered: tumours arising from the undersurface of the tentorium without involvement of the major venous sinuses; those involving one or more of the following structures, the straight sinus, torcula herophili or the lateral sinus; and tumours extending into the supratentorial compartments, so-called cerebello-occipital tumours.

The authors find the best way of approaching these neoplasms is with the patient in the sitting position with the head flexed and the usual precautions against air embolus being observed.

The mode of access to the tumour will depend on its origin, whether anterior or posterior on the tentorium. In the latter site the capsule will probably present as soon as the dura is opened. In the former a semicircular excision (with its base on the tentorium) of the upper folia of the cerebellar hemisphere down to the capsule will be required.

The interior of the tumour is excised in the usual fashion.

The capsule is removed in segments to expose the attachment.

When this is confined to the tentorial leaf the latter is incised and then a complete circumferential incision is made around the tumour between tantalum clips, bearing in mind that there may be large venous channels within the tentorium itself.

When the attachment spreads onto the straight sinus, torcula herophili or the lateral sinus it is best dealt with by coagulation.

If the attachment is discrete to the lateral sinus it is possible to excise a segment of the wall in the same fashion as with the parasagittal tumour. However, it is probably easier and certainly safer to excise the affected portion of the sinus completely.

Before embarking on this procedure it should be ascertained from the arteriogram that both lateral sinuses are patent, and that a preliminary test compression of the sinus with forceps is shown not to raise the local venous pressure unduly. However, with controlled respiration this test is not completely reliable and despite a satisfactory response on compression impaired venous drainage may sometimes arise postoperatively and produce oedema with raised pressure. If excision is decided upon, the sinus is separated from the bone and displaced forwards and then the incision carried out as described for the blocked sagittal sinus from a parasagittal tumour. Significant extension of a posterior fossa tentorial tumour up into the supratentorial compartment will be recognized preoperatively by the CT scan and arteriography.

Occasionally a large tumour may elevate and stretch the tentorium sufficiently even to deform the occipital horn without actual penetration. This may be misleading.

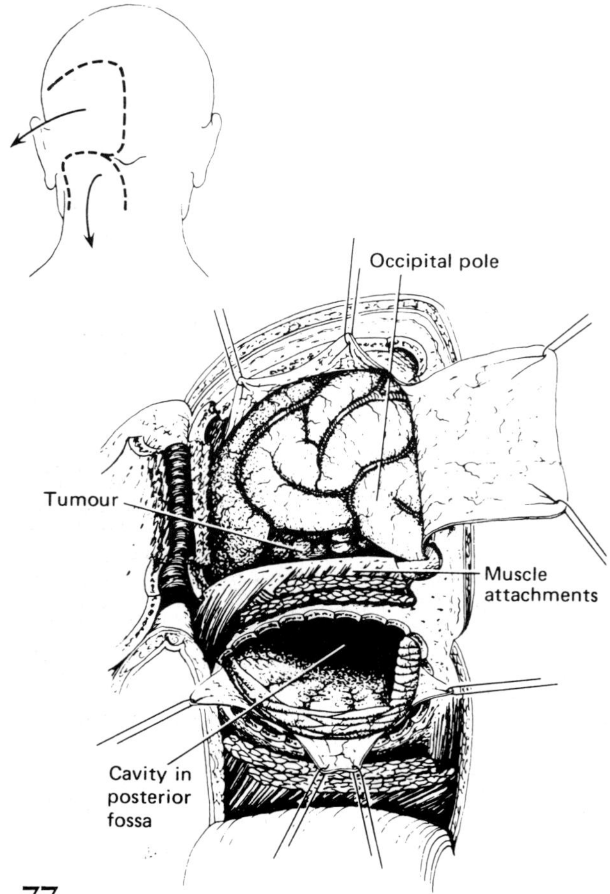


77

# 77

When a true extension through the tentorium is present, rather than attempting removal of the occipital portion entirely from below, it may be best to make an additional bone flap above the tentorium, preserving the rim of bone bearing the muscle anchorage. This will permit a better muscle closure.

The alternative procedure is to extend the suboccipital decompression above the superior curved line by making a medial and a lateral burr hole 1 inch (2.5 cm) above this line and freeing the resulting quadrilateral area of bone with saw cuts extending between the two burr holes and also from each of them down into the suboccipital craniectomy. The block of bone is replaced later using retaining perforating wire sutures.

The suboccipital portion of the tumour is dealt with first, to leave a large cavity lying above the cerebellum. Now working from above it is relatively easy to depress the supratentorial portion of neoplasm downwards and out of the evocative occipital lobe into the cavity below with a minimum of dissection, under direct vision, and then to excise it with a circumferential incision through the tentorium.

## TUMOURS OF THE CLIVUS AND BASI-OCCIPUT

These tumours are amongst the most difficult in neurosurgical practice. They are often insidious in onset, a single cranial nerve palsy being present for many years before symptoms of neuraxial compression or raised intracranial pressure supervene; sometimes they pursue a course of progressive paralysis of a wide group of cranial nerves from the oculomotor nerves to the nerves of the pharynx and vocal cords and their close relationship with the cranial nerves and the branches of the basilar artery together with their relative inaccessibility make the removal a hazardous process.

# 78a, b & c

The route of access depends on the precise situation of the tumour. Possibly the commonest are apical petrous and clivus tumours which are, as their names imply, offset to one side. These may very well involve both surfaces of the petrous bone straddling the petrous pyramid and invading the medial part of the middle fossa supratentorially. In the lower part of the clivus, the tumours may extend into the upper cervical canal through the foramen magnum and closely involve the vertebral artery, the basilar bifurcation and the posterior cranial nerves.

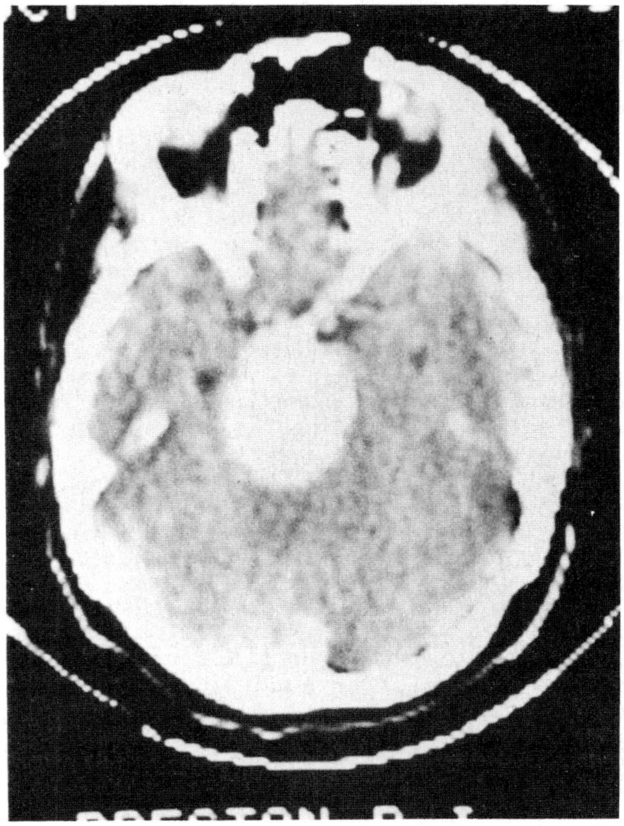

78a

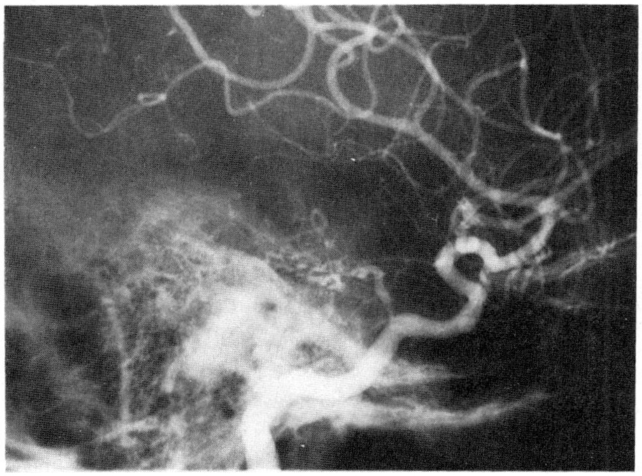

78b

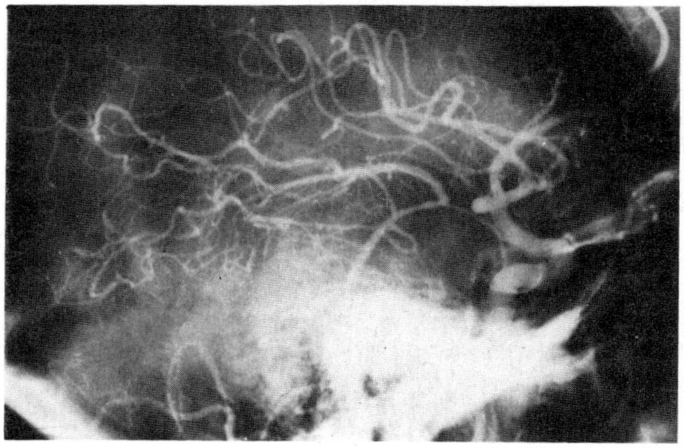

78c

*Figure 78. Axial tomography (enhanced) of a high clivus meningioma (a). The blood supply of this meningioma from the meningohypophyseal branches of the internal carotid artery; a grossly hypertrophied meningohypophyseal trunk is clearly visible (b). The arterial displacement of the basilar artery and posterior communicating artery by the meningioma is shown in (c).*

## APICAL PETROUS TUMOURS

# 79

Probably the best method of approach for these tumours is one providing access to the middle and posterior cranial fossae. The approach preferred by one of the authors has been a combined small supratentorial flap in the middle cranial fossa centred above the ear, its posterior limb being prolonged into the posterior fossa. The base of the petrous pyramid is drilled away with the inevitable opening of numerous mastoid cells, and the middle and posterior cranial fossae opened. The surgeon may then elect to divide the lateral sinus if a complete torcula herophili has been demonstrated by careful angiography, or alternatively, to pass forwards of the junction of lateral and sigmoid sinuses and divide the superior petrosal sinus in the dural opening to obtain access to both the middle and posterior fossae. This second approach, while favoured by some distinguished surgeons, provides less access than straightforward division of the lateral sinus since it inevitably restricts the posterior access available from retraction of the posterior divided portion of the tentorium. Whichever route is employed, however, Labbé's vein is carried back with the posterior portion of the tentorium and lateral sinus and drains across the torcula to the other side. Self-retaining retraction on the under aspect of the temporal lobe and on the superior aspect of the cerebellum provides unparalleled access to the tentorial hiatus and to both aspects of the petrous bone. Indeed, the brain may be said to open like a book. Provided the torcula herophili is complete and Labbé's vein rigorously protected even a dominant lateral sinus may be safely divided. Where the torcula is incomplete, however, division of the lateral sinus is extremely hazardous and will result in venous infarction of the posterior part of the temporal lobe which in the dominant hemisphere will produce a crippling dysphasia.

The side of approach will be determined by the offset of the tumour from the midline.

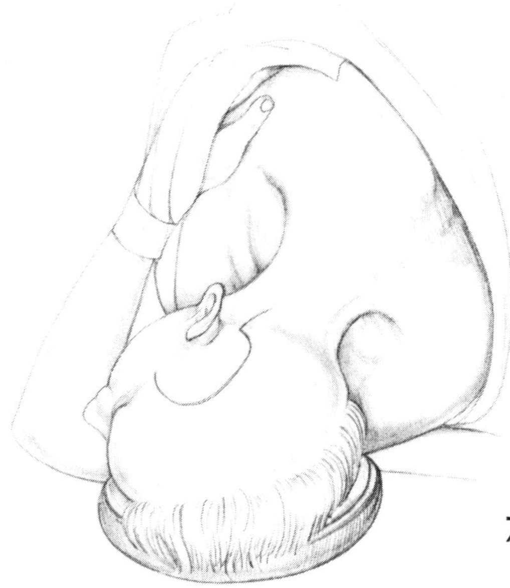

79

*Figure 79. The 'park bench' position and incision for combined supratentorial and infratentorial approach.*

## Incision and exposure

# 80

The scalp flap is turned from in front of the ear just above the zygomatic process, passing upwards and backwards as shown to curve forwards towards the asterion. It is then prolonged downwards and backwards towards the foramen magnum though it is never necessary to pass as low as the foramen itself. The supratentorial flap can be cut through three or four burr holes, the posterior being just above the lateral sinus. The most important burr hole should be made with the aid of the Hall drill and should be low in the middle fossa over the knee of the sigmoid to lateral sinus junction, enabling the bone flap to be prolonged into the posterior fossa across the sinuses. Alternatively, the supratentorial bone flap may be flush with the floor on the lateral sinus, and extension into the posterior fossa made by craniectomy. It is vital in this approach that the bone removal reaches the posterior face of the mastoid in the posterior fossa and the floor of the middle fossa supratentorially. Mastoid air cells are temporarily closed with wax and more effectively closed with a temporal fascia graft at the close of the procedure.

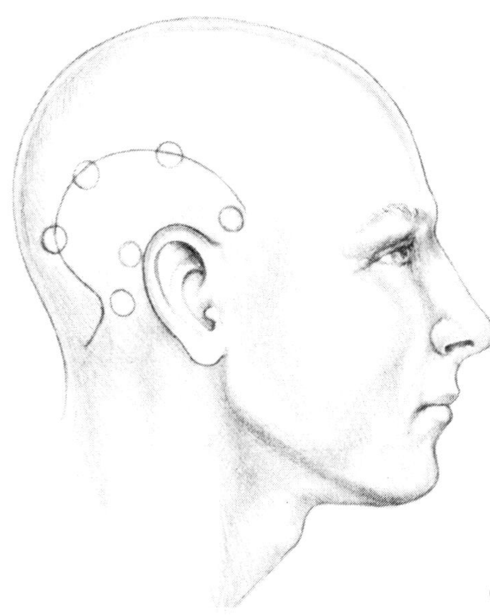

80

*Figure 80. Lateral view of the incision for the combined supratentorial and infratentorial approach with the site of burr holes shown.*

# 81

The supratentorial dura is opened just sufficiently to enable delineation of the upper margin of the lateral sinus, and the small flap hinged inferiorly may be turned back over the bone edge at this stage. The infratentorial dura is opened along the lower border of the sinus with a T-shaped extension to enable flaps to be retracted, and the surface of the cerebellum and posterior face of the petrous bone are exposed. The lateral sinus is then divided between white silk ligatures and division pursued to the medial edge of the tentorium. Labbé's vein and the posterior tentorial flap are then elevated with a subtemporal retractor and the vein protected with cottonoid. As the tentorium is divided medially it is essential that microscopic techniques are employed to protect the fourth cranial nerve.

The usual apical petrous and clivus meningioma extends towards the midline from medial to the fifth cranial nerve. However, it may encircle the fifth nerve or may lie entirely below it. Alternatively, it may extend well above the fifth nerve across the top of the dorsum sellae or lateral to it into Meckel's cave or into the cavernous sinus. Not infrequently it remains on the surface of the dura, crossing the petrous apex onto the superior surface of the petrous bone as a supratentorial mass. The major hazards in such a tumour are its close relationship to the fifth and oculomotor nerves, to the orbit, and to the branches of superior cerebellar and posterior cerebral arteries. The basilar artery is seldom adherent, but is usually in contact, and the degree of adhesion of the mass to the brain-stem itself is highly variable.

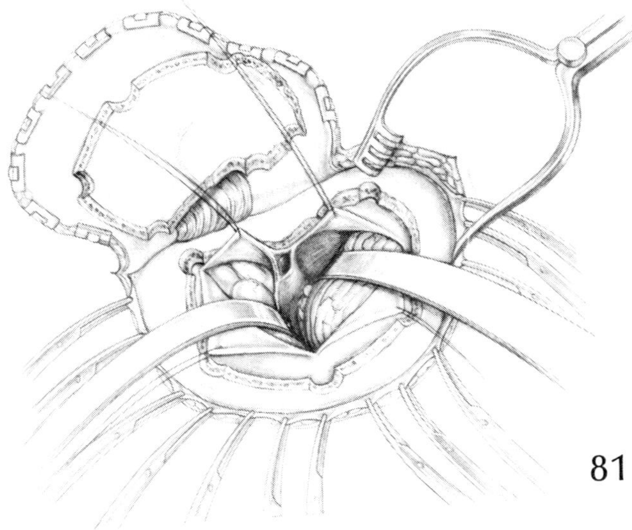

81

*Figure 81. The exposure by the combined supratentorial and infratentorial approach after division of the lateral sinus whose anterior end is shown as if it were open. Cerebellar and midtemporal retraction is performed as indicated.*

# 82

It is essential at an early stage to identify as far as possible the cranial nerves present in the field. The bulk of the tumour may make this very difficult, but as a rule the clival tumours will run true to type and be carried medial to the nerves in the internal auditory meatus and to the ninth, tenth and eleventh cranial nerves if they extend sufficiently far downwards on the clivus. Their relationship to the two sixth nerves is extremely variable and these nerves often prove very difficult to identify until the tumour has been almost completely removed.

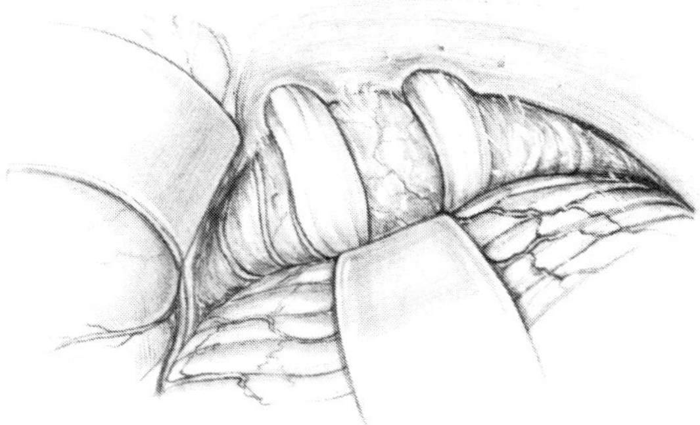

82

*Figure 82. Exposure by the combined approach of a clivus meningioma anterior to the fifth and the bundle of the seventh and eighth nerves which are shown. Linear streaks above the fifth nerve are branches of the superior cerebellar artery.*

## Removal of the tumour

# 83

A portion of the surface of the tumour may be coagulated, and with the combined supratentorial and infratentorial approach it is usually possible to reach a fair segment of the surface of the tumour above the fifth cranial nerve. In lower tumours it may be necessary to pass below the fifth cranial nerve and quite frequently it may be necessary to work both above and below the nerve as a tumour is exenterated. Commonly, hooks, rongeurs, the CUSA on relatively high power, and suction coagulation are the tools employed; cutting loops in such restricted access may be highly dangerous.

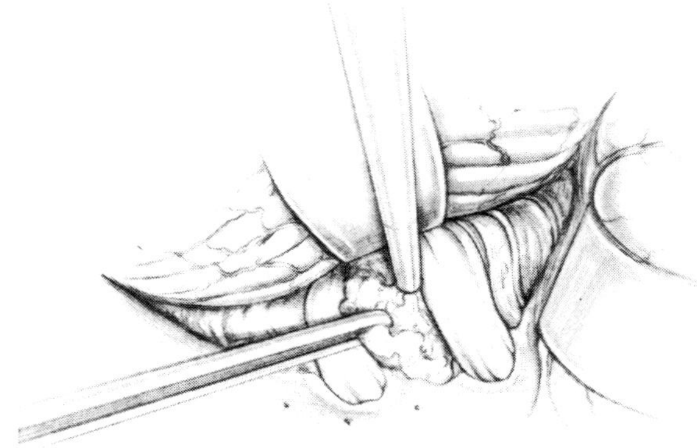

83

*Figure 83. Commencement of dissection of the clivus meningioma between the fifth and the seventh and eighth nerves.*

The use of the operating microscope is mandatory.

The blood supply of these tumours arises from the meningohypophyseal branches of the internal carotid artery and penetrates the tumour usually just medial to the entrance to Meckel's cave. If this fact is remembered then coagulation in this area and careful dissection early on will result in the remainder of the tumour being relatively bloodless. However, branches from the ascending pharyngeal artery along the inferior border of the porus acousticus and branches through the clivus from the ascending pharyngeal at a lower level may need to be coagulated as the tumour is excised.

The tumour is exenterated progressively and rotated gently against the clivus while the exposed surface and its contact with the brain-stem are carefully separated. Small venous attachments to the stem are coagulated using the bipolar coagulator, and the position of the major brain-stem vessels borne in mind. Superiorly the posterior cerebral artery may be used as a guide to the basilar, and the basilar artery then followed down from above, ensuring that none of its perforating branches pull away with the capsule of the tumour.

As with every meningioma, with progressive wedge excision of portions of the capsule, mobilization of the remainder of the tumour becomes easier as it is freed from the stem and the contralateral side is usually resected without difficulty. Once again, the position of the major cranial nerves must be remembered and finally the attachment of the tumour to the clivus may be heavily coagulated. In recent years some authorities have recommended the use of the neodymium-YAG laser, the penetration of which enables more deep sterilization of the clival attachment, but it is the author's experience that few of these tumours recur if a radical or complete excision has been performed onto the dural attachment in the first instance.

## Haemostasis and closure

It will usually be desirable to carry out resection of such tumours with moderate hypotension, and this must be reversed during closure. Small vessels entering the tumour from the bone on the clivus, particularly the meningohypophyseal vessels, may arrest with gentle coagulation at hypotension and reopen as the blood pressure rises. Coagulation of their bony orifices with a blunt hook inserted into the orifice may very well achieve complete haemostasis, but it is often wise to wax the origin of arterial supply through the clivus heavily and to cover it with Surgicel before closure.

The tentorium is not sutured and the defect produced by division of the lateral sinus is best covered by temporal fascia or some dural substitute. The remainder of the temporal fascia may be detached from the supratentorial bone, leaving the bone attached only by muscle, and the temporal fascia folded down over the surface of the open mastoid air cells.

The supratentorial convexity dura, which has been opened by no more than a linear incision, is closed and the bone flap attached with at least one perforating stitch and multiple pericranial sutures. It is best, if postoperative drainage is used, that dependent drainage without suction be used since a considerable area of brain may be covered with poor dural repair. If the fifth nerve has been affected or, as is commonly the case, is traumatized in the course of the removal, consideration should be given to at least temporary tarsorrhaphy. If the facial nerve has also been involved, particularly if the tumour has encircled and destroyed almost all the cranial nerves on one side, then a permanent lateral tarsorrhaphy is mandatory.

## LOWER CLIVAL TUMOURS

In many instances, these tumours present an insuperable problem. By the time they present they have frequently involved the neural supply of the larynx and pharynx on one side and may have encased the vertebral artery at its point of entry to the skull or distally. Even if they have not destroyed the nerves, their situation medial to the finely spread network of branches of ninth, tenth and eleventh nerves means that their removal carries a very high risk of damage to these nerves with consequent dangers of inhalation, consequent on pharyngeal paralysis in the postoperative period. There are occasional optimistic reports in the literature of removal of these tumours by a transoral approach, but the restricted access provided by this route means that excision is almost invariably incomplete.

The preferred route for approach to these tumours is posterolateral and because of the hazards to respiration it is usually wise to carry this out in the 'park bench' position with the head rotated towards the floor and the intracranial tension controlled by every available manoeuvre.

The incision is made posterolaterally from above the lateral sinus to the foramen magnum or below as described and it is essential that the bone removal be carried right forward to flush with the posterior face of the petrous bone. Inferiorly, the bone removal will need to proceed at least as far as the hypoglossal emissary foramen with its accompanying vein, and perhaps as far as the lateral margin of the jugular foramen. It may be necessary to remove the lateral half or more of the arch of the atlas and it is necessary to identify the vertebral artery before extensive lateral removal of bone in the region of the foramen magnum.

The dural opening should be made in a long-stemmed 'Y', the superior extent of the exposure reaching preferably as far as the junction of lateral and sigmoid sinuses, since this enhances the ease of cerebellar retraction greatly. A fixation post is placed in the bone at or above the level of the lateral sinus.

Initially, dissection should be pursued in the foramen magnum, identifying the posterior cranial nerves as far as possible and dividing by bipolar coagulation the irritating small vein which often joins the floccular area of the cerebellum to the dura just posterior to the tenth cranial nerve. The vertebral artery below the tumour and if possible the posterior inferior cerebellar artery should be identified at this stage and the capsule of the tumour approached from an angle which is convenient, considering the relationship of the cranial nerves and vessels. It is sometimes helpful to maintain the capsule intact where it is crossed by the fan of posterior cranial nerves, working as far as possible within the tumour and freeing it from the medial vascular structures before freeing the cranial nerves laterally with the tumour exenterated and pressing the shelf of retained capsule medially into the exenterated cavity. Even so, damage to these tender nerves is a constant hazard.

Having freed the ipsilateral cranial nerves, the base of the tumour on the basi-occiput should be heavily coagulated and the opposite side of the capsule then investigated. If the tumour has extended to involve the contralateral posterior cranial nerves, no attempt should be made to excise this portion of the capsule at the initial operation. Ipsilateral damage to the posterior cranial nerves will carry a considerable risk of postoperative inhalation and respiratory problems, but bilateral damage renders these problems almost insuperable and certainly inevitable. It may be necessary to delay a second approach possibly from the other side for many months until the ipsilateral nerves have recovered. In many instances, the removal of the bulk of the tumour, especially in old patients, will have to be accepted.

The sixth cranial nerves have a particularly irritating relationship to tumours which involve the middle portion of the clivus. Only with careful microscopic dissection may they be preserved, but like the other motor nerves to the orbit the degree of recovery which even a heavily traumatized oculomotor nerve will show is astonishing, and the sixth nerve is no exception.

## Closure of the wound

Particularly where residual tumour remains it is often wise to leave the dura open. Mastoid air cells should be carefully closed with a mixture of bone dust and fibrin glue. Sheets of Surgicel soaked in such fibrin glue act as a comfortable closure, particularly over the region of the foramen magnum, where closure may be not only difficult, but unwise. The muscles and fasciae are closed in layers with white silk or some other suitable suture material, and the wounds left undrained.

Illustrations by D. Peace, M. E. Barry and Barbara Hyams

# Operative approaches to the lateral ventricles (supratentorial intraventricular tumours)

**Albert L. Rhoton Jr** MD
R. D. Keene Family Professor and Chairman, Department of Neurological Surgery, University of Florida College of Medicine, Gainesville, Florida, USA

The lateral ventricles are the site of deep lesions that are commonly treated using micro-operative techniques. They also provide deep cavities through which the third ventricle and basal cisterns may be approached. The neural and vascular relationships that provide the basis for optimizing the results obtained with intraventricular operations are reviewed before describing the individual operative approaches.

## Neural relationships

## 1a & b

Each lateral ventricle is a C-shaped cavity found deep within the cerebrum. The walls of each ventricle are formed predominantly by the thalamus, septum pellucidum, corpus callosum, caudate nucleus and fornix[1,2].

The thalamus is located in the centre of each lateral ventricle. The body of the lateral ventricle is above the thalamus, the atrium and occipital horn are posterior to the thalamus, and the temporal horn is inferolateral to the thalamus.

The caudate nucleus is an arched, C-shaped, cellular mass that wraps around the thalamus and constitutes an important part of the wall of each lateral ventricle. Its head bulges into the lateral wall of the frontal horn and body of the lateral ventricle. Its body forms part of the lateral wall of the atrium, and its tail extends from the atrium into the roof of the temporal horn.

The fornix is another C-shaped structure that wraps around the thalamus in the wall of the ventricle. In the body of the lateral ventricle, the body of the fornix is in the lower part of the medial wall; in the atrium, the crus of the fornix is in the medial part of the anterior wall; in the temporal horn, the fimbria of the fornix is in the medial part of the floor. The body of the fornix crosses the thalamus approximately half-way between the medial and lateral edge of the superior surface of the thalamus: the part of the thalamus lateral to the body of the fornix forms the floor of the body of the lateral ventricle and the part medial to the fornix forms part of the roof of the velum interpositum and third ventricle. The crus of the fornix crosses the pulvinar approximately midway between the medial and lateral edge of the pulvinar: the part of the pulvinar lateral to the crus of the fornix forms part of the anterior wall of the atrium and the part medial to the fornix forms part of the anterior wall of the quadrigeminal cistern. The fimbriae of the fornix pass below the inferolateral part of the thalamus just lateral to the medial and lateral geniculate bodies. The part of the thalamus medial to the fimbria forms the roof of the ambient cistern. The body of the fornix separates into two columns that arch along the superior and anterior margins of the foramen of Monro.

The corpus callosum, which forms the largest part of the ventricular walls, contributes to the wall of each of the five parts of the lateral ventricle. The rostrum of the corpus callosum is situated below and forms the floor of the frontal horn. The bundle of fibres in the genu called the forceps minor forms the anterior wall of the frontal horn. The genu and the body of the corpus callosum form the roof of both the frontal horn and the body of the lateral ventricle. The splenium contains a large fibre bundle, the forceps major, which forms a prominence called the bulb in the upper part of the medial wall of the atrium. Another fibre tract, the tapetum, which arises in the posterior part of the body and splenium of the corpus callosum, sweeps laterally and inferiorly to form the roof and lateral wall of the atrium and the temporal horns. The tapetum separates the fibres of the optic radiations from the temporal horn.

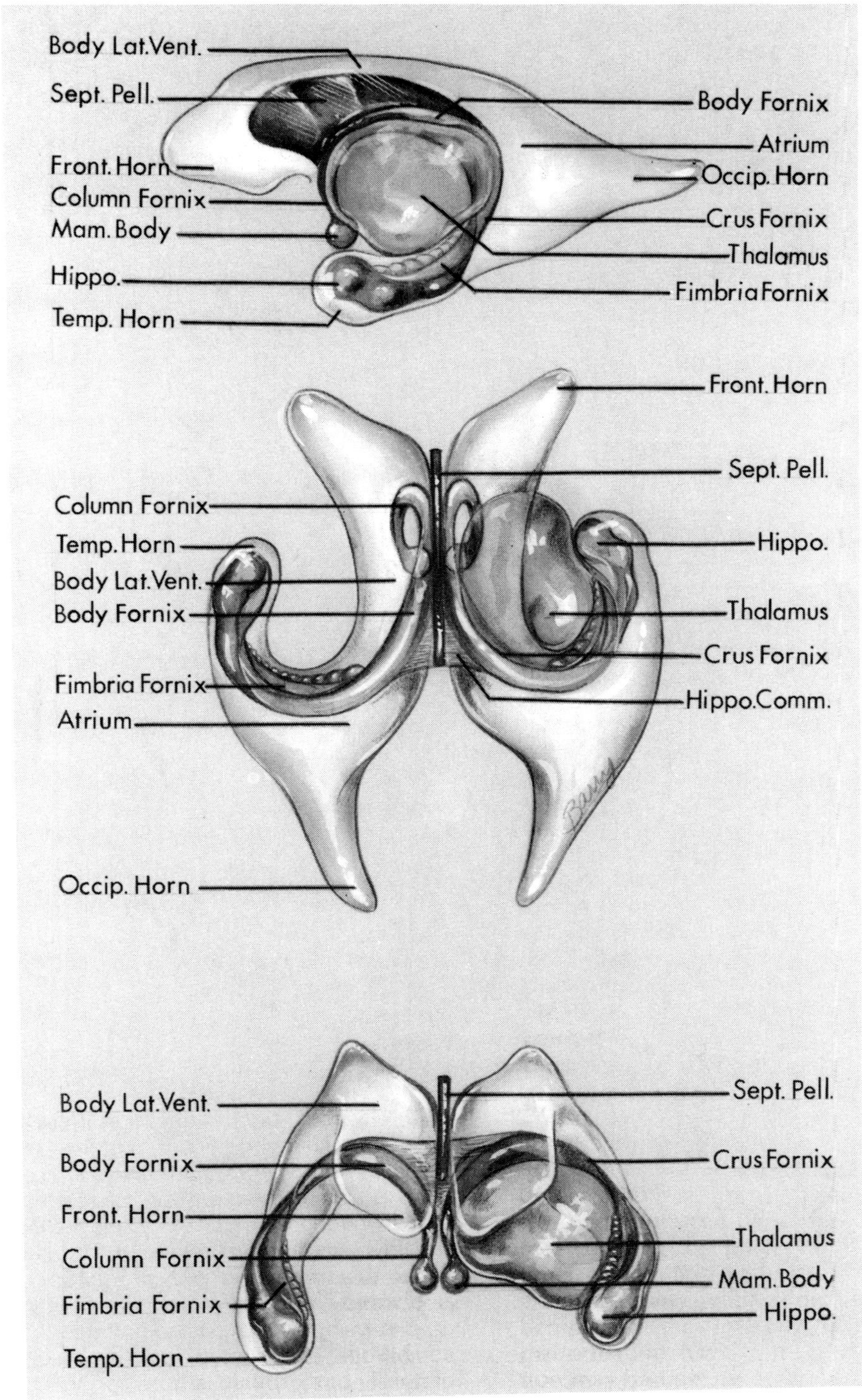
Body Lat.Vent.
Sept. Pell.
Front. Horn
Column Fornix
Mam. Body
Hippo.
Temp. Horn
Body Fornix
Atrium
Occip. Horn
Crus Fornix
Thalamus
Fimbria Fornix
Front. Horn
Sept. Pell.
Column Fornix
Temp. Horn
Body Lat.Vent.
Body Fornix
Fimbria Fornix
Atrium
Occip. Horn
Hippo.
Thalamus
Crus Fornix
Hippo.Comm.
Body Lat.Vent.
Body Fornix
Front. Horn
Column Fornix
Fimbria Fornix
Temp. Horn
Sept. Pell.
Crus Fornix
Thalamus
Mam. Body
Hippo.

1a

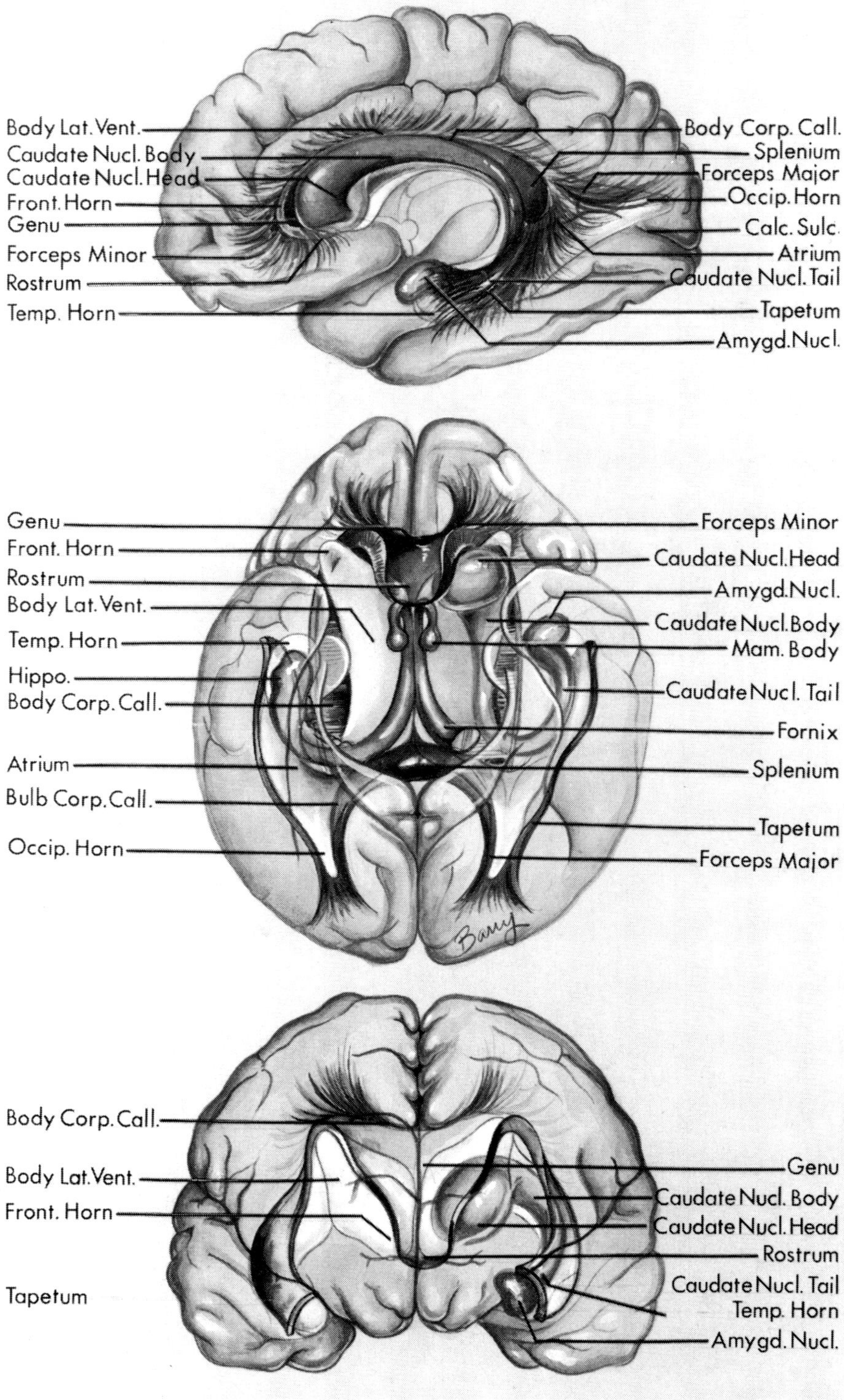
Body Lat. Vent.
Caudate Nucl. Body
Caudate Nucl. Head
Front. Horn
Genu
Forceps Minor
Rostrum
Temp. Horn
Body Corp. Call.
Splenium
Forceps Major
Occip. Horn
Calc. Sulc.
Atrium
Caudate Nucl. Tail
Tapetum
Amygd. Nucl.
Genu
Front. Horn
Rostrum
Body Lat. Vent.
Temp. Horn
Hippo.
Body Corp. Call.
Atrium
Bulb Corp. Call.
Occip. Horn
Forceps Minor
Caudate Nucl. Head
Amygd. Nucl.
Caudate Nucl. Body
Mam. Body
Caudate Nucl. Tail
Fornix
Splenium
Tapetum
Forceps Major
Barry
Body Corp. Call.
Body Lat. Vent.
Front. Horn
Tapetum
Genu
Caudate Nucl. Body
Caudate Nucl. Head
Rostrum
Caudate Nucl. Tail
Temp. Horn
Amygd. Nucl.

1b

# 2a–d

The septum pellucidum, which is composed of paired laminae, separates the frontal horns and bodies of the lateral ventricles in the midline. There may be a cavity, the cavum septum pellucidum, in the midline between the laminae of the septum pellucidum.

The close relationship of the internal capsule to the lateral wall of the frontal horn and body of the lateral ventricle is often forgotten when planning operative approaches to the ventricles. The anterior limb of the internal capsule, which is located between the caudate and lentiform nuclei, is separated from the frontal horn by the head of the caudate nucleus. The posterior limb, which is situated between the thalamus and the lentiform nucleus, is separated from the body of the lateral ventricle by the thalamus and body of the caudate nucleus. However, the genu of the internal capsule comes directly to the ventricular surface and touches the wall of the lateral ventricle immediately lateral to the foramen of Monro in the interval between the caudate nucleus and the thalamus.

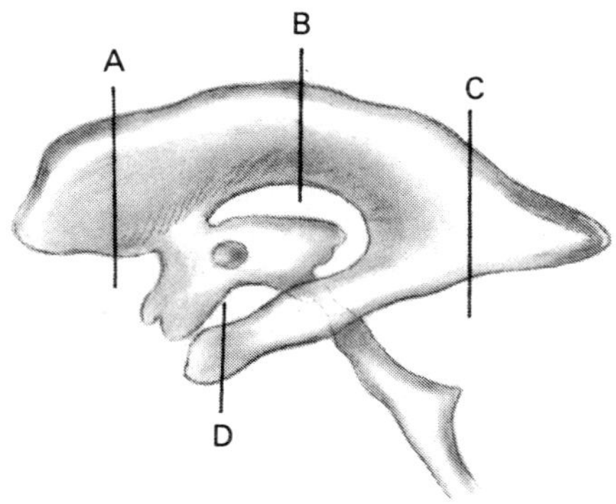


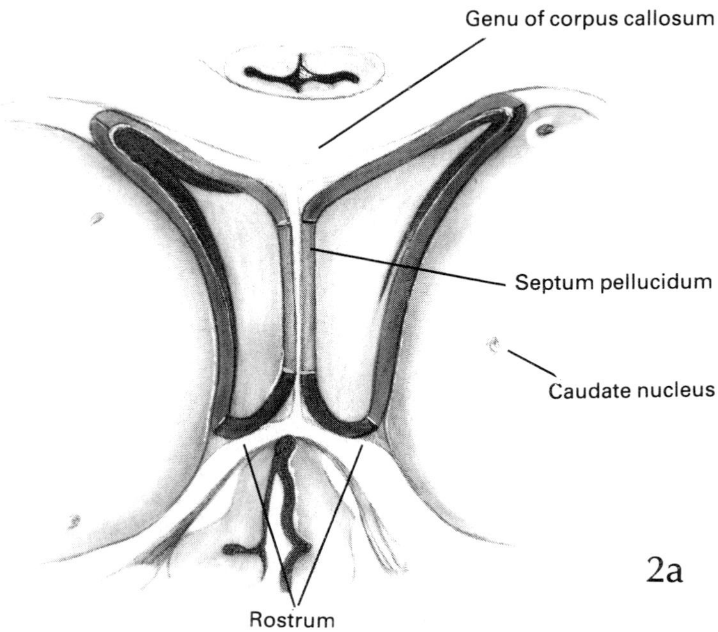


2a

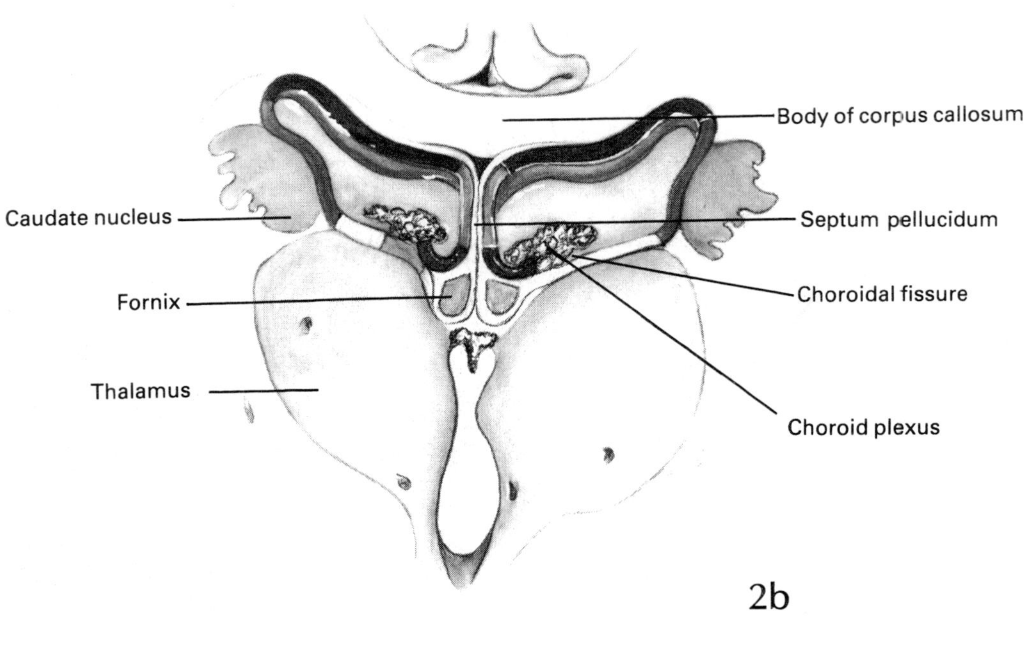


2b

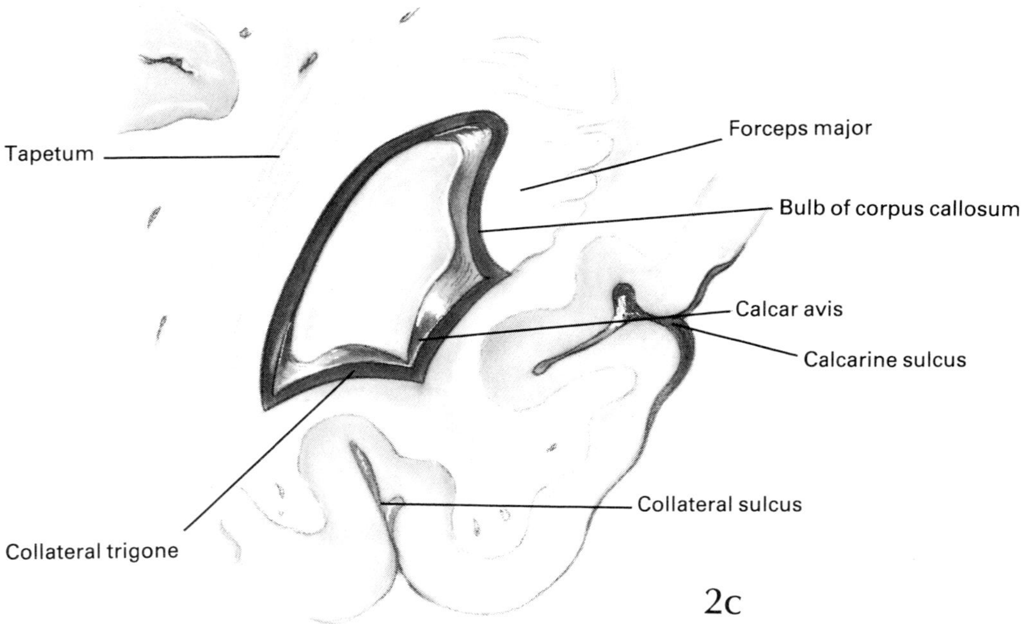
Tapetum
Forceps major
Bulb of corpus callosum
Calcar avis
Calcarine sulcus
Collateral sulcus
Collateral trigone

2c

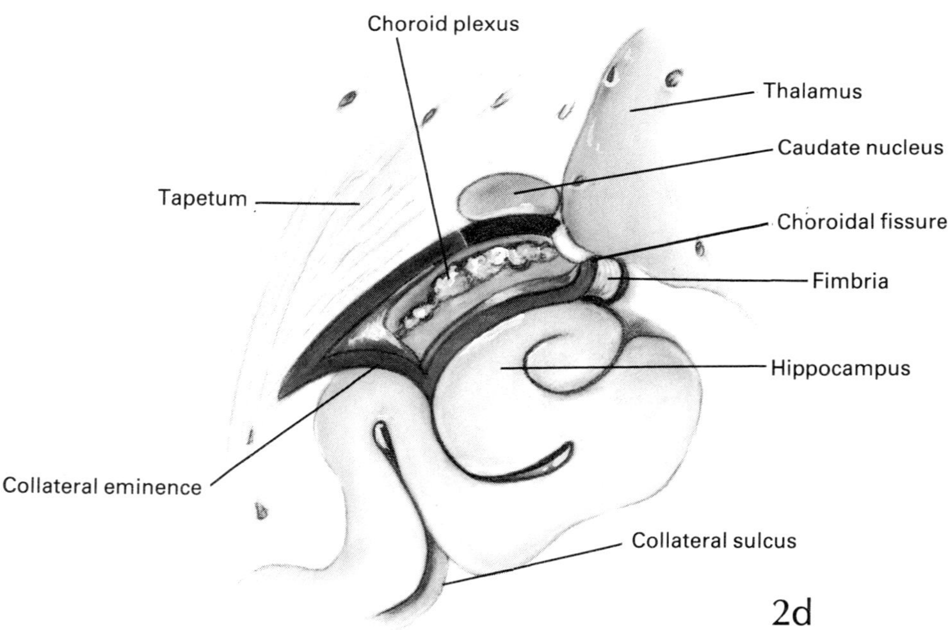
Choroid plexus
Thalamus
Caudate nucleus
Tapetum
Choroidal fissure
Fimbria
Hippocampus
Collateral eminence
Collateral sulcus

2d

## VENTRICULAR WALLS

### Frontal horn

Cross sections through the ventricle at various places are shown in *Illustration 2*. The frontal horn, the part of the lateral ventricle located anterior to the foramen of Monro, has a medial wall formed by the septum pellucidum, an anterior wall formed by the genu of the corpus callosum, a lateral wall composed of the head of the caudate nucleus, and a narrow floor formed by the rostrum of the corpus callosum. The columns of the fornix, as they pass anterior and superior to the foramen of Monro, are in the posteroinferior part of the medial wall.

### Body

3a, b & c

The body of the lateral ventricle extends from the posterior edge of the foramen of Monro to the point where the septum pellucidum disappears and the corpus callosum and fornix meet. The roof is formed by the body of the corpus callosum, the medial wall by the septum pellucidum above and the body of the fornix below, the lateral wall by the body of the caudate nucleus, and the floor by the thalamus. The caudate nucleus and thalamus are separated by the striothalamic sulcus, the groove in which the stria terminalis and the thalamostriate vein course.

### Atrium and occipital horn

The atrium and occipital horn together form a roughly triangular cavity, with the apex posteriorly in the occipital lobe and the base anteriorly on the pulvinar. The roof of the atrium is formed by the body, splenium and tapetum of the corpus callosum. The medial wall is formed by two roughly horizontal prominences which are located one above the other. The upper prominence, called the bulb of the corpus callosum, overlies and is formed by the large bundle of fibres called the forceps major, and the lower prominence, called the calcar avis, overlies the deepest part of the calcarine sulcus. The lateral wall has an anterior part formed by the caudate nucleus and a posterior part formed by the fibres of the tapetum. The anterior wall has a medial part composed of the crus of the fornix and a lateral part formed by the pulvinar of the thalamus. The floor is formed by the collateral trigone, a triangular area that bulges upward over the posterior end of the collateral sulcus.

The occipital horn extends posteriorly into the occipital lobe from the atrium. It varies in size from being absent to extending far posteriorly in the occipital lobe and it may vary in size from side to side. Its medial wall is formed by the bulb of the corpus callosum and the calcar avis, the roof and lateral wall are formed by the tapetum, and the floor is formed by the collateral trigone.

### Temporal horn

The temporal horn extends forward from the atrium below the pulvinar into the medial part of the temporal lobe and ends blindly in an anterior wall that is situated immediately behind the amygdaloid nucleus. The floor of the temporal horn is formed medially by the hippocampus, the smooth prominence overlying the hippocampal formation, and laterally by the collateral eminence, the prominence overlying the collateral sulcus that separates the parahippocampal and occipitotemporal gyri on the inferior surface of the temporal lobe. The roof is formed medially by the inferior surface of the thalamus and the tail of the caudate nucleus, and laterally by the tapetum of the corpus callosum. The medial wall is little more than a narrow cleft, the choroidal fissure, situated between the inferolateral part of the thalamus and the fimbria of the fornix.

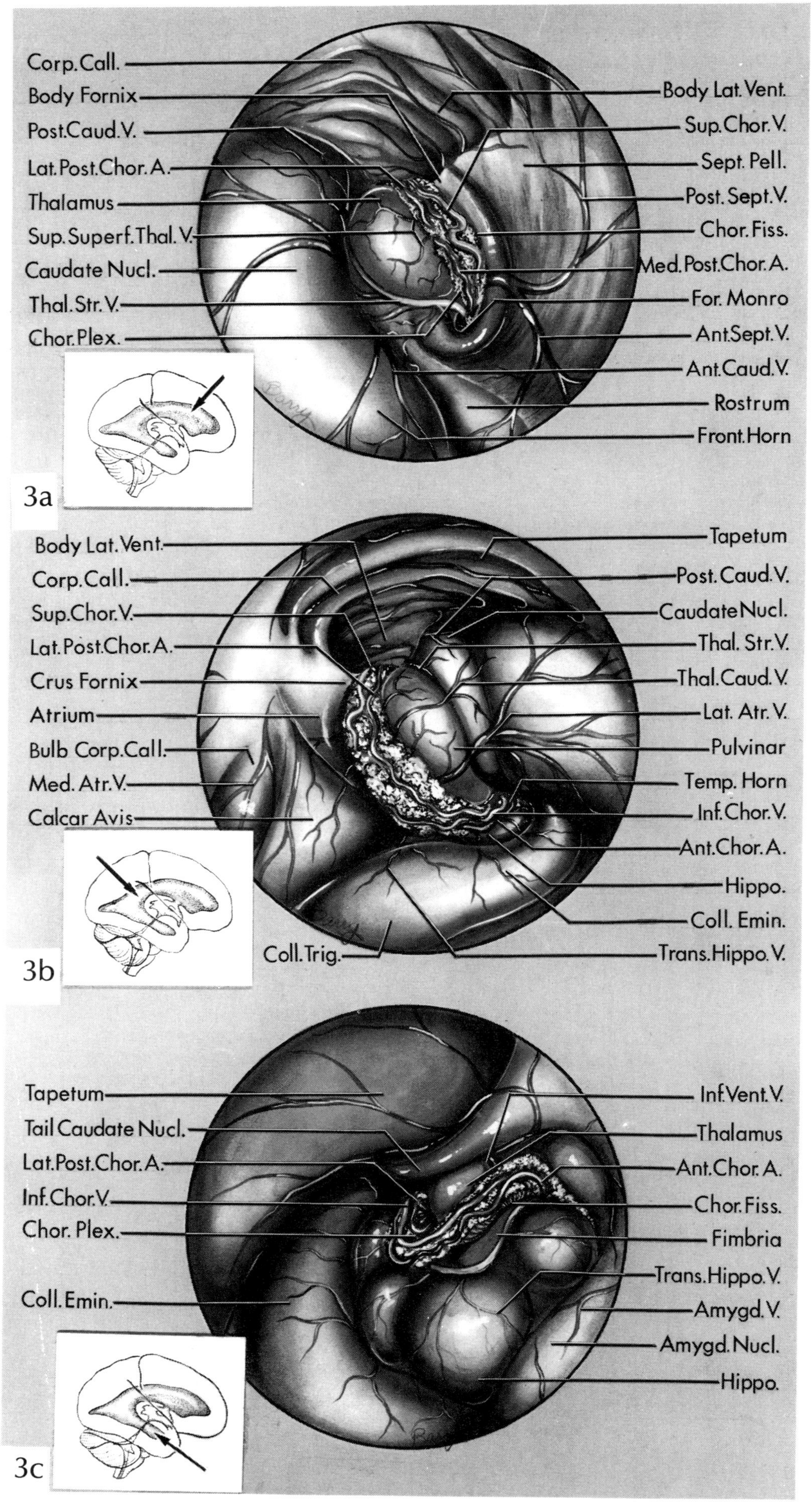
Corp.Call.
Body Fornix
Post.Caud.V.
Lat.Post.Chor.A.
Thalamus
Sup.Superf.Thal.V.
Caudate Nucl.
Thal.Str.V.
Chor.Plex.
Body Lat.Vent.
Sup.Chor.V.
Sept. Pell.
Post. Sept.V.
Chor. Fiss.
Med.Post.Chor.A.
For. Monro
Ant.Sept.V.
Ant.Caud.V.
Rostrum
Front.Horn
3a
Body Lat.Vent.
Corp.Call.
Sup.Chor.V.
Lat.Post.Chor.A.
Crus Fornix
Atrium
Bulb Corp.Call.
Med. Atr.V.
Calcar Avis
Tapetum
Post. Caud.V.
Caudate Nucl.
Thal. Str.V.
Thal.Caud.V.
Lat. Atr.V.
Pulvinar
Temp. Horn
Inf.Chor.V.
Ant.Chor.A.
Hippo.
Coll. Emin.
Coll.Trig.
Trans.Hippo.V.
3b
Tapetum
Tail Caudate Nucl.
Lat.Post.Chor.A.
Inf.Chor.V.
Chor. Plex.
Coll.Emin.
Inf.Vent.V.
Thalamus
Ant.Chor.A.
Chor.Fiss.
Fimbria
Trans.Hippo.V.
Amygd.V.
Amygd.Nucl.
Hippo.
3c

## CHOROID PLEXUS AND CHOROIDAL FISSURE

# 4

The choroid plexus in the lateral ventricle has a C-shaped configuration that parallels the fornix[1,3]. It is attached along the choroidal fissure, the narrow C-shaped cleft that is situated between the fornix and the thalamus. The choroid plexus from each lateral ventricle extends through the foramen of Monro and is continuous with the two parallel strands of choroid plexus in the roof of the third ventricle. In the atrium, the choroid plexus forms a prominent triangular tuft called the glomus. The edges of the thalamus and fornix bordering the choroidal fissure have small ridges called the taeniae that anchor the choroid plexus to the fornix and thalamus. The taenia on the thalamic side is called the tenia choroidea. The taenia on the forniceal side of the fissure is called the tenia fornicis except in the temporal horn where it is referred to as the tenia fimbriae.

The choroidal fissure extends in a C-shaped arc from the foramen of Monro through the body, atrium and temporal horn to its inferior termination, called the inferior choroidal point, which is located just behind the uncus and amygdaloid nucleus and just lateral to the lateral geniculate body[1]. The choroidal fissure is divided into body, atrial and temporal parts. The body portion of the choroidal fissure is situated in the body of the lateral ventricle between the body of the fornix and the thalamus. The velum interpositum, through which the internal cerebral veins course, is located on the medial side of the body portion of the fissure in the roof of the third ventricle. The velum interpositum and the roof of the third ventricle can be exposed by opening through the choroidal fissure from the body of the ventricle. The atrial part is located in the atrium of the lateral ventricle between the crus of the fornix and the pulvinar. The quadrigeminal cistern, the pineal region and the posterior portion of the ambient cistern can be exposed by opening through the fissure from the atrium. The temporal part is situated in the temporal horn between the fimbria of the fornix and the inferolateral surface of the thalamus. The structures in the ambient and posterior part of the crural cisterns can be exposed by opening through the choroidal fissure from the temporal horn. The fissure is the thinnest site in the wall of the lateral ventricle bordering the basal cisterns and the roof of the third ventricle.

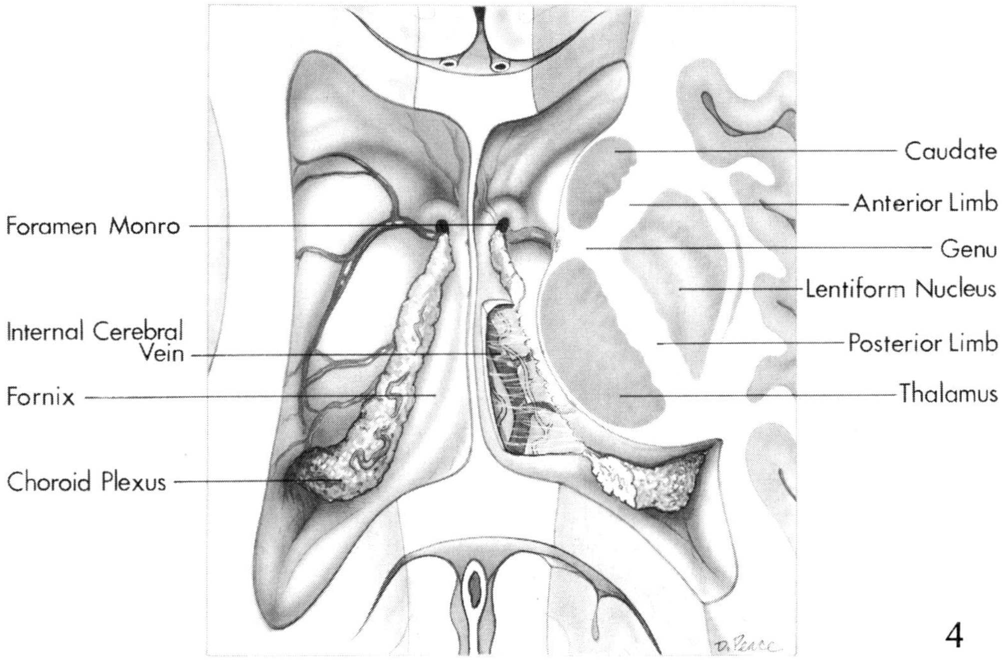


4

## VELUM INTERPOSITUM

The velum interpositum is located in the roof of the third ventricle below the body of the fornix and between the superomedial surfaces of the thalami[4]. The upper and lower walls of the velum interpositum are formed by the two membranous layers of tela choroidea in the roof of the third ventricle. The upper wall is formed by the layer that is attached to the lower surface of the fornix and the hippocampal commissure. The anterior part of the lower wall is attached to the small ridges on the free edge of the striae medullaris thalami. The posterior part of the lower wall is attached to the superior surface of the pineal body. The internal cerebral veins arise in the anterior part of the velum interpositum just behind the foramen of Monro and they exit the velum interpositum above the pineal body to enter the quadrigeminal cistern, where they join the great vein.

# 5a–g

A comparison of the left and right transchoroidal and transforniceal routes to the third ventricle is shown in *Illustrations 5a* and *b*. In *Illustration 5a* the superior part of the cerebral hemispheres has been removed to expose the frontal horns, bodies and atria of the lateral ventricles. The choroid plexus is attached along the choroidal fissures. The structures forming the walls of the lateral ventricle include the corpus callosum, fornix, thalamus, septum pellucidum and the caudate nucleus. The anterior septal, anterior caudate and superior choroidal veins join the thalamostriate veins near the foramen of Monro. A thalamocaudate vein crosses the walls of the left lateral ventricle. A right transchoroidal approach to the third ventricle is shown in *Illustration 5b*. The right choroidal fissure is opened by incising along the tenia fornicis. The fornix is retracted to the left in order to expose the paired internal cerebral veins which course through the velum interpositum. The anterior septal, thalamostriate, superior choroidal and posterior septal veins empty into the right internal cerebral vein. The medial posterior choroidal arteries course in the velum interpositum with the internal cerebral veins. A layer of tela choroidea is located above and below the internal cerebral veins. The lower layer of tela choroidea is opened to expose the third ventricle, massa intermedia, habenular and posterior commissures and choroid plexus in the third ventricle (*c*). A left transchoroidal approach to the third ventricle in the same specimen is shown in *Illustration 5d*. The left choroidal fissure is opened by incising along the tenia fornicis and the fornix is retracted toward the left side. The internal cerebral veins are separated (*e*) and the lower layer of tela choroidea is opened to expose the third ventricle. A transforniceal approach to the third ventricle is shown in the same specimen (*f*). The velum interpositum is opened by incising the body of the fornix in the midline along the direction of its fibres. The upper layer of tela choroidea is opened to expose the internal cerebral veins and the medial posterior choroidal arteries in the velum interpositum. The anterior commissure is exposed in the anterior part of the third ventricle. The lower layer of tela choroidea is opened to expose the interior of the third ventricle (*g*).

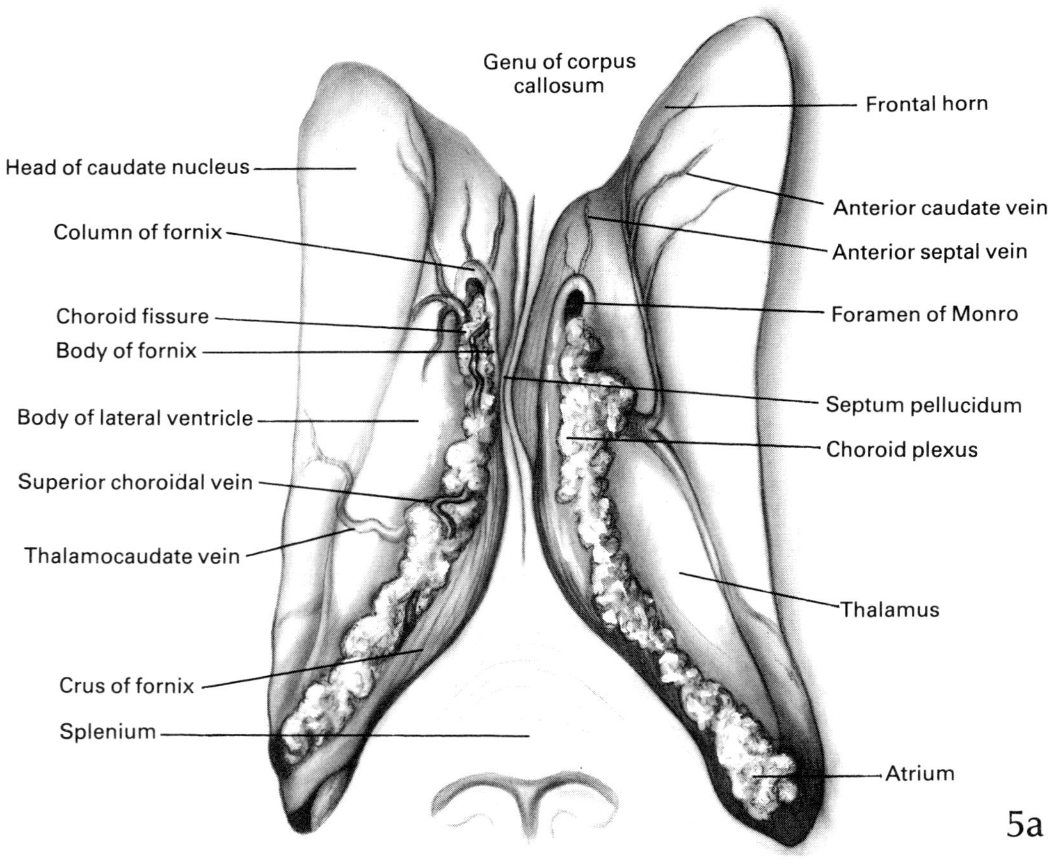


5a

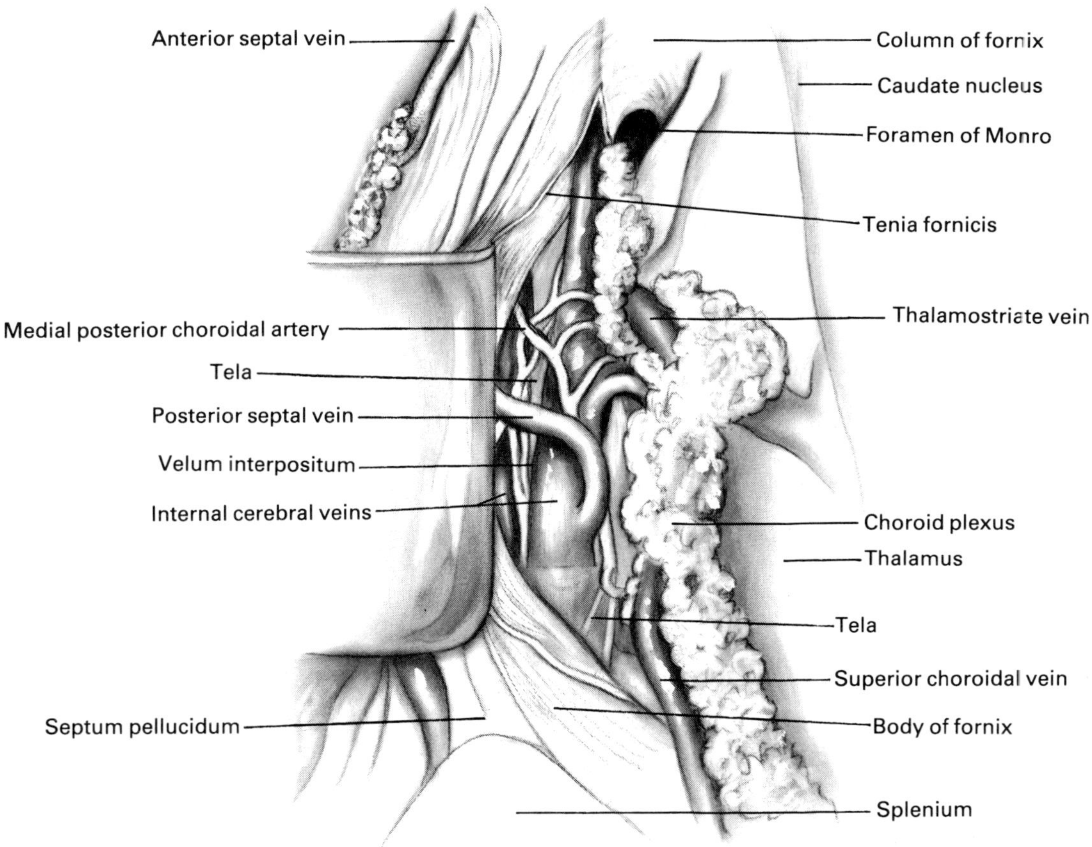
Anterior septal vein
Column of fornix
Caudate nucleus
Foramen of Monro
Tenia fornicis
Thalamostriate vein
Medial posterior choroidal artery
Tela
Posterior septal vein
Velum interpositum
Internal cerebral veins
Choroid plexus
Thalamus
Tela
Superior choroidal vein
Septum pellucidum
Body of fornix
Splenium

5b

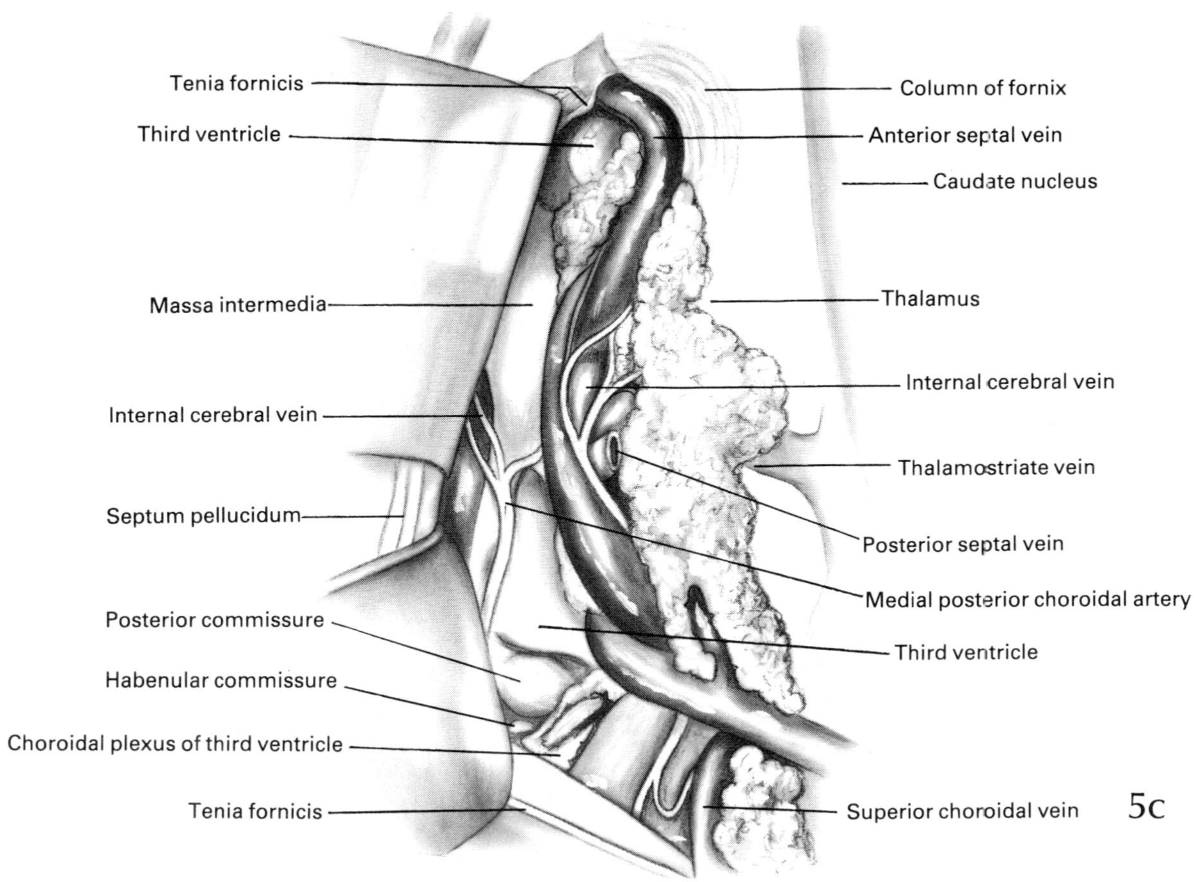
Tenia fornicis
Column of fornix
Third ventricle
Anterior septal vein
Caudate nucleus
Massa intermedia
Thalamus
Internal cerebral vein
Internal cerebral vein
Thalamostriate vein
Septum pellucidum
Posterior septal vein
Medial posterior choroidal artery
Posterior commissure
Third ventricle
Habenular commissure
Choroidal plexus of third ventricle
Tenia fornicis
Superior choroidal vein

5c

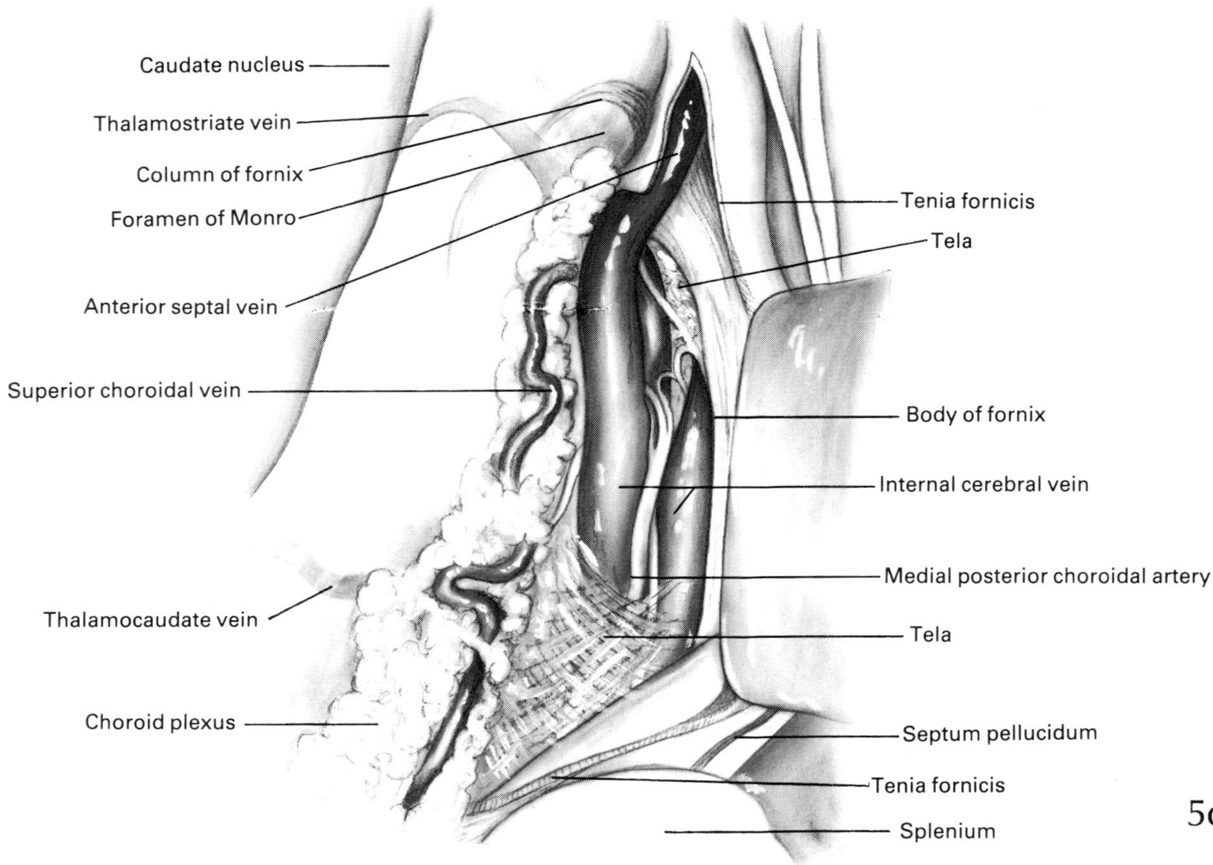
Caudate nucleus
Thalamostriate vein
Column of fornix
Foramen of Monro
Anterior septal vein
Superior choroidal vein
Thalamocaudate vein
Choroid plexus
Tenia fornicis
Tela
Body of fornix
Internal cerebral vein
Medial posterior choroidal artery
Tela
Septum pellucidum
Tenia fornicis
Splenium

5d

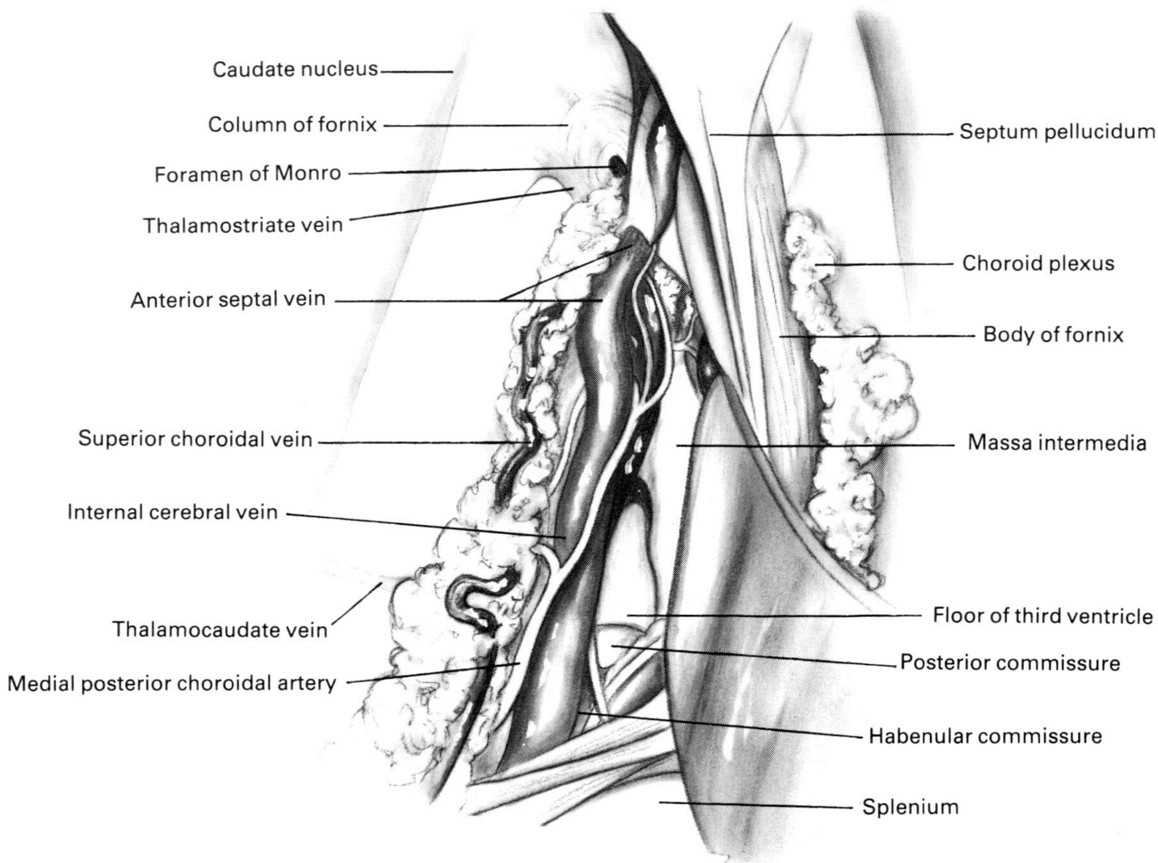
Caudate nucleus
Column of fornix
Foramen of Monro
Thalamostriate vein
Anterior septal vein
Superior choroidal vein
Internal cerebral vein
Thalamocaudate vein
Medial posterior choroidal artery
Septum pellucidum
Choroid plexus
Body of fornix
Massa intermedia
Floor of third ventricle
Posterior commissure
Habenular commissure
Splenium

5e

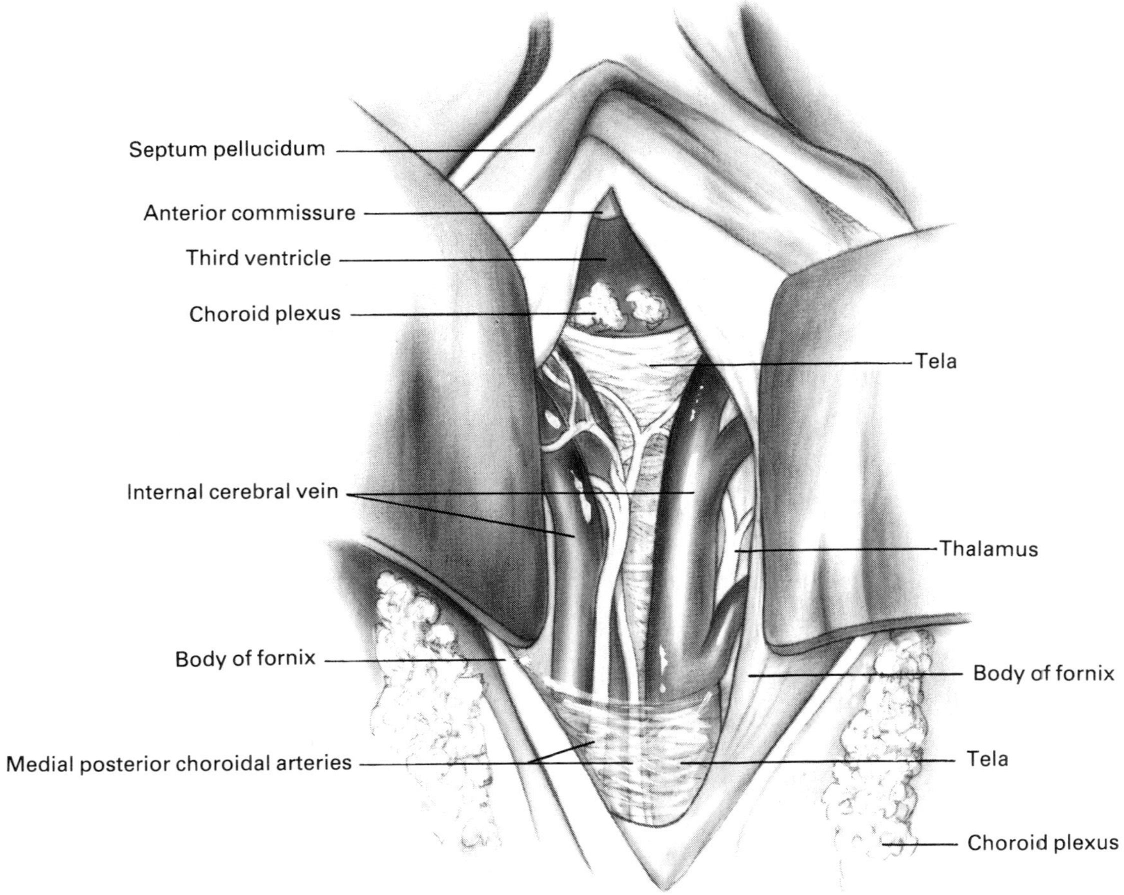


5f

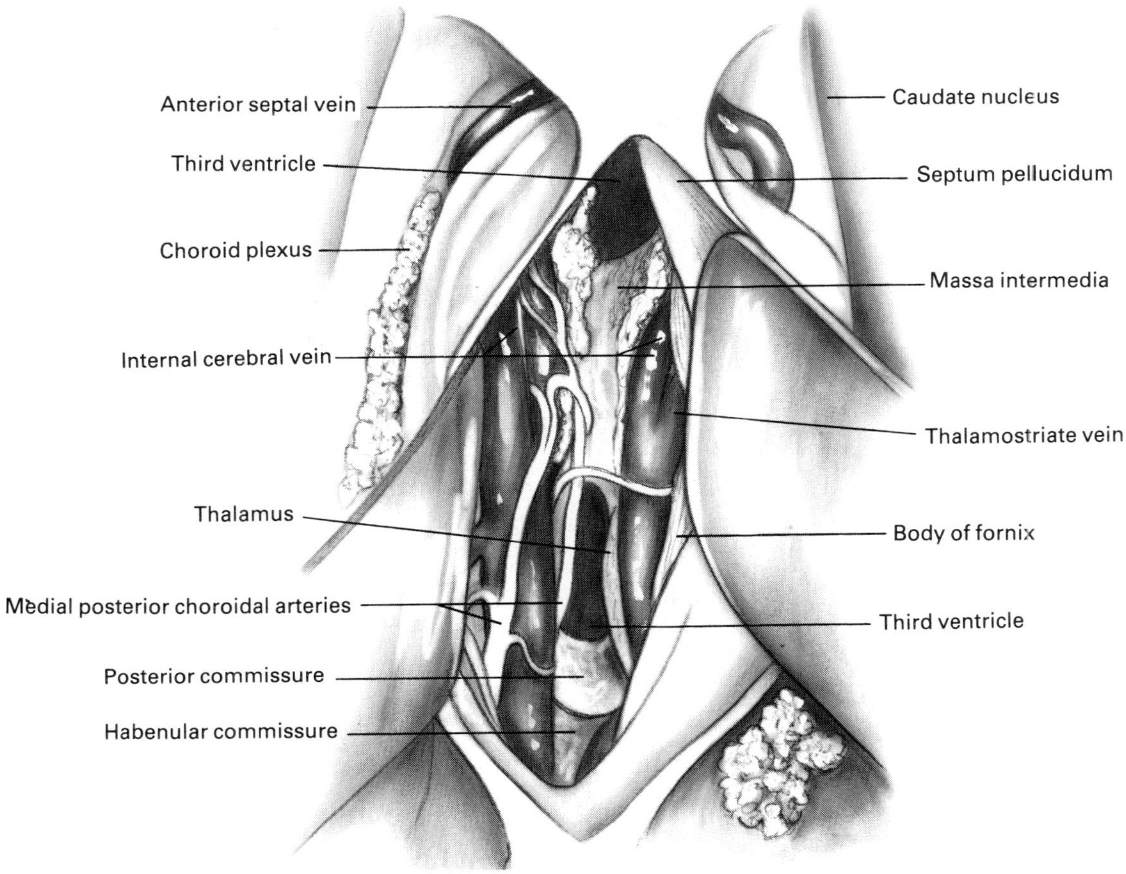


5g

Figures 5a–g are reprinted by permission of the publisher from 'Microsurgical anatomy of the choroidal fissure' by Cohen, *Surgical Neurology*, volume 30, pp. 50–53. © 1988 Elsevier Science Publishing Co., Inc.

## Tentorial and cisternal relationships

### 6

The lateral ventricles are situated above the tentorial incisura, the triangular space situated between the free edges of the tentorium and the dorsum sellae[5]. The midbrain is situated in the centre of the incisura. The area between the midbrain and the free edges is divided into an anterior incisural space located in front of the brain stem, paired middle incisural spaces situated lateral to the midbrain, and a posterior incisural space located behind the midbrain. The frontal horns are located above the anterior incisural space. The bodies of the lateral ventricles are located directly above the central part of the incisura, where they sit on and are separated from the central part of the incisura by the thalamus. The atria are located above the posterior incisural space, and the temporal horns are situated superolateral to the middle incisural space. The three incisural spaces contain some of the basal cisterns, and are so intimately related to the lateral ventricles that some operative approaches to the basal cisterns situated within the incisura are directed through the lateral ventricles.

The anterior incisural space, which is situated anterior to the midbrain, extends obliquely upward around the optic chiasm to the area below the rostrum of the corpus callosum and the floor of the frontal horn. This space contains the interpeduncular and chiasmatic cisterns and the cisterna lamina terminalis.

The middle incisural space is located between the temporal lobe and the midbrain. The temporal horn extends into the medial part of the temporal lobe lateral to the middle incisural space and ends approximately 4 cm from the anterior pole of the temporal lobe. The crural and ambient cisterns are situated medial to the temporal horn in the middle incisural space. The crural cistern is located between the cerebral peduncle and the uncus. The ambient cistern is bounded medially by the midbrain, above by the pulvinar and laterally by the parahippocampal and dentate gyri. The ambient cistern opens laterally through the choroidal fissure into the temporal horn.

The posterior incisural space lies below the atria of the lateral ventricles and contains the quadrigeminal cistern. The quadrigeminal cistern has an anterior wall formed by the quadrigeminal plate and pineal body, a roof formed by the lower surface of the splenium, and lateral walls formed by the part of the pulvinars located just lateral to the pineal body, and the cortical areas located below the splenium. The atrium is separated from the quadrigeminal cistern by the crus of the fornix and the cortical gyri located in the lateral wall of the posterior incisural space.

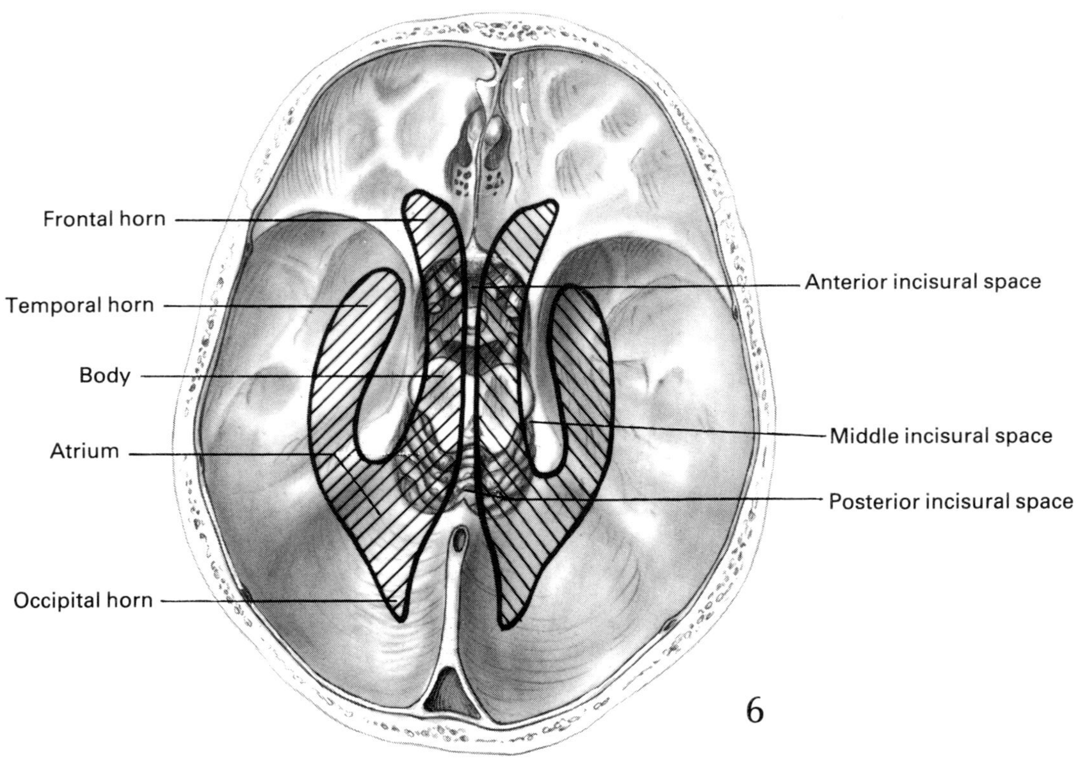


6

## Arterial relationships

# 7

Arterial relationships of the lateral ventricles are shown in *Illustration 7* in lateral (top), superior (middle), and anterior (lower) views. Each part of the lateral ventricle has surgically important arterial relationships: all of the arterial components of the circle of Willis are located in the anterior incisural space below the frontal horns and bodies of the lateral ventricles. The internal carotid arteries bifurcate into the anterior and middle cerebral arteries in the area below the frontal horns, and give rise to the anterior choroidal arteries, which send branches through the choroidal fissures to the choroid plexus. The posterior part of the circle of Willis and the apex of the basilar artery are situated below the thalami and bodies of the lateral ventricles. The anterior cerebral arteries pass around the floor and anterior wall of the frontal horns to reach the roof of the frontal horns and bodies; the posterior cerebral arteries pass medial to the temporal horns and atria in the ambient and quadrigeminal cisterns and give rise to the posterior choroidal arteries, which supply the choroid plexus in the temporal horns, atria and bodies[1, 3, 5].

The arteries most intimately related to the lateral ventricles and choroidal fissures are the choroidal arteries which supply the choroid plexus in the lateral and third ventricles. They arise from the internal carotid and posterior cerebral arteries in the basal cisterns and reach the choroid plexus by passing through the choroidal fissures. The most common pattern is for the anterior choroidal artery to supply a portion of the choroid plexus in the temporal horn and atrium; the lateral posterior choroidal arteries to supply a portion of the choroid plexus in the atrium, body and posterior part of the temporal horn; and the medial posterior choroidal arteries to supply the choroid plexus in the roof of the third ventricle and part of that in the body of the lateral ventricle.

The anterior choroidal artery arises from the internal carotid artery, courses between the cerebral peduncle and uncus and below the optic tract, passes through the choroidal fissure near the inferior choroidal point, and courses along the medial border of the choroid plexus in the temporal horn.

The lateral posterior choroidal arteries range in number from one to six branches and arise in the ambient and quadrigeminal cisterns from the posterior cerebral artery. They pass laterally around the pulvinar and through the choroidal fissure to reach the choroid plexus in the temporal horn, atrium and body.

The medial posterior choroidal arteries arise as one to three branches from the proximal part of the posterior cerebral artery in the interpeduncular and crural cisterns; they encircle the midbrain medial to the main trunk of the posterior cerebral artery, turn forward at the side of the pineal gland to enter the roof of the third ventricle, and course in the velum interpositum adjacent to the internal cerebral veins. They supply the choroid plexus in the roof of the third ventricle and sometimes pass through the foramen of Monro or choroidal fissures to supply the choroid plexus in the lateral ventricles.

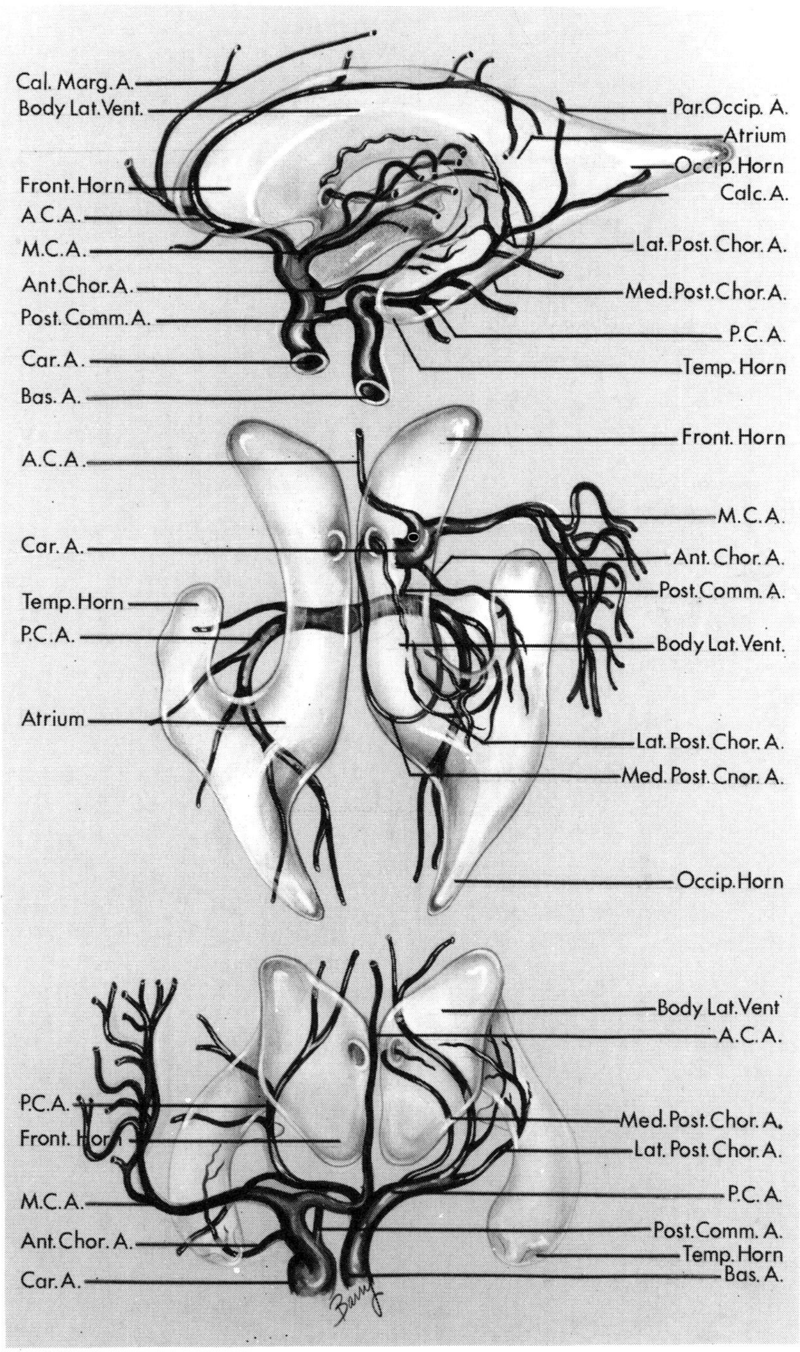
Cal. Marg. A.
Body Lat. Vent.
Front. Horn
A C.A.
M.C.A.
Ant. Chor. A.
Post. Comm. A.
Car. A.
Bas. A.
Par. Occip. A.
Atrium
Occip. Horn
Calc. A.
Lat. Post. Chor. A.
Med. Post. Chor. A.
P.C.A.
Temp. Horn
A.C.A.
Car. A.
Temp. Horn
P.C.A.
Atrium
Front. Horn
M.C.A.
Ant. Chor. A.
Post. Comm. A.
Body Lat. Vent.
Lat. Post. Chor. A.
Med. Post. Cnor. A.
Occip. Horn
P.C.A.
M.C.A.
Ant. Chor. A.
Car. A.
Body Lat. Vent
A.C.A.
Med. Post. Chor. A.
Lat. Post. Chor. A.
P.C.A.
Post. Comm. A.
Temp. Horn
Bas. A.

7

# Venous relationships

## 8

The venous relationships of the lateral ventricles are shown in *Illustration 8* in lateral (top), anterior (middle) and superior (lower) views. The deep venous system of the brain collects into channels that course in a subependymal location through the walls of the lateral ventricles and pass through the margins of the choroidal fissure to reach the internal cerebral, basal and great veins[1,4,6]. In general, the veins draining the frontal horn and body of the lateral ventricle drain into the internal cerebral vein as it courses through the velum interpositum; those draining the temporal horn drain into the segment of the basal vein coursing through the ambient cistern; and the veins from the atrium drain into the segments of the basal, internal cerebral and great veins coursing through the quadrigeminal cistern.

During operations on the lateral ventricles, the veins provide orientating landmarks more commonly than the arteries because the arteries in the ventricular walls are small and poorly seen, but the veins are larger and are easily visible through the ependyma. These venous landmarks are especially helpful in the presence of hydrocephalus, when the normal angles between the neural structures disappear.

The ventricular veins are divided into medial and lateral groups based on whether they course through the thalamic or forniceal side of the choroidal fissure: the lateral group passes through the thalamic or inner side of the fissure, and the medial group passes through the outer or forniceal circumference of the fissure. The veins comprising the medial and lateral groups frequently join near the choroidal fissure to form a common stem before terminating in the large veins in the velum interpositum and basal cisterns.

The medial group of veins in the frontal horn and body is formed by the anterior and posterior septal veins, and the lateral group consists of the thalamostriate, thalamocaudate, and anterior and posterior caudate veins. The veins of the lateral group are larger than those of the medial group. The veins in the lateral group penetrate the tenia choroidea to reach the velum interpositum.

The anterior septal veins course in the frontal horn on the septum pellucidum and the posterior septal veins course on the septum pellucidum in the body. They terminate by penetrating the junction of the fornix and septum pellucidum to enter the velum interpositum where they join the internal cerebral vein. The anterior caudate veins course on the lateral wall of the frontal horn and terminate near the foramen of Monro in the thalamostriate vein. The posterior caudate veins originate at the lateral edge of the body of the ventricle and course across the caudate nucleus to terminate in the thalamostriate or thalamocaudate veins.

The thalamostriate vein passes forward in the sulcus between the caudate nucleus and thalamus towards the foramen of Monro, where it turns sharply posterior through the posterior margin of the foramen of Monro and enters the velum interpositum to join the internal cerebral vein. The angle formed by the junction of the thalamostriate and internal cerebral veins, called the venous angle, as seen on the lateral view of the cerebral angiogram, approximates the site of the foramen of Monro. In some cases, this venous angle will not approximate the site of the foramen of Monro because the thalamostriate vein passes through the choroidal fissure well behind the foramen of Monro. If the thalamostriate vein is small or absent, the thalamocaudate vein will drain the same area. The thalamocaudate vein courses medially across the caudate nucleus and thalamus behind the posterior extent of the thalamostriate vein and passes through the margin of the choroidal fissure well behind the foramen of Monro. It ends in the internal cerebral vein.

The medial group of veins in the atrium and occipital horn consists of the medial atrial veins, and the lateral group is composed of the lateral atrial veins. The medial atrial veins course forward on the medial wall of the atrium and occipital horn, and pass through the margin of the choroidal fissure to terminate within the velum interpositum or quadrigeminal cistern by joining the internal cerebral, basal or great vein. The lateral atrial veins course forward on the lateral wall of the atrium to reach the anterior wall, where they turn medially on the posterior surface of the pulvinar and pass through the choroidal fissure to reach the quadrigeminal cistern, where they join the internal cerebral, basal, or great veins. The medial and lateral atrial veins may join near the choroidal fissure to form a common trunk called the common atrial vein.

The lateral group in the temporal horn is formed by the inferior ventricular and amygdalar veins and the medial group is formed by the transverse hippocampal veins. The inferior ventricular vein arises in the posterior and lateral part of the roof of the temporal horn, courses anterior and medially, exits the temporal horn just behind the inferior choroidal point and joins the basal vein. The amygdalar vein courses across the ventricular surface of the amygdaloid nucleus and terminates in the inferior ventricular or basal vein. The transverse hippocampal veins are a group of very fine veins that course medially across the hippocampal formation and collateral eminence. They penetrate the attachment of the fimbria to the hippocampus to enter the ambient cistern, where they empty into tributaries of the basal vein.

The superior and inferior choroidal veins are the largest veins on the choroid plexus. The superior choroidal vein runs forward on the choroid plexus in the body of the lateral ventricle and terminates near the foramen of Monro in the internal cerebral vein or its tributaries. The inferior choroidal vein courses anteriorly in the temporal horn along the inferior end of the choroidal plexus and terminates by passing through the choroidal fissure near the inferior choroidal point to terminate in the basal vein or its tributaries. The superior and inferior choroidal veins frequently anastomose on the choroid plexus in the atrium.

The venous relationships in the quadrigeminal cistern medial to the atria are the most complex in the cranium because the internal cerebral, basal and great veins, and many of their tributaries converge on this area. The internal cerebral veins originate just behind the foramen of Monro and course posteriorly within the velum interpositum. The union of the paired internal cerebral veins to form the great vein may be located above or posterior to the pineal body and inferior or posterior to the splenium. The basal vein is formed on the anterior perforated substance below the frontal horn; it proceeds posteriorly between the midbrain and temporal lobe to drain the walls of the crural and ambient cisterns, and terminates within the quadrigeminal cistern by joining the internal cerebral or great vein. The great vein passes below the splenium to enter the straight sinus at the tentorial apex.

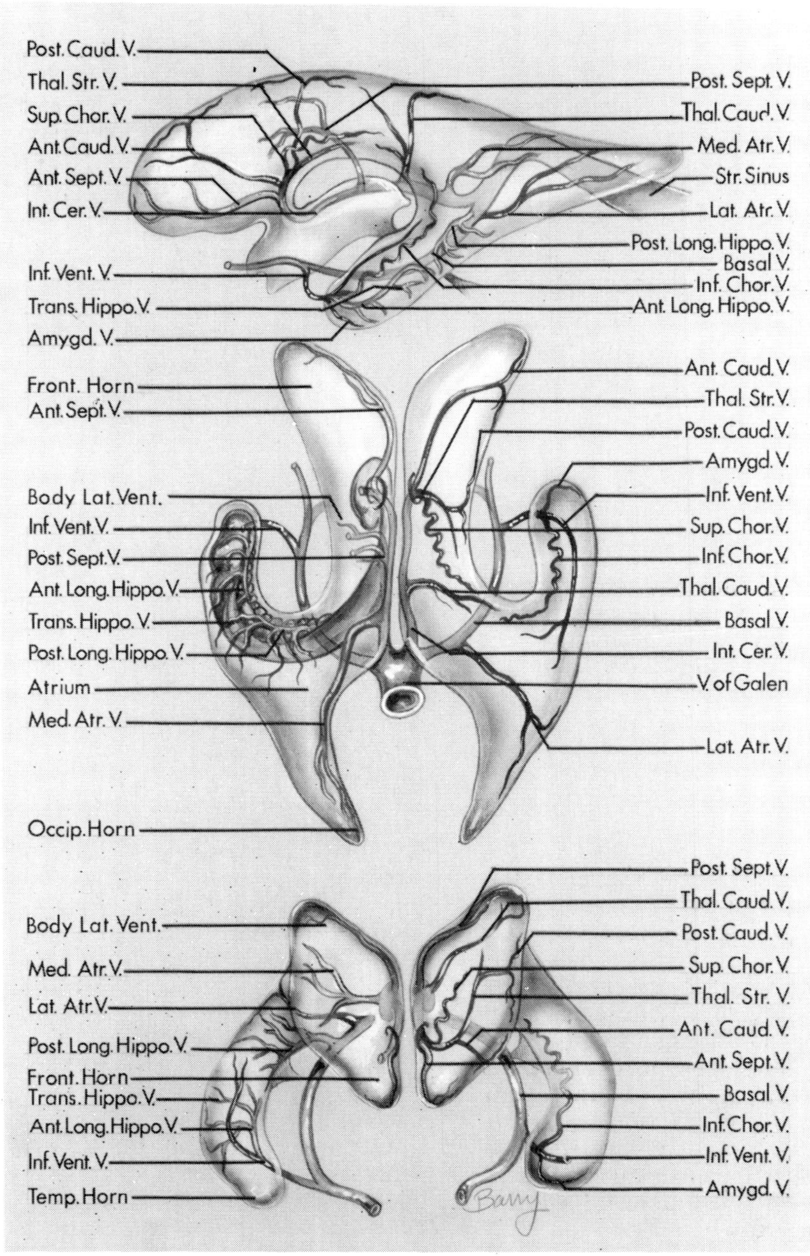


8

# Possible operative approaches

# 9

The selection of the best operative approach to a lesion in the lateral ventricles is determined by the site of the lesion, the size of the lateral ventricles and the relationships of the lesion to the third ventricle and basal cisterns. Various surgical approaches are shown in the illustration, the site of the skin incision (solid line) and the bone flap (interrupted line) being shown for each approach. This section reviews some general principles applicable to all of the operative approaches to the lateral ventricles.

## Neural incisions

It is impossible to reach the lateral ventricles without opening some neural structures. The surgical approaches to the lateral ventricle may require cortical incisions in the frontal, parietal or temporal lobes, and the anterior or posterior part of the corpus callosum; division or displacement of the fornix; and opening of the choroidal fissure and septum pellucidum. The brain may be retracted to expose an external wall of the ventricle such as the corpus callosum, but the wall must then be incised to reach the ventricle. After reaching the lateral ventricles, another neural incision through a site such as the fornix, or opening of the choroidal fissure, is needed to expose those lesions which extend into the third ventricle or the basal cisterns.

When opening the choroidal fissure, it is better to open through the tenia fornicis and tenia fimbriae than through the tenia choroidea, as fewer arteries and veins pass through these (*see Illustration 10d*). The branches of the medial and lateral posterior and anterior choroidal arteries enter the ventricle, and the thalamostriate, thalamocaudate, lateral atrial and inferior ventricular veins exit the ventricle by passing through the tenia choroidea. None of the choroidal arteries or the major ventricular veins pass through the tenia fornicis or the tenia fimbriae. Opening through the choroidal fissure in the body of the ventricle will expose the velum interpositum and the roof of the third ventricle; opening through it in the atrium will expose the quadrigeminal cistern and the pineal region; opening through it in the temporal horn will expose the crural and ambient cisterns.

The incision and retraction of neural structures in order to reach the lateral ventricles produces variable results: in some cases there has been no deficit, and in others the deficit has been transient or permanent or has resulted in the loss of life. Structures sacrificed with variable results include the anterior and posterior parts of the corpus callosum and various parts of the fornix. Callosal incisions have resulted in disorders of the interhemispheric transfer of information, visuospatial transfer, the learning of bimanual motor tasks, and memory, and also in deficits such as alexia, apraxia and astereognosis[7–9]. The cerebral retraction and cortical incisions needed for the anterior and posterior transcallosal approaches have caused convulsions, hemiplegia, mutism, impairment of consciousness, and visual field loss[10–12]. Manipulation of lesions extending into the walls of the third ventricle may cause hypothalamic dysfunction as manifested by disturbances of temperature control, respiration, consciousness and hypophyseal secretion; also, visual loss owing to damage of the optic chiasm and tracts, and memory loss owing to injury to the body and columns of the fornix may occur [11, 13]. Dissection medial to the atrium in the area of the quadrigeminal plate may cause disorders of eye movement, oedematous closure of the aqueduct of Sylvius, blindness from oedema in the colliculi or geniculate bodies, and extraocular palsies due to oedema of the nuclei of the nerves or the central pathways in the brain stem[14, 15].

Opening the choroidal fissure carries the risk of damaging the fornix. However, unilateral damage to the fornix produces no deficit and damage to the forniceal fibres from both hemispheres does not usually produce a permanent memory loss[16–19]. This is evidence that lesions in the crus and hippocampal commissure have a more deleterious effect on memory than lesions in the body or columns[20, 21]. Opening the temporal part of the choroidal fissure risks damaging the fimbria and hippocampal formation. However, unilateral damage of the hippocampal formation produces no deficit[20–23].

## Arterial considerations

Intraventricular tumours and arteriovenous malformations are commonly supplied by the choroidal arteries. The fact that the choroidal arteries converge on and pass through the choroidal fissure assists in identifying this fissure. Opening through the fissure in the body of the ventricle will expose the medial posterior choroidal arteries in the velum interpositum and the roof of the third ventricle; opening through the fissure in the atrium will expose the medial and lateral posterior choroidal arteries in the quadrigeminal cistern and the pineal region; and opening through it in the temporal horn will expose the anterior, and the medial and lateral posterior choroidal arteries in the ambient cistern.

Other arteries which may also be exposed in removing tumours of the lateral ventricle are the anterior cerebral and anterior communicating arteries in the region of the frontal horns and bodies, the posterior part of the circle of Willis, the apex of the basilar artery and the proximal part of the posterior cerebral arteries in the area medial to the temporal horns, the distal part of the posterior cerebral arteries in the area medial to the atria, and branches of both the anterior and the posterior cerebral arteries in the roof of the bodies and atria. Extreme effort should be made to avoid sacrificing any of these arteries. Occlusion of the perforating branches of these arteries at the anterior part of the circle of Willis is likely to result in disturbances of memory and personality, and occlusion of those at the posterior part of the circle of Willis is more likely to result in disorders in the level of consciousness.

## Venous considerations

The ventricular veins provide valuable landmarks in directing the operator to the foramen of Monro and choroidal fissure during operations on the ventricles. This is especially true if hydrocephalus, as commonly occurs with ventricular tumours, is present, because the borders between the neural structures in the ventricular walls become less distinct as the ventricles dilate.

The number of veins sacrificed when approaching a ventricular lesion should be kept to a minimum because of the undesirable consequences of their loss. Obliteration of the deep veins, including the great, basal and internal cerebral veins and their tributaries, and the bridging veins from the cerebrum to the dural sinuses, is inescapable in reaching and removing some tumours in or near the ventricles. Before sacrificing these veins, one should try placing them under moderate or even severe stretch (accepting the fact that they may be torn) if it will allow satisfactory exposure and yield some possibility of the veins being saved. Before sacrificing the basal, internal cerebral and great veins, one should attempt to work around them or displace them out of the operative route, or try dividing only a few of their small branches, which may allow the displacement of the main trunk out of the operative field.

Sacrifice of branches of the superficial and deep venous systems has produced inconsistent deficits. Dandy[14, 15] noted that one internal cerebral vein could be sacrificed without effect, and on a few occasions both veins and even the great vein of Galen could be ligated without any apparent disturbance of function on recovery. Alternatively, it seems that injury to this venous network may cause diencephalic oedema, mental symptoms, coma, hyperpyrexia, tachycardia, tachypnoea, miosis, rigidity of limbs and exaggeration of deep tendon reflexes[24–26]. Occlusion of the thalamostriate and other veins at the foramen of Monro may cause drowsiness, hemiplegia, mutism and haemorrhagic infarction of the basal ganglia[10]. Obliteration of veins coursing between the cerebrum and the superior sagittal sinus anterior or posterior to the Rolandic vein, as may be required in the transcallosal approaches, although usually not causing a deficit, may be accompanied by hemiplegia[27]. Sacrifice of the internal occipital vein or the bridging veins from the occipital pole to the superior sagittal or transverse sinuses may cause hemianopia[26].

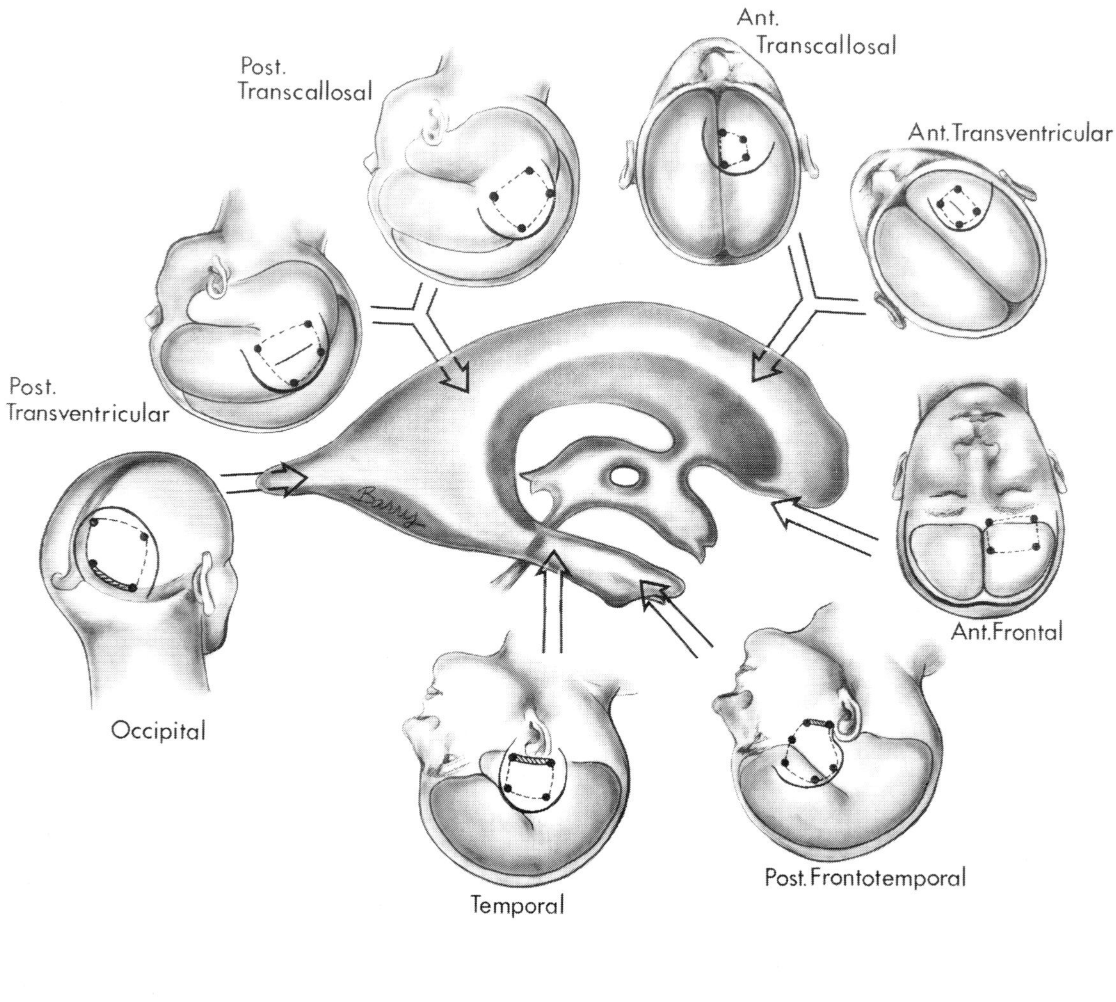


9

# Operative approaches

The routes to the lateral ventricles are divided into anterior, posterior and inferior approaches. The anterior approaches are directed to the frontal horn and body of the lateral ventricle. The posterior approaches are directed to the atrium and the inferior approaches are directed to the temporal horn.

## Anterior approaches

# 10a–i

Lesions within the frontal horn and anterior portion of the body of the lateral ventricle are most commonly reached by the anterior transcallosal or anterior transcortical approaches. The transcallosal approach is easier to perform than the transcortical approach if the ventricles are of a normal size or are minimally enlarged. On occasion an anterior frontal approach may be combined with an approach along the adjacent part of the interhemispheric fissure to reach the anterior wall and floor of the frontal horn.

### *Anterior transcallosal approach*

This approach is suitable for reaching lesions located within the frontal horn and body of the lateral ventricle, and for exposing the anterosuperior part of the third ventricle through the lateral ventricle[2, 27, 28]. The patient is positioned supine with the head elevated 20–30°. A right frontal horse-shoe or a Souttar skin incision is used (*a*). The right frontal bone flap, extending to the lateral edge of, or across the sagittal sinus, is centred on the coronal suture. The dura is opened with the base on the sagittal sinus. The cortical veins entering the superior sagittal sinus are protected: some, usually no more than one, may have to be divided in order to retract the medial surface of the right frontal lobe away from the falx. The arachnoid membrane, encountered deep to the free edge of the falx, is opened. The right and left cingulate gyri, which face each other, are separated to expose the corpus callosum and the anterior cerebral arteries. The approach is directed between the pericallosal arteries, although some of their branches may cross the midline above the corpus callosum.

The part of the corpus callosum above the foramen of Monro is split in the midline. An incision 3 cm in length extending forward into the genu provides satisfactory access to both lateral ventricles. When the ventricle is opened, either by the transcallosal or transventricular approach, the foramen of Monro is found by following the attachment of the choroid plexus and the thalamostriate vein anteriorly since both converge on this foramen (*b*). The opening into the lateral ventricle may expose the frontal horn and body on the same or opposite side of the cranial exposure, but the anatomy makes this obvious. A simple rule for finding whether the left or right lateral ventricle has been exposed is to determine whether the thalamostriate vein is to the left or right side of the choroid plexus: the left lateral ventricle has been opened if the thalamostriate vein is further to the patient's left side than the choroid plexus: the right lateral ventricle has been entered if the thalamostriate vein is further to the patient's right side than the choroid plexus. Opening the septum pellucidum will provide access to the opposite lateral ventricle and to the opening of the foramen of Monro into both lateral ventricles. Entry into a cavity between the leaves of the septum pellucidum may be confusing until one realizes that no intraventricular structures are present (*c*).

The close relationship of the genu of the internal capsule to the foramen of Monro should be borne in mind when retracting the walls of the lateral ventricle. The genu of the internal capsule touches the wall of the ventricle in the area lateral to the foramen of Monro near the anterior pole of the thalamus. Care should be exercised in retracting this area since a thin brain spatula could easily cut into the ventricular wall in this critical region.

An incision is made anteriorly through one column of the fornix at the anterosuperior edge of the foramen of Monro only if it is needed in order to explore a deeper portion of the anterior part of the third ventricle (see *Illustration 10b, '1 and 2'*). To prevent the complications associated with sectioning the fornix, Hirsch *et al.*[10] sectioned the thalamostriate vein at the posterior margin of the foramen of Monro rather than damaging the fornix to enlarge the opening into the third ventricle. However, this may cause drowsiness, hemiplegia and mutism owing to haemorrhagic infarction of the basal ganglia[11].

Routes through the lateral ventricles to the anterior part of the third ventricle (other than by incising the ipsilateral column of the fornix), are by the transforniceal approach, in which the body of the fornix is split in the midline in the direction of its fibres to expose the velum interpositum (see *Illustration 10b, '2'*). The transchoroidal approach, in which the choroidal fissure is opened by incising along the tenia fornicis, can also be used (see *Illustration 10b, '3'*), thus allowing the fornix to be pushed to the opposite side in order to expose the structures in the roof of the third ventricle (see *also Illustration 5*)[16, 29–31]. The transchoroidal and transforniceal approaches have the advantage of giving access to the central portion of the third ventricle behind the foramen of Monro by displacing, rather than transecting, the fibres in the fornix. When using the approach through the corpus callosum the transforniceal and transchoroidal openings provide a satisfactory view into the third ventricle. When the approach through the middle frontal gyrus is used the transchoroidal approach provides a better view into the third ventricle than the transforniceal route. It is both easier and safer to direct the transchoroidal approach through the tenia fornicis than through the tenia choroidea because larger vessels pass through the tenia choroidea than through the tenia fornicis. The transchoroidal approach is especially well suited to lesions that are fed by the terminal branches of the choroidal arteries.

In the transchoroidal approach, the third ventricle is exposed by opening the choroidal fissure along the tenia fornicis and displacing the fornix to the opposite side, after which the roof of the third ventricle is entered by opening the layers of tela choroidea. Opening through the velum interpositum in the interval between the internal cerebral veins allows a more extensive exposure of the third ventricle than if the third ventricle is exposed between the ipsilateral internal cerebral vein and the thalamus. It is often necessary to sacrifice some of the branches of the internal cerebral vein if the third ventricle is entered on the lateral side of the internal cerebral vein. However, the roof of the third ventricle can commonly be entered without sacrificing any branches of the internal cerebral veins if the approach is directed between these veins. After opening the lower layer of tela choroidea, the choroid plexus in the roof of the third ventricle, the sulcus limitans, massa intermedia and the floor of the third ventricle are encountered.

### *Anterior transcortical approach*

This approach is suitable for lesions in the anterior part of the lateral ventricle and the anterosuperior part of the third ventricle, especially if the tumour is situated predominantly in the lateral ventricle on the side of the approach. It is more difficult to expose the anterior part of the lateral ventricle on the side opposite to the approach through the transcortical than through the transcallosal approach. The transcortical approach is facilitated if the lateral ventricles are enlarged.

With the patient supine, the head is rotated slightly to the side opposite the frontal lobe through which the ventricle is to be approached. The scalp and bone flaps are positioned over the central part of the middle frontal gyrus. If the approach is through the dominant hemisphere, care is taken to place the cortical incision above and anterior to the expressive speech centres on the inferior frontal gyrus and anterior to the precentral motor strip. The dilated frontal horn is reached through a small cortical incision located in the long axis of the middle frontal gyrus. Once inside the ventricle the landmarks and approaches to the third ventricle are the same as those described for the transcallosal approach. The removal of a colloid cyst by this technique using an incision in the ipsilateral column of the fornix is shown in *Illustrations 10d and e*.

The colloid cyst is first aspirated with a needle through the foramen of Monro. It may be necessary to divide the column of the fornix to enlarge the foramen of Monro, although it is frequently possible to perform the entire operation without such division. It is extremely important that if the division of one column of the fornix is undertaken, the other column must be left intact lest recent memory disturbances occur. Grumous material within the cyst is then removed using suction, perhaps with the addition of forceps extraction (*e*). In the case of a very large colloid cyst, an approach through the choroidal fissure may be preferable (*f,g*). A colloid cyst that obstructs the foramen of Monro may be further exposed by opening the choroidal fissure along the attachment of the choroid plexus to the fornix (*f*). This exposes the internal cerebral veins and medial posterior choroidal arteries behind the foramen of Monro. *Illustration 10g* shows the final remnant of the attachment of the cyst to the choroidal plexus being coagulated.

Elaboration of this exposure by opening the septum pellucidum to expose both frontal horns and bodies of both lateral ventricles is shown in *Illustration 10h*. In *Illustration 10i* the body of the fornix has been split in the midline to expose the third ventricle, and the internal cerebral veins and the medial posterior choroidal arteries in the roof of the third ventricle. This transfornical approach is suitable for exposing lesions located in the third ventricle behind the foramen of Monro.

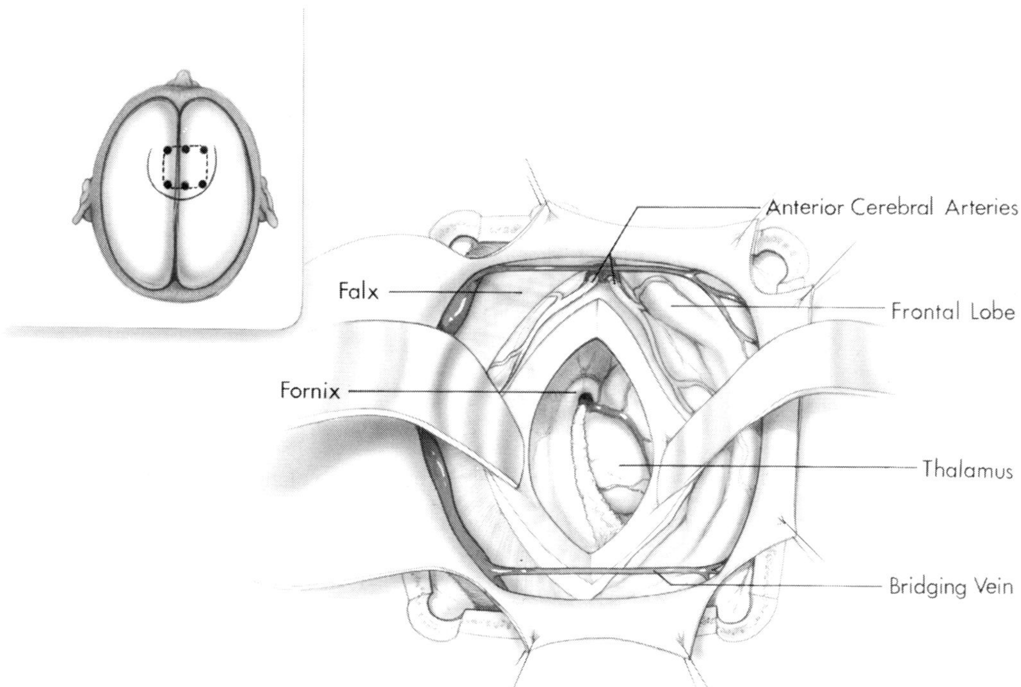


10a

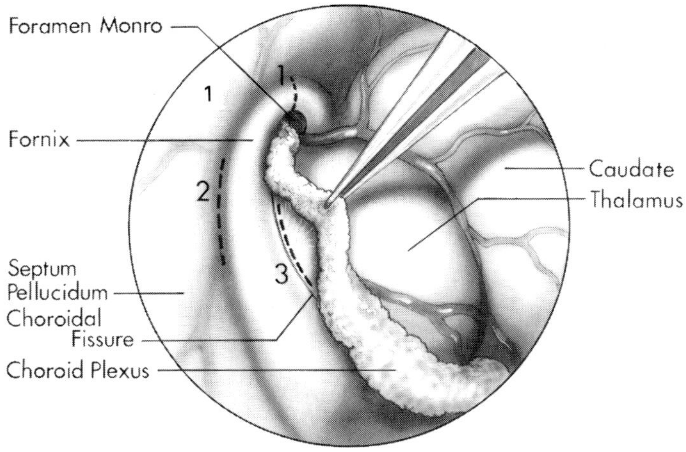


10b

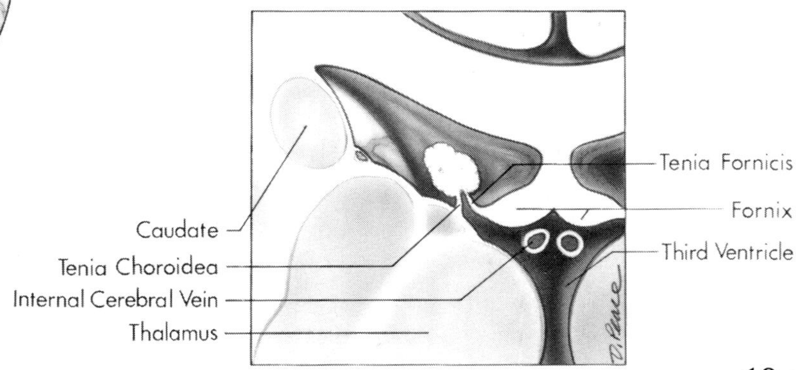


10c

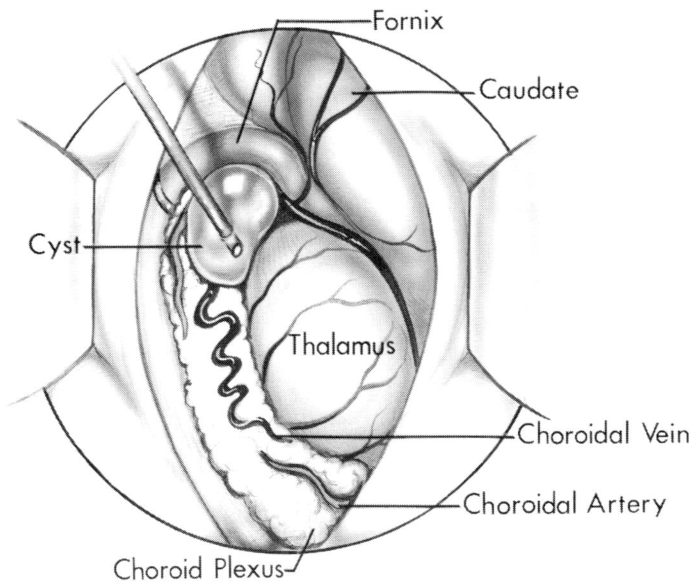


10d

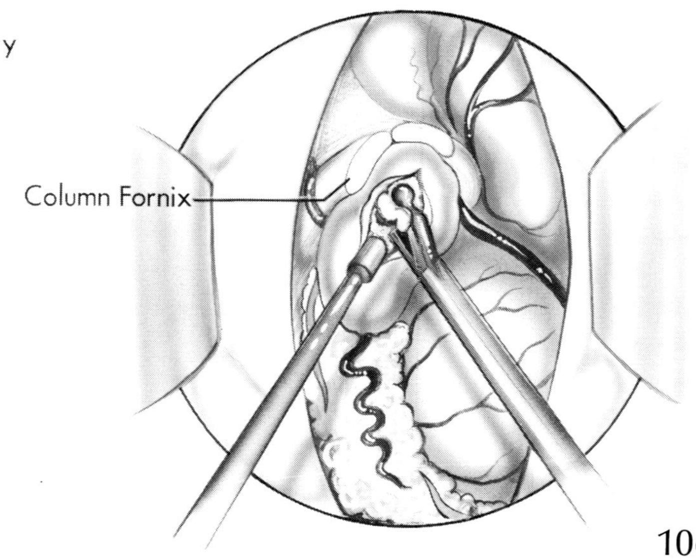


10e

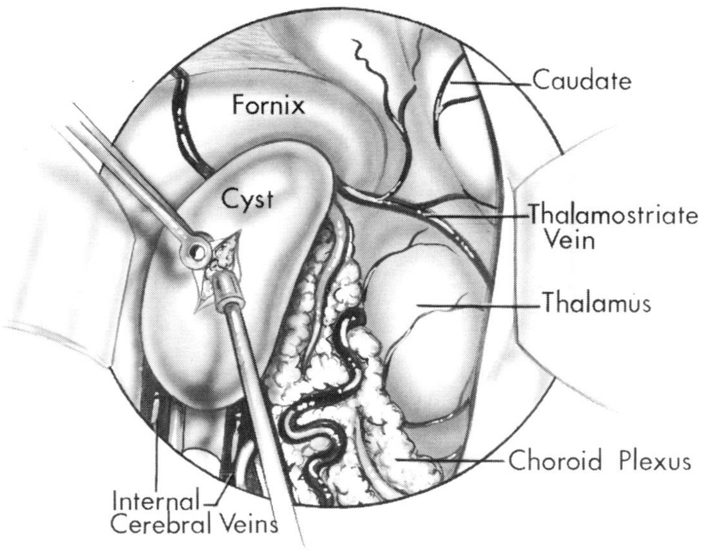


10f

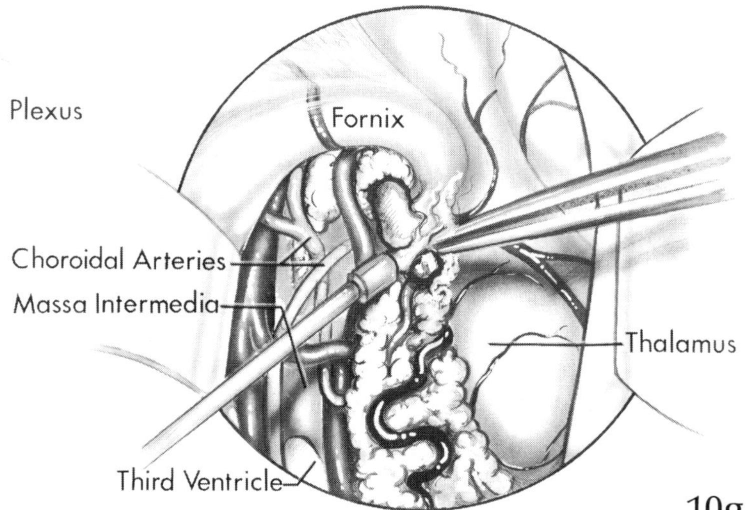


10g

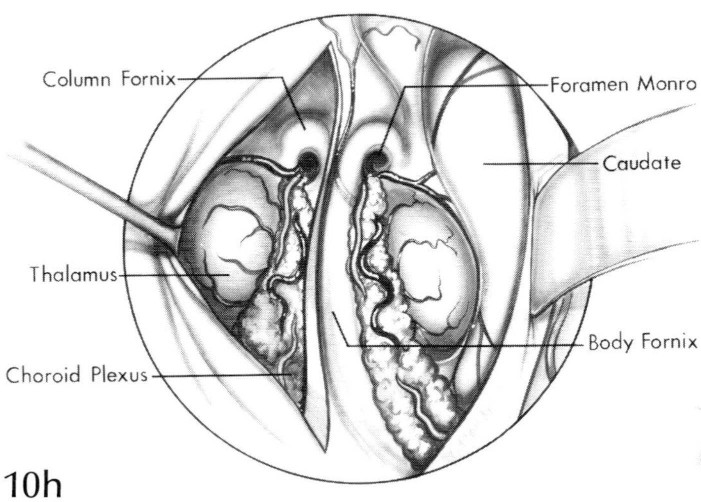


10h

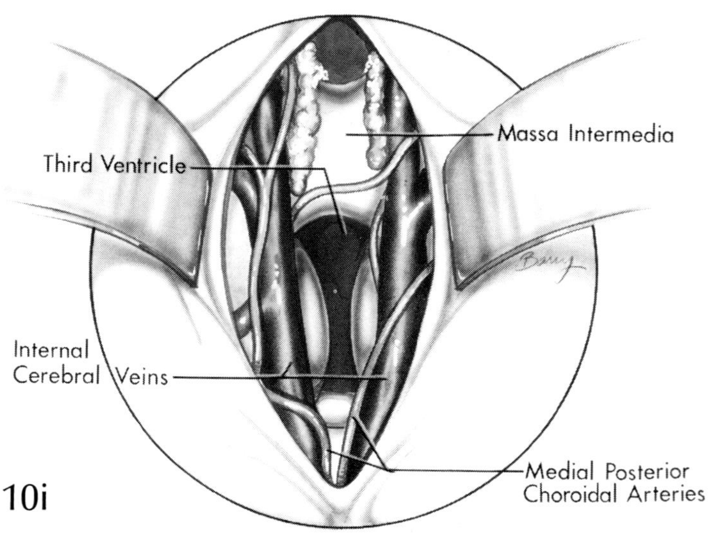


10i

# 11a–e

The position of the scalp flap (*a*), normal lateral ventricular anatomy (*b*), and the details of the third ventricle following opening of the choroid fissure (*c*) are illustrated.

A choroid plexus papilloma has been exposed using the transcortical approach (*d*). The illustration inset shows the site of the tumour and the position of the head for the operation. The tumour should be removed with the aid of an ultrasonic aspirator and extra suction since these are often extremely vascular lesions. The last remnant of the tumour is then removed from its attachment to the choroid plexus (*e*).

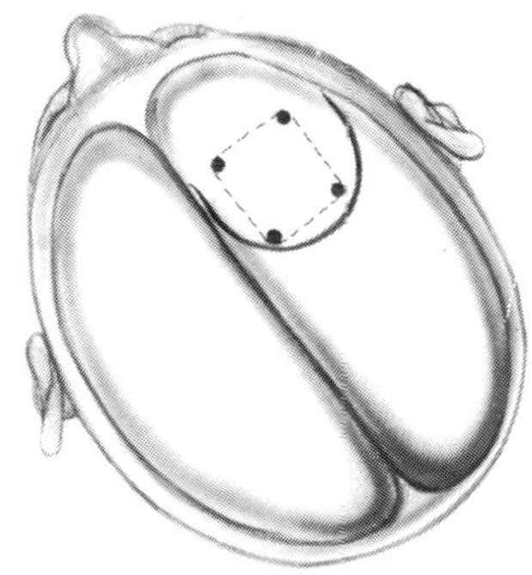

11a

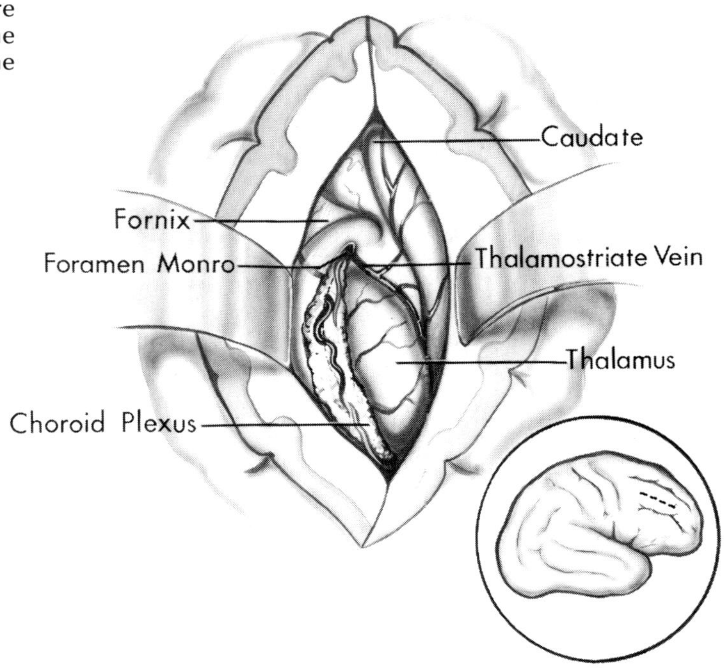


11b

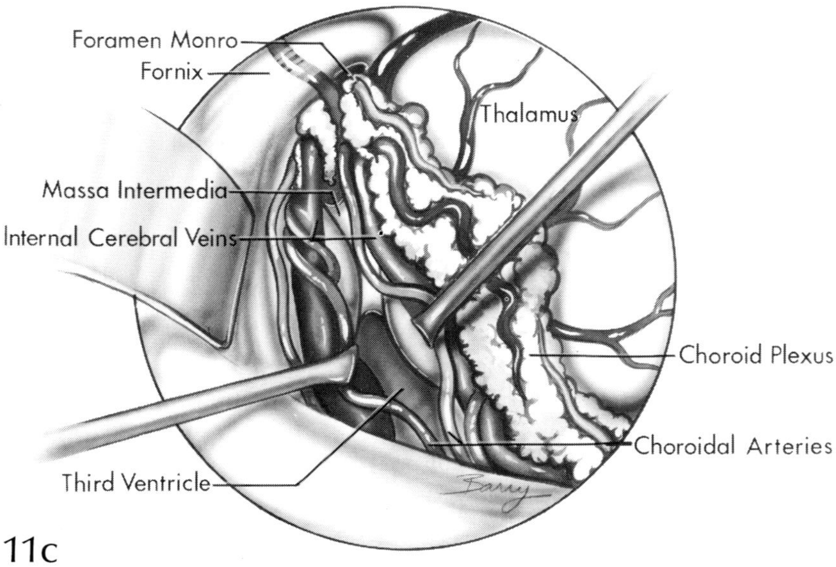
Foramen Monro
Fornix
Thalamus
Massa Intermedia
Internal Cerebral Veins
Choroid Plexus
Choroidal Arteries
Third Ventricle

11c

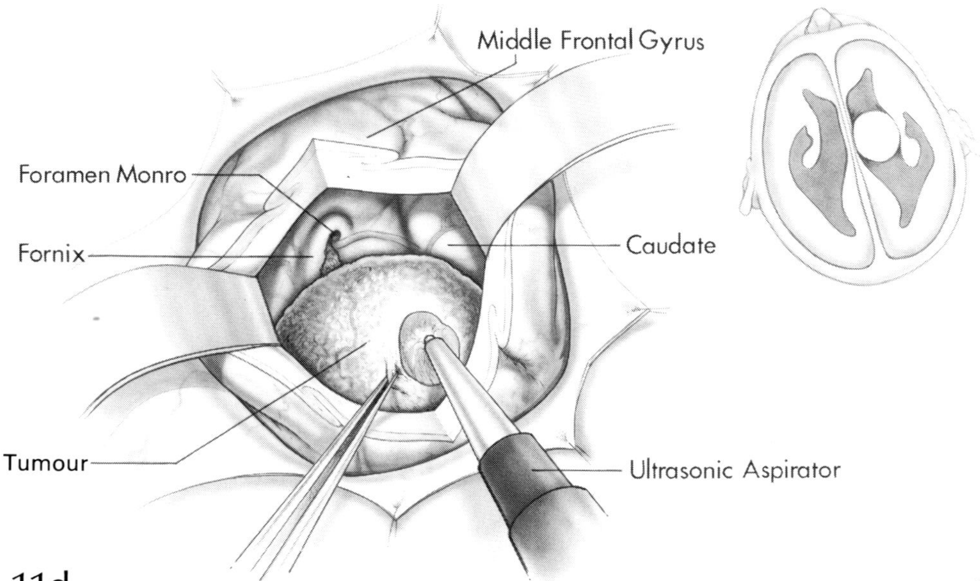
Middle Frontal Gyrus
Foramen Monro
Fornix
Caudate
Tumour
Ultrasonic Aspirator

11d

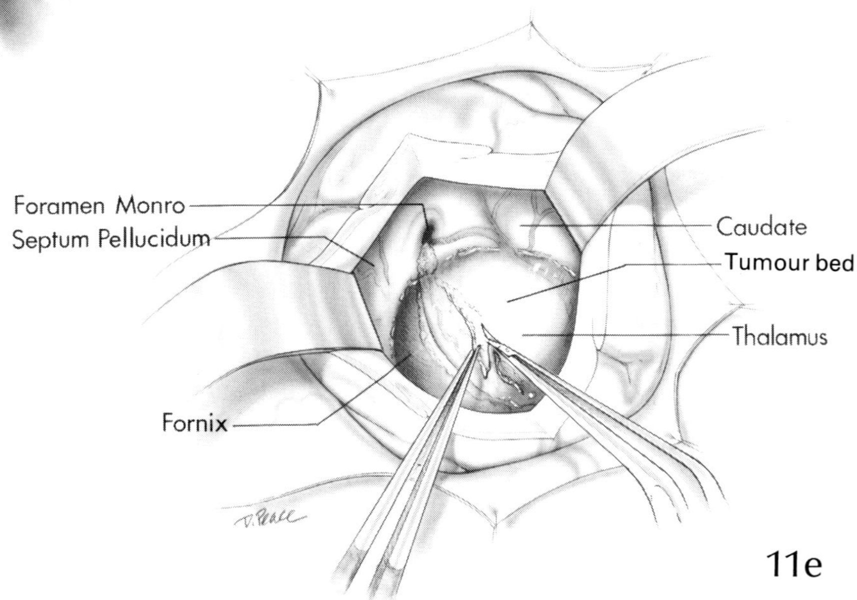
Foramen Monro
Septum Pellucidum
Caudate
Tumour bed
Thalamus
Fornix

11e

# 12a–e

*Anterior frontal approach*

The anterior frontal approach may be considered for a lesion involving the floor and lower part of the anterior wall of the frontal horn that extends into the third ventricle behind the lamina terminalis[1, 32]. This approach is not suitable for reaching a lesion in the body of the lateral ventricle or in the third ventricle behind the foramen of Monro.

The patient is positioned supine with the face looking directly upward. A Souttar scalp incision is used (*a*). A unilateral bone flap extending to the edge of the superior sagittal sinus is elevated. The lower margin of the flap is positioned just above the supraorbital ridge if the lesion is in the rostrum and adjacent part of the lamina terminalis, but it would be placed higher if the lesion is located in the lower part of the genu of the corpus callosum. The dura is opened with the base on the superior sagittal sinus. The orbital surface of the frontal lobe is elevated and the arachnoid is opened to expose the optic nerves and chiasm, lamina terminalis and the anterior cerebral and anterior communicating arteries (*b*). The olfactory nerves may need to be divided above the cribriform plate to expose the area above the optic chiasm. The medial surface of the frontal lobe is retracted away from the falx to expose the rostrum and genu of the corpus callosum. One or two small bridging veins entering the superior and inferior sagittal sinus may need to be sacrificed in order to retract the frontal pole away from the falx. The arachnoid in the depths of the interhemispheric fissure is opened to expose the anterior cerebral arteries and their bifurcation into the pericallosal and callosomarginal arteries. The corpus callosum is exposed between the anterior cerebral arteries. Care should be taken to avoid occluding the perforating branches of the anterior communicating artery which extend into the walls of the third ventricle to supply columns of the fornix. A vertical incision beginning in the lamina terminalis and extending upward into the rostrum will expose a lesion in the floor of the frontal horn or straddling the lateral and third ventricular sides of the foramen of Monro (*c*). The landmarks within the ventricle have already been described.

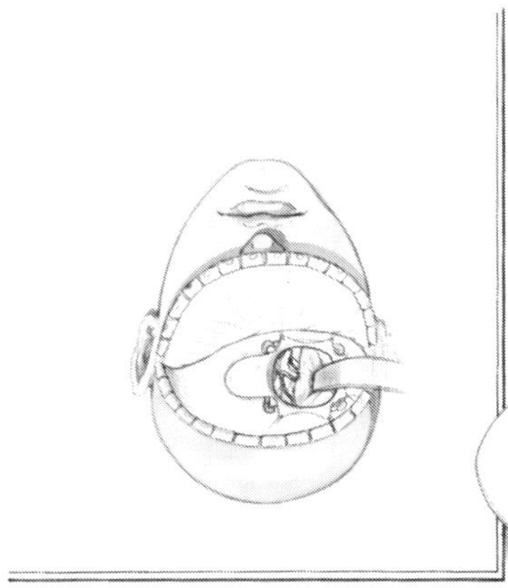

12a

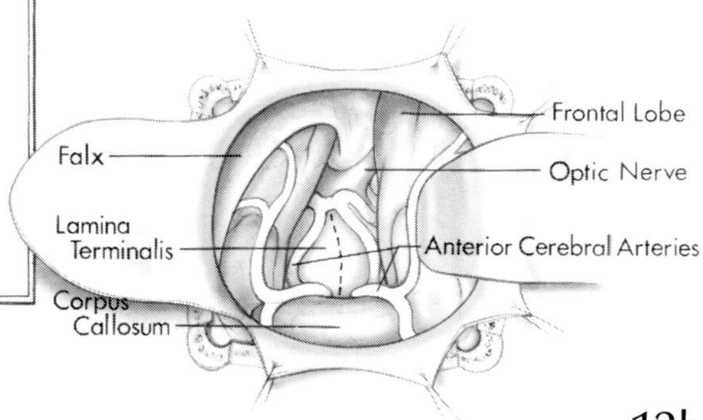


12b

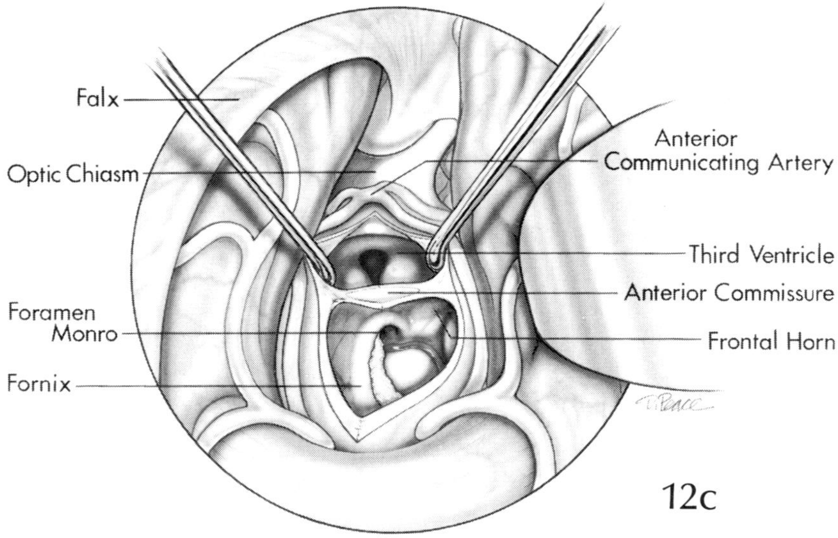
Falx
Optic Chiasm
Anterior Communicating Artery
Third Ventricle
Anterior Commissure
Foramen Monro
Frontal Horn
Fornix

12c

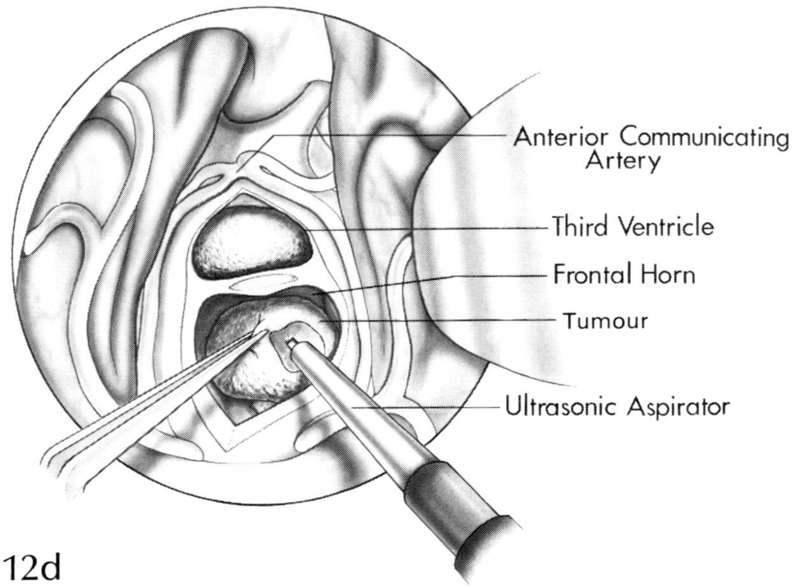
Anterior Communicating Artery
Third Ventricle
Frontal Horn
Tumour
Ultrasonic Aspirator

12d

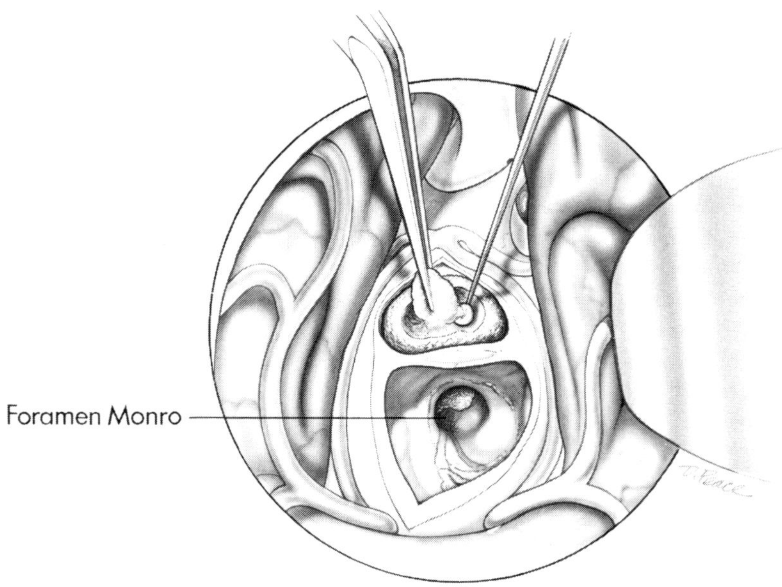
Foramen Monro

12e

## Posterior approaches

Lesions situated within the posterior part of the body and the atrium are most commonly exposed using a posterior transcortical approach. Selected lesions may be exposed by the posterior transcallosal or the occipital approaches. The transcallosal approach is considered if the lesion involves the splenium of the corpus callosum and extends into the ventricle from the roof or the upper part of the medial wall of the atrium. The approach directed along the occipital pole is used if the lesion arises in the medial wall of the atrium and extends into the ventricle and quadrigeminal cistern from the medial wall. Pineal tumours are removed by a posterior transventricular approach directed through the medial wall of the atrium. However, this area is very narrow and is heavily vascularized and this makes it difficult to approach these tumours by this route[33]. The occipital–transtentorial approach and the infratentorial–supracerebellar approaches are most commonly used for exposing pineal tumours.

### *Posterior transcortical approach*

# 13a–i

This is the preferred approach to a lesion situated entirely within the atrium or arising in the region of the glomus of the choroid plexus (*a*). Opening through the choroidal fissure from the atrium exposes the quadrigeminal cistern and pineal region. The transchoroidal approach to the quadrigeminal cistern is most commonly used for arteriovenous malformations or vascular tumours located behind the pulvinar in the region of the choroidal fissure.

The patient is positioned in the three-quarter prone position with the face turned toward the floor and the parietal area to be operated on uppermost (*b*). A high posterior parietal bone flap, centred behind the postcentral gyrus over the superior parietal lobule, is elevated (*c*). The cortex is incised in the long axis of the superior parietal lobule, preferably in a sulcus crossing the lobule (*d,e*). The atrium is also approached through cortical incisions in the superior and middle temporal gyri and the temporoparietal junction. However, exposing the atrium through the temporoparietal area may cause a homonymous visual field deficit owing to the interruption of the optic radiations in either hemisphere, disturbances of visuospatial function in the non-dominant hemisphere, and aphasia and agnostic disorders in the dominant hemisphere[2, 5, 34]. Opening through the middle temporal gyrus might be considered for a lesion in the dominant hemisphere. However, cortical mapping during surgery has revealed an occasional extension of the speech representative into the middle temporal gyrus[35]. When approaching through the superior parietal lobule the ventricle is entered above the junction of the body and crus of the fornix. This approach exposes the glomus of the choroid plexus. The medial and lateral atrial veins are seen converging on the choroidal fissure (*f*). The arterial supply of lesions in this area is predominantly from the lateral posterior choroidal arteries. This approach is illustrated (*h,i*) in the removal of a meningioma from the atrium of the lateral ventricle, a common site. The bulk of the tumour is removed using an ultrasonic aspirator (*h*) and the last remnant is removed with its attachment to the choroid plexus being coagulated (*i*). An alternative route to the atrium or trigone of the lateral ventricle is through the inferior temporal gyrus. Separation of the fibres of the tapetum produces a surprisingly small homonymous field deficit which frequently clears completely, and remaining low in the hemisphere prevents disturbances of visuospatial or speech function even in the dominant hemisphere. The lower the approach, the more readily accessible is the anterior choroidal supply to tumours arising in the trigonal region and it is possible to slip beneath such tumours as meningiomas in the trigone by this route, after partially de-bulking them, to pick up the medial blood supply from the lateral posterior choroidal vessels.

To reach the quadrigeminal cistern the choroidal fissure is opened by retracting the glomus of the choroid plexus laterally and incising along the tenia fornicis with a fine knife. Care is taken to avoid damaging the lateral posterior choroidal arteries that course medial to the choroidal fissure. Retracting the crus medially and posteriorly exposes the quadrigeminal cistern and the caudal portion of the ambient cistern (*g*). Retraction should be carefully applied as it may damage the calcar avis and underlying visual cortex. Retraction of the pulvinar should be minimized in order to prevent language and speech disturbances in the dominant hemisphere. If the pulvinar bulges too far posteriorly, a supplemental horizontal incision in the medial wall of the atrium behind the crus may be needed in order to avoid retraction of the pulvinar. However, extending this incision posteriorly into the calcar avis will cause a visual field deficit. The opening into the quadrigeminal cisterns may also be obtained by making an arcuate incision along the direction of the fibres in the crus of the fornix. This incision should spare the contralateral half of the fornix. However, avoiding the contralateral half of the fornix is easier in this area than in the body of the ventricle because the crura have separated at the level of the atrium.

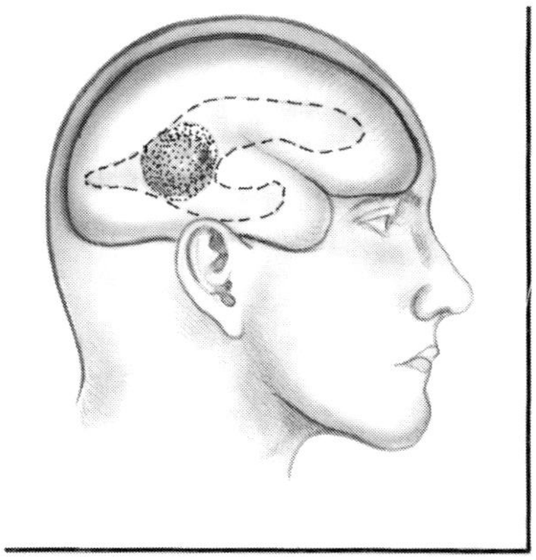

13a

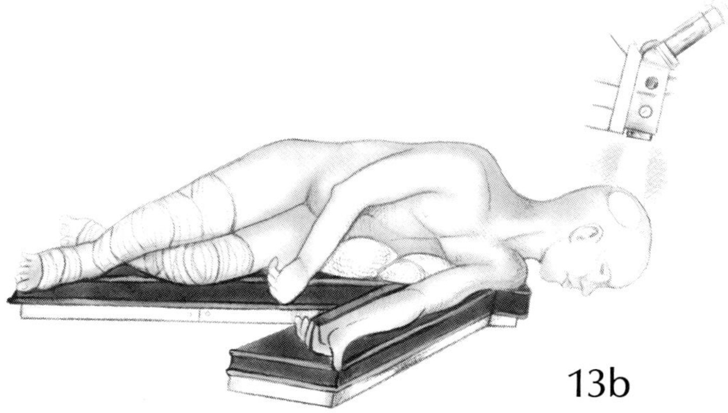

13b

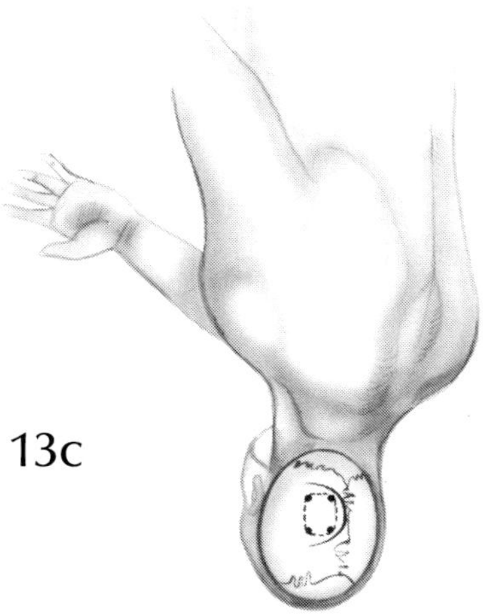

13c

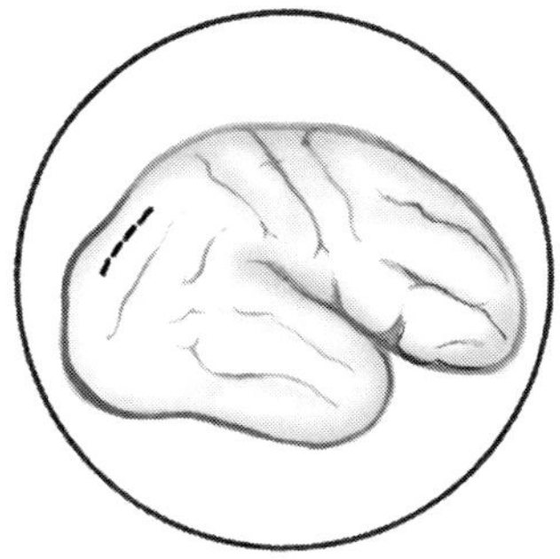

13d

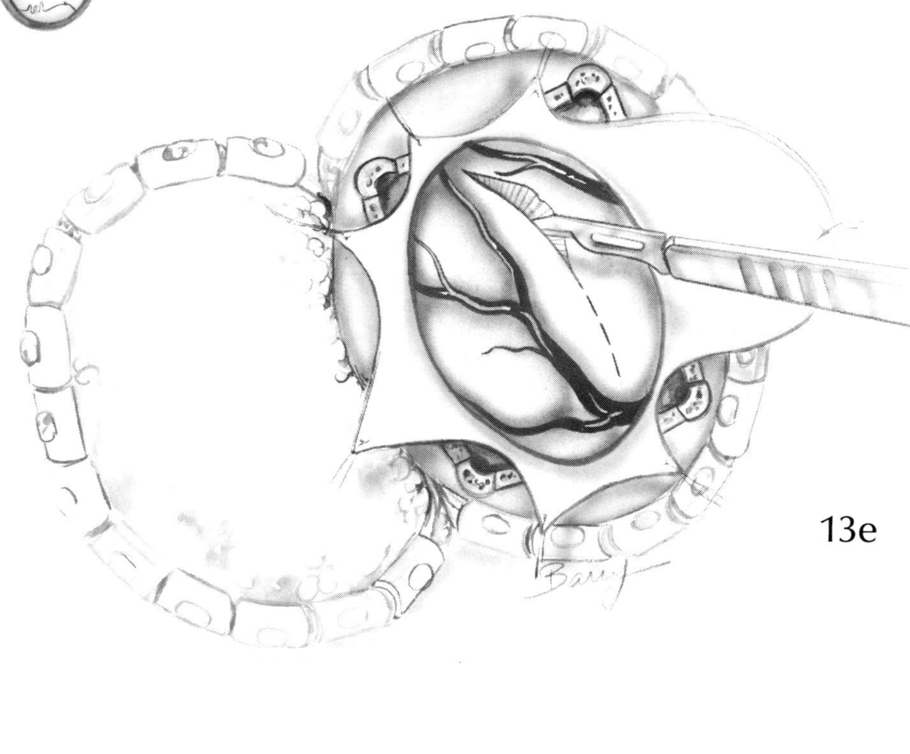

13e

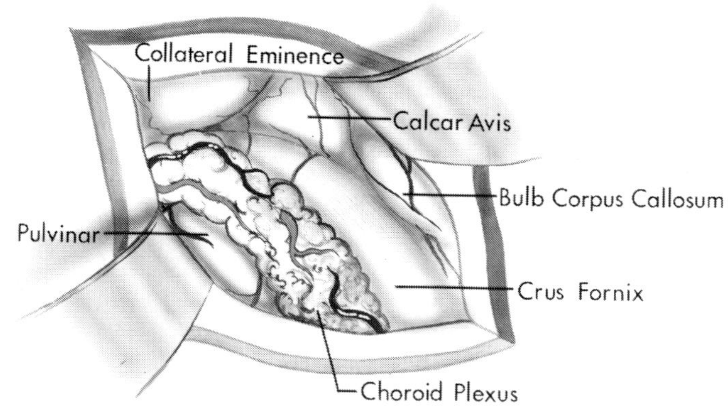


13f

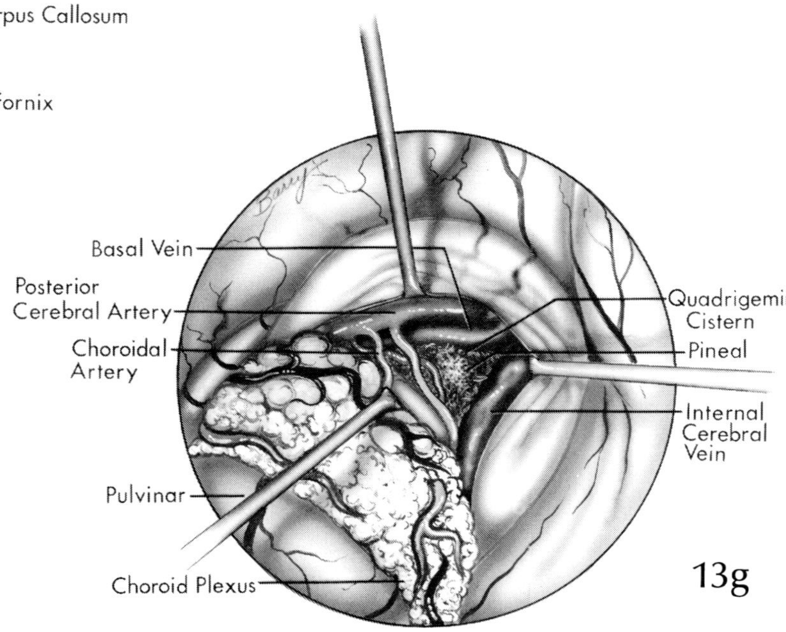


13g

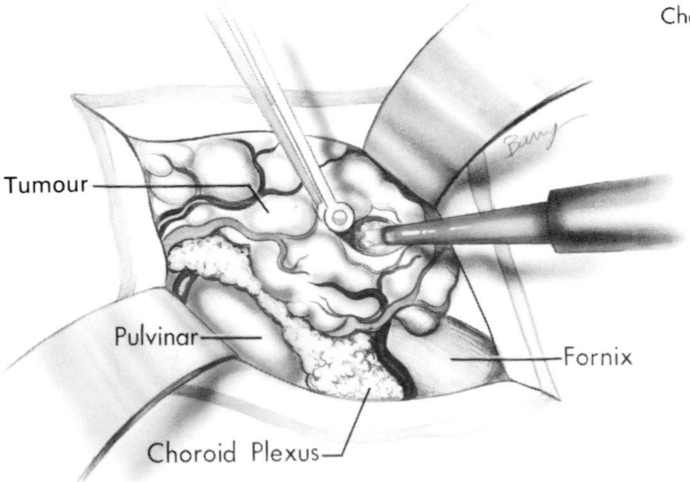


13h

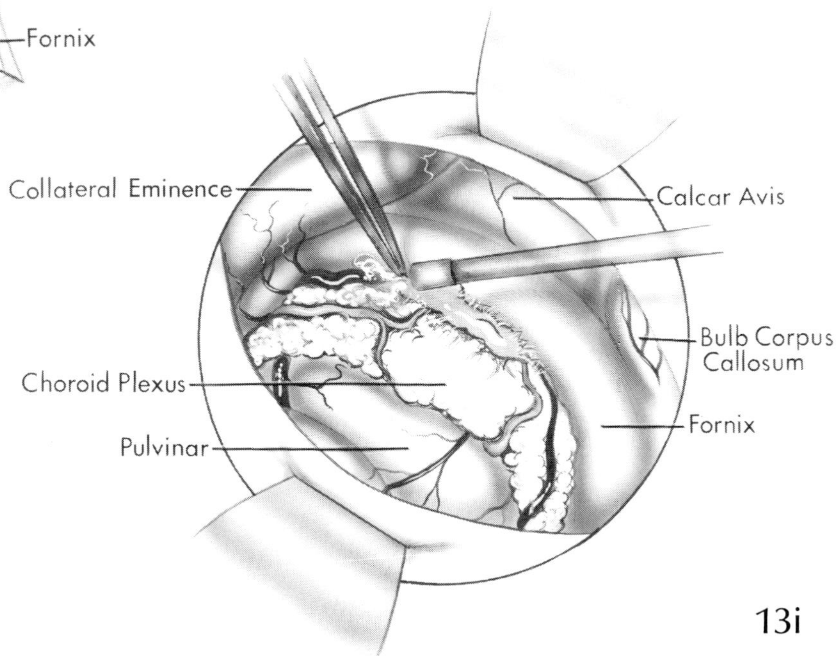


13i

### *Posterior transcallosal approach*

# 14a–f

This approach is best suited to lesions that arise in the splenium and extend into the atrium rather than those situated entirely within the atrium[36]. The patient is positioned in the three-quarter prone position with the face toward the floor and the parietal region to be operated on uppermost (*a*). The parieto-occipital scalp flap and the craniotomy extend up to or across the superior sagittal sinus and have their anterior margin behind the postcentral gyrus. The dura is opened with the pedicle reflected toward the sagittal sinus. A bridging vein entering the superior sagittal sinus posterior to the Rolandic vein may need to be divided so that the hemisphere may be retracted away from the falx. Opening the arachnoid below the falx will expose the distal branches of the anterior cerebral arteries and occasionally the splenial branches of the posterior cerebral arteries. Opening the posterior part of the corpus callosum in the midline will expose the pineal region and the posterior part of the third ventricle (*b*). For the approach to the atrium an incision is made in the cingulate gyrus behind the posterosuperior part of the corpus callosum. This cortical incision is directed obliquely forward through the lateral part of the splenium to enter the atrium just above the bulb of the corpus callosum (*c*). It should be remembered that the ventricles have started to deviate laterally at this point. The landmarks within the ventricle are described in the section on the posterior transcortical approach. The approach is directed lateral to the junction of the internal cerebral veins with the great vein. Dandy[14, 15] resected the great and internal cerebral veins and the straight sinus in this region in some cases without neurological dysfunction. However, every effort should be made to spare these venous structures because their obliteration may cause major deficits. The use of this approach in the removal of a glioma of the forceps major is shown (*d–f*). The tumour is removed with an ultrasonic aspirator. The choroid plexus and pulvinar are pushed forward by the tumour (*e*). After the tumour has been removed, and with incision of the corpus callosum, the internal cerebral veins in the roof of the third ventricle and the quadrigeminal cistern are exposed (*f*). Residual tumour is of course present in the corpus callosum.

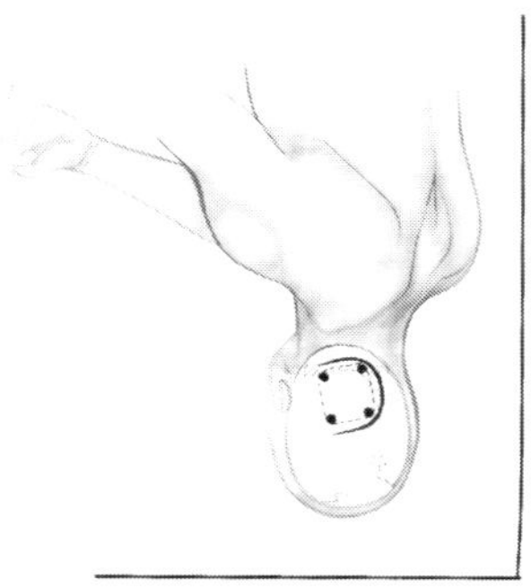

14a

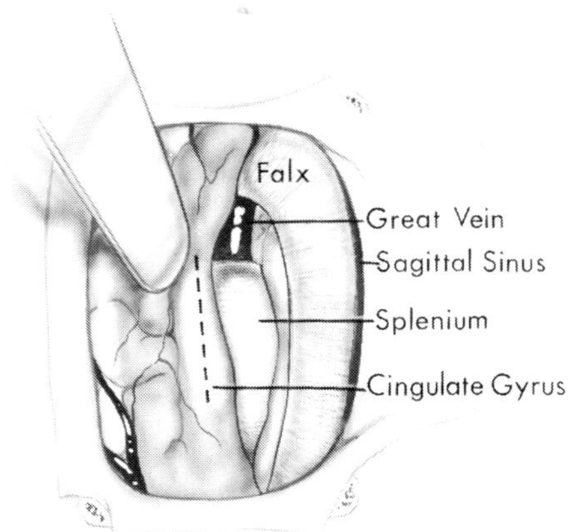


14b

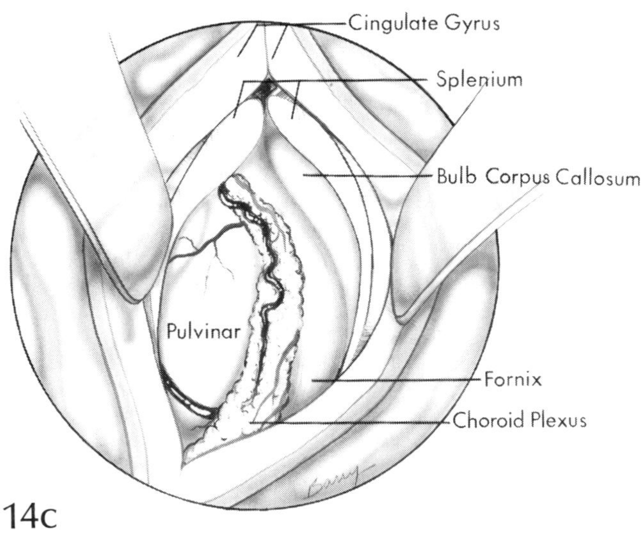


14c

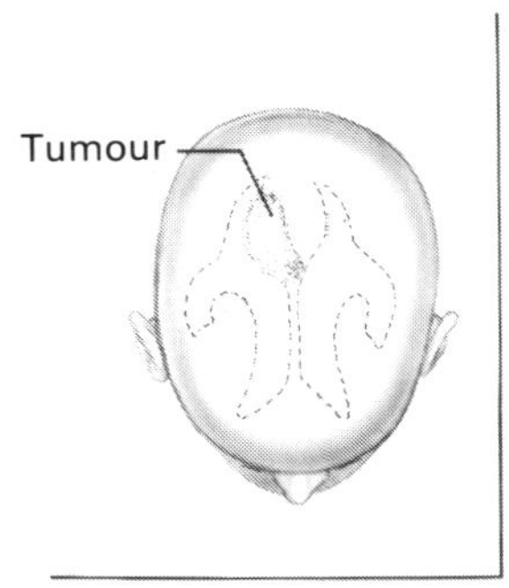


14d

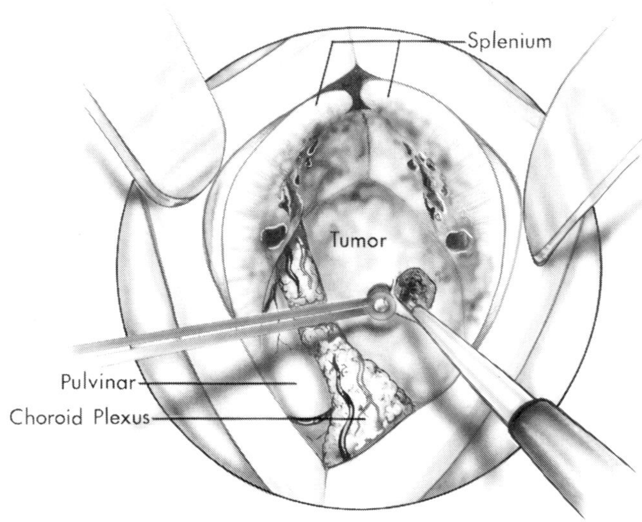


14e

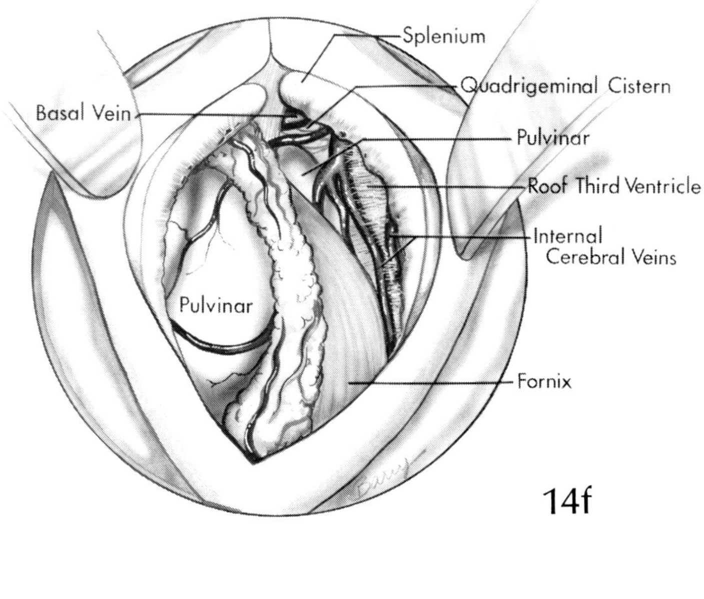


14f

*Occipital approach*

# 15a–f

This approach is suitable for approaching tumours that arise in the medial wall of the atrium and extend in the atrium or quadrigeminal cistern from the medial wall[37]. These lesions may be situated in the region of the atrial part of the choroidal fissure, in the posteromedial part of the pulvinar or in the region of the calcar avis and bulb of the corpus callosum. In order to use this approach, the lesion should come through the medial wall of the atrium to the cisternal surface. It might also be considered for a lesion such as an arteriovenous malformation in which it is desirable to expose the feeding choroidal arteries in the quadrigeminal cistern before exposing the lesion in the ventricle.

The patient is positioned in a semi-sitting or three-quarter prone position with the occipital area to be operated on uppermost and the face turned toward the floor. The occipital scalp flap and craniotomy are placed so that they will extend to the edge of, or across, the transverse and sagittal sinuses and the torcula (*a*). The dura is opened using two flaps, one based on the superior sagittal sinus and the other on the transverse sinus (*b*). The inferomedial aspect of the occipital pole is retracted superiorly and laterally. The occipital lobe can usually be retracted superolaterally without sacrificing any bridging veins because there are infrequently bridging veins between the medial occipital pole and the transverse, straight and superior sagittal sinuses (*c*). The arachnoid over the ambient and quadrigeminal cisterns is opened. The internal occipital vein, which usually crosses from the anteromedial surface of the occipital lobe to the quadrigeminal cistern, is transected if necessary to expose the tumour. Division of this vein, however, may produce a homonymous hemianopia which is often permanent, and, particularly in the approach to the pineal body, strenuous effort should be made to preserve the internal occipital vein. The ventricle is exposed by opening through the isthmus of the cingulate gyrus in front of the calcarine sulcus (*d*). The opening enters the medial wall of the atrium behind the choroidal fissure. The tumour should extend into the cortical area near the junction of the vein of Galen and straight sinus for this approach to be successful. The branches of the posterior cerebral artery and its bifurcation into the calcarine and parieto-occipital branches course medial to the tumour. The lateral posterior choroidal arteries pass through the choroidal fissure in this area and the medial posterior choroidal arteries and basal vein will be seen beside the pineal body. The lower portion of the splenium is divided, if necessary, to reach a lesion in the medial wall of the atrium near the crus of the fornix. The quadrigeminal plate, trochlear nerve, superrior cerebellar artery and the precentral cerebellar vein may be seen in the depths of the exposure. *Illustration 15e* shows a malformation situated in the choroid plexus exposed by opening the medial wall of the atrium behind the choroidal fissure. In *Illustration 15f* the choroidal arteries that feed the malformation have been coagulated and divided and the last draining vein from the malformation obliterated with bipolar coagulation.

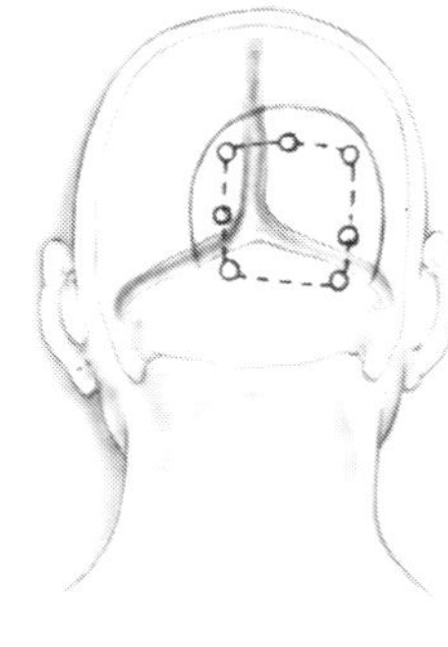

15a

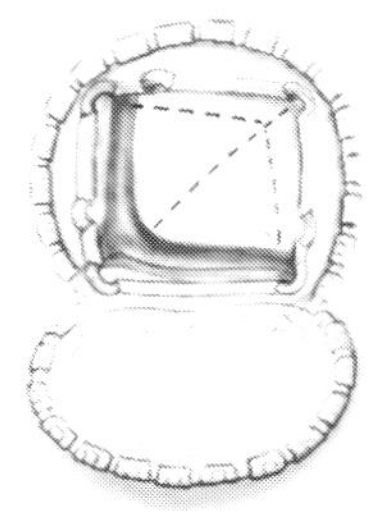

15b

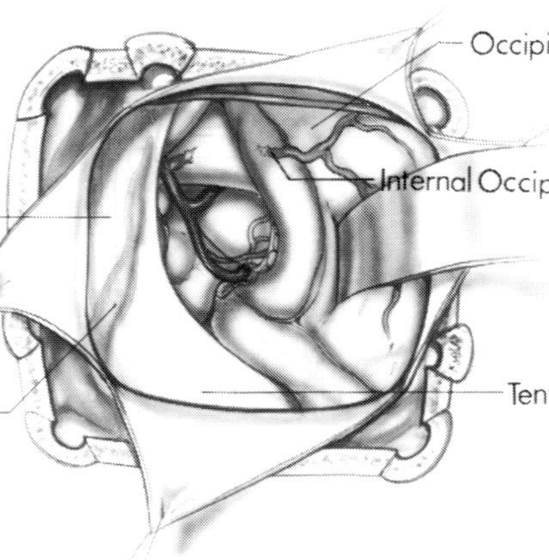


15c

## Inferior approaches

The inferior approaches are the posterior frontotemporal, transtemporal and subtemporal approaches. The posterior frontotemporal approach exposes the anterior pole of the temporal lobe and permits the anterior part of the temporal horn to be exposed through a small cortical incision or a temporal lobectomy. The transtemporal and subtemporal exposures are performed through a temporal craniotomy centred above the ear and permit the full length of the temporal horn to be opened through cortical incisions on the lateral or inferior surfaces of the temporal lobe.

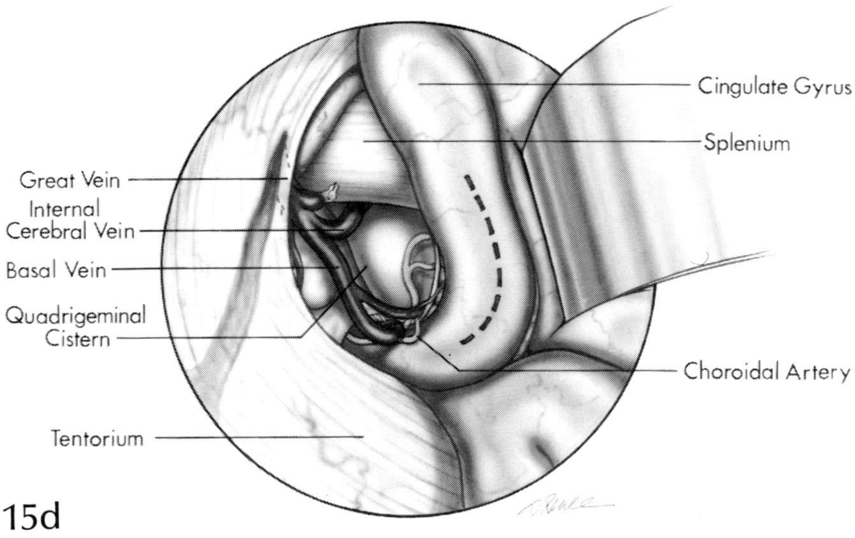
Cingulate Gyrus
Splenium
Great Vein
Internal Cerebral Vein
Basal Vein
Quadrigeminal Cistern
Choroidal Artery
Tentorium

15d

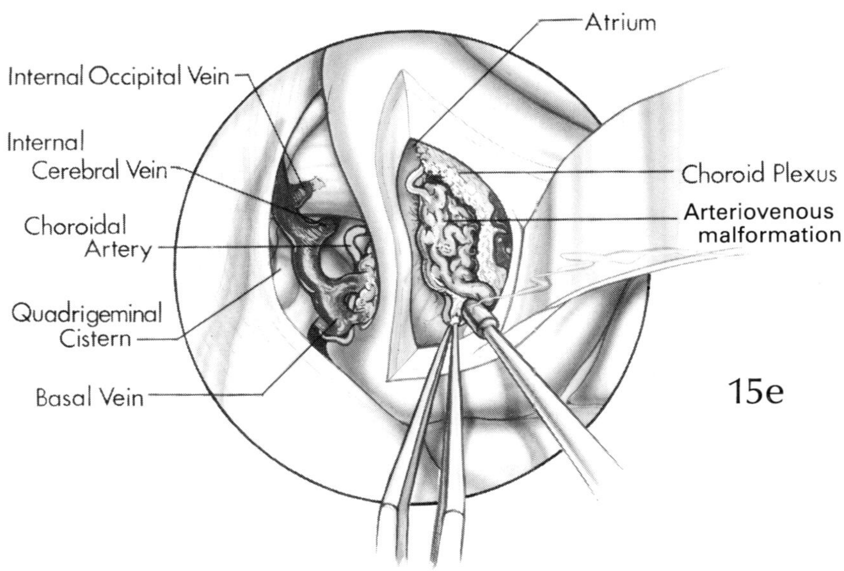
Atrium
Internal Occipital Vein
Internal Cerebral Vein
Choroidal Artery
Quadrigeminal Cistern
Basal Vein
Choroid Plexus
Arteriovenous malformation

15e

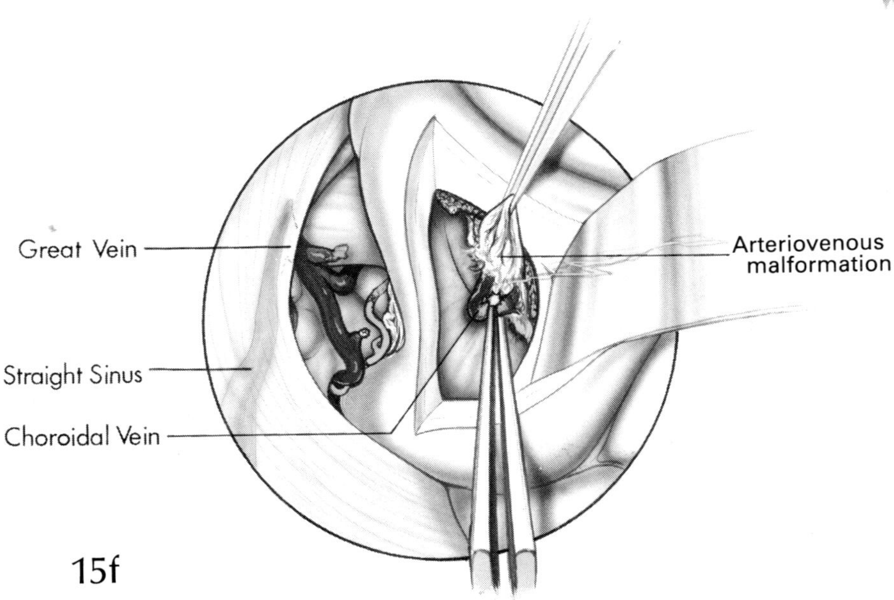
Great Vein
Straight Sinus
Choroidal Vein
Arteriovenous malformation

15f

*Posterior frontotemporal approach*

# 16a–e

The posterior frontotemporal approach is used for a lesion involving the anterior portion of the temporal horn that can be exposed through a temporal lobectomy or a small cortical incision in the anterior part of the temporal lobe. The patient is placed supine with a sandbag under the shoulder on the side to be operated on. The head is tilted slightly backward and turned 45° away from the side of the operation (*a*). The scalp incision begins in the frontal area and extends in a question mark configuration back to the area above the ear, and then downward to the zygoma in front of the ear. The scalp, temporalis muscle, temporalis fascia and pericranium are reflected as a single layer. A free frontotemporal bone flap that will expose the anterior half of the lateral surface of the temporal lobe is elevated and the lateral aspect of the sphenoid ridge is removed with a rongeur or a drill. The dura is opened with the main flap pulled anterior–inferior along the region of the pterion. After opening the dura a decision is made as to whether to enter the temporal horn through a cortical incision or through a temporal lobectomy. The cortical incision is selected if the lesion is strictly localized to the region of the tip of the temporal horn. The temporal lobectomy is considered if the lesion involves not only the tip of the temporal horn, but extends into the temporal lobe in front of the temporal horn (*b*). For the transcortical approach, the lower part of the middle temporal gyrus or the upper part of the inferior temporal gyrus is opened in the long axis of the gyrus and the incision is directed backward through the temporal lobe to the anterior part of the temporal horn.

To use a temporal lobectomy the vertical incision through the temporal lobe should be situated no more than 5 cm from the temporal tip in order to avoid the optic radiations; the horizontal incision paralleling the sylvian fissure should be directed medially through the lower part of the superior temporal gyrus or the upper part of the middle temporal gyrus. Medially, an incision through the superior temporal gyrus will encounter the pia arachnoid on the medial surface of the lower lip of the sylvian fissure that covers the lower branches of the middle cerebral artery as they course over the insula. This incision paralleling the sylvian fissure is extended anteriorly and medially into the anterior pole of the temporal lobe just below the sylvian fissure and sphenoid ridge. The depths of the cortical incision will encounter the uncus and the parahippocampal gyrus which are removed using subpial dissection with fine suction in order to avoid injury to the perforating branches of the middle cerebral and anterior choroidal arteries that pass through the anterior perforated substance to supply the internal capsule. The cortical incision extending around the temporal tip can often be completed without sacrificing the major sylvian veins that enter the sphenoparietal sinus just below the edge of the sphenoid ridge. These approaches will expose the anterior part of the temporal horn as far back as the site where the anterior choroidal artery passes through the choroidal fissure. The prominence over the hippocampus and the collateral eminence will be seen in the floor of the temporal horn and the inferior ventricular vein may be seen in the roof (*c*). The amygdaloid nucleus lies directly anterior and slightly above the tip of the temporal horn and is directly lateral to the cisternal surface of the uncus. Opening through the amygdaloid nucleus and uncus will expose the structures in the crural cistern. This approach is sufficiently anterior that it does not permit more than minimal opening of the choroidal fissure to expose the ambient cistern.

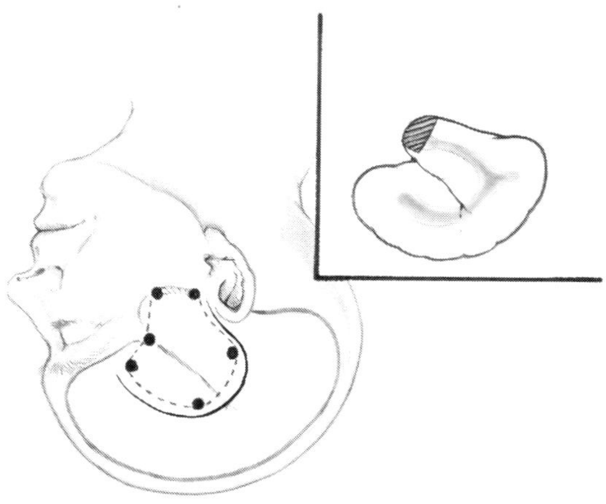

16a

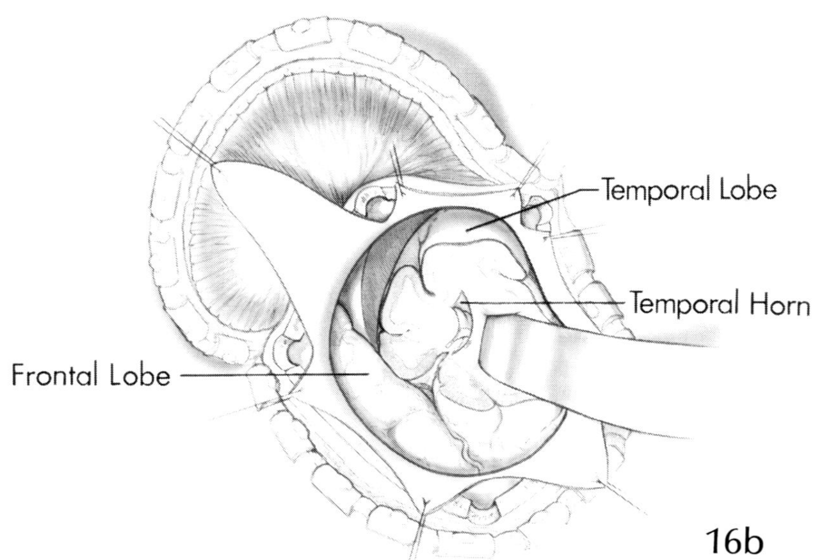


16b

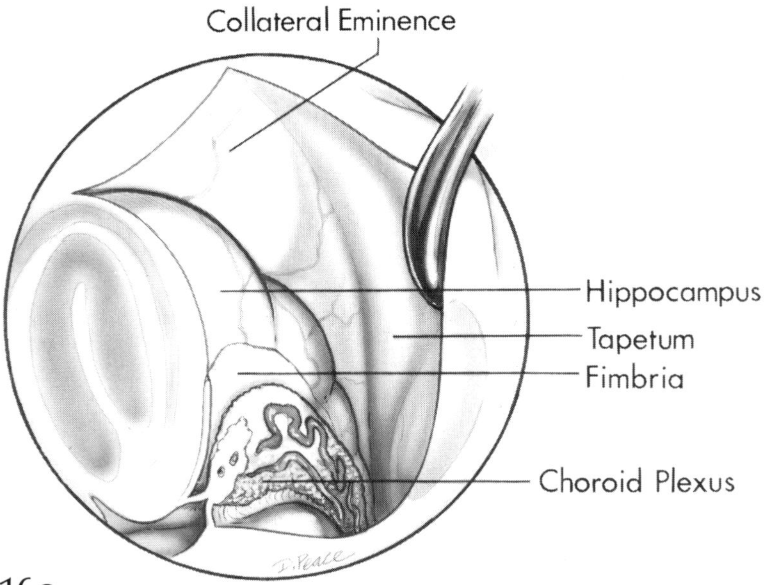
Collateral Eminence
Hippocampus
Tapetum
Fimbria
Choroid Plexus

16c

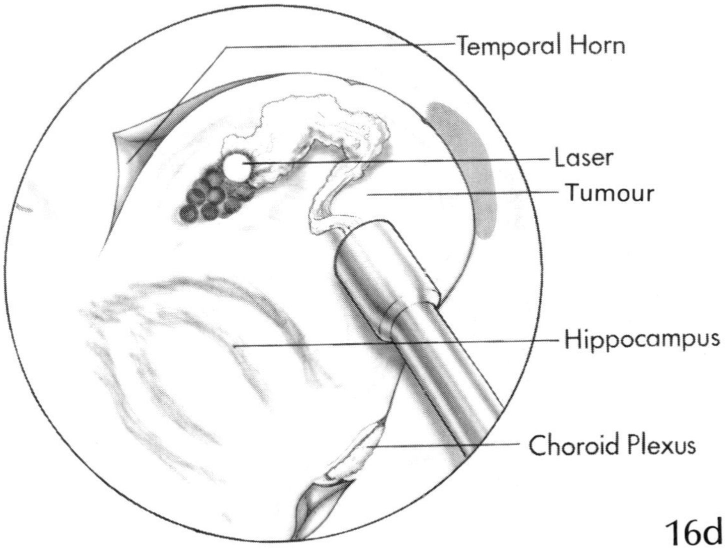
Temporal Horn
Laser
Tumour
Hippocampus
Choroid Plexus

16d

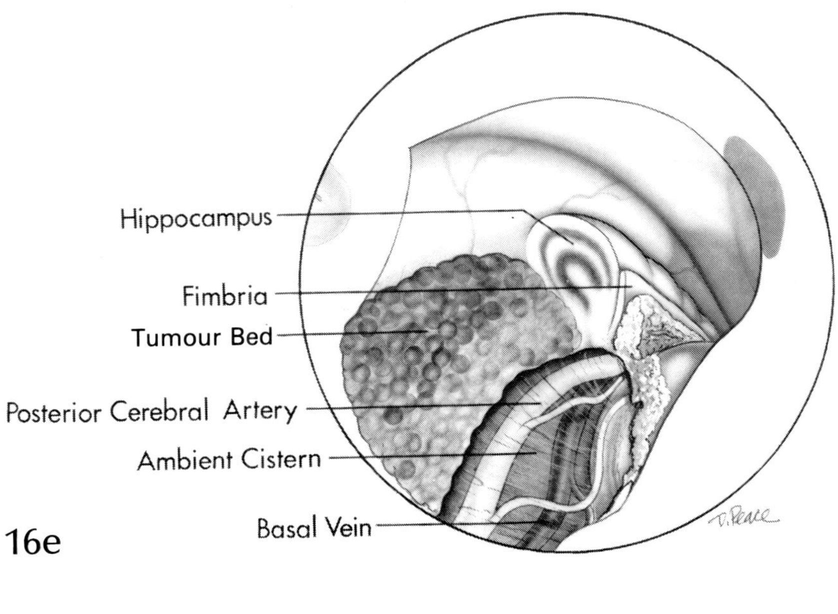
Hippocampus
Fimbria
Tumour Bed
Posterior Cerebral Artery
Ambient Cistern
Basal Vein

16e

*Transtemporal and subtemporal approaches*

# 17a–d

A temporal craniotomy and a transtemporal or subtemporal cortical incision are used for a lesion in the middle or posterior one-third of the temporal horn and for selected lesions in the ambient and crural cisterns.

For the temporal craniotomy centred above the ear, the patient is positioned supine with the shoulder on the side of the lesion elevated, and the head tilted 60–80° away from the side of the operation. The scalp incision extends from above the zygoma anterior to the ear to the area above the ear, and then posteriorly and downward to the region of the asterion posterior to the ear (*a*). The scalp, temporalis muscle, temporalis fascia and pericranium are reflected as a single layer. It is important that the bone flap be cut low or that a small craniectomy be carried out down to the floor of the fossa. This may well open mastoid air cells and care must be taken not to open the attic of the middle ear. Transient deafness from effusion of fluid into the middle ear may well follow this approach. The temporal horn may be exposed using a cortical incision in the middle temporal gyrus anterior to the optic radiations in the non-dominant hemisphere and the inferior temporal gyrus in the dominant hemisphere. An alternative, and often preferable, route that minimizes the possibility of damage to the optic radiations and speech centres is the subtemporal route, in which an incision is made in the inferior temporal or occipitotemporal gyrus on the inferior surface of the temporal lobe or through the collateral sulcus. The risk of haemorrhage, venous infarction and oedema of the temporal lobe is reduced by avoiding occlusion of the bridging veins, especially the vein of Labbé. The opening into the temporal horn will expose the choroidal fissure and the branches of the anterior and lateral posterior choroidal arteries as they enter the choroid plexus (*c*). The choroidal fissure is opened by incising along tenia fimbriae, so avoiding damage to the vessels that pass through the tenia choroidea. Opening the choroidal fissure between the tenia fimbriae and the choroid plexus permits the arteries and veins that pass through the tenia choroidea to be retracted upward with the choroid plexus. This exposes the posterior cerebral and the anterior and posterior choroidal arteries, and the basal vein without extensive retraction of the temporal lobe (*d*). The approach is especially useful for exposing arteriovenous malformations of the temporal horn, hippocampus and medial part of the temporal lobe that are fed by the arteries entering, and drained by the veins leaving, the choroidal fissure[38]. The transchoroidal approach to the basal cisterns reduces the risks of injury to the vein of Labbé and the swelling and haematoma of the temporal lobe that may result from the extensive retraction required to reach the ambient cistern by the subtemporal extracerebral approach.

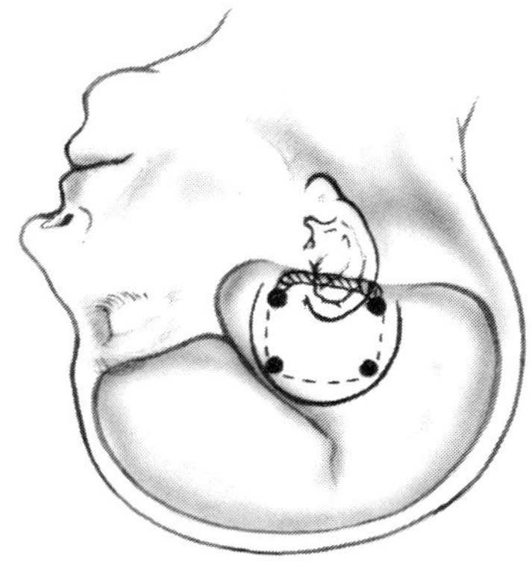

17a

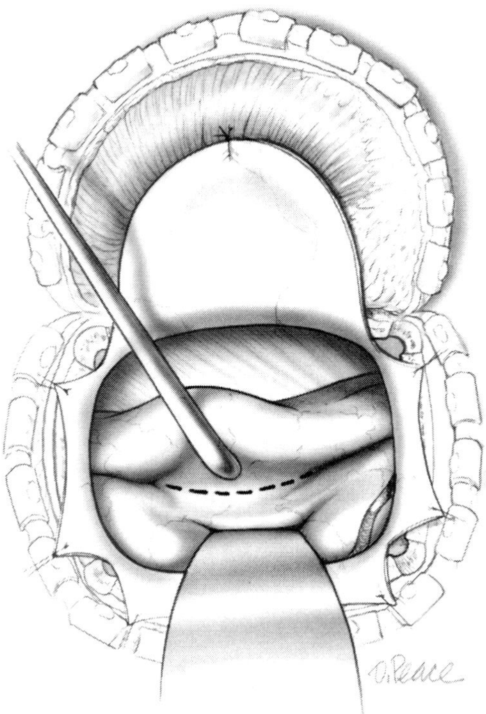

17b

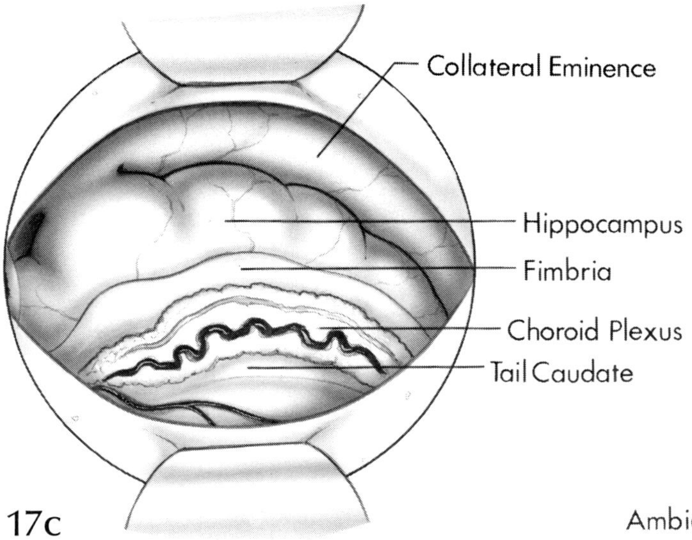


17c

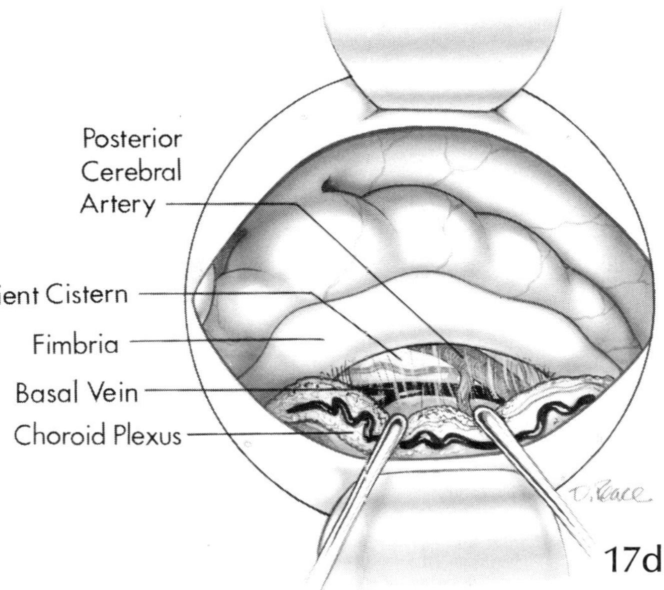


17d

## Selection of operative approaches

Lesions within the anterior portion of the lateral ventricle are most commonly reached by the anterior transcallosal and anterior transcortical approaches. This anterior transcallosal approach is suitable for lesions in the frontal horn and body of the lateral ventricle, and for reaching the anterosuperior part of the third ventricle through the lateral ventricle. The transcallosal approach is easier to perform than the transcortical approach if the ventricles are of a normal size or are minimally enlarged. This anterior transcortical approach is suitable for reaching tumours in the anterior part of the lateral ventricle and the anterosuperior part of the third ventricle, especially if the tumour is situated predominantly in the lateral ventricle on the side of the approach. It is more difficult to expose the lateral ventricle on the opposite side through the transcortical than through the transcallosal approach. The transcortical approach is facilitated if the lateral ventricles are enlarged. Routes through the lateral ventricles to the anterior part of the third ventricle, other than by incising the ipsilateral column of the fornix, are by the transforniceal approach in which the body of the fornix is split longitudinally in the midline, or by the transchoroidal approach in which the choroidal fissure is opened, so allowing the fornix to be pushed to the opposite side in order to expose the structures in the roof of the third ventricle. The transchoroidal and transforniceal approaches have the advantage of allowing access to the central portion of the third ventricle behind the foramen of Monro by displacing, rather than transecting, the fibres in the fornix. The transforniceal and transchoroidal routes provide a satisfactory view into the third ventricle when the ventricle is exposed through the corpus callosum. On the other hand, the transchoroidal opening provides a better view into the third ventricle than the transforniceal approach when the ventricle is exposed through the middle frontal gyrus.

An anterior frontal approach may infrequently be considered for a lesion that involves the region of the rostrum and lower half of the genu of the corpus callosum or that extends from the rostrum into the third ventricle behind the lamina terminalis.

The posterior transcortical approach is the preferred route for exposing lesions situated entirely within the atrium or arising in the glomus of the choroid plexus. Selected lesions may be exposed by the posterior transcallosal or the occipital approaches. The transcallosal approach is considered for a lesion that arises in the splenium and extends into the ventricle from the roof or the upper part of the medial wall of the atrium. The occipital approach directed along the falacotentorial junction is used if the lesion arises in the medial wall of the atrium or extends from the atrium to the cisternal surface of the medial wall.

The temporal horn may be approached by the posterior frontotemporal, temporal or subtemporal approach. The posterior frontotemporal approach is used for a lesion involving the anterior portion of the temporal horn which can be exposed through a small cortical incision in the anterior part of the temporal lobe or through a temporal lobectomy. The temporal and subtemporal routes to the temporal horn are used for lesions in the middle or posterior third of the temporal horn or for selected lesions in the cisterns medial to the temporal horn. The subtemporal route using a cortical incision in the occipitotemporal gyrus on the inferior surface of the temporal lobe is preferred. The opening into the temporal horn will expose the choroidal fissure. Opening through the choroidal fissure in the temporal horn will provide a transventricular view of the posterior cerebral artery and basal vein in the ambient cistern.

## References


1. Nagata, S., Rhoton, A. L. Jr, Barry, M. (1988) Microsurgical anatomy of the choroidal fissure. Surgical Neurology (in press)
2. Spencer, D. D., Collins, W. F. (1982) Surgical management of lateral intraventricular tumors. In: Schmidek, H. H., Sweet, W. M., eds. Operative Neurosurgical Techniques. Indications, methods and results. New York: Grune & Stratton, pp. 561–574
3. Fujii, K., Lenkey, C., Rhoton, A. L. Jr (1980) Microsurgical anatomy of the choroidal arteries: lateral and third ventricles. Journal of Neurosurgery, 52, 165–188
4. Rhoton, A. L. Jr (1987) Microsurgical anatomy of the third ventricular region. In: Apuzzo, M. L. F., ed. Surgery of the Third Ventricle. Baltimore: Williams & Wilkins, pp. 92–166
5. Timurkaynak, E., Rhoton, A. L. Jr, Barry, M. (1986) Microsurgical anatomy and operative approaches to the lateral ventricles. Neurosurgery 19, 685–723
6. Ono, M., Rhoton, A. L. Jr, Peace, D., Rodriquez, R. J. (1984) Microsurgical anatomy of the deep venous system of the brain. Neurosurgery 15, 621–657
7. Preilowski, B. F. (1972) Possible contribution of the anterior forebrain commissures to bilateral motor coordination. Neuropsychologia 10, 267–277
8. Van Wagenen, W. P., Herren, R. Y. (1940) Surgical division of commissural pathways in the corpus callosum: relation to the spread of epileptic attack. Archives of Neurology and Psychiatry 44, 740–759
9. Zaidel, D., Sperry, R. W. (1974) Memory impairment after commissurotomy in man. Brain 97, 263–272
10. Hirsch, J. F., Zouaoui, A., Renier, D., Pierre-Kahn, A. (1979) A new surgical approach to the third ventricle with interruption of the striothalamic vein. Acta Neurochirurgica 47, 135–147
11. McKissock, W. (1951) The surgical treatment of the colloid cyst of the third ventricle: a report based upon twenty-one personal cases. Brain 74, 1–9
12. Poppen, J. L., Reyes, V., Horrax, G. (1953) Colloid cysts of the third ventricle: report of seven cases. Journal of Neurosurgery 10, 242–263
13. Olivecrona, H. (1987) Colloidal cysts of the third ventricle. In: Olivecrona, H., Tonnis, W., eds. Handbuch der Neurochirurgie. Berlin: Springer-Verlag, Vol. 4, pp. 101–109
14. Dandy, W. E. (1921) An operation for the removal of pineal tumors. Surgery, Gynecology and Obstetrics 33, 113–119
15. Dandy, W. E. (1936) Operative experience in cases of pineal tumor. Archives of Surgery 33, 19–46
16. Apuzzo, M. L. J., Giannotta, S.L. (1987) Transcallosal interforniceal approach. In: Apuzzo, M. L. J., ed. Surgery of the Third Ventricle. Baltimore: Williams & Wilkins, pp. 354–380
17. Horel, J. A. (1978) The neuroanatomy of amnesia. A critique of the hippocampal memory hypotheses. Brain 101, 403–445
18. Penfield, W., Milner, B. (1958) Memory deficit produced by bilateral lesions in the hippocampal zone. Archives of Neurology and Psychiatry 79, 475–497
19. Sweet, W. H., Talland, G. A., Ervin, F. R. (1959) Loss of recent memory following section of the fornix. Transactions of the American Neurological Association 84, 76–82
20. Ehni, G., Ehni, B. (1987) Considerations in transforaminal entry. In: Apuzzo, M. L. J., ed. Surgery of the Third Ventricle. Baltimore: Williams & Wilkins, pp. 326–353
21. Garretson, H. D. (1987) Memory in man: a neurosurgeon's perspective. In: Apuzzo, M. L. J., ed. Surgery of the Third Ventricle. Baltimore: Williams & Wilkins, pp. 209–212
22. Heilman, K. M., Sypert, G. W. (1977) Korsakoff's syndrome resulting from bilateral fornix lesion. Neurology 27, 490–493
23. Woolsey, R. M., Nelson, J. S. (1975) Asymptomatic destruction of the fornix in man. Archives of Neurology 32, 566–568
24. Bailey, P. (1934) Peculiarities of the intracranial venous system and their clinical significance. Archives of Neurology and Psychiatry 32, 1105
25. Kunicki, A. (1960) Operative experiences in 8 cases of pineal tumor. Journal of Neurosurgery 17, 815–823
26. Stern, W. E., Batzdorf, U., Rich, J. R. (1971) Challenges of surgical excision of tumors in the pineal region. Bulletin of the Los Angeles Neurological Society 36, 105–118
27. Shucart, W. A., Stein, B. M. (1978) Transcallosal approach to the anterior ventricular system. Neurosurgery 3, 339–343
28. Stein, B. M. (1982) Transcallosal approach to third ventricular tumors. In: Schmidek, H. H., Sweet, W. H., eds. Operative Neurosurgical Techniques. Indications, Methods and Results. New York: Grune & Stratton, pp. 575–584
29. Apuzzo, M. L., Chikovani, O. K., Gott, P. S. *et al.* (1982) Transcallosal, interforniceal approaches for lesions affecting the third ventricle: surgical consideration and consequences. Neurosurgery 10, 547–554
30. Lavyne, M. H., Patterson, R. H. Jr. (1987) Subchoroidal trans-velum interpositum approach. In: Apuzzo, M. L. J., ed. Surgery of the Third Ventricle. Baltimore: Williams & Wilkins, pp. 381–397
31. Viale, G.L., Turtas, S. (1980) The subchoroid approach to the third ventricle. Surgical Neurology 14, 71–74
32. Rhoton, A. L. Jr, Yamamoto, I., Peace, D. (1981) Microsurgery of the third ventricle: part 2. Operative approaches. Neurosurgery 8, 357–373
33. Van Wagenen, W. P. (1931) A surgical approach for the removal of certain pineal tumors: report of a case. Surgery, Gynecology and Obstetrics 53, 216–220
34. Brodal, A. (1981) Neurological Anatomy in Relation to Clinical Medicine. 3rd ed. New York: Oxford University Press, pp. 832–841
35. Ojemann, G. A. (1979) Individual variability in cortical localization of language. Journal of Neurosurgery 50, 164–169
36. Horrax, G. (1937) Extirpation of a huge pinealoma from a patient with pubertas praecox: a new operative approach. Archives of Neurology and Psychiatry 37, 385–397
37. Poppen, J. L. (1966) The right occipital approach to a pinealoma. Journal of Neurosurgery 25, 706–710
38. Heros, R. C. (1982) Arteriovenous malformations of the medial temporal lobe: surgical approach and neuroradiological characterization. Journal of Neurosurgery 56, 44–52

Illustrations by Angela Christie

# Intracranial approach to tumours in the area of the sella turcica

**Lindsay Symon** TD, FRCS
Professor of Neurosurgery, Gough-Cooper Department of Neurological Surgery, Institute of Neurology, National Hospitals for Nervous Diseases, London, UK

## Indications

The most frequent indication for surgery in this group of tumours is embarrassment of the visual pathways. Less frequently, raised intracranial pressure, either from tumour bulk or from obstruction of the third ventricle by the tumour with the production of internal hydrocephalus, may bring the patient to surgery. Where the suprasellar extension is regular in shape and not too large, many surgeons will now advocate its removal by the trans-sphenoidal route. Detailed comparison of the two approaches is not appropriate here but it may be stated briefly that where the sphenoidal air sinus is absent or awkwardly structured, where the suprasellar extension appears to have a relatively narrow waist separating it from its intrasellar component, or where extension of the adenoma in the suprasellar space has occurred in more than one direction, then the transcranial route is preferred. We treat almost all cases presenting with visual compression by the transcranial approach.

### Endocrine-active tumours

Hormone-producing tumours confined to the pituitary fossa without evidence of extrasellar extension are best dealt with by a trans-sphenoidal approach. The intracranial route may be chosen at the discretion of the individual surgeon. While the intracranial approach is also possible for ablation of the pituitary gland in the treatment of disseminated carcinomatosis or in the management of severe diabetes mellitus, the trans-sphenoidal route is much less disturbing for these seriously ill patients, and particular indications such as an absence of the sphenoidal air sinus would be necessary to justify a transcranial approach. This approach is perfectly feasible but generally more difficult than the trans-sphenoidal approach which should commonly be preferred.

## Investigations

Appropriate endocrine tests are indicated where a mass in the area of the sella turcica may be thought to have embarrassed pituitary or hypothalamic function. Baseline cortisol levels, prolactin, and growth hormone are commonly estimated but few endocrinologists will recommend stress testing in the preoperative phase. Detailed tests of the endocrine axis, adrenal, and thyroid glands may be left until the postoperative period.

### SPECIFIC RADIOLOGICAL INVESTIGATIONS

### Plain X-rays of the skull

With the increasing availability of computerized tomograms, plain X-rays of the skull are often overlooked. A good lateral X-ray of the pituitary fossa, with tomography if necessary, is mandatory in any case of visual failure, and overlooking this very simple rule has cost many patients appreciable visual function.

### Computerized axial tomography

CT scanning is now generally available and is often the first investigation employed in screening patients with visual failure. Scans with and without contrast are essential. A pituitary tumour has a density frequently similar to that of the brain and may be missed completely on plain scans, although if the pentagon of the suprasellar cistern is scrutinized in a basal cut one will often find that this well-marked space is missing, suggesting that it has been filled by a mass. The degree of contrast uptake in suprasellar tumours is widely variable, but pituitary tumours will usually enhance to some degree and comparison of the unenhanced and enhanced scans will reveal the presence of the mass. Quite frequently, a tumour enhances briskly and the diagnosis is not in doubt. The mixed calcification of a craniopharyngioma may also be evident.

Modern (fourth generation) scanners with excellent reconstructive capabilities in the coronal and sagittal planes have much advanced the detailed analysis of parasellar masses, and such special techniques as contrast cisternography have largely been superseded. Even close-cut fourth generation reconstructions, however, have been overtaken by magnetic resonance imaging.

### Magnetic resonance scanning

This is now the preferred technique for the elucidation of the detail of parasellar anatomy in such masses. In my experience, the clarity of picture is the best obtainable since air encephalography was abandoned, and of course the simplicity and reliability of the technique is unsurpassed. Perhaps the only disadvantage compared with CT scanning is the inability to enhance with contrast, and this alone would justify continued CT scanning in an endeavour to aid the prediction of the probable nature of the tumour.

Magnetic resonance scans should be obtained in sagittal and coronal planes when the extrasellar extensions of the mass will be clearly delineated. Both spin echo and inversion recovery images are commonly employed, the weighting factors depending on the particular resonance laboratory. Thus it is important that the surgeon discuss the characteristics of these images with the technicians who produce them.

### ANGIOGRAPHY

In my view, bilateral carotid angiography should always be performed, although some now proceed on the basis of intravenous digital subtraction techniques. Involvement of the carotid vessels in sellar or parasellar tumours constitutes the main source of surgical morbidity, and the surgeon should be aware of it before embarking on operation. The rare case of aneurysm of the internal carotid artery masquerading as a true intrasellar mass may be hinted at by specific destruction of the inner end of the sphenoidal wing on plain anteroposterior views, or by sharp bony loss in the sellar walls; however, this may scarcely be evident and only angiography will reveal the true nature of the tumour. Cross-compression angiography from a single side may be insufficient to outline the cavernous carotid on the opposite side, and if any doubt exists, bilateral carotid angiography should be performed. Where a craniopharyngioma is to be approached by the subtemporal route in an attempt at complete excision, vertebral angiography with visualization of the top of the basilar and thalamoperforating vessels is usually wise.

When modern imaging techniques are unavailable it may be appropriate to supplement the findings of angiography by selective air encephalography of the basal cisterns, both to outline the mass itself (if necessary in lateral and anteroposterior tomograms) and to indicate the position of the chiasm and the anterior part of the third ventricle. Hypocycloidal tomography with air encephalography will produce especially accurate definition. In most clinics, however, air encephalography has been abandoned.

## Preoperative management

Whatever the preoperative endocrine testing may indicate, it is important to place the patient on high-dose steroids several days preoperatively. The standard technique using 4 mg dexamethasone 6-hourly is commonly employed. Should the preoperative prolactin level be very high, many endocrinologists will already have placed the patient on bromocriptine (up to 7.5 mg per day) or other suitable prolactin antagonists. More commonly, however, the final decision for or against bromocriptine treatment may be left until the adenoma has been excised and the endocrine effects of such excision assessed.

### Anaesthesia

Standard endotracheal anaesthesia is employed with continuous blood pressure monitoring and monitoring of end-tidal carbon dioxide. It is unwise to overventilate elderly patients with pituitary tumours, in the presence of extensive brain atrophy, or even if the mild hydrocephalus commonly associated with pituitary tumours is present, as extensive displacement of basal structures may result during surgery if overventilation is employed, and delayed recovery of consciousness at the least may result.

## The anterior approach to the sella turcica

This approach is indicated for the suprasellar extension of the usual pituitary tumour, pituitary adenoma, and for meningiomas of the jugum sphenoidale. It is also indicated occasionally for cases of craniopharyngioma in which the chiasmal elevation is considerable, and preoperative assessment of the position of the optic recess of the third ventricle indicates that accessibility to over half the anterior area of the mass may be achieved beneath the anterior margin of the chiasm between the two optic nerves. This precondition in craniopharyngiomas is rare, and the anterior approach cannot be recommended for attempted radical excision of these tumours.

# The operation

The patient is positioned on his back with the head turned 20° to the left side. Right-handed surgeons will generally prefer to operate under the right hemisphere, which has the additional advantage of being, as a rule, the non-dominant hemisphere. Only where extensive lateral involvement in the left parasellar area is likely, with the tumour spreading lateral to the line of the carotid artery on the left, should a directly left-sided approach be employed.

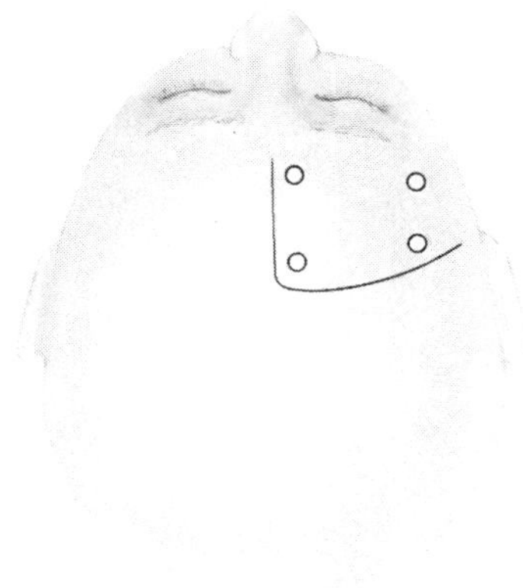

1a

## 1a & b

A small, cosmetically acceptable scalp flap commonly employed is illustrated, but a cosmetic bifrontal scalp flap behind the hairline may be used. A four-burr-hole bone flap is cut and hinged on the anterior part of the temporal muscle. The anterior medial burr hole should be in the midline and, if possible, should avoid the frontal sinus. Where the frontal sinuses are large it may be wiser to breach them formally and repair them with a graft of pericranium or lyophilized dura which may be held in place with cyanoacrylate glue. The lateral frontal burr hole should be just behind the zygomatic process of the frontal bone and on the floor of the frontal fossa. The posterior medial burr hole need not be on the midline and, particularly in the elderly with extensive hyperostosis frontalis interna, avoiding the lateral margin of the sagittal sinus will prevent troublesome bleeding if the dura is torn. The flap is cut with a Gigli guide and saw as described elsewhere, but if an air drill is used, the lateral frontal burr hole should be employed as the starting point of the flap reflection.

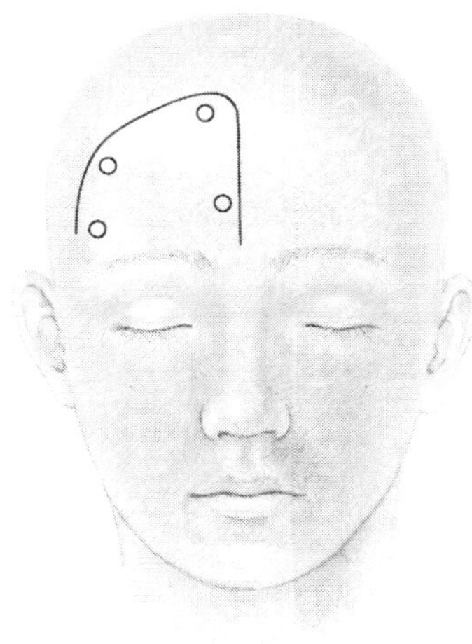

1b

# 2

Extradural haemostasis is effected with hitching stitches and waxing of cut bone edges. The dura is opened through a curved subfrontal incision with a re-entrant directed towards the temporal fossa, and the dural flaps held back with stay sutures. A variety of self-retaining retractors are presently available, from the complete head ring attached to the patient developed by Sugita, through an external bar fixed to the operating table, to the straightforward skull-mounted double Yaşargil post. The author prefers the last of these, as it enables slight movement of the head during surgery to adjust the angle of sight of the operator, without the necessity of removing and replacing the retractors. Double self-retaining retraction is best employed, the first retractor passing downwards and medially along the top of the orbital roof with final fixation of this retractor being deferred until the chiasmal cistern is open. At this point a second retractor may be used to retract the lateral frontal zone and to open up the inner end of the sylvian fissure. Particular care is necessary in the use of this retractor, since it is placed directly above the right optic nerve and if disturbed may produce inadvertent compression of the nerve. Retractor insertion should be directed downwards and medially along the top of the orbital roof to identify the olfactory tract first. It is usually wise to divide the olfactory tract behind the olfactory bulb to prevent troublesome bleeding if later in the operation the bulb is avulsed from its bed. The olfactory tract may then be followed back to the point at which it crosses the sphenoidal wing, where the optic nerve will be found. However displaced the nerve is, its point of entry to the canal will be close to the crossing of the wing by the olfactory tract. Working medially along the jugum sphenoidale, it is usually wise at this point to breach the arachnoid of the chiasmatic cistern. The presenting face of a chromophobe adenoma will then be evident.

It is perfectly possible to conduct transcranial pituitary surgery by direct vision, but the majority of surgeons have now adopted the operating microscope routinely for basal surgery, and in the author's view this is strongly to be recommended. Following the placement of retraction and the opening of the chiasmal cistern, therefore, the operating microscope should be brought in, to aid further dissection. Dissecting to the left, one will pick up the left optic nerve. With a large subfrontal extrasellar extension of the pituitary tumour, the tumour itself may impede the dissection to the left at this stage. In dealing with the average chromophobe adenoma, the tumour should be aspirated in the hope that decompression of a cyst may aid the subsequent surgery. The capsule of the adenoma should then be opened in a circular or cruciate fashion after any large veins on its surface have been carefully coagulated with bipolar diathermy. It is wise to exenterate the tumour in a planned fashion, first creating a cavity in the centre of the mass by sucking down into the main part of the sella with a large sucker, then working to the left where the surgeon's oblique line of sight will enable him to define the carotid artery and left optic nerve and to develop a plane outside the adenoma capsule in the left parasellar zone.

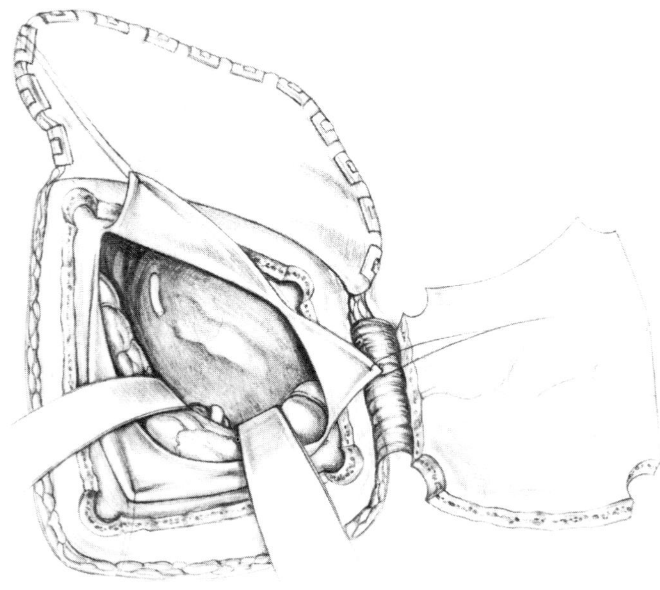

2

The surgeon should concentrate on thinning down the mass of tumour beneath the line of the capsule now evident to him and, working gradually into the midline, the capsule is freed from the region of the third ventricle by gentle traction downwards and inwards into the decompressive cavity already made. The hypophyseal stalk may be identified and separated from the top of the adenoma, or a portion of capsule may be left in relation to the stalk. With the use of the operating microscope it is often possible to identify residual normal pituitary tissue which has a relatively bright orange colour, quite different from the dull grey of the average chromophobe adenoma. Often a distinct piece of normal appearing pituitary will lie at the foot of the stalk and this, together with a small portion of capsule, may be preserved. It may then be quite possible, despite a radical excision of the adenoma, to maintain normal pituitary function after operation; this, particularly in young patients, may be eminently desirable. The most troublesome portion of resection of the capsule of a pituitary adenoma is that part lying in the right parasellar area above and behind the optic nerve; however, careful dissection with angled suckers will usually suffice to clear this corner. Dissection in the right parasellar area should not be undertaken until the right carotid artery has been identified, usually by splitting the chiasmal arachnoid over the top of the right optic nerve and laterally into the medial sylvian fissure. In very large adenomas which have extended posteriorly, either without or within the cavernous sinus towards the apex of the petrous bone, it may be advantageous to make a further small incision in the cavernous sinus dura just lateral to the internal carotid artery. Using this method, quite massive tumours within the cavernous sinus may be dissected. With the clearance of the suprasellar area, curved suction may be passed from the suprasellar opening into the lateral opening and complete clearance of tumour beneath the right optic nerve and between the site of the two curves of the carotid siphon can be achieved. The dangers of this approach are damage to the third nerve but the opening of the sylvian fissure in the presence of the large tumour mass will usually enable the surgeon to identify this nerve with preliminary decompression of the mass. Transient third-nerve palsy may occur but, provided the nerve is left in continuity, complete recovery is the rule. Where the adenoma is very hard and adherent to the third ventricle, it may prove impossible to dissect its apex, but in my experience, this is extremely rare. In cases of large extension involving multiple excrescences above the line of the capsule, particular care should be exercised as the capsule is divided, lest portions of the anterior cerebral complex are enveloped in tumour. In these circumstances, microscopic dissection and the use of self-retaining retractors is essential.

## Hypophysectomy by the anterior route for acromegaly or in pituitary ablation for carcinoma and diabetes

An approach similar to that described for chromophobe adenoma is best. In these extremely ill patients, it may be wise to use dehydrating agents (mannitol 40–60 g intravenously) to obtain maximal ease of retraction. Careful visualization of both optic nerves and the hypophyseal stalk is essential and the hypophyseal stalk should be divided below a tantalum clip close to its insertion into the diaphragma sellae. The insertion of the hypophyseal stalk may be used as the point of entry into the sella, the opening into the diaphragma is then enlarged with an arachnoid knife and blunt curettes are used to separate the hypophysis, preferably in fairly large pieces. It is important that if electrical coagulation is used, it should be confined to the sellar structures themselves and not to the hypophyseal portal system of veins on the pituitary stalk. After excision of the hypophysis, coagulation of the wall of the sella with a pledget soaked in a protein coagulating agent such as Zenker's solution may be used. However, the danger of leakage of such solutions into the subarachnoid space cannot be overemphasized. Some authors have completed the hypophysectomy by filling the empty sella with bone wax impregnated with yttrium-90, to continue the destruction of residual pituitary tissue.

## The temporal approach for resection of craniopharyngioma

Where radical excision of a craniopharyngioma is to be attempted, this approach provides the least difficulty in a highly complex and dangerous field. Essential preliminary investigations include carotid and vertebral angiography to outline not only the displacement of major carotid branches, but also the position of both the posterior communicating artery and the anterior choroidal artery, and the perforating vessels to the mamillary body and thalamus which arise from the posterior communicating artery. Where intracranial pressure is grossly raised it may be necessary to visualize the third ventricle with contrast, which is best introduced through a frontal burr hole into one lateral ventricle. Iohexol is commonly employed.

With the development of modern fourth generation CT scanning with sagittal and coronal reconstruction, and more particularly since the more widespread availability of magnetic resonance scanning, the necessity for air studies in the management of these tumours has been substantially reduced.

The clarity of definition of magnetic resonance scans has greatly added to the safety of dissection of such tumours. CT scanning with and without contrast, however, provides valuable information about the likely nature of the tumour, cystic and calcifying areas being usually identifiable.

Where intracranial pressure is grossly raised and there is massive hydrocephalus, formal operation to remove the mass may be preceded either by temporal ventricular drainage (see chapter on 'Control of intracranial tension', pp. 1–11) or by the formal establishment of a ventriculoperitoneal shunt.

## The operation

# 3

A frontotemporal flap should be employed. The basic approach is along the sphenoidal wing with access to the anterior temporal fossa to enable a limited temporal lobe resection. The bone flap is fashioned around the outer end of the sphenoidal wing, utilizing a spectacle or keyhole burr hole on the wing itself. The flap is broken down on the central part of the temporalis muscle and a small excision of bone in the anterior part of the temporal fossa may further improve access.

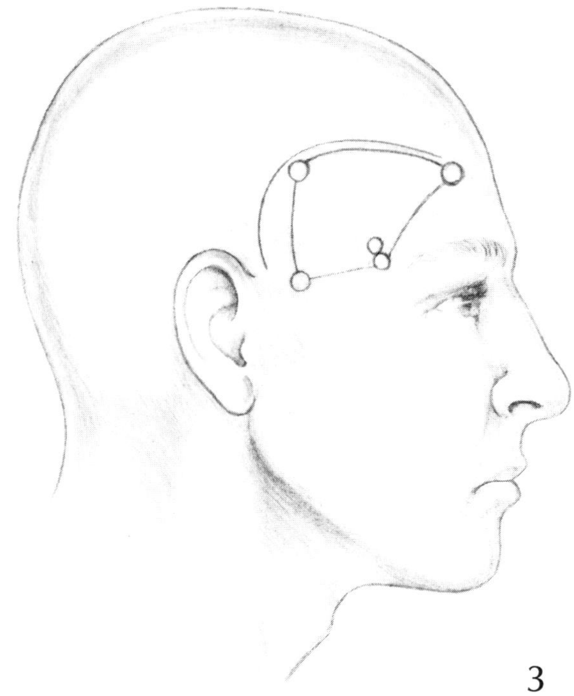

3

# 4a & b

The dura should be opened through an asymmetrical Y-incision as indicated, and dissection initially pursued subfrontally to define the olfactory tract and optic nerve. It is then wise to divide the major veins entering the sphenoparietal sinus from the temporal lobe and to resect the anterior 1.0–1.5 inches (25–38 mm) of the temporal lobe to expose the third nerve and tentorium. Self-retaining retraction and the use of the operating microscope are mandatory from this point on. It is the author's practice to place the support post of the Yaşargil double self-retaining retractor on the posterosuperior angle of the bone flap, although methods of external fixation of these retractors may be employed. The advantage of skull-mounted retraction is that the head may be moved slightly in the course of surgery without having to replace the retractors. The preferred retractor positions are an anterior retractor retracting the cut surface of the superior temporal gyrus just behind the line of the middle cerebral artery (direct pressure on this vessel should be avoided), with a second retractor retracting posteriorly on the posterior cut stem of the temporal lobe. This enables the space between the posterior cut surface of the temporal lobe and the tentorium to be opened and facilitates dissection in the interpeduncular cistern. The downward extension of the craniopharyngioma will be evident medial to the carotid artery and frequently extends right down into the interpeduncular cistern so that a considerable area of this surface of the mass is available below the posterior communicating artery.

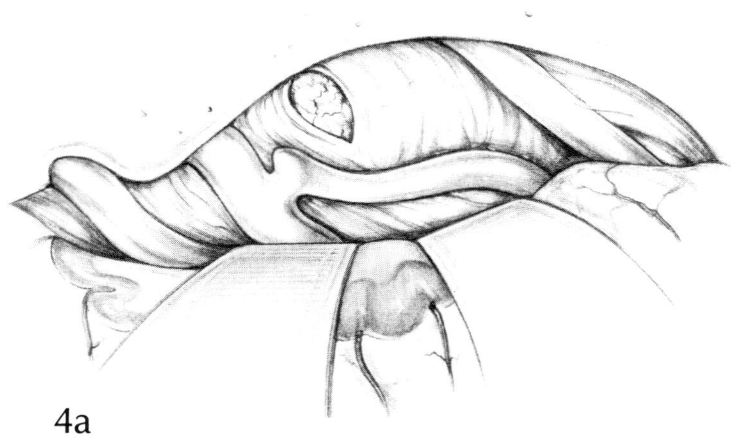

4a

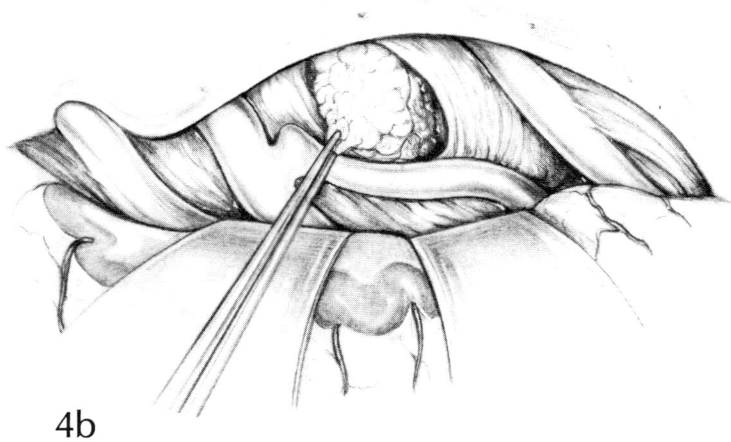

4b

It may be necessary to dissect above the posterior communicating artery between this vessel, its perforating vessels and the anterior choroidal artery; accurate knowledge of the positions of these vessels will have been obtained from preoperative angiography. Dissection of the posteroinferior portion of the mass should be attempted first. The position of the main trunk of the basilar artery and of the posterior cerebral artery and its branches should be identified. Neither of these vessels are commonly enveloped in tumour, but the basilar artery is usually pressed backwards by the posterior margin of the craniopharyngioma. At this point decompression of the craniopharyngioma should be commenced, the capsule of the tumour entered and this downward posteroinferior extension gutted and gently drawn up from the interpeduncular cistern. An attempt should then be made to work from the interpeduncular cistern along the posterior part of the wall of the third ventricle. Adhesion of the mass to the floor is frequently less evident than further anteriorly, but separation of the mass from the floor of the third ventricle may be difficult, and the cavity of the third ventricle may be entered. In these long lasting masses, however, the floor of the third ventricle is grossly thinned and seems to consist only of glial membrane, the nuclear masses having been pushed laterally by the expansion of the tumour. It is also evident that the hypothalamic nuclei have an astonishing capacity for recovery of function, and that provided one side of the hypothalamus is relatively undamaged, the inevitable trauma on the side of dissection need not present an undue hazard. As dissection round the periphery of the mass proceeds, the centre of the mass should be broken up by a variety of techniques. It is important to steady the mass of the tumour while this central disintegration is attempted, using either blunt hooks or low monopolar coagulation on a fine sucker which will often enable suction removal of soft parts of the tumour in the interstices of calcium, with the consequent mobilization of fairly large and apparently resistant portions of calcified tumour. The ultrasonic dissector is sometimes helpful, although access is so restricted and the field so narrow that the present bulk of most of these instruments limits their use. The most difficult dissection frequently lies anterosuperiorly, in the region of the posterior part of the chiasm, and it may be impossible to excise the tumour from this area completely. The anterior portion of the exposure in front of the optic nerve may be employed to displace the anterior part of the capsule of the mass from in front, while the dissection is pursued with gentle traction from behind.

High-dose preoperative and postoperative steroids are essential. Dexamethasone 4 mg 6-hourly should be commenced several days before surgery, together with a suitable anti-convulsant. Sodium valproate is commonly preferred in doses of 200–500 mg three times a day.

The development of diabetes insipidus postoperatively is the rule following such radical excision, but the assessment of plasma electrolytes and osmolality and the use of desamino-D-arginine vasopressin (DDAVP), a synthetic anti-diuretic, has eased the management of this previously serious complication. It is important in postoperative management to resume oral fluid administration as soon as possible, and also to avoid the contradictory use of intravenous fluid and DDAVP at the same time, the fluid load tending to increase renal excretion while the DDAVP is given to suppress it. In our practice, intravenous fluid is discontinued as soon as the patient is conscious. If levels of consciousness are inadequate for complete oral alimentation, a nasogastric tube should be passed.

The early phase of diabetes insipidus may be succeeded by a phase of fluid retention attributed to inappropriate ADH secretion, characterized by low serum osmolality, fluid retention, brain swelling, and in the worst cases, the development of convulsions. This is possibly the most dangerous postoperative state at the present time. It is therefore extremely important to avoid fluid overload, and safer to run the patient slightly dry. Seizures, which, as with any other major craniotomy, may occur at any time postoperatively are best controlled by the use of intravenous chlormethiazole, with due attention to the fluid load necessary to carry the drug.

The main cause of morbidity and mortality in the radical excision of craniopharyngioma results from injury to the carotid artery or major perforating vessels. Small infarcts in the thalamus from thrombosis of one of the perforating branches of the posterior communicating artery are not uncommon but the risk is much reduced by use of the operating microscope and careful preoperative angiography. Adhesion to the carotid arteries on the same or the opposite side is a common cause for the abandonment of an attempted radical excision.

Illustrations by Barbara Hyams

# Surgery for posterior fossa tumours

**C. B. T. Adams** MChir, FRCS
Consultant Neurosurgeon, The Radcliffe Infirmary, Oxford, UK

## Introduction

Posterior fossa tumours present with either focal neurological signs (from either cranial nerves, cerebellum or brain stem) or raised intracranial pressure. The age of the patient often indicates the pathology. In the first decade, cystic cerebellar astrocytomas and medulloblastomas are common. Haemangioblastomas are found in the second and third decades, while metastatic tumours occur more often from the fourth decade onwards. Meningiomas are found particularly in middle-aged females. Acoustic neuromas have a wide age incidence and often elude diagnosis until a very late stage. Indeed, acoustic neuromas will continue to be the commonest cause of blindness secondary to papilloedema from raised intracranial pressure until the lay public and medical profession cease to regard unilateral deafness as an inevitable consequence of ageing.

CT scanning with contrast enhancement is the investigation of choice. Lumbar puncture should be avoided if there is any evidence from the history or physical examination of a posterior fossa mass. Vertebral angiography is indicated if the clinical features and CT scan suggest a haemangioblastoma, while the suspicion of an acoustic neuroma will indicate audiological and caloric tests.

## Principles of surgery

The posterior fossa contains more vital structures in less accessible sites than any other part of the body. Thus, posterior fossa surgery demands particular care to facilitate access to the tumour as well as extreme care in the handling of tissues. These demands are met by reducing intracranial pressure, by careful and precise positioning of the patient, specialized anaesthesia[1] and by the use of microsurgical techniques.

### Reduction of intracranial pressure

Intracranial pressure should be reduced both preoperatively and during the operation. Obstructive hydrocephalus is a common cause of raised intracranial pressure in these patients. The easiest and safest method of reducing intracranial pressure in these circumstances is to introduce a ventriculo-atrial or peritoneal shunt. If the tumour is lateralized, then obviously the opposite lateral ventricle should be shunted lest this incision interferes with the subsequent posterior fossa surgery. The danger of upward herniation through the tentorial notch following the shunt has in the author's opinion been unduly stressed, for he has never seen this happen in these circumstances. The alternative is to introduce a ventricular drain at the time of surgery, but this not only introduces the possibility of infection in the postoperative period but may also lead to the development of an acute supratentorial subdural haematoma, especially if the sitting position is used. This complication is announced by a sudden and unexpected discomforting bulging of the posterior fossa accompanied by marked venous bleeding. The preoperative course of dexamethasone may be of considerable use where there is oedema of the cerebellum, as is commonly seen with metastatic tumours.

There are several helpful manoeuvres which the surgeon can use to reduce intracranial pressure during the operation. The position of the patient and reduction of venous pressure are of great importance and will be discussed further. If there is a cystic component, as with a haemangioblastoma or astrocytoma, then the cyst should be tapped as soon as possible. If the dura is drum-tight and thus too tight to open, then the cyst should be tapped transdurally before formal opening of the dura itself.

On opening the dura, the cerebellum may bulge alarmingly even in the absence of an obstructive hydrocephalus. This should be countered quickly by finding a subarachnoid cistern, either the cisterna magna or the cerebellopontine angle cistern, either of which may be opened to release cerebrospinal fluid (CSF). Mannitol or other such agents have little place in the surgery of the posterior fossa. Avoiding hypercapnia and jugular compression are of course essential.

## Position of patient

Sitting the patient up with the head flexed allows good exposure, particularly for midline lesions, as well as improving CSF and venous drainage. This is the position of choice for midline tumours, but since it is associated with two particular dangers, hypotension and air embolism[2], it should be avoided in hypertensive or arteriopathic patients. An arterial line for continuous blood pressure and ECG monitoring is essential. The incidence of air embolism is inversely proportional to the experience of the anaesthetist and surgeon. Thus, the sitting position should only be used with a midline incision through the avascular ligamentum nuchae. The position should allow elevation of the legs, which may be bound, to reduce venous stasis. Precordial Doppler monitoring is the most sensitive and important indicator of air embolism available and should be in position. The anaesthetist should have immediate access to the neck to allow jugular compression. End-tidal carbon dioxide and atrial catheterization are further techniques sometimes used to diagnose and treat air embolism. However, most important is dialogue between the surgeon and anaesthetist. A bloodless field should not be a cause of self-satisfaction but should indicate a danger of imminent air embolism. The surgeon can often see an open vein and counter air embolism by immediately flooding the field with Ringer's solution and requesting jugular compression. The latter should be carried out after each stage of the exposure, the particularly dangerous phases being the stripping or cutting of the suboccipital muscles and the bone removal. Immediate waxing of the diploic spaces of the bone is essential. If air embolism occurs, then aspiration of air through the right atrial catheter is sometimes useful. If the venous pressure is dangerously low, then posterior fossa exposure must be carried out while the anaesthetist gently squeezes the jugular veins in the neck.

## Microsurgical techniques

In the author's opinion, very few posterior fossa procedures should be performed without microsurgical techniques, that is to say, the operating microscope, bipolar coagulation and microsurgical instrumentation. These allow minimal retraction of the cerebellum, magnification and illumination, all of which facilitate gentle surgical technique. The time-honoured procedure of excising the lateral third of the cerebellum to gain access to the cerebellopontine angle is unnecessary these days, and a large acoustic neuroma does not require incision of the tentorium, as has been advocated in the pre-microscope era. Retraction should at all times be as gentle as possible and it is worth remembering that the capillary circulation in the tissues adjacent to the retractor is the critical factor in the production or avoidance of tissue damage. The Yasargil type of retractor is particularly convenient in conjunction with the microscope but it should be relaxed periodically whenever retraction is not strictly necessary. A pattie or lintine strip should *always* be placed on that part of the brain against which the retractor is applied.

A motorized operating table is particularly helpful, allowing the tumour to be rotated around the microscope as well as permitting rapid alteration of the patient's position. This is especially useful when removing cerebellopontine tumours.

The microsurgical technique used in the posterior fossa does not differ from that used elsewhere. The author's practice is to hold a carefully regulated narrow-bore sucker in the left hand while using bipolar coagulation or microscissors in the right. The assistant at this stage is superfluous but he/she and the scrub nurse are best positioned on the surgeon's right to allow the microscope stand to be positioned on the left.

In general, malignant tumours should be removed by excising the obviously pathological tissue and not transgressing into the surrounding cerebellar white matter. Metastases, cystic cerebellar astrocytomas and haemangioblastomas should be excised by working in the normal, but possibly oedematous, white matter of the cerebellum. The microscope allows vessels to be seen, coagulated and cut, so preventing the difficult problem of having to deal with a torn vessel that has retracted into the surrounding brain substance.

## Choice of approach

Posterior fossa tumours are conveniently divided into those arising in or near the midline, those arising laterally in or near the cerebellopontine angle and the much rarer large tumours extending to both areas. The approach to midline tumours is different from that towards laterally placed tumours.

# MIDLINE EXPOSURE

## Position of patient

### 1

The aim is to place the suboccipital bone in the vertical plane. Overflexion of the chin may cause airway obstruction and must be avoided. Pin fixation of the head is very useful. The legs should be elevated and bound with a compression bandage. It is important that the head be strictly positioned in the midline, without rotation, to allow the surgeon to find and maintain the midline avascular plane of the ligamentum nuchae.

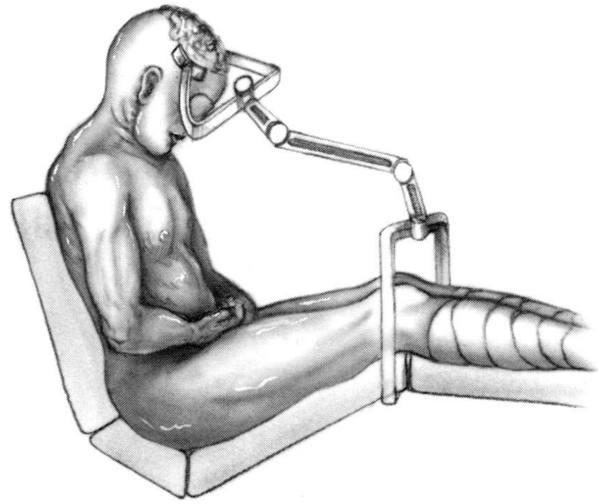

1

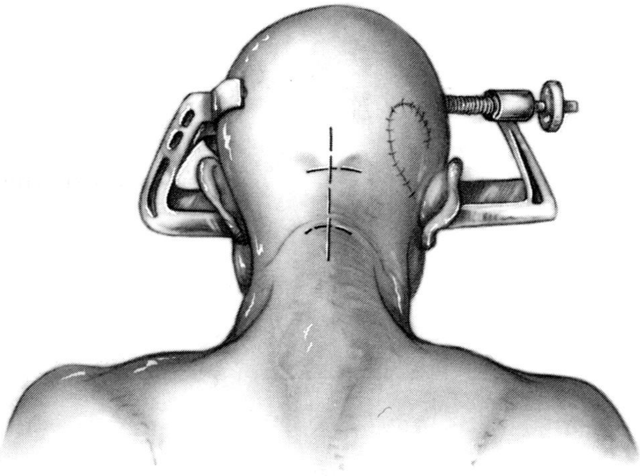

2

## The operation

### The incision

### 2

An incision is made in the midline extending from 3 cm above the external occipital protuberance to approximately 3 cm below the spine of the axis.

# 3

The skin is undermined and Raney clips are applied. The avascular plane of the ligamentum nuchae is found and opened with cutting diathermy. This is deepened until the occipital bone is exposed.

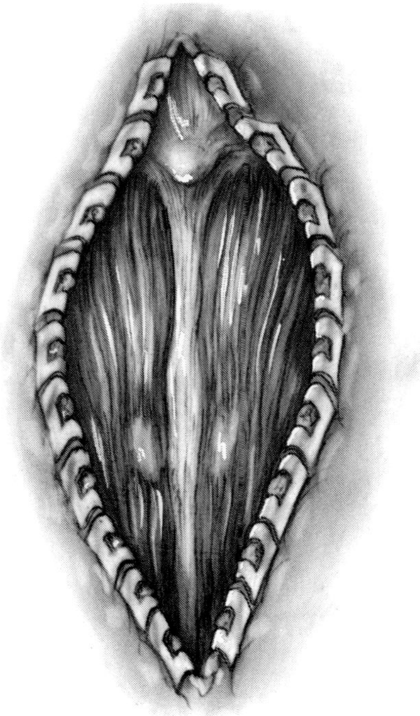

3

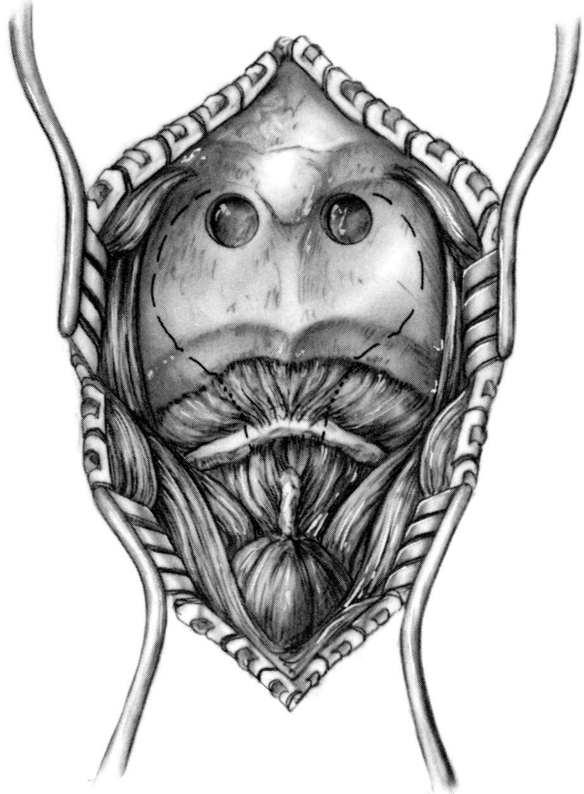

4

# 4

The arch of the atlas is then defined and exposed. The vertebral artery is related to the upper surface of the lateral part of the arch of the atlas. Two landmarks warn the surgeon of the artery's proximity. First, a 'dead space' is encountered adjacent to the medial aspect of the artery. Secondly, a plexus of veins immediately surrounds the artery itself.

If particular access is required laterally, then the suboccipital muscles may be detached on one side just below the superior nuchal line, making sure there is an adequate rim of muscle and fascia to allow reapproximation at the end of the operation. This manoeuvre requires extensive undermining of the skin on that side but is a very useful method of obtaining extensive exposure of one side of the posterior fossa, especially in children.

## Craniectomy

# 5

Two burr holes are made on either side of the midline over the transverse sinuses. It is far easier to work from above downwards than vice versa. Wilm's, then Horsley's bone rongeurs are used to open up and extend the burr holes to form the craniectomy. Careful and quick waxing of the bone is essential, especially near the occipital protuberance which contains large diploic channels. The bone is thick over the venous sinuses, midline and rim of the foramen magnum, but thinner elsewhere. The arch of the atlas is removed by one or two bites with the Horsley rongeurs. This is advisable in most instances to prevent postoperative tonsillar coning but may be dispensed with if the tumour is large and cystic.

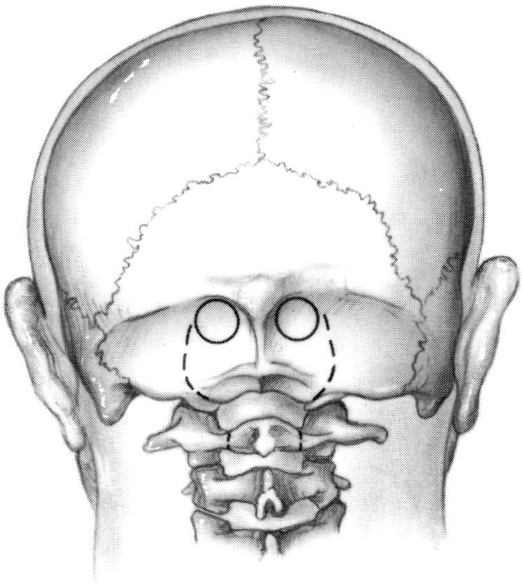

5

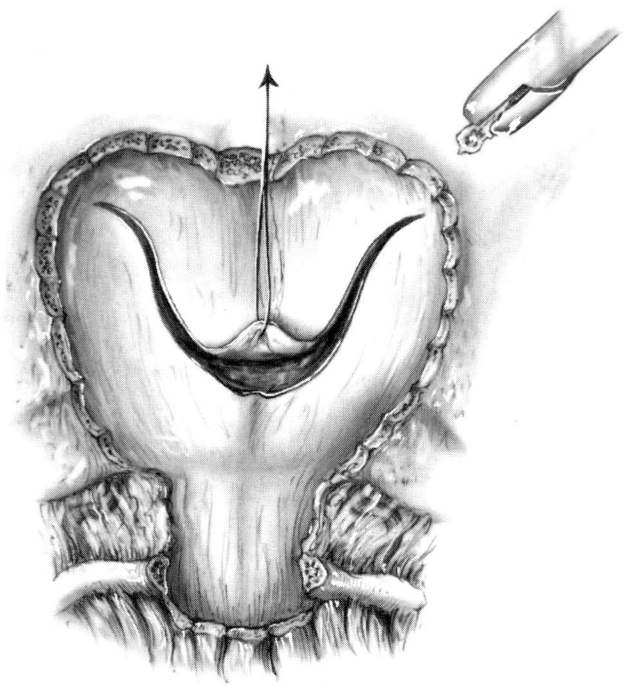

6

## Dural opening

# 6

The dura is opened as an inverted 'U', with a midline extension caudally across the foramen magnum to below the level of the arch of the atlas. The initial dural incision is best made with scissors while the extension is most easily achieved with a tenotome after a pattie has been introduced into the subdural space overlying the cranio-cervical junction.

7

A small unnamed dural artery requires coagulation on each side. The dura in the region of the vermis may contain large venous channels which must be coagulated or ligated. Sometimes there is a prominent fold, the falx cerebelli. The craniovertebral junction also contains large venous channels and so it is essential to coagulate the edges of the dura in this region even though they are not obviously bleeding in the sitting position.

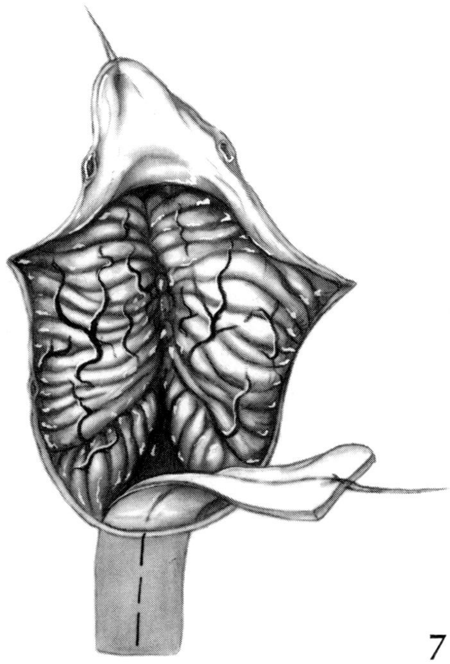

7

## Removal of tumour

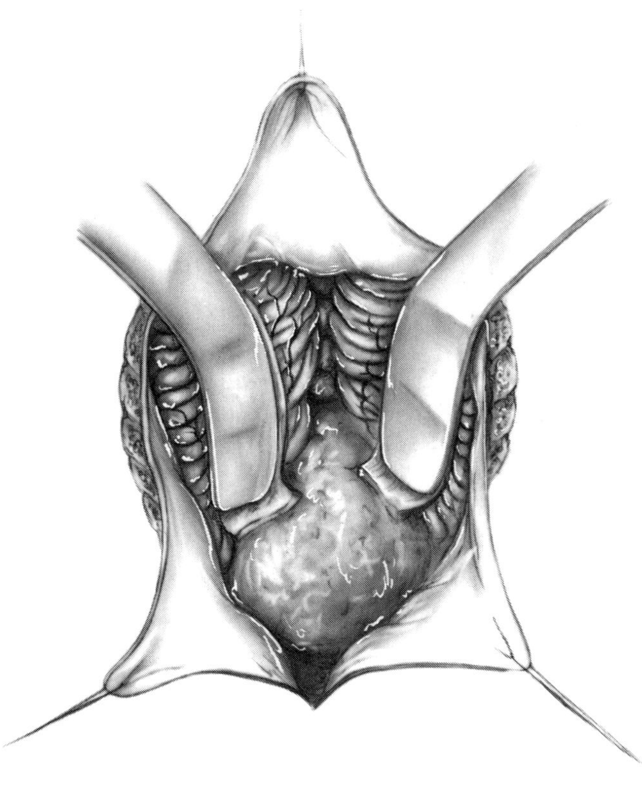

8

8

If the midline tumour is not obviously visible, the arachnoid should be opened and the tonsils gently parted. One can then look up to the fourth ventricle through the foramen of Magendie. Often the tumour will be seen bulging into this ventricle. The floor of the fourth ventricle is sacrosanct and must not be damaged in any way. It should be covered with a cellolite pattie at the first opportunity. A pattie should also be placed in the cisterna magna to prevent blood trickling down the spinal canal. If still no lesion is found, then the inferior vermis of the cerebellum is split, keeping strictly to the midline to avoid damage to the dentate and other cerebellar nuclear masses. Self-retaining retractors are now inserted on each side of the cut vermis to allow microsurgical techniques to be used from this stage onwards. If a hemispheric lesion is found, then the folia should be carefully inspected. They are often expanded and stretched over the lesion. A transverse incision along the line of the cerebellar folia is then made. If the lesion is in or adjacent to the superior surface of the cerebellum, adjacent to the tentorium, then the veins bridging the cerebellum, transverse sinuses and tentorium must be coagulated and cut. Access here demands that the craniectomy has to be taken sufficiently high and also that the head and neck of the patient are sufficiently flexed. An alternative route in these circumstances is from above by way of a right occipital craniotomy and incising the tentorium. This is especially useful for small arteriovenous malformations on the superior surface of the cerebellum.

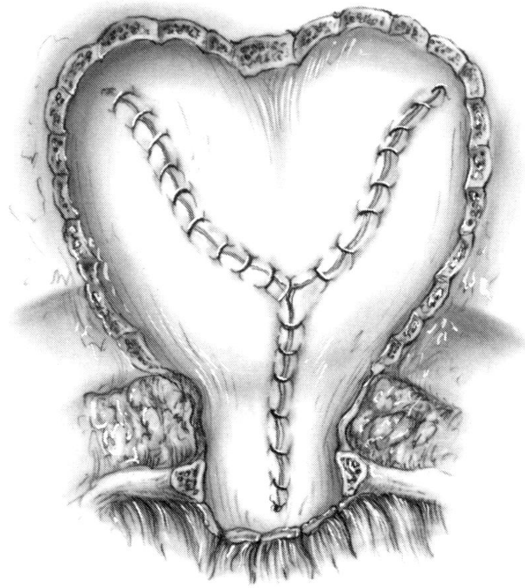

9

### Closure

## 9 & 10

Careful haemostasis is essential. The author prefers the systolic blood pressure to be over 100 mmHg before coming out. The cut surfaces of the cerebellum should be covered with absorbable cellulose (e.g. Surgicel, Ethicon, UK). This expands postoperatively, so should never be packed into a cavity. Irrigation with Ringer's solution will detect any bleeding points. The dura cannot usually be closed (unless the tumour is hemispheric and has a large cystic component). The dural defect is covered with a sheet of Surgicel, which in 3 months becomes a fibrous membrane. The muscles are carefully checked for bleeding points and then closed with absorbable sutures. Note that, as the ligamentum nuchae is triangular in shape, the first suture is at the apex of the triangle while subsequent layers of sutures become longer as one works superficially. The skin, which is in effect the base of the triangle, is closed carefully in two layers without drainage.

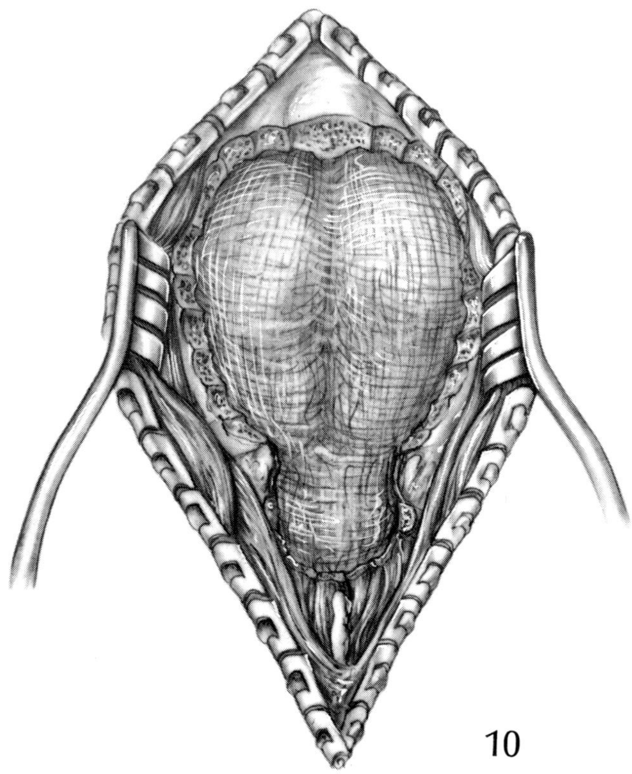

10

# Postoperative care

Postoperative care does not differ from that after other cranial operations. Postoperative haematomas are particularly hazardous in this region and may present with sudden apnoea.

## EXAMPLE: HAEMANGIOBLASTOMA OF THE CEREBELLUM

# 11

Haemangioblastoma is an example of a cerebellar tumour which usually arises near the midline and which is suitable for removal through a midline exposure with the patient in a sitting position. Such tumours are the commonest posterior fossa tumours in the second and third decade of life. Their cell of origin is debatable. They do not occur above the tentorium and, although usually cerebellar and cystic, they may occasionally be solid and arise in the brainstem or spinal cord. They are benign but have a propensity to have a multifocal origin, especially when familial (von Hippel Lindau syndrome). Polycythaemia may also be a concomitant feature. In such patients, repeated haemangioblastomas occur but arise at various sites from both sides of the cerebellum. Occasionally, especially after repeated operations, local invasion of extracerebellar tissues may occur.

The typical haemangioblastoma consists of a cyst containing yellow-tinged fluid in which there is a 'cherry-red' nodule. This is the highly vascular tumour which secretes the cyst fluid. The nodule itself has to be removed. The tumour usually has several feeding arteries and large red draining veins but the circulation is not unusually rapid as in arteriovenous malformation. Hence, early filling veins are not usually seen on angiography, in contradistinction to arteriovenous malformations.

However, from a technical point of view it is important, as with arteriovenous malformations, to remove the arterial input at an early stage of the excision and delay taking the major draining vein until the end. Failure to do this will result in a rapidly swelling engorged and bleeding tumour – a particularly alarming situation when the tumour is solid and in the brainstem, and a situation which can only be resolved by rapidly enucleating the tumour. Usually, however, removing a haemangioblastoma is one of the easiest tasks that faces a surgeon in the posterior fossa.

The diagnosis is usually apparent on the CT scan, the only other cystic tumour being cystic cerebellar astrocytoma. It is always advisable to carry out vertebral angiography to demonstrate the 'cherry-red' nodule. There may be more than one, but the symptomatic nodule will be associated with the cyst. Whether to remove other asymptomatic nodules at this stage depends on their accessibility as well as the ease of finding them when unassociated with a cyst.

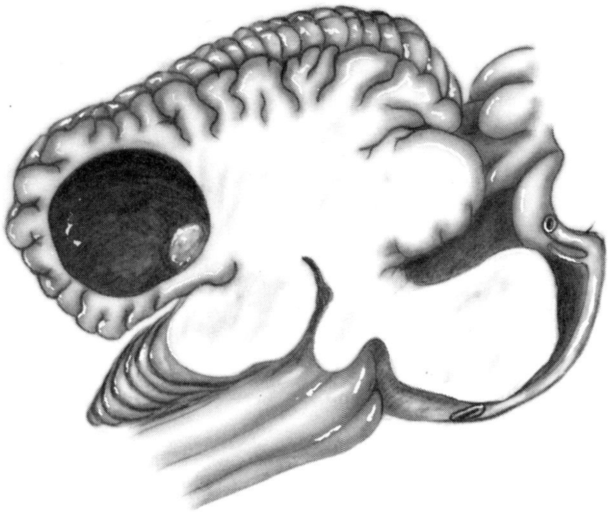

11

## Position of patient and incision

If, as is usually the case, the haemangioblastoma cyst and nodule are near the midline, then the patient is operated upon in a sitting position (*see Illustration 1*) through a midline exposure. If necessary, a lateral muscle cut is made just below the superior nuchal line, in the direction of the tumour, to provide more lateral exposure. Less often the tumour is laterally placed; the lying 'park bench' position is then more appropriate. If there is severe hydrocephalus, prior shunting is advisable. If, despite this, the dura on exposure is 'drum-hard' and unsafe to open, then a small nick should be made in the dura and a brain needle inserted into the cyst to slacken off the posterior fossa structures before opening the dura. With this cystic tumour, it is feasible to make a small cruciate dural incision immediately overlying the cyst which allows the dura to be resutured without difficulty at the end of the operation.

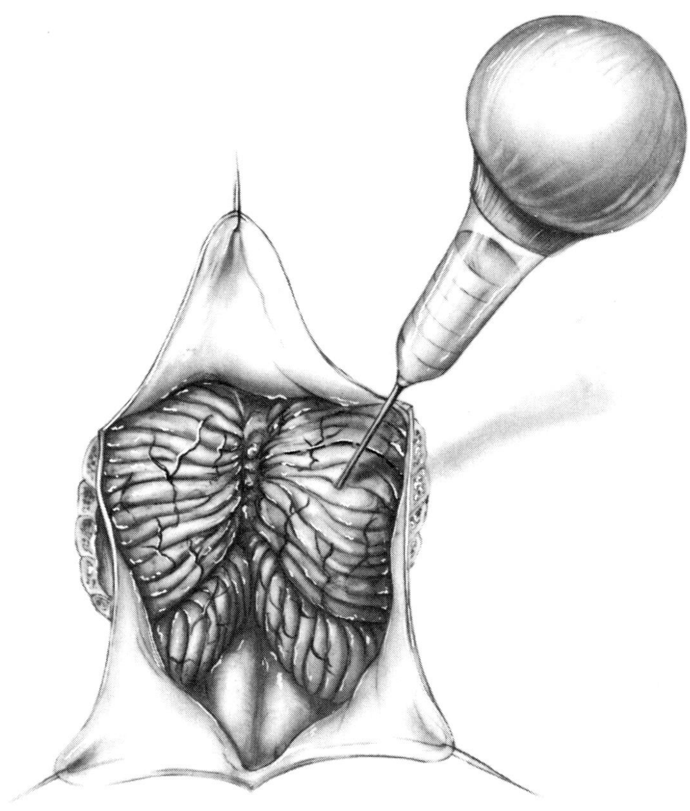

12

### Exposure

# 12 & 13

On exposure of the appropriate part of the cerebellum, the folia overlying the tumour will be seen to be expanded, stretched and rather whiter in colour. Feeding arteries or draining veins may also be seen. If the cyst has not already been tapped transdurally, then it should be tapped at this stage to slacken off the cerebellum. It is inadvisable to remove more than is necessary at this stage. A transverse incision along the folia nearest to the most superficial part of the cyst is then made. Obviously, this incision must avoid the tumour nodule should this also be superficially placed. The cerebellar cortex is coagulated and cut in the usual fashion and the white matter incised using a fine metal sucker with the diathermy applied to the handle of the sucker. A gush of typical clear yellow fluid greets the surgeon on entering the cyst if not too much fluid has been aspirated previously. At this stage, the microscope and self-retaining retractor are introduced. It is important to examine all areas of the cyst carefully to find the nodule and any others that may be present.

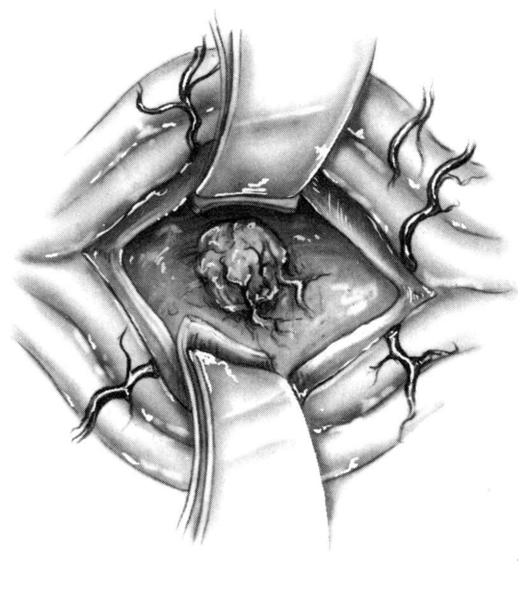

13

## Excision of tumour

# 14 & 15

The operating microscope and bipolar coagulation should be used to remove the tumour. The excision is usually carried out from within the cyst, but if the tumour arises from the exposed cerebellum then the excision is even more straightforward. It is advisable to stay within normal cerebellar white matter and to identify, if possible, the main draining vein at an early stage in order to preserve it until last. With cystic tumours this is less important than with solid tumours, not only because the cyst allows easier working conditions but also because the nodules are invariably smaller by the time symptoms arise by virtue of the cyst rather than the nodule.

By dissecting around the normal white matter and avoiding at all costs the vascular tumour tissue, the major vessels can be easily identified, coagulated and cut. If there is any doubt about the completeness of the coagulation, then the vessel should be 'half cut' to check haemostasis before completing section of the vessel. This avoids the problem of having to chase bleeding vessels which have retracted into the surrounding and hitherto normal brain. After the nodule has been excised, haemostasis is carefully checked and the tumour bed covered with a layer of Surgicel.

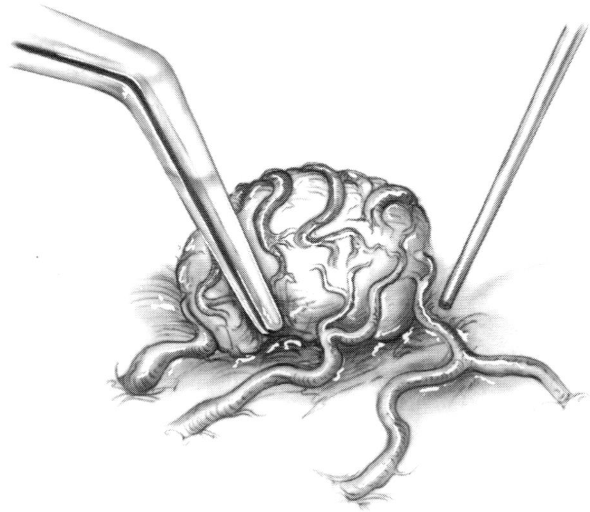

14

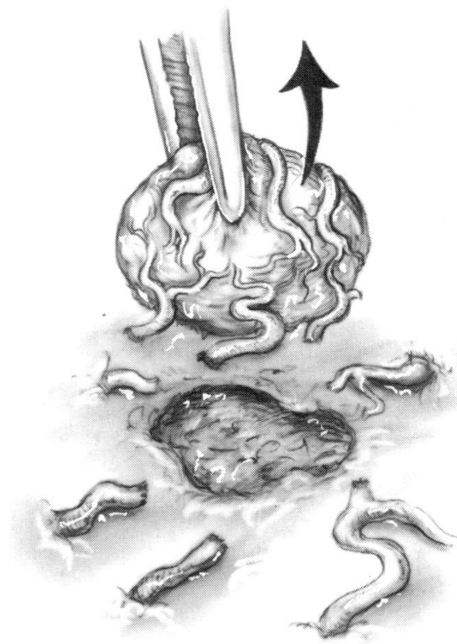

15

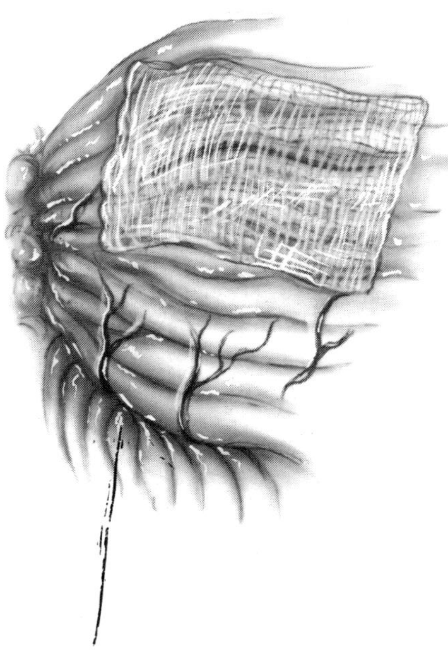

16

## Closure

# 16

Because of the presence of a cyst it is usually feasible to close the dura. This allows quicker postoperative recovery by avoiding serosanguinous fluid from muscles to permeate the subarachnoid pathways. If the dura is under tension because of cerebellar swelling, then it is better to leave the dura open and to remove the posterior arch of the atlas.

# LATERAL CEREBELLOPONTINE ANGLE TUMOURS

## Position of patient

## 17 & 18

The author has tried various approaches and positions for gaining access to the cerebellopontine angle but finds the lying or 'park bench' position to be the best. Lengthy microsurgical procedures are much less tiring if the surgeon is sitting, and moreover sitting over the patient, rather than if the patient is in the sitting position. Also, the danger of air embolism, greater with incisions off the midline, is best avoided by lying the patient down and not using the sitting position.

Great care must be taken with positioning of the patient. The head is fixed with pins. The mastoid process is horizontal, the table tilted head-up about 30°. The overlying shoulder is strapped down to open up the angle between the retromastoid area and the neck. A rolled-up towel is placed under the thorax just below the underlying axilla to minimize pressure on the brachial plexus. The underlying arm is strapped to pull the area of the radial groove (above the elbow) away from the operating table. This area is also well padded. Two patients experienced temporary radial nerve palsies before we took these precautions. It is important *not* to flex the head but to keep it in the neutral position. Finally, the trunk of the patient is fixed to the back rest and other areas of the table with elasticated strapping. Test rotation of the table is carried out to ensure that the patient is firmly attached. The motorized table is an important adjunct. By rotating or tilting the table, the appropriate part of the tumour can be brought into view without significantly moving the microscope or oneself. An operating chair is used once the microscope has been introduced.

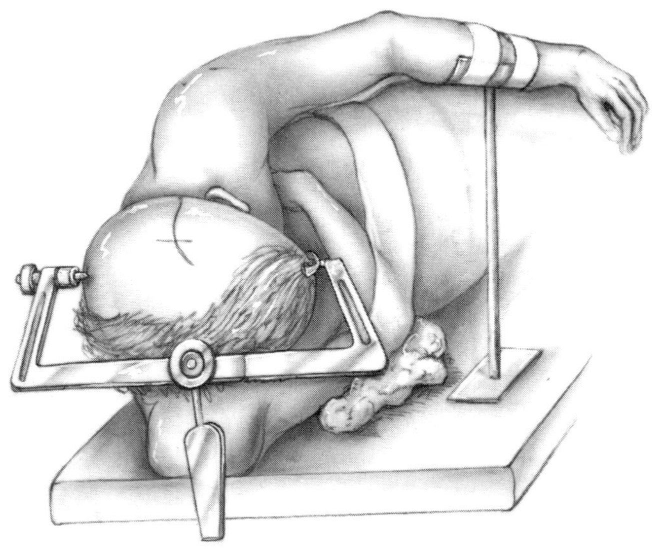

17

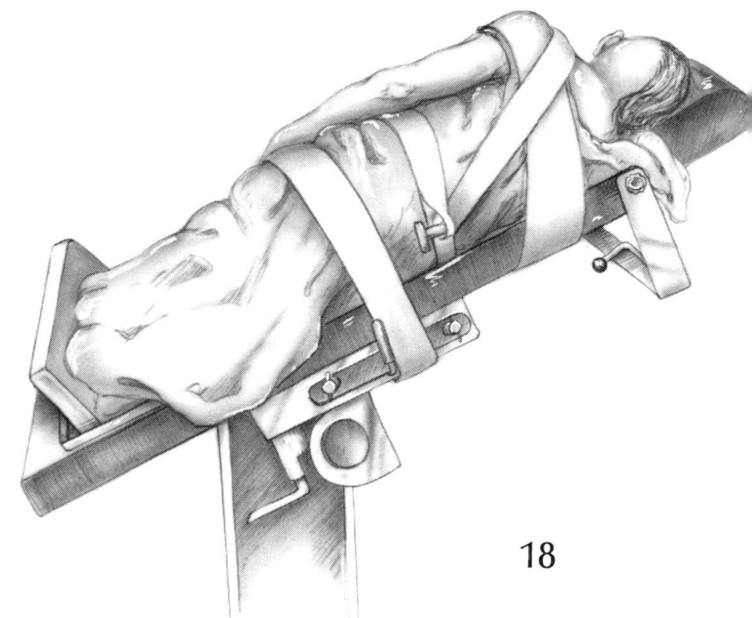

18

# The operation

## The incision

## 19

The incision must expose the sigmoid sinus and the distal third of the transverse sinus.

The sinuous incision is placed one finger's breadth behind the mastoid process. This produces good exposure especially if access is required towards the base of the skull. However, it entails more muscle cutting and more postoperative pain. For small angle tumours or access to cranial nerves V to XI, an alternative, smaller, quicker and less painful incision is quite adequate. This is placed over the distal half of the transverse sinus and extends at a right angle over the mastoid process to its tip (mastoid–nuchal line incision).

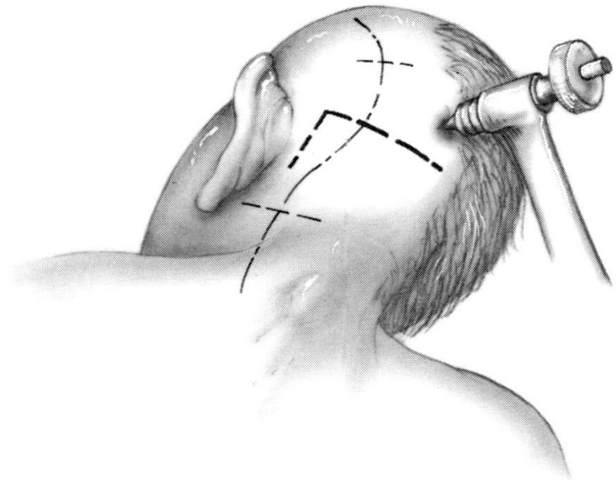

19

## 20

Both incisions allow exposure of the mastoid process, the lateral part of the superior nuchal line as well as the occipital bone between these landmarks and the foramen magnum. The occipital artery is seen and coagulated at the digastric groove. The mastoid emissary vein, a useful landmark, must be cut and the foramen plugged with wax. Great care is taken to avoid damage to the vertebral artery when using the sinuous retromastoid incision.

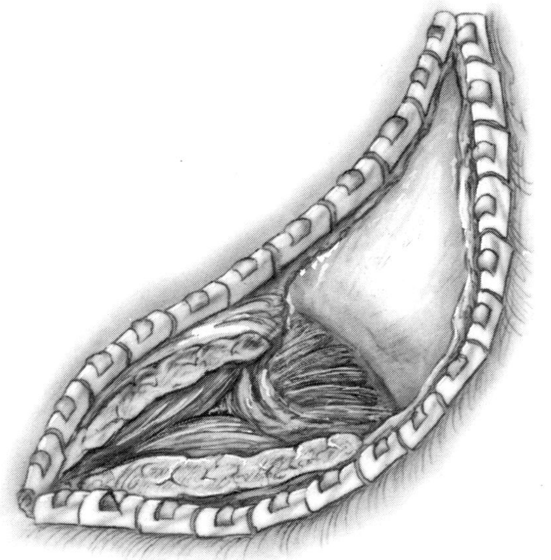

20

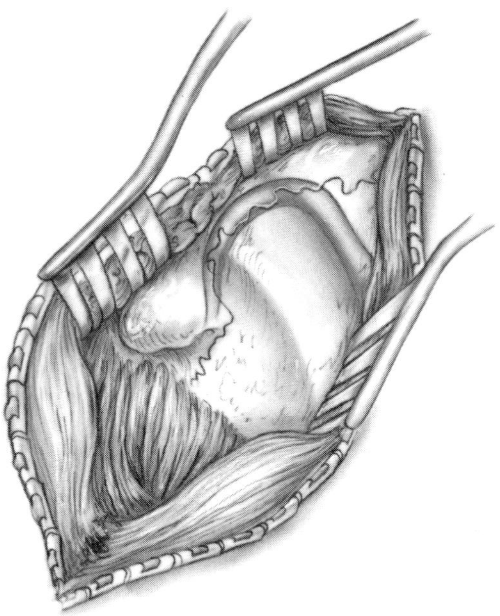

21

## 21

This will not arise with the small right-angle incision. The vertebral artery is avoided by sticking closely to the occipital bone by using cutting diathermy to undermine the muscle from the occiput before cutting more superficially. Also, the arch of the atlas should be felt for at frequent intervals. The artery is in danger once all the muscles (especially those of the suboccipital triangle) have been cut. As mentioned earlier, the vertebral artery is surrounded by a 'dead space' and a plexus of veins, and these will be encountered before the artery itself. It is not necessary to expose the artery although some surgeons make a point of doing so. Scissor dissection rather than diathermy should be used at this stage.

Since the stylomastoid foramen is quite near with this exposure, care must be taken to avoid damaging the facial nerve before even entering the posterior fossa.

## Craniectomy

# 22

Three burr holes are made, the first over the distal transverse sinus, which is indicated by the lateral extent of the lambdoid suture. Further burr holes may be made over the cerebellum and over the mastoid process, although the latter should not penetrate the inner cortical bone of the skull overlying the sigmoid sinus. Using rongeurs, the dura is exposed. This is extremely thin over the sigmoid sinus, and often it is easier to expose the medial edge of this sinus by working alternately from the transverse sinus above and the distal sigmoid sinus below, meeting at the point of entry of the mastoid emissary vein. A Watson-Cheyne dissector is often more useful than a smooth Adson for dissecting this thin dura off the sigmoid sinus. The craniectomy is about 5 cm in diameter.

Penetration of a venous sinus should not cause alarm; any venous bleeding can be stopped by Surgicel, pressure and patience. Often a little bone wax can be applied to the adjacent bone and pattie, thus exerting the necessary pressure and obviating the surgeon's need for much patience. The opened mastoid air cells must be carefully and completely waxed to prevent postoperative CSF rhinorrhoea.

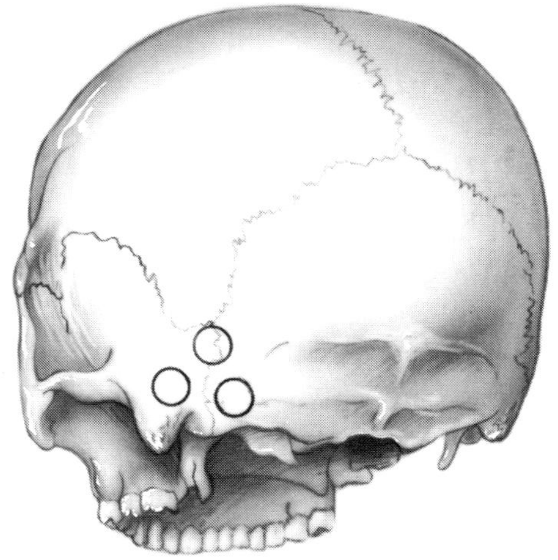

22

## Dural opening

# 23

The first dural incision should be made to the angle between the transverse and sigmoid sinuses, and then further incisions made to form a cruciate incision. The dural flaps are retracted by stay sutures.

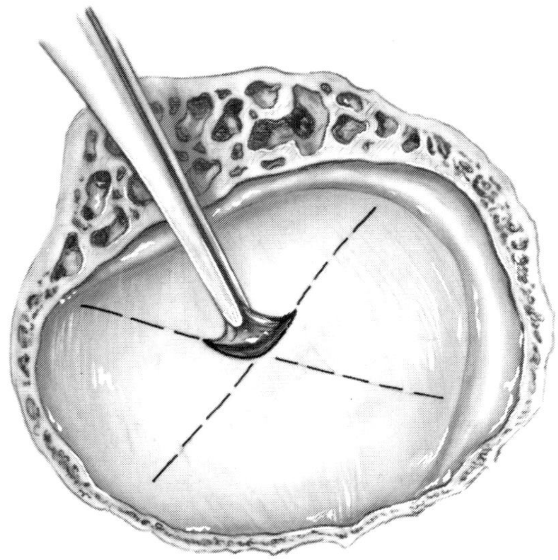

23

# 24

Two measures to protect the cerebellum are of great importance at this stage. First, the exposed cerebellum is covered by a sheet of Surgicel. Secondly, a pattie is tucked under the medial dural fold. Otherwise this edge cuts into the cerebellum even with gentle retraction. At this stage, the cerebellum may bulge rather alarmingly, but this can be counteracted by introducing the operating microscope and opening a subarachnoid cistern, either laterally or inferiorly, near the vagal group of nerves.

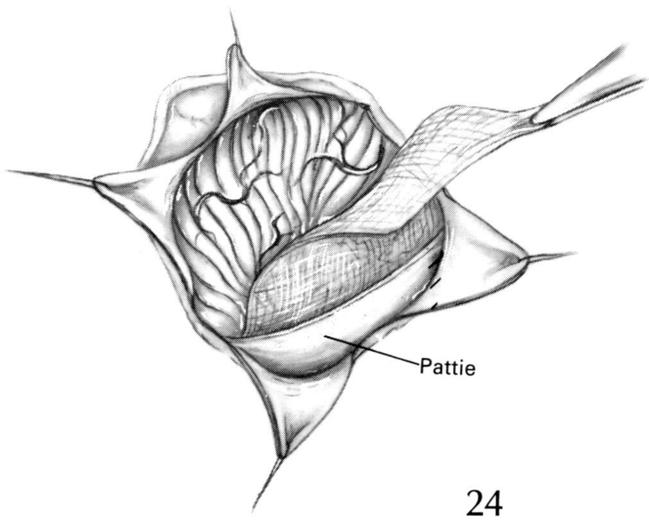


24

## Exposure of cerebellopontine angle

Even with this lateral exposure it is necessary to work around the posterolateral margin of the cerebellum. It is essential always to note the presence or absence of a draining vein from the cerebellum to the transverse sinus, for if present this will surely rupture during even gentle cerebellar retraction. The motorized operating table is of great help at this stage since, by rotating the table (and patient) well forward, it is possible to work around this posterolateral margin of the cerebellum under direct vision. Having reached the petrous bone, the surgeon then gradually rotates the patient backwards towards himself, thus allowing exposure of the cerebellopontine angle, the tentorial notch (and IVth nerve) above and the spinal accessory nerve below.

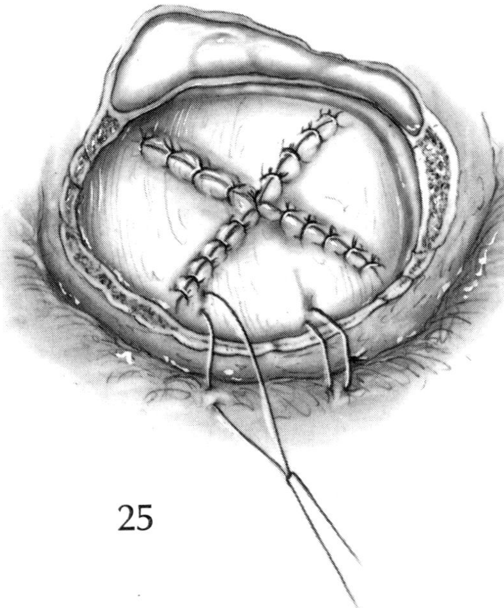

25

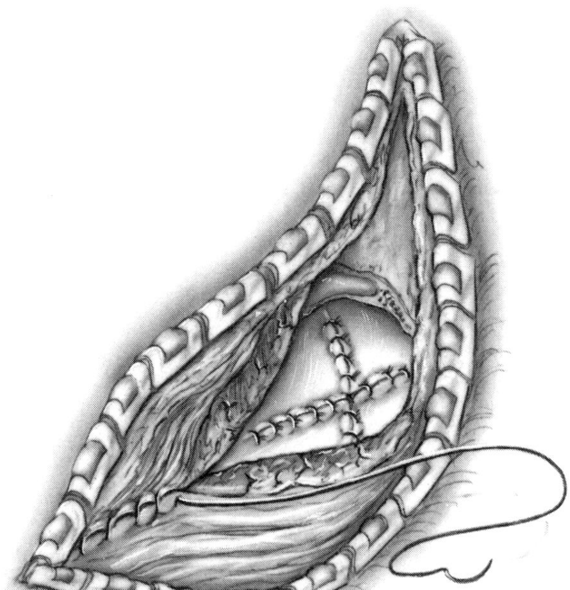

26

## Removal of tumour

Removal of an acoustic neuroma will be described in detail below. If there is doubt about the tumour type, the first structures to define are the VIIth and VIIIth cranial nerves. Meningioma, epidermoid cyst and a glioma mushrooming out of the brainstem or lateral recess of the fourth ventricle are all possibilities. A fusiform aneurysm of the basilar artery is not infrequent and should be considered when finding a rather 'rigid' and yellowed mass. The principles of dealing with these tumours do not differ from elsewhere.

## Closure

## 25

The dura should be closed if possible to reduce the risk of CSF rhinorrhoea via the mastoid air cells. This poses no problem if a benign tumour has been removed. If there is much cerebellar swelling, then the dura must be left open and covered with a sheet of Surgicel. If the dura is very slack, then one or two 'hitch' stitches should be put in to prevent postoperative extradural haemorrhage.

## 26

The muscle should be checked carefully for bleeding and closed in layers without drainage. The smaller, right-angled incision requires only a single layer of muscle sutures (and these, unlike the old-fashioned crossbow incision, are under no strain or tension). The skin is closed in two layers without drainage.

## EXAMPLE: REMOVAL OF AN ACOUSTIC NEUROMA

Removal of an acoustic neuroma is perhaps the most difficult operation in neurosurgery. The aim of the operation is total removal of the tumour with preservation of the facial nerve and even the cochlear nerve[3–5]. Partial, intracapsular removal should be considered nowadays only in the elderly or very disabled. The ability of the surgeon to preserve the facial nerve depends primarily on the size of the tumour and also on the consistency and vascularity of the tumour. The facial nerve is curiously resistant to distortion. A patient may have no evidence of lower motor neurone facial weakness (best shown by delayed or absent blink despite what neurological books state) yet at operation the nerve may be stretched and distorted often beyond identification and preservation despite use of the operating microscope. However, occasionally, a remarkably distinct facial nerve bundle may be found with a large tumour.

Obviously, the surgeon's task is greatly facilitated if the tumour is small. Thus early diagnosis must be encouraged and this requires that both the public as well as primary care doctors and ENT specialists regard unilateral hearing loss as due to an acoustic neuroma until proved otherwise. Caloric and brainstem auditory evoked potential tests should be carried out, followed by CT scanning and meatography. Acute vertigo, once thought never to be caused by an acoustic neuroma, may indeed be the presenting feature of this tumour.

### Anatomy

# 27

Successful acoustic neuroma surgery depends on an intimate knowledge of the pathological anatomy. There are three particular aspects that require emphasis: first, the relationship of the components of the auditory nerve to each other, especially in the internal auditory meatus (IAM); secondly, the blood supply of the tumour; and finally, but most importantly, the relationship of the tumour to the surrounding arachnoid.

Acoustic neuromas are misnamed, for they arise from the vestibular nerve, especially the superior vestibular nerve, usually just medial to the lip of the internal auditory meatus. The lateral, distal part of the internal auditory meatus may be divided into four quadrants (with the skull in the head-up position) so that each quadrant is occupied by a nerve. The facial nerve is in the anterior and superior quadrant, while the cochlear nerve is anterior and inferior. These are often inseparable when both are flatted by neuroma. Posteriorly, the meatus is occupied by the vestibular nerves, inferior and superior each in the appropriate quadrant. The blood supply of acoustic tumours comes from two directions. Medially the tumour is supplied by the internal auditory artery and other branches of the anterior inferior cerebellar artery (AICA). It is especially important to realize that the AICA may loop onto the lower pole of the tumour, giving off branches to the tumour capsule, then leave to supply the brainstem. These branches must be coagulated and cut; but failure to preserve the AICA may lead to brainstem infarction. It is useful to note the very varied relationship of the AICA to the VIIth and VIIIth nerves when exploring this area for hemifacial spasm and thereby imagine the various relationships this artery may have to the facial nerve in the presence of an acoustic neuroma. Not infrequently, the AICA is substituted by a branch of the posterior inferior cerebellar artery (PICA). All one can say is that the anatomy is not constant and the surgeon has to be vigilant. When trying to preserve hearing when removing a small acoustic neuroma, it is necessary to preserve the internal auditory artery supplying the inner ear.

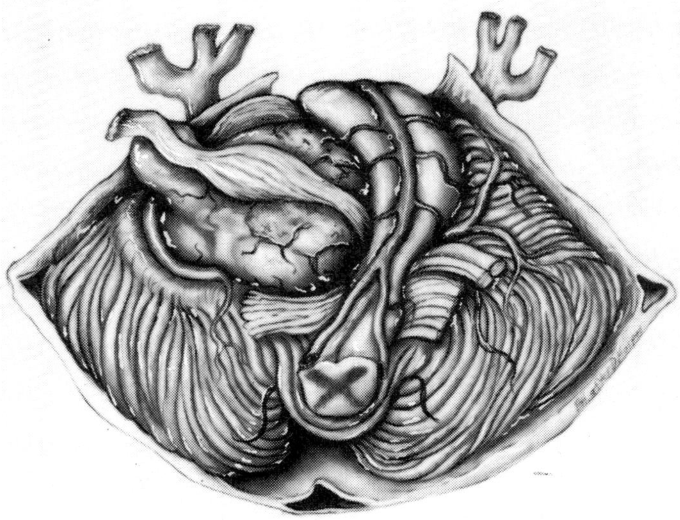

27

The lateral blood supply enters the tumour through the dura surrounding the internal auditory meatus. This originates from the external carotid artery and may be considerable. (In the past, when angiography was done for acoustic neuromas, a tumour 'blush' was occasionally seen with an external carotid injection of dye.) The vascularity of these tumours can be extremely troublesome. Hypotension is very useful but the surgeon can help himself by coagulating and cutting the dural attachment around the rim of the internal auditory meatus although the most anterior part cannot be cut until the facial nerve has been identified. Very often it is the vascularity as much as the size of the tumour that determines whether or not the facial nerve can be preserved.

# 28

The craft of surgery depends on 'getting in the right plane'. It is the knowledge of the distribution of the arachnoid that allows the surgeon to find and maintain that correct plane, not only to dissect the tumour away from the brainstem but also to preserve the facial nerve. In normal circumstances, an elongated funnel of arachnoid enters the meatus surrounding the VIIth and VIIIth cranial nerves as well as the internal auditory artery.

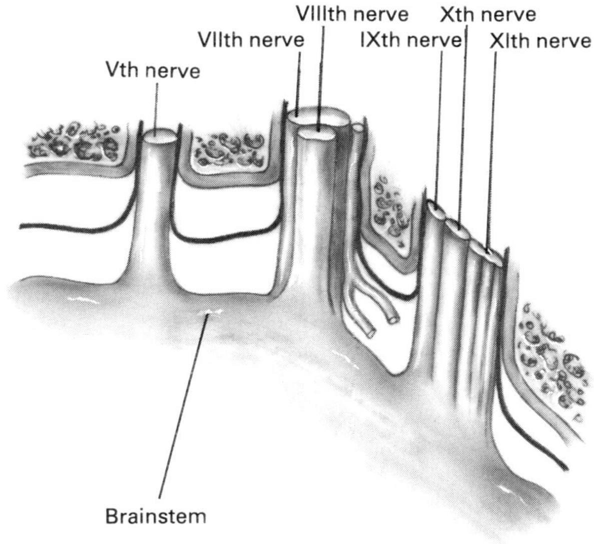


28

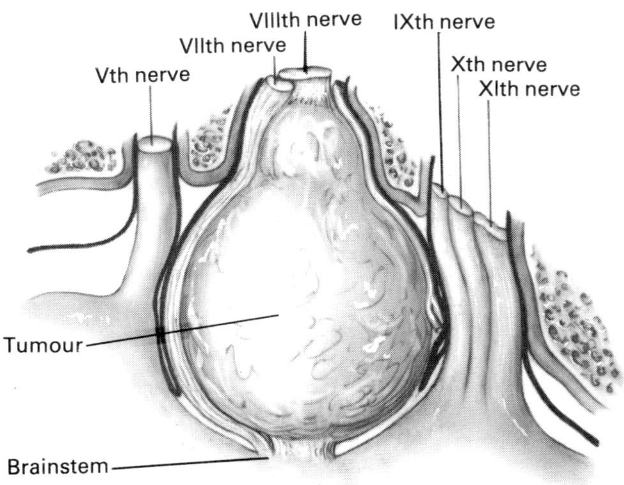


29

# 29

When an acoustic neuroma develops, it is initially surrounded by the arachnoid except for its point of attachment to the brainstem by the VIIIth nerve. Further enlargement and indentation into the cerebellum and brainstem moulds the arachnoid as shown. This has at least three important consequences for the surgeon. First, the facial nerve is expanded and incorporated into the arachnoid sheath adjacent to the meatus. Secondly, the lateral part of the tumour is surrounded by a double layer of arachnoid, and here the cerebellum is easily teased away by obtaining the plane between these two layers. Thirdly, the brainstem and adjacent cerebellum is bereft of arachnoid; the right plane is between the pia and the tumour capsule. The *only* point of attachment of the tumour is where the VIIIth nerve enters the brainstem.

## Position of patient and incision

These have been described already (see p. 336). Either incision may be used. In general, the less traumatic right-angled (mastoid–nuchal line) incision is entirely satisfactory for the smaller acoustic tumour while larger tumours are better approached through the retromastoid incision. Having opened the dura, particular care must be taken to protect the cerebellum. The microscope is introduced and a subarachnoid cistern found and opened to release CSF in order to slacken the cerebellum. Usually it is easiest to go to the inferior pole of the tumour and open the cistern surrounding the vagal group of nerves. With smaller tumours, the cistern around the petrosal vein and Vth nerve is more accessible. Just occasionally, an acoustic tumour has an arachnoid 'cap' or cyst containing xanthochromic (high-protein) CSF, which is usefully evacuated.

## Removal of tumour

As removal of a large acoustic tumour is the most difficult operation in neurosurgery, it will be described in some detail. The tumour is removed in eight stages. The actual order may be varied in some respects. For instance, with a medium-sized or smaller tumour the author finds the medial end of the facial nerve at the third stage (as described) before the plane becomes obscured by blood. When dealing with a larger tumour and/or oedematous cerebellum, it is advisable to carry out stage 4 before stage 3.

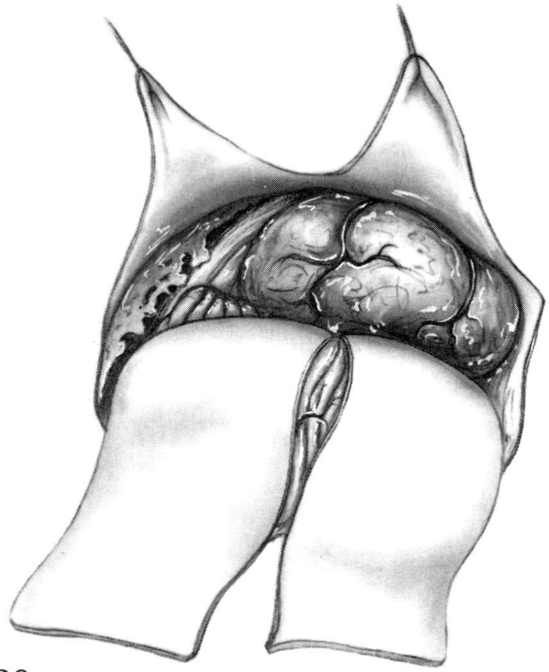

30

*Stage 1*

# 30

The first step is to expose as much of the tumour as possible by gently dissecting the cerebellum away. This entails finding the plane between the two layers of the arachnoid. The petrosal vein is seen and may be preserved, but with large tumours, inevitably it has to be coagulated and cut. It is better to do this now than to avulse it from the superior petrosal sinus, which is more difficult to deal with (by using Surgicel and pattie pressure). At all times, the cerebellum must be protected by patties and the retractor released whenever possible.

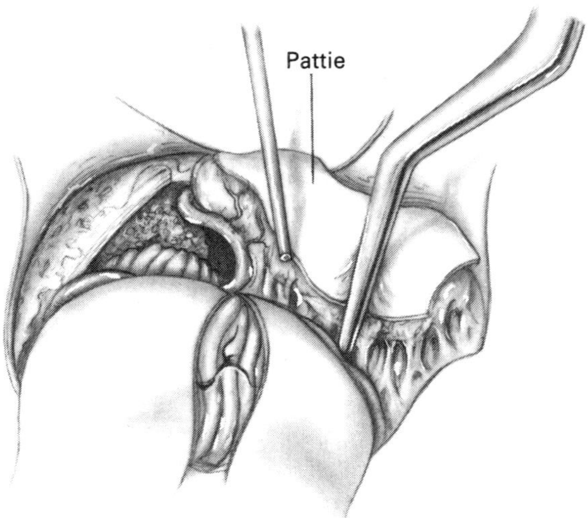


31

*Stage 2*

# 31

The second step is to find and protect the IXth, Xth and XIth cranial nerves. Like the Vth nerve, these have a separate arachnoid sleeve distinct from the tumour and VIIth nerve and so can be gently dissected away and protected, preferably with a cellolite pattie. At this stage, the AICA (or PICA substitute) is found looping onto the lower pole of the tumour. Its branches to the tumour must be carefully coagulated and cut to allow the vessel to be gently dissected off the tumour and likewise protected by a pattie. The VIth nerve is seen further anteriorly near the vertebral artery.

*Stage 3*

By rotating the table towards the surgeon, it is possible at this stage to work around to the junction of the cerebellum and brainstem and so find the medial end of the facial nerve. There are four landmarks to this nerve.

1. The flocculus of the cerebellum. This must be retracted to reveal the second landmark.
2. The vein of the lateral recess of the fourth ventricle. This drains into the petrosal vein.
3. The choroid plexus protruding out of the lateral recess of the fourth ventricle through the foramen of Luschka.
4. Immediately in front of the choroid plexus is the attachment of the VIIIth nerve to the brainstem. *This is the only (non-vascular) structure that can be cut.* If in doubt, cutting should be delayed unless one is sure of the anatomy. The cochlear nerve is seen coursing along the inferior pole of the tumour. The origin of the IXth nerve is nearby as well. The facial nerve is seen immediately anterior and inferior to the VIIIth nerve attachment. It is greyer than the underlying brainstem and may be extremely flattened as it passes upwards and laterally. The AICA or internal auditory artery may run between the facial nerve and the tumour. If seen, a small micropattie should be placed on the facial nerve origin as a marker to which to return.

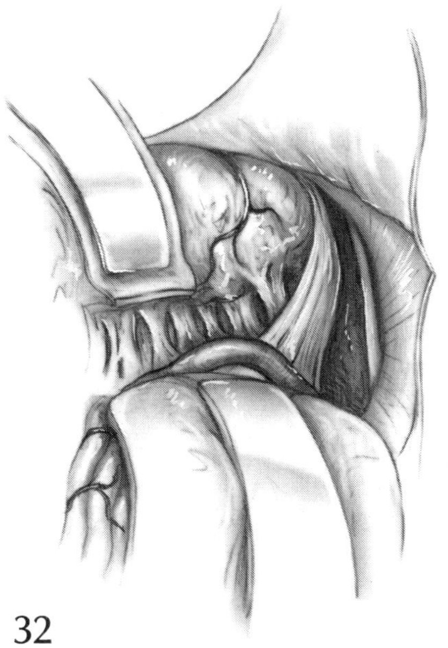

32

# 32

The dissection is now continued towards the upper pole. The plane between tumour and brainstem must be meticulously maintained. It is a matter of experience and judgement as to which veins belong to the brainstem or tumour capsule. Arterial bleeding indicates the plane has been lost. If this happens, the surgeon should tuck in a piece of Surgicel and move elsewhere to find the correct plane before working back to where the plane has been lost. It is particularly helpful to place a pattie on the tumour itself, gently pulling tumour away from brain. Every tumour is different with regard to its consistency and vascularity and the surgeon has to adapt his technique for these variations.

*Stage 4*

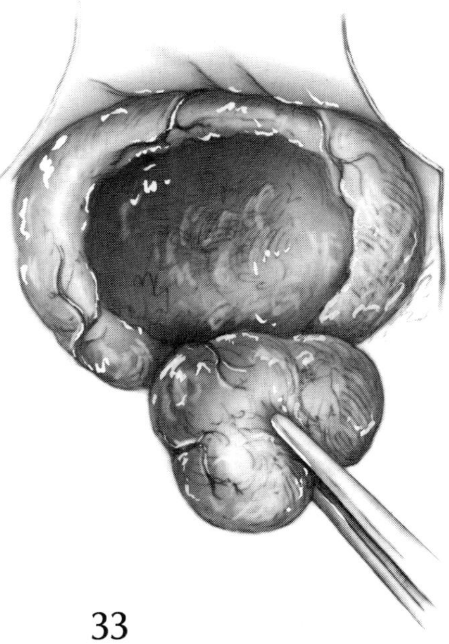

33

# 33

The next stage is to hollow out the tumour. With large tumours this should precede stage 3. As much as possible of the posterior surface of the tumour is exposed, avoiding the upper and lower poles where the facial nerve may be. Using bipolar coagulation, the surface is coagulated and cut into. The tumour is typically butter-yellow in appearance and is usually soft. Occasionally, cystic degeneration occurs. Bleeding can be reduced by coagulation and squeezing the tumour tissue with bipolar forceps before cutting with scissors, rather than the traditional method of scraping out the tumour with a surgical spoon. If available, an ultrasonic aspirator may be of help at this stage. The softer the tumour, the larger is the 'capsule' that must be left for fear of penetrating into surrounding structures. Having carried out stage 3, the surgeon can determine how much of the interior area of the tumour it is safe to remove, for he has a direct method of assessing the thickness of the capsule in relation to the consistency of the remaining capsule. After haemostasis of the more obvious bleeding vessels, using coagulation or Surgicel, the cavity is packed with wool in saline. Induction of hypotension is particularly helpful at this stage.

*Stage 5*

## 34

The internal auditory meatus is then brought into view by rotating the table forward as much as possible. The dura adjacent to the meatus containing pathological vessels is coagulated and incised.

A curved dissector defines the meatus, and the adjacent bone is drilled away to expose the dura lining the meatus. A cutting burr is used to begin with and a diamond burr to remove remnants of the bone. Two important points are: (*1*) to remove nearby patties to avoid sudden and traumatic avulsion of the pattie (and adjacent structures) caught in the drill; and (*2*) to protect the adjacent structures by holding (in one's left hand) the sucker with the tip near the drill end. It is essential always to make sure the drill has stopped rotating before removing it from the wound. It is important to continue drilling until the lateral extent of the meatus is reached, to avoid leaving tumour behind.

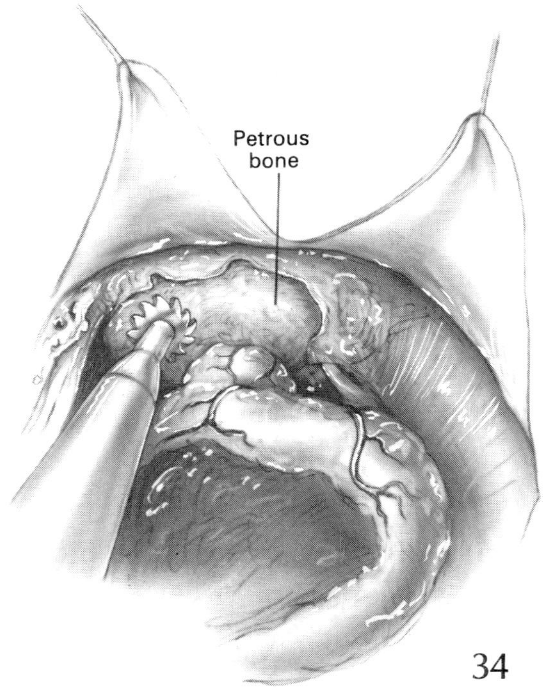


34

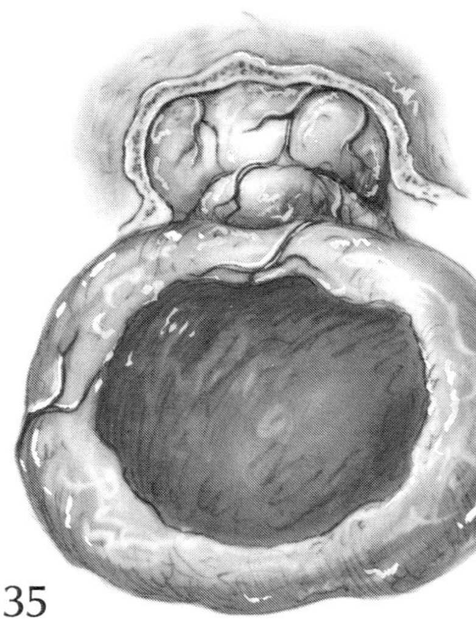

35

## 35

The dural lining is then incised and the meatal tumour and vestibular nerves are removed. The facial nerve, placed anterior and superiorly, is distinct from the tumour and is at this stage fairly easily defined and preserved. A pattie and, later, a retractor should be placed on the meatal tumour, pulling it towards the surgeon (*see Illustration 36*). The facial nerve is markedly stretched into a gossamer-thin membrane merged with the arachnoid at this point just medial to the entrance to the meatus. The surgeon needs patience, determination, and hypotension at this stage to preserve the facial nerve. He needs to know that the nerve can usually be preserved and that this is the most difficult phase.

*Stages 6 and 7*

## 36

Having defined the lateral part of the facial nerve, the next step is to cut the dural attachment of the tumour around the internal auditory meatus, thus cutting off this source of blood supply to the tumour. The surgeon then moves to the upper and lower poles of the tumour and continues gentle dissection of the tumour capsule from surrounding structures. The Vth nerve is easily preserved, having its own arachnoid sheath. The bulk of the tumour is gradually reduced by excising chunks of redundant tumour capsule, always careful to avoid areas where the facial nerve may be attached. It is helpful to place a pattie on the tumour and gently dissect this away from the brain rather than vice versa. The facial nerve is usually anterior, but may be displaced as far as the lower or upper poles of the tumour and the surgeon must be aware of these variations. Eventually one is left with a small amount of tumour attached to the facial nerve.

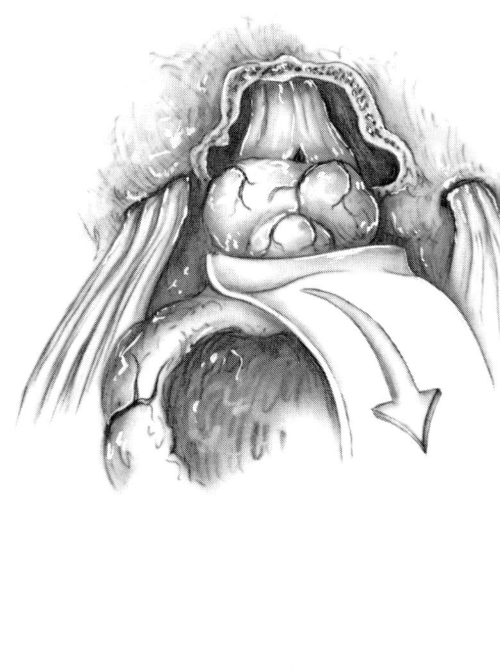

36

*Stage 8*

## 37

The final stage is to tease the remaining tumour off the facial nerve by working from all directions. The elongated facial nerve adds to the difficulties by preventing dissection from a fixed structure. Patties placed on the exposed facial nerve reduce this mobility. It is remarkable how a stretched membranous facial nerve becomes a respectable nerve bundle by the end of the operation. If it is impossible to preserve the facial nerve over the summit of the tumour, then it is worth approximating the two ends with a single stitch. Failing that, the author proceeds to a facio-accessory anastomosis and a lateral tarsorrhaphy a few days later.

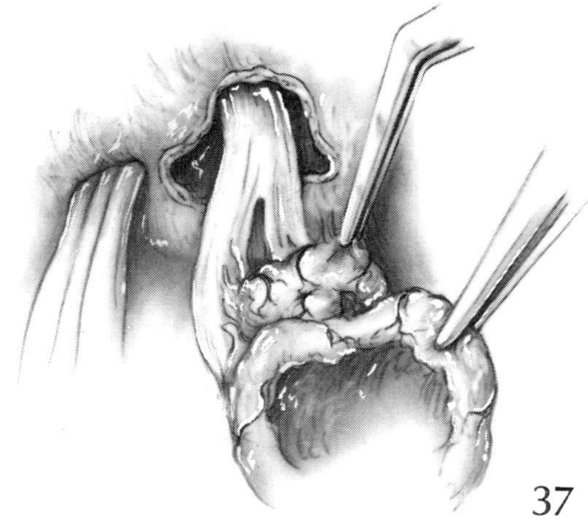

37

## 38

Finally, a piece of muscle is placed in the meatus. This reduces the chances of CSF rhinorrhoea via a small mastoid air cell opened during the meatal exposure. The patties are gently removed and any bleeding points sealed with bipolar coagulation or Surgicel. The hypotension should be reversed before dural closure. Haemostasis must be obsessional, for not only is evacuation of a postoperative clot following this operation far more difficult and hazardous to the cranial nerves that have been so carefully preserved, such a clot is also far more likely to give rise to long-term sequelae from subtle, or not so subtle, brainstem damage.

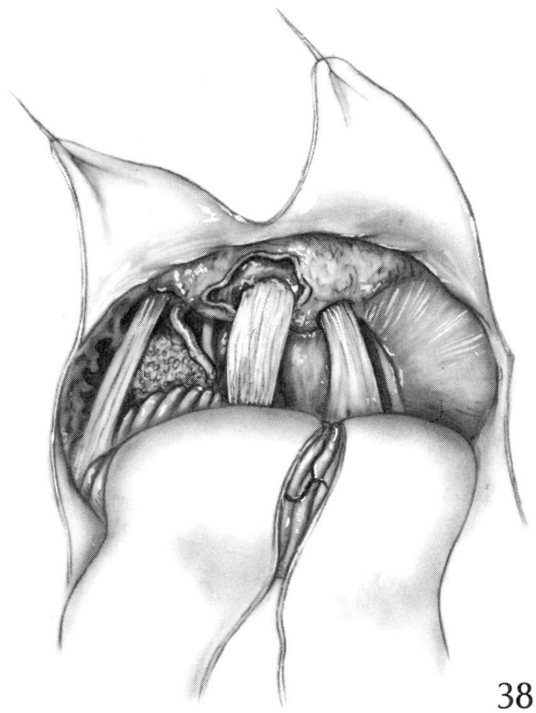

38

## Postoperative care

The patient should not be allowed fluid by mouth for at least 24 hours, and then only if palatal movement is satisfactory. Voice and swallowing go together so that, if a patient is phonating well postoperatively, swallowing will also be satisfactory. Failure to swallow for more than a few days is an indication for tracheostomy to prevent aspiration pneumonia. After 2–3 months, adaptation occurs but this may be aided by injecting Teflon (El du Pont, UK) paste into the paralysed vocal cord. The danger of postoperative haematoma has already been discussed. The clot may be in the tumour cavity or extradurally.

CSF rhinorrhoea via the mastoid air cells and Eustachian tube may occur. This is most easily stopped by asking an ENT surgeon to carry out a mastoidectomy and packing the middle ear and mastoid cavities. In the rare patient with preserved hearing, re-exploration of the posterior fossa and meatus would have to be advised instead.

With tumours up to 2 or 3 cm in diameter, the facial nerve may not only be intact but functioning. If the nerve has been preserved, then 6–9 months may elapse before function returns. The first sign of this is return of tone to the resting face so that the drooping mouth becomes horizontal on the weak side. If the nerve cannot be preserved, then the author advises a facio-accessory anastomosis and lateral tarsorrhaphy, preserving the upper eyelashes, a few days postoperatively. Other surgeons use a facio-hypoglossal anastomosis but to the author it seems better to avoid adding a weak tongue to a weak face; moreover, patients find facial movements on tongue movement off-putting. After an accessory nerve anastomosis it is important to instruct the patient to carry out shoulder girdle exercises. After 9 months or so, facial movements occur and the patient can, with the aid of daily practice in front of a mirror, obtain quite acceptable facial movement while tensing the shoulder girdle.

# EXTENSIVE TUMOURS: ACCESS TO BOTH THE MIDLINE AND THE CEREBELLOPONTINE ANGLE

## 39

On rare occasions, it may be necessary to obtain exposure from the midline to the cerebellopontine angle. This may be achieved by a hockey-stick incision, starting over the mastoid process and running along the superior nuchal line and down the midline. This may be used with the patient sitting. Alternatively, if the patient is in the lying position, the retromastoid incision can be placed more medially, midway between the mastoid process and the midline. As long as the principles enunciated above are followed, the surgeon need not, nor should he, be hide-bound by particular incisions.

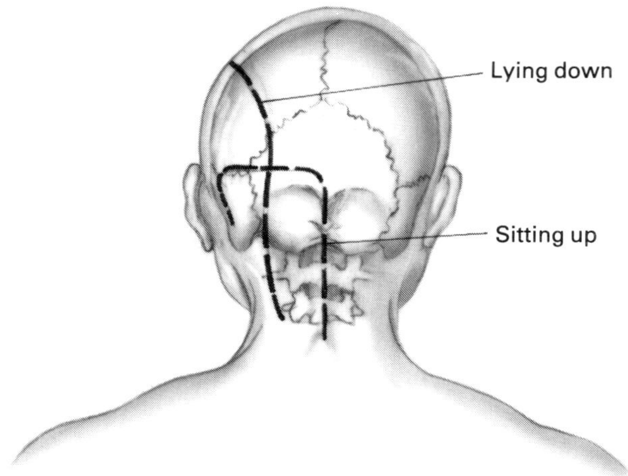


39

### References

1. Frost, E. A. M. (1984) Some inquiries in neuroanaesthesia and neurological supportive care. Journal of Neurosurgery, 60, 673–686

2. Matjasko, J., Petrozza, P., Cohen, M., Steinberg, P. (1985) Anaesthesia and surgery in the seated position: analysis of 554 cases. Neurosurgery, 17, 695–702

3. DiTallio, M. V., Malkasian, D., Rand, R. W. (1978) A critical comparison of neurosurgical and otolaryngological approaches to acoustic neuromas. Journal of Neurosurgery, 48, 1–12

4. Ojemann, R. G., Levine, R. A., Mongomery, W. M., McGaffigan, P. (1984) Use of intraoperative auditory evoked potentials to preserve hearing in unilateral acoustic neuroma removal. Journal of Neurosurgery, 61, 938–948

5. Malis, L. I. (1975) Microsurgical treatment of acoustic neuromas. In: Microneurosurgery, H. Handa (ed.). Baltimore, MD., University Park Press

Illustrations by Robert N. Lane

# Translabyrinthine and transtentorial removal of acoustic nerve tumours

**T. T. King** FRCS
Consultant Neurosurgeon, The London Hospital, London, UK

**A. W. Morrison** FRCS, DLO
Consultant Ear, Nose and Throat Surgeon, The London Hospital, London, UK

## Introduction

The success, limited though it was, achieved by Cushing and Dandy established the posterior fossa or retrosigmoid approach as the standard neurosurgical method for removing acoustic nerve tumours, a position that was unchallenged until the reintroduction by House in 1964 of the translabyrinthine operation[1]. This is different in three ways: the approach lies in front of the sigmoid sinus, it depends on the removal of a portion of the petrous bone, and it makes the cerebellopontine angle accessible to otorhinolaryngologists. Its advent was not welcomed by neurosurgeons, who have largely ignored it. However, meanwhile its originators have acquired the largest experience of acoustic nerve tumours ever published[2].

## Preoperative

### Indications

The use of this technique is largely a matter of personal taste. It has, however, two contraindications. If hearing and speech discrimination are good preoperatively and the tumour is small (1 cm or so in diameter), an attempt should be made to preserve hearing, and, as this is incompatible with the translabyrinthine operation, the posterior fossa approach is necessary. The other contraindication is coexistent middle ear or mastoid infection or an old mastoid cavity. In the occasional case, not always recognized preoperatively, where the tumour arises from the facial nerve and extends into the petrous bone along the facial canal, the translabyrinthine approach has a clear advantage because it allows exposure of the intrapetrous part of the nerve. This ability to follow the nerve into its bony canal is also of value with acoustic nerve tumours since, if the nerve has been divided but its central end is recognizable, the distal end can be mobilized out of petrous bone to effect an end-to-end anastomosis or, if a graft is necessary, the length required will be shorter.

For the rest, the larger the tumour, the more advantageous the translabyrinthine operation, because exposure and retraction of the cerebellum are minimized and the deepest part of the cerebellopontine angle, around the fifth nerve and tentorial hiatus, is more easily accessible. In small tumours (up to 1–2 cm in diameter), there is not much to choose between the two if the patient has no useful hearing.

The translabyrinthine approach may be used for other types of cerebellopontine angle tumours, especially meningiomas, but its use needs discrimination. Meningiomas lateral to the meatus are best approached through the posterior fossa. Those on a level with it can be satisfactorily dealt with by the translabyrinthine operation, provided that the patient is deaf. When the tumour arises from the posterior surface of the petrous bone medial to the meatus, the posterior fossa approach is unsatisfactory and a translabyrinthine approach, combined if necessary with division of the tentorium, is more suitable. The exposure in such difficult cases may be improved by transposing the facial nerve backwards from its canal in the petrous bone and removing the cochlear and medial portion of the petrous pyramid. Jugular neurinomas can be managed through the labyrinth if they do not extend into the jugular foramen, but if the diagnosis is clear preoperatively, which it may not be, a retrosigmoid approach is to be preferred.

The special disadvantages of the translabyrinthine approach are that it involves a field unfamiliar to the neurosurgeon, who consequently needs to cooperate with an otologist; that it is more time-consuming, the petrous bone dissection adding 1½–2 hours to the duration of the operation; that the approach is relatively narrow, although this can be overcome by experience and by attention to certain points described below; and most seriously, that it is liable to postoperative cerebrospinal fluid (CSF) leaks through the Eustachian tube and nose.

## Investigations

The neuro-otological diagnosis of acoustic nerve tumours is beyond the scope of this chapter. However, it is important to have a good idea of the size of the tumour before the operation, upon which depend the risks and difficulties of the operation and the chances that the facial nerve or hearing may be preserved, points about which the patient will be anxious to have information. Neuroradiology provides the answer to this, with computerized axial tomography, in its most refined form, allowing most tumours to be seen directly, although with intrameatal growths it may be necessary to inject air into the cerebellopontine angle cistern to outline the tumour. Nuclear magnetic resonance (NMR) scanning, although not at present freely available, is superior to CT in showing growths of all sizes, even those confined to the meatus, as the petrous bone gives no signal and does not obscure the image of the tumour.

## Anaesthesia

General anaesthesia through an endotracheal tube and controlled ventilation are essential, as ideal operating conditions are necessary in such a restricted exposure. In large tumours, ventricular drainage and intravenous mannitol are used, but they are unnecessary if the tumour is less than 2 cm in diameter. Continuous recording of the arterial blood pressure through a catheter inserted for preference in the dorsalis pedis artery, and of the ECG allows sudden fluctuations in blood pressure and pulse rate to be detected. They signal a need for caution by the surgeon but not for abandonment of the operation. The duration of the procedure makes it likely that the patient's temperature will fall, hypothermia then causing delay in recovery from anaesthesia and anxiety to the surgeon and anaesthetist. Some warming blanket or device should therefore be used.

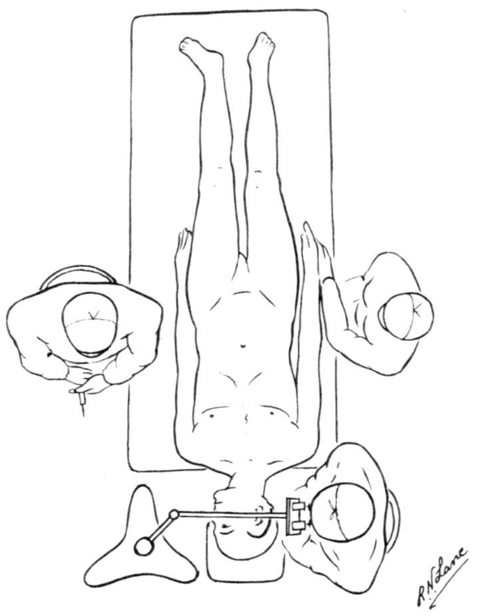

1

# 1

## Position of patient

The patient is placed in the supine position with the head turned about 45° to the opposite side. Too much rotation should be avoided, as this could obstruct the great veins in the neck. A little elevation of the head-end of the table will help to reduce venous pressure. Before starting the craniotomy, a piece of fascia about 5 × 5 cm and a lump of fat are cut from the right thigh. Before draping the patient's head the surgeon should check that the instrument table is placed well towards the patient's feet. Its upper margin should not be placed more cranially than the patient's costal margin or it will cause obstruction when the surgeon is trying to look up towards the apex of the cerebellopontine angle. The surgeon sits behind the patient's head, and the microscope should be on the opposite side. The anaesthetist is on the patient's left side and the theatre sister on his right, irrespective of the side of the tumour.

# The operation

## The incision

### 2

For large tumours, a ventricular catheter is inserted into the ipsilateral frontal horn and allowed to drain when the translabyrinthine dissection is completed. The incision, which is shaped like an inverted hockey stick, is made. It starts just below the tip of the mastoid process, runs upwards parallel with the posterior aspect of the pinna and about 2 cm behind its root, reaches a point on the lateral aspect of the scalp about three fingers' breadth above and behind the tip of the pinna, and then curves forward into the temporal fossa, sufficiently far to outline a scalp flap which, when turned forwards, will expose the outer end of the external auditory canal.

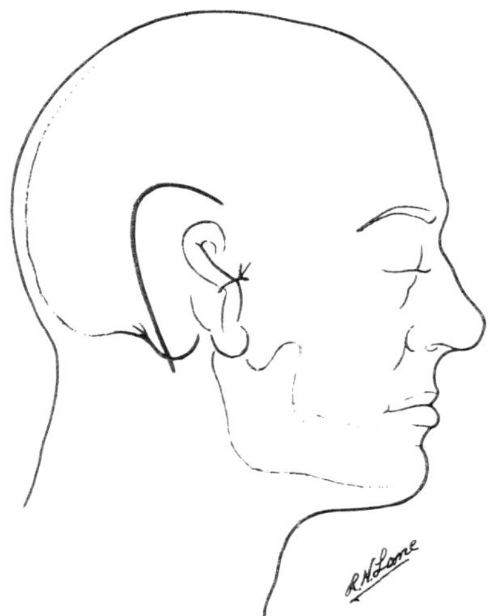

2

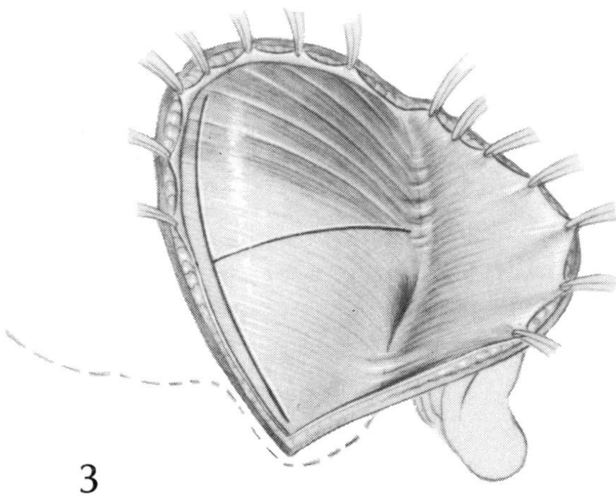

3

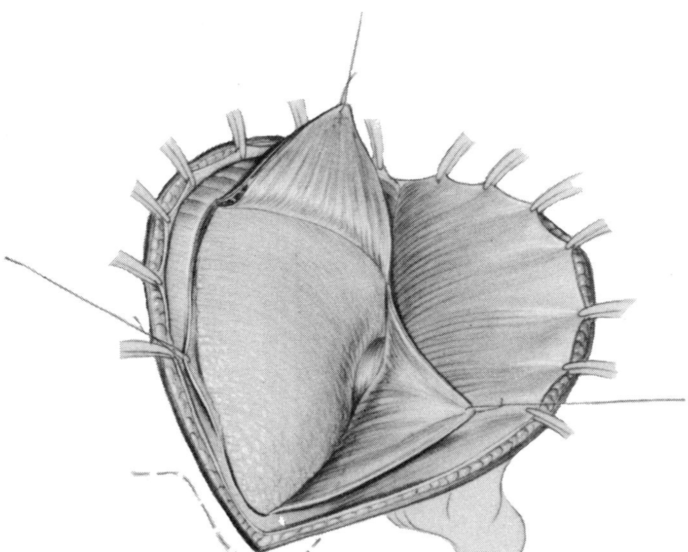

4

### 3 & 4

A T-shaped incision is made in the pericranium over the mastoid process and temporalis muscle, outlining two triangular flaps, the lower of which is turned forwards until the edge of the external auditory meatus is exposed. Above the external auditory canal, soft tissue should be cleared from the bone as far forwards as possible so that bone removal can be carried out along the roof of the meatus until the middle ear cavity is reached.

## Translabyrinthine dissection

# 5

The otologist now carries out the bone dissection, the details of which are described in the *Ear* volume of this series and will not be dealt with here. It is necessary, however, to emphasize the points which allow removal of a large tumour to be accomplished through a relatively small opening. The cortical mastoidectomy is of first importance because it can be extended freely whereas, deeper in, anatomical obstructions such as the jugular bulb and facial nerve restrict bone removal. By making the surface opening large – and especially by carrying it upwards over the inferior 2 cm or so of the temporal lobe, backwards over the sigmoid sinus and forwards above the external auditory meatus – the angle or arc through which instruments, and the surgeon's line of vision, can be directed into the depth of the wound is greatly increased. For instance, when working on the lower pole of the tumour, the surgeon looks downwards from above the patient's head, retracting the edge of the temporal dura upwards with the shanks of his instruments, and, when looking towards the petrous apex, the fifth nerve, he treats the exposed sigmoid sinus similarly. If the cortical opening is not quite big enough, it may prove difficult, especially towards the end of the operation, for instruments to penetrate into the depths of the wound. The surgeon will then need to stop and remove the obstructing ledge of bone, a somewhat irritating digression from the main procedure. Bevelling the edges of the mastoidectomy opening is a further aid to exposure.

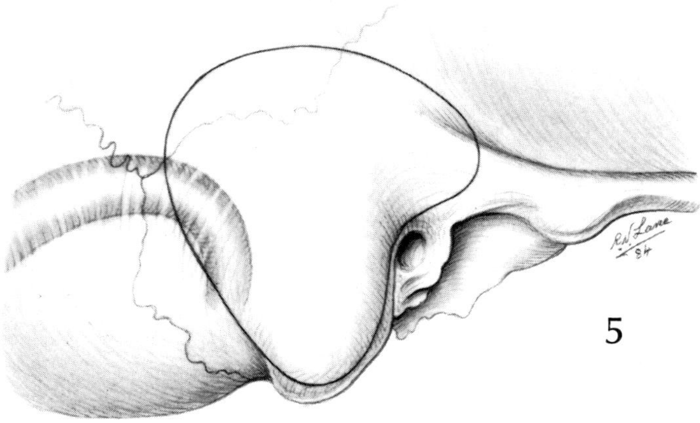

5

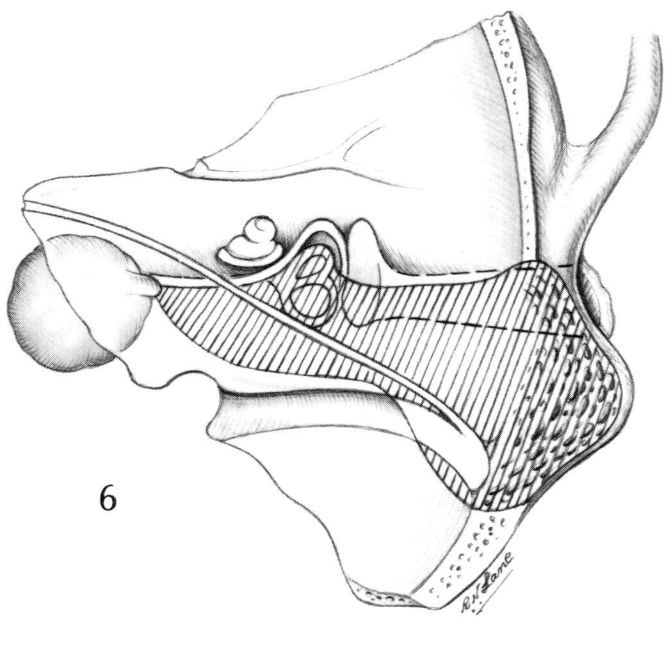

6

# 6

The petrous excavation is limited anteriorly by the posterior wall of the external auditory meatus and the descending portion of the facial nerve, both of which are left covered by a thin layer of bone and, in the deepest part of the opening, by the internal auditory meatus itself. Posteriorly, the dura of the posterior fossa between the sigmoid sinus laterally and the internal porus acusticus medially and from the superior petrosal sinus above to the jugular bulb below is cleared of bone, and the petrosal sinus and an area of middle fossa dura in front of it are also exposed. Initially, a thin layer of bone is left over all these structures in order to protect them and minimize bleeding until the internal auditory meatus has been fully opened from its lateral end to the rim of the porus. When exposing the internal meatus, as much bone should be removed from the roof and floor as is judged safe, keeping in mind the proximity of the facial nerve above and the jugular bulb below. The dissection is completed by the removal of the thin shell of bone overlying the dura of the posterior fossa, and the petrosal and sigmoid sinuses. The jugular bulb, however, is not denuded as it may bleed awkwardly.

# 7 & 8

Access to the cerebellopontine angle is afforded through the internal auditory meatus and the posterior fossa dura lateral to it.

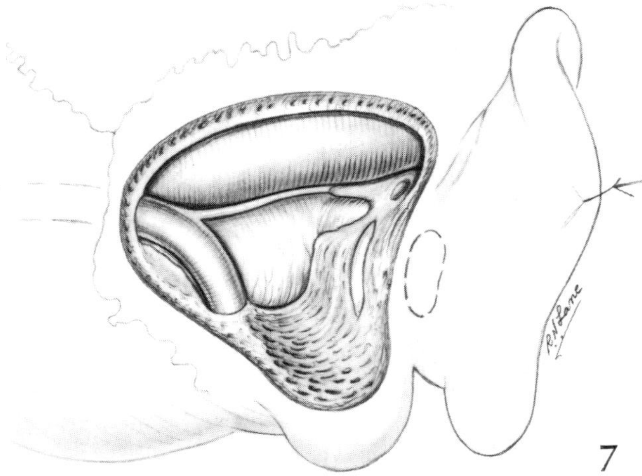

7

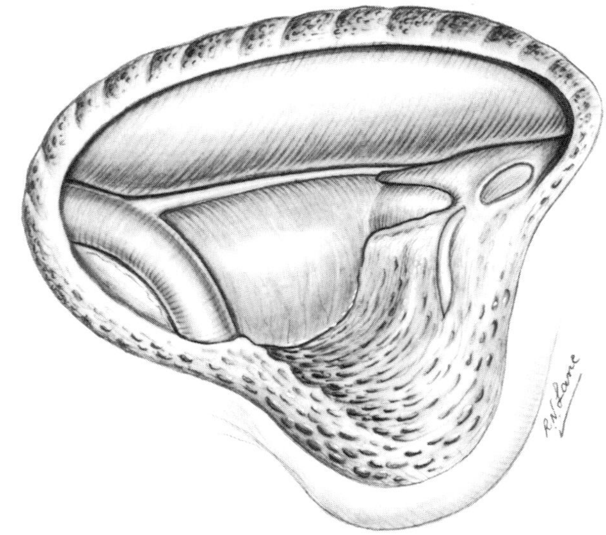

8

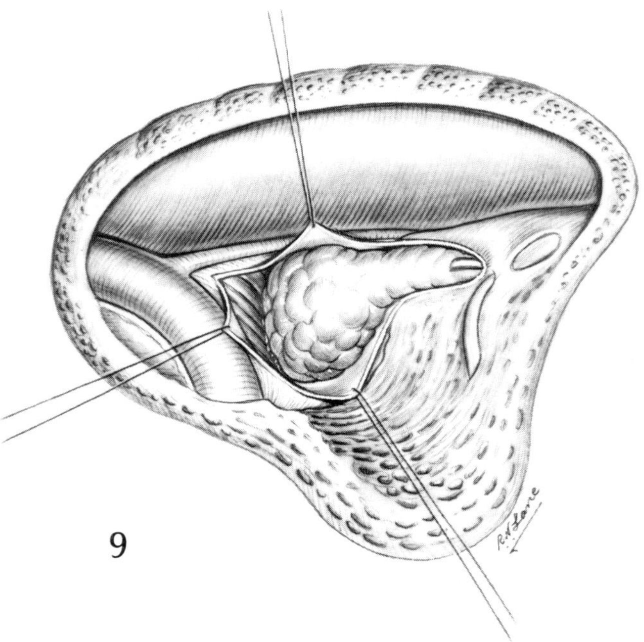

9

## Dural opening

# 9

This is begun by the otologist, who incises the dura of the meatus from the medial to the lateral end. It is obviously important to develop the plane between the dura, which is always very thin, and the tumour, avoiding the serious error of entering into an extradural plane, which would prevent identification of the facial nerve. The superior vestibular nerve, which is found laterally where it enters the vestibule of the inner ear, is divided and turned back to expose the facial nerve immediately anterior to it.

# 10

The tumour is then retracted backwards by the tip of a sucker placed on a small pattie, the plane between it and the facial nerve being thus opened up, and the nerve is followed medially by division of adhesions and arachnoidal strands with microscissors. The sucker should have a double channel, the second providing continuous saline irrigation which will wash blood away from the area being dissected. Sharp dissection is preferable to blunt throughout the operation, especially along the facial nerve, as it is gentler and more accurate. Inferiorly, the cochlear nerve is similarly progressively exposed. It is rare for the tumour to be entirely confined to the meatus, even intracanalicular growths extending a short distance through the porus as a rule. The posterior fossa dura therefore needs to be opened in almost all cases and this is the usual point for the neurosurgeon to take over. The incision in the meatal dura is carried through the toughened rim of the porus, where arachnoid, dura and tumour are fused, and thence laterally into the posterior fossa to the edge of the sigmoid sinus. Radiating cuts are added to produce superior, inferior and lateral flaps, which are retracted by fine sutures weighted with artery forceps. This exposes the tumour in the angle medially and a small area of cerebellum laterally, both still covered by arachnoid.

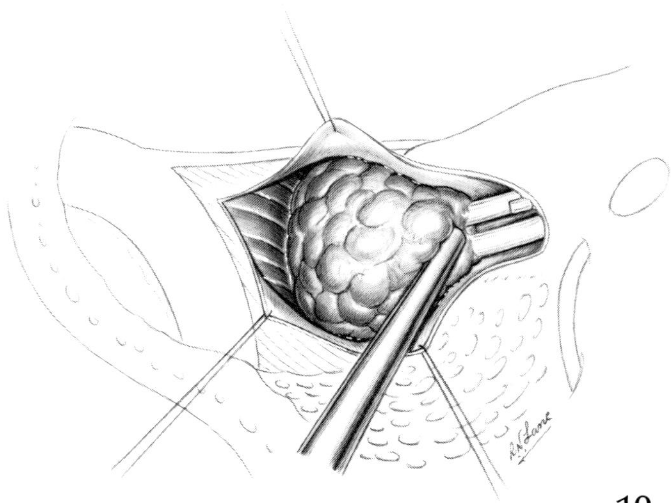

10

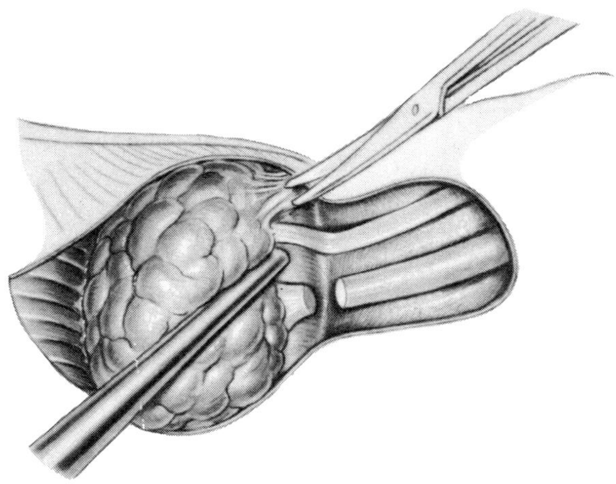

11

# 11

The dural opening is sufficient to allow removal of tumours of any size. Except in the very smallest intracanalicular ones, the next step is to free the tumour from the margins of the porus acusticus, to which it is always densely adherent, and to enter the plane between tumour and arachnoid in which the removal of the tumour has to be carried out. It is best to start inferiorly, both because the facial nerve is not at risk here and because opening the cistern below the porus allows CSF to escape, giving more room. The arachnoid is put on stretch by pushing the tumour backwards with the sucker and then divided with sharp-tipped microscissors. The lower pole of the tumour is found by following the subarachnoid plane below the porus until the medullary cistern is reached. The uppermost fibres of the ninth nerve are usually seen but the remaining nerves of the jugular foramen are not exposed, an advantage of this approach. The choroid plexus of the lateral recess is fairly easily seen with a little retraction or, if the tumour is larger, after reduction of the growth; it is an important reference point whose position should be marked with a small square of Silastic (Dow Corning, UK) sheeting.

## Removal of tumour in cerebellopontine angle

# 12

If the tumour is small (less than 1 cm in diameter), removal is straightforward. The facial nerve is followed to a point where it is no longer in contact with the tumour, and the tumour is then freed from its remaining arachnoidal attachments, often in one piece, without the need for any reduction in its size by gutting.

Larger tumours (ranging from 1 cm to 3 or 4 cm in diameter) are removed by progressive and persistent reduction in the size of the tumour, mainly by hollowing out its inside, alternating with dissection under direct vision along the capsule. The latter is carried out from four directions. The tumour is separated anteriorly from the facial nerve; superiorly from underneath the tentorium, the arachnoid, the petrosal vein (preservation of which is a matter of convenience rather than principle as its importance lies only in its tendency to bleed severely if torn) and the trigeminal nerve; inferiorly, in the medullary cistern, from the ninth nerve and the choroid plexus of the lateral recess medial to which the central end of the facial and acoustic nerves are found; and posteriorly from the cerebellum and middle cerebellar peduncle (*see Illustration 13*).

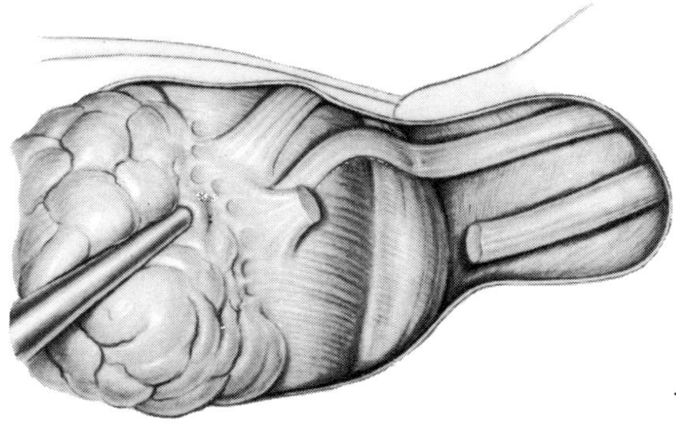

12

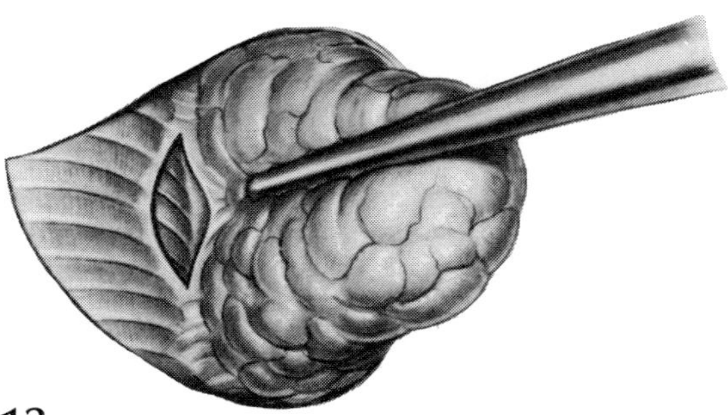

13

# 13

First, the arachnoid around the margins of the visible tumour is incised, allowing entry to the subarachnoid plane. This incision runs from the upper margin of the porus round the top of the tumour to the cerebellum, where it turns down to run along the groove between brain and tumour, turning forwards inferiorly to reach the arachnoid incision already made below the porus. The surface of the tumour thus demarcated is diathermied and as large a window as possible is cut in it to allow gutting to be started. This may be done with a sucker and pituitary rongeur, but is much easier with a special instrument such as the House–Urban rotary dissector or the Cavitron ultrasonic aspirator. Both are expensive, but save much time and effort in what can be a very exhausting operation for the surgeon by combining the two functions of fragmentation and aspiration in a single instrument and one hand. The tumour should, at this stage, be hollowed out as much as the surgeon dare without perforating its deep surface. This will allow the capsule to be easily retracted centrally, away from the surrounding tissues, by the tip of a sucker while adhesions between the two are divided by scissors. The facial nerve can be followed centrally, the upper pole dissected away from the fifth nerve, and the tumour separated posteriorly from the cerebellum, middle cerebellar peduncle and brainstem. Each portion of the tumour so mobilized should be immediately removed by whatever method has been used for gutting, as it is essential to consolidate each gain so that the tumour is gradually and somewhat tediously reduced in size until the brainstem is reached. The last piece of tumour to be removed is usually attached to the central end of the cochlear nerve, which is divided to free it.

# 14 & 15

## Anomalous position of facial nerve

In some cases the facial nerve is displaced almost directly upwards medial to the porus by a piece of tumour which insinuates itself beneath it and extends up towards the petrous apex. This makes the facial nerve very vulnerable to injury because it is more superficial and also because mobilization of the upper pole of the tumour has to be performed by working deep to the facial nerve. This arrangement can be predicted early if the nerve is found to lie along the roof of the meatus.

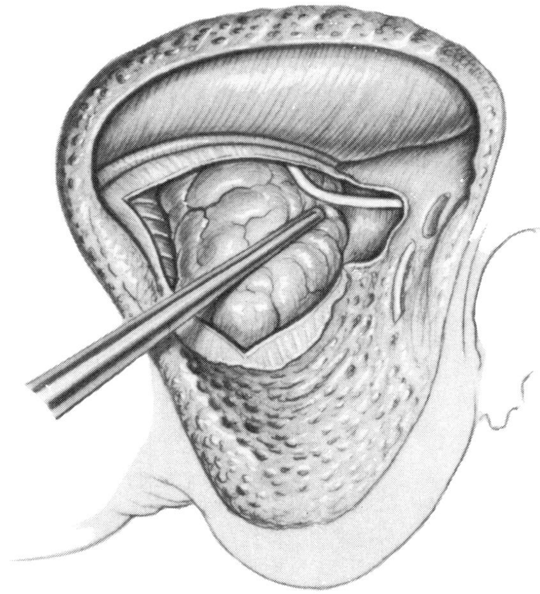

14

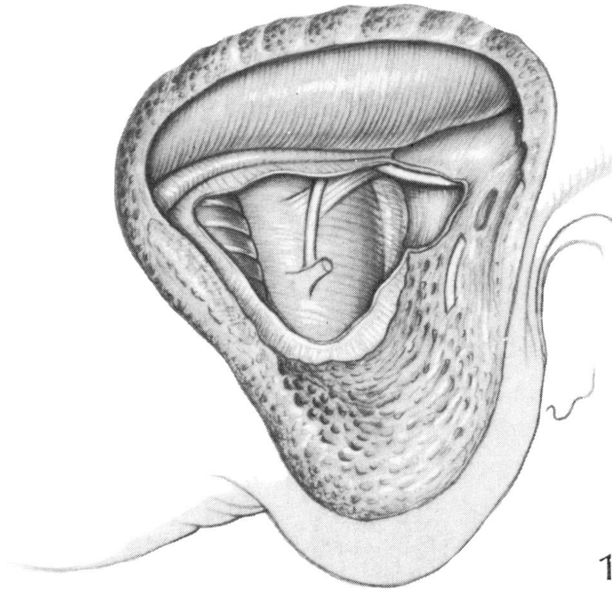

15

# 16

## Extension of exposure

Criticism of the restricted exposure afforded by the translabyrinthine operation has been met by devising ways of expanding it. This can be done either by dividing the sigmoid sinus or by cutting the tentorium. Neither is necessary for acoustic nerve tumours if the cortical mastoidectomy is made large enough. Division of the superior petrosal sinus and tentorium may, however, be useful in a meningioma arising medial to the porus, especially if it perforates the tentorium. An incision is made in the dura of the middle fossa just in front of the superior petrosal sinus, which is divided between haemoclips. The tentorium may be incised into the hiatus by elevating the temporal lobe[3].

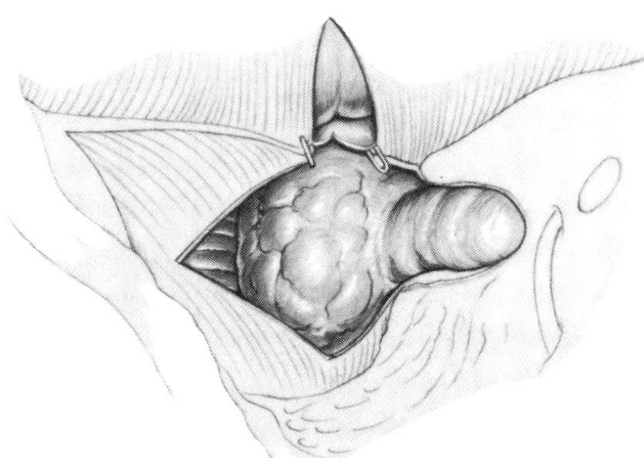

16

### Closure

Careful haemostasis is essential, as postoperative haematomas are likely to have catastrophic consequences, especially as no decompression is provided. Before closure, the blood pressure is allowed to rise to a normal level and any blood transfusion is completed. All obvious bleeding is stopped, but the wound should be left open for about half an hour, packed with cotton wool or patties soaked in hydrogen peroxide, before deciding that it is safe to close. The middle ear cavity is packed with fat, and the piece of fascia lata which was cut earlier is then laid across the opening into the middle ear and may be glued down, preferably with a biological glue. A second layer of fascia may be laid across the first and the pyramidal cavity left by the bone removal filled with fat.

## Postoperative care

As soon as he is awake the patient should be nursed in a semi-sitting position. Antibiotics and steroids are given for 5 days. If the facial nerve has been destroyed, the eye should be carefully protected by a shield and it may be necessary to do a lateral tarsorrhaphy. If the facial nerve is known to be intact but the patient has a complete paralysis postoperatively, it is advisable to wait at least 6 months for evidence of recovery before contemplating any further procedure. If the nerve is known to be destroyed, a faciohypoglossal anastomosis is done about 10 days after the operation.

## Complications

As with any attempt to remove an acoustic nerve tumour, haematoma formation in the operative cavity and infection are important complications. The most frequent and troublesome sequel, and one to which this technique is peculiarly liable, is the development of a CSF leak through the middle ear and into the nose via the Eustachian tube. The method described above for sealing the middle ear cannot be completely relied upon to prevent this complication. Occasionally, the graft seems to shift postoperatively although the use of glue would be expected to reduce this possibility. It may be that in some cases a leak develops directly through the medial wall of the middle ear, either via air cells opening directly there or, perhaps, through dislocation of the stapes, which would allow the vestibule to open directly into the middle ear. Leaks usually become evident early in the postoperative period and, in our experience, almost always require reoperation. This may be done through the original incision, but if this fails it is best to operate through the posterior fossa and cover the remains of the internal auditory meatus with a large fascial graft.

In the extended operation, in which the temporal lobe is exposed, epilepsy is an important complication, its frequency being as high as 20 per cent[4]. Prophylactic anticonvulsants and avoidance of wide exposure of the temporal lobe may help to reduce its incidence.

### *References*


1. House, W. F. (1964) Monograph. Transtemporal bone microsurgical removal of acoustic neuromas. Archives of Otolaryngology, 80, 597–756

2. House, W. F., Luetje, C. M. (1979) Acoustic tumors, 2 vols. University Park Press. Baltimore

3. Morrison, A. W. and King, T. T. (1973) Experiences with a translabyrinthine transtentorial approach to the cerebellopontine angle. Technical Note (1973). Neurosurgery, 38, 382–390

4. Cabral, R., King, T. T., Scott, D. F. (1976) Incidence of postoperative epilepsy after a transtentorial approach to acoustic nerve tumours. Journal of Neurology, Neurosurgery and Psychiatry, 39, 665

Illustrations by Barbara Hyams

# Glomus tumours

**A. D. Cheesman** FRCS
Consultant Otolaryngologist, Charing Cross Hospital, London; Royal National Throat, Nose and Ear Hospital, London, UK

**Lindsay Symon** TD, FRCS
Professor of Neurosurgery, Gough-Cooper Department of Neurological Surgery, Institute of Neurology, National Hospitals for Nervous Diseases, London, UK

The management of these tumours has for many years been controversial. Initial attempts at surgical resection were often curtailed by significant complications and many clinicians felt that they should be treated by radiotherapy. Unfortunately, early attempts at irradiation were also followed by complications such as necrosis of the temporal bone and adjacent brain. Furthermore, both clinical and histological studies have shown that radiotherapy results only in a decreased growth rate and rarely gives a complete cure. Over the last decade there have been enormous advances in the surgical management of glomus tumours. These have been based on a better understanding of tumour behaviour and a better knowledge of the complex anatomy of the skull base, and have been helped by advances in both radiology and anaesthesia.

## Anatomy

The anatomy of the jugular foramen is complex and its understanding is essential for safe surgery in this region. It must be studied from both the intracranial and extracranial aspects.

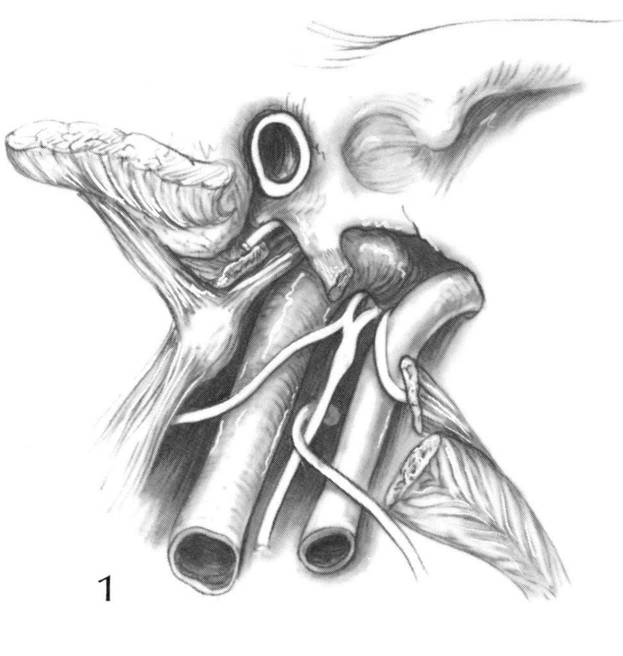

1

### 1

The illustration shows an extracranial view of the jugular foramen. The sternomastoid and digastric muscles have been cut to show the underlying lateral process of the atlas and styloid processes. The styloid muscles have been divided to show the structures of the jugular foramen beneath. The internal carotid artery is situated anteromedially where it enters the carotid canal. The glossopharyngeal nerve leaves the foramen in a notch anteriorly and curves laterally round the carotid artery, passing forward to the pharyngeal plexus deep to the styloid muscles. The accessory and vagus nerves leave the medial compartment of the foramen, the accessory nerve passing anterior to the internal jugular vein towards the anterior border of the sternomastoid muscle. The vagus nerve lies in the posterior part of the carotid sheath between the artery and vein. The internal jugular vein arises from the posterior compartment and enters the carotid sheath just in front of the lateral process of the atlas. A very prominent lateral process often restricts exposure here. The facial nerve, after leaving the stylomastoid foramen, makes an acute angle anteriorly to enter the posterior aspect of the parotid gland. The hypoglossal nerve is closely related to the jugular vein as it leaves the anterior condylar canal medial to the jugular foramen and passes posterolateral to the vagus and internal carotid before passing forward deep to the digastric muscle to the tongue.

# 2a, b & c

An intracranial view of the jugular foramen is illustrated. The structures of importance here are the nerves, as the venous component continues extradurally in the sigmoid sinus, but it is important to remember that the jugular bulb may present without a bony covering in the floor of the internal meatus. The areas of bone removed in the posterolateral approach are indicated.

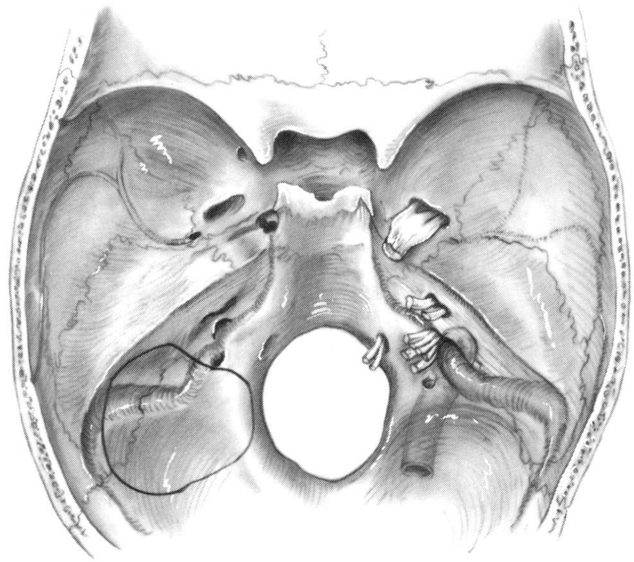

2a

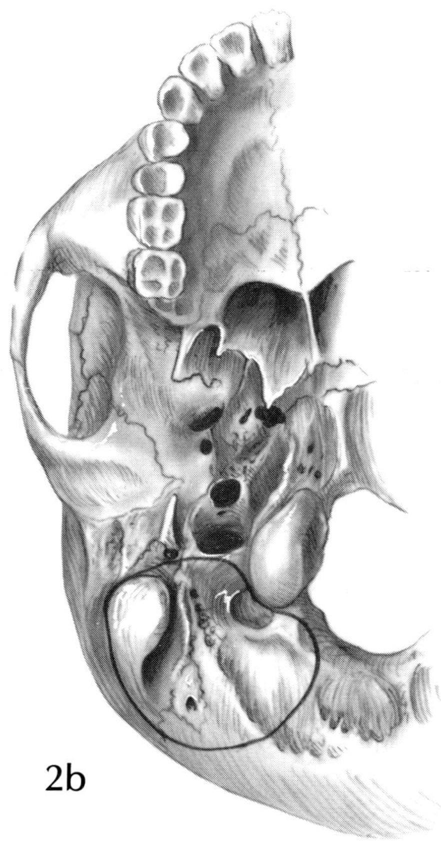

2b

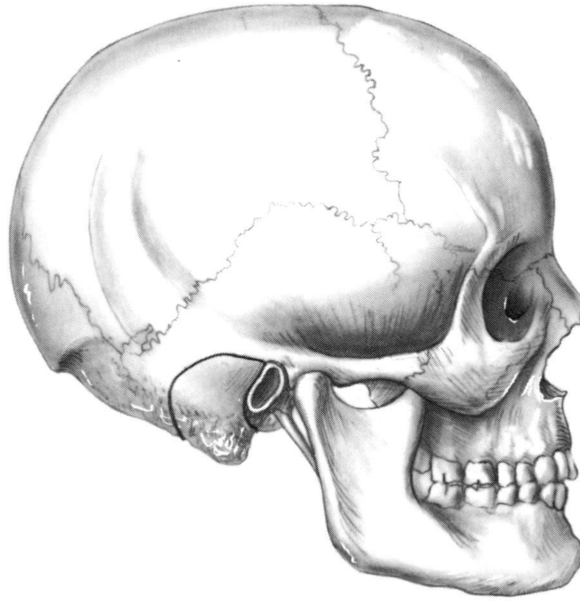

2c

**Classification**

# 3a–d

Various classifications have been proposed, but that of Fisch *et al.* is the most useful clinically.

*a*. Type A. Tumours localized to the middle ear cleft (glomus tympanicus tumours)

*b*. Type B. Tympanomastoid tumours with no destruction of bone in the infralabyrinthine compartment of the temporal bone.

*c*. Type C. Tumours invading and destroying bone in the infralabyrinthine region with extension towards the petrous apex.

*d*. Type D. Tumours with intracranial extension.

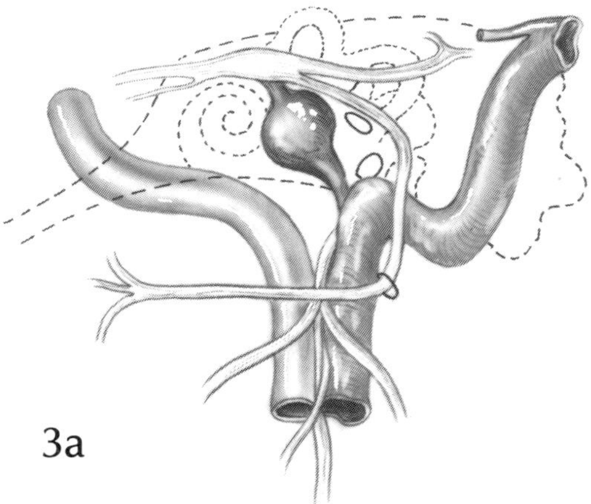

3a

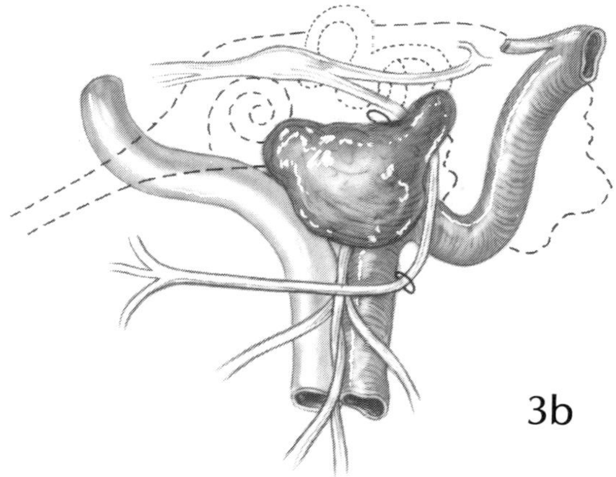

3b

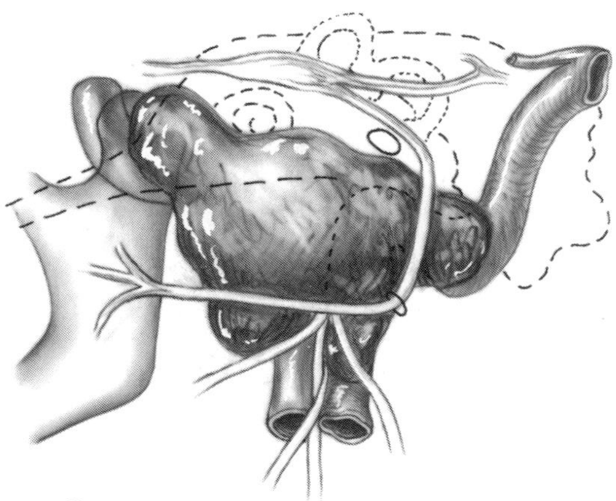

3c

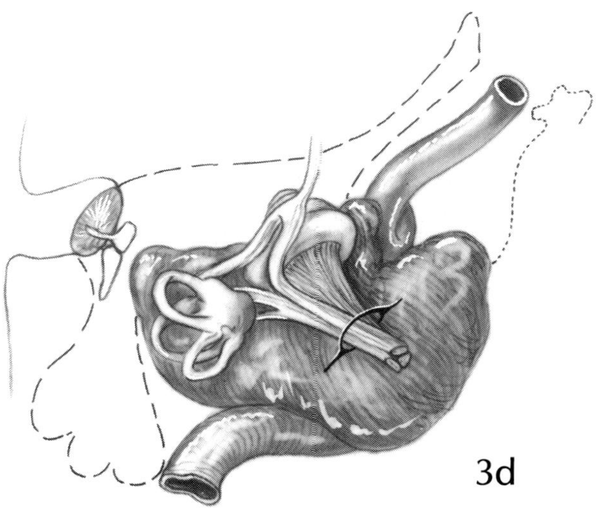

3d

## Investigations

Careful neuro-otological examination with full audiometry is essential in each case, but it is also important to investigate every case both endocrinologically and radiologically.

### *Endocrine investigation*

A small number of glomus tumours secrete vasoactive hormones and it is important to detect these preoperatively by measuring the vanillylmandelic acid levels in a 24-hour collection of urine. (The normal level is up to 7 mg/24 hours.)

### *Radiological investigation*

# 4 & 5a–d

Modern imaging techniques are capable of accurately defining the true extent of the tumour and the use of ultraselective angiography can indicate the main arterial supply to the tumour.

Initial screening is carried out with high resolution CT scanning to show both bone destruction and soft tissue tumour.

*Illustration 4* shows the diagnostic pathway in establishing the type of glomus tumour. Axial scans are performed initially and the jugular foramen is studied to see whether it is enlarged and if its cortex is eroded.

An axial scan of an abnormally high jugular bulb showing smooth well corticated enlargement of the bulb is seen in *Illustration 5a;* and an axial scan of a glomus jugulare tumour with an enlarged bulb and eroded cortex is seen in *Illustration 5b.*

If the jugular bulb has normal dimensions, coronal CT scans are necessary to investigate any middle ear mass further. *Illustration 5c* is a coronal scan showing an aberrant carotid artery. It demonstrates an anterior cut showing absent bone over the carotid canal.

A coronal scan showing a glomus tympanicus tumour is seen in *Illustration 5d.* The carotid canal is intact.

Although CT scanning is the method of choice, magnetic resonance imaging (MRI) provides additional supplementary information in a non-invasive manner. MRI with Gadolinium enhancement demonstrates any soft tissue extension into the neck or posterior fossa optimally. It is also the best method of detecting recurrence following surgery.

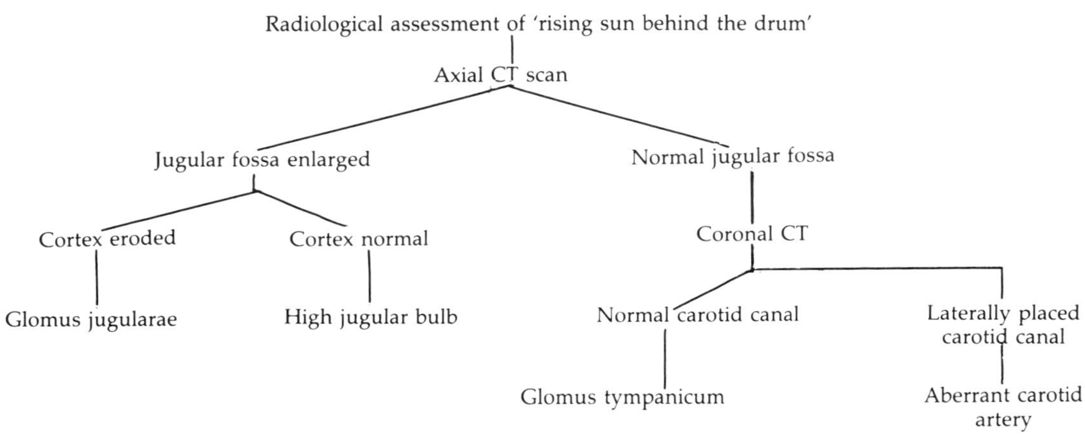


4

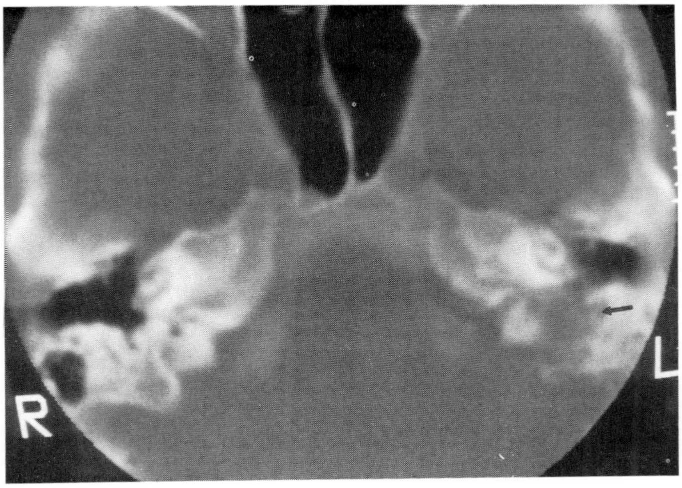


5a

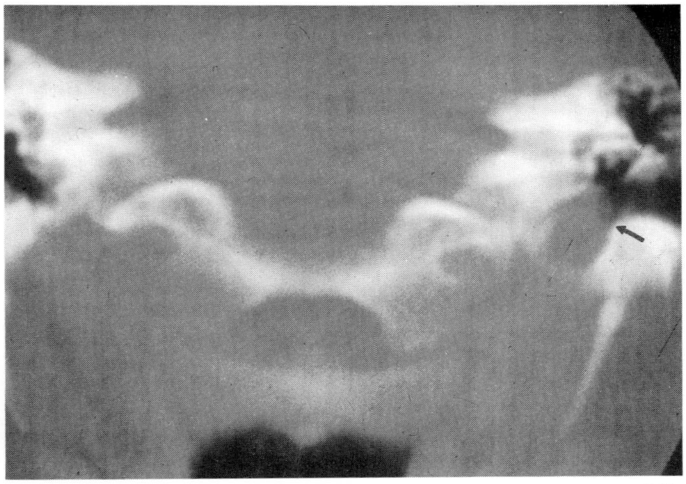

5b

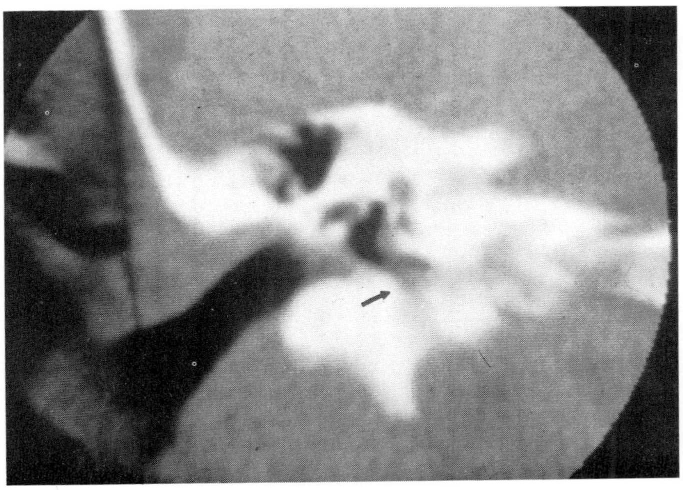

5c

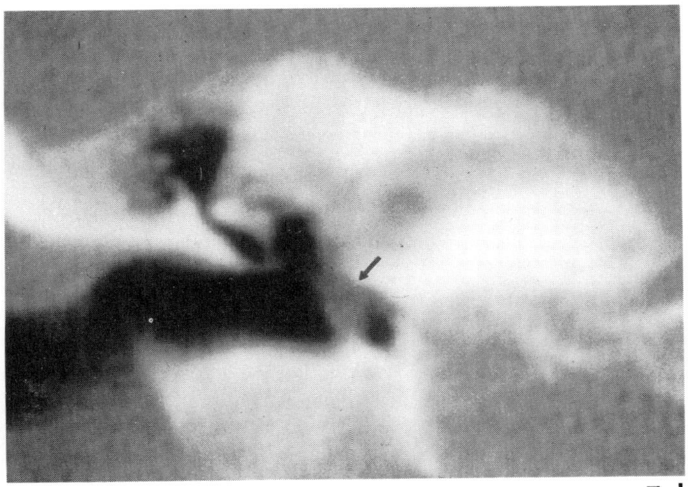

5d

*Angiography*

Retrograde venography may demonstrate occlusion of the jugular bulb by tumour, but this information has limited surgical value. Digital subtraction angiography can confirm the vascular nature of the tumour and may demonstrate occlusion of the bulb but again this has limited surgical value. Ultraselective arteriography is of considerable value in the preoperative assessment as it can define the individual vessels supplying the tumour, and can indicate whether there is any direct supply from the internal carotid and vertebral vessels. However, most importantly, it allows preoperative embolization of the tumour using emboli of absorbable gelatin foam or other suitable material. This is performed some 4–5 days before the planned resection under light anaesthesia and in our experience greatly decreases blood loss.

## Treatment options

It is now possible to define various treatment options for the management of glomus tumours. However, each case must be carefully assessed before deciding treatment and consideration also given to the therapeutic skills available. Surgical resection by an inexperienced surgeon is more likely to result in serious complication than irradiation, particularly with type C and D tumours.

*No treatment*

Glomus tumours often present in the sixth and seventh decades and tend to grow slowly. Consequently, if in an elderly patient the tumour is not very extensive and the symptoms minimal, no treatment is indicated. Follow-up with CT scans is easily performed and accurate.

*Radiotherapy*

Most surgeons will agree that an elderly or infirm patient with a symptomatic, growing tumour should be treated solely with radiotherapy, but it must be remembered that some 40 per cent of tumours continue to grow after radiotherapy.

*Surgical resection*

The objectives of surgery must be total resection of the tumour, if possible. This should ideally be achieved without increasing the patient's neurological deficit.

# The operations

The exact type of operative procedure depends on the type of tumour as shown by the radiological assessment: type A tumours can usually be excised by a permeatal approach; type B tumours can be removed by a combined approach tympanoplasty procedure with an extended posterior tympanotomy; type C tumours need some form of skull base resection to include the jugular bulb such as the lateral or posterolateral approach. Type D tumours need the combination of skull base resection and a posterior fossa exploration such as is given by the posterolateral approach.

We have used three different surgical procedures.

1. Transmeatal approach (Shambaugh's hypotympanotomy)
2. Lateral approach (Fisch's infratemporal fossa approach)
3. Posterolateral approach.

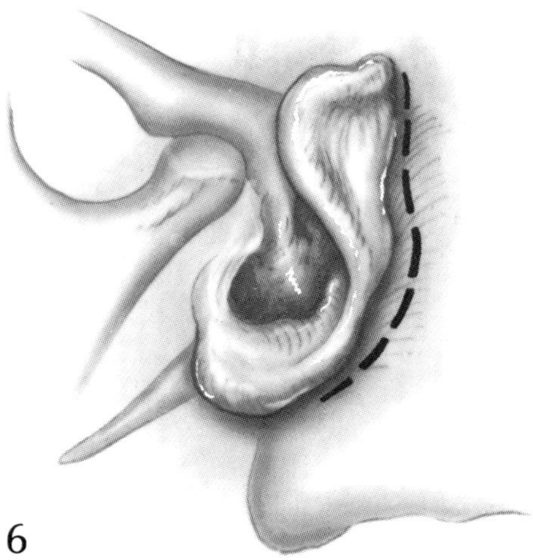

6

## TRANSMEATAL APPROACH

### 6

Some small glomus tympanicus tumours can be removed via a standard tympanotomy. If the margins of the tumour cannot be seen through the drum, a postaurale approach should be used as it allows the operation to be extended easily into either the mastoid segment or the neck to control the jugular venous circulation if problems are encountered.

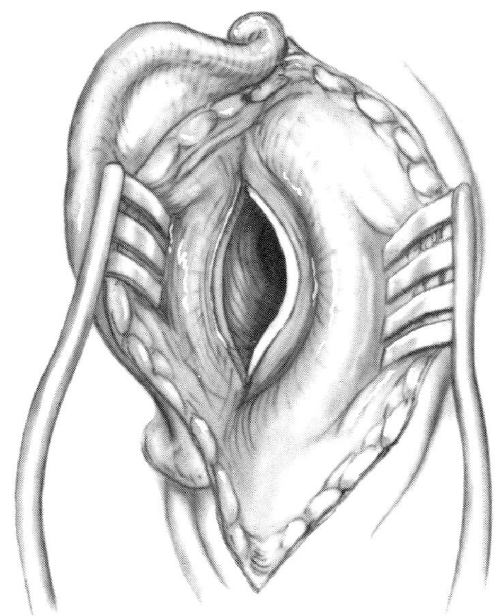

7

### 7

The postaurale incision is extended superiorly to obtain temporalis fascia. It extends inferiorly down to the mastoid tip. The meatal skin is mobilized from the bone superiorly, posteriorly and inferiorly. The meatus is then opened by an incision at the junction of the bony and cartilaginous meatus, giving direct vision of the drum.

# 8

A large tympanomeatal flap is raised posteriorly and reflected forward to give excellent exposure of the middle ear and the tumour in the hypotympanum.

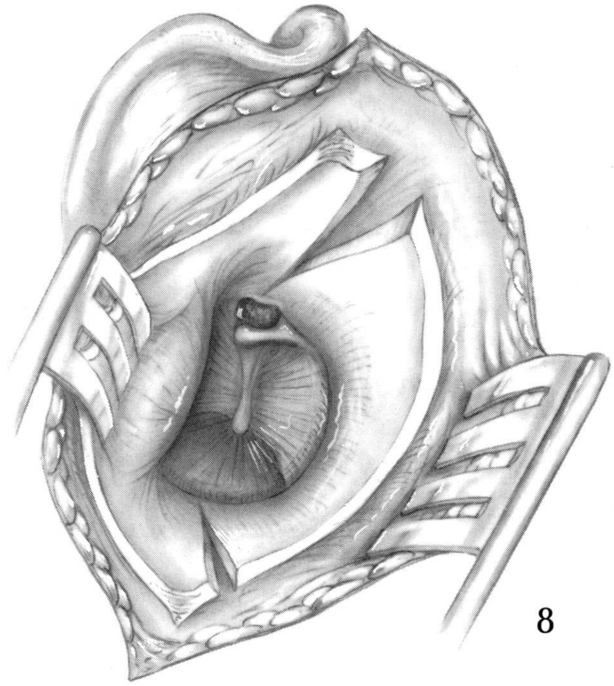

8

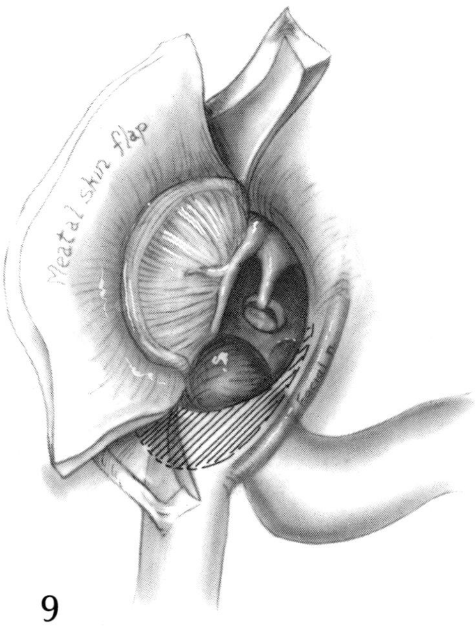


9

# 9

Complete exposure of the tumour and the associated jugular bulb is obtained by removing the outer wall of the hypotympanum with a diamond burr. If it is necessary to extend the bone removal to include the inferior part of the posterior wall, care must be exercised to avoid damage to the facial nerve which may be lateral to the annulus in about 10 per cent of temporal bones.

# 10

Additional exposure for anteriorly based tumours may be obtained by dissecting the drum free of the malleus handle. The tumour is then mobilized with small cotton wool balls soaked in topical adrenaline 1:1000. It can usually be excised with little bleeding but occasionally the associated artery needs to be coagulated with bipolar diathermy. To ensure complete removal the tumour bed should be smoothed with the diamond burr. Very occasionally the tumour is attached to an exposed jugular bulb which may be torn during the removal. The bleeding which results can be controlled temporarily with a pack, but permanent control requires ligation of the internal jugular vein in the neck and clipping the sigmoid sinus in the mastoid segment. Following this, residual bleeding from the inferior petrosal sinus can usually be controlled by Surgicel (Ethicon, UK) packing.

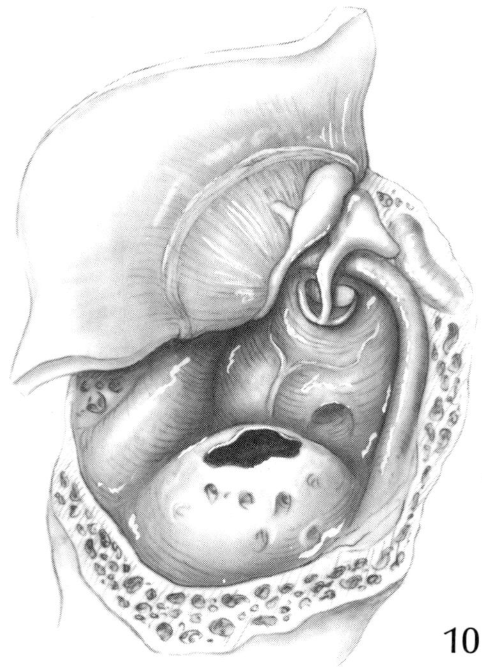

10

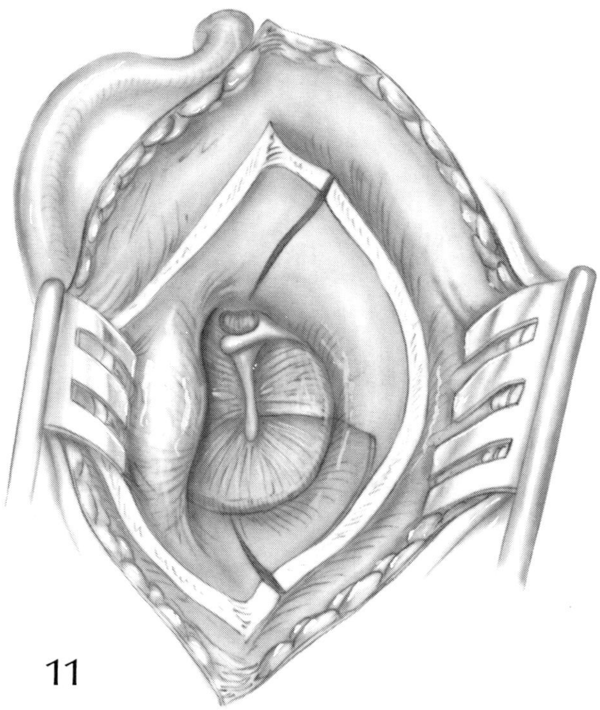

11

# 11

The bony defect inferiorly is reinforced with an underlay temporalis fascia graft which will also repair any tears in the drum. The deep meatus is packed with Sterispon (Allen & Hanbury's, UK) soaked in topical antibiotic solution and then a BIPP pack is placed laterally. The packing is removed after 10 days.

## LATERAL APPROACH (INFRATEMPORAL FOSSA APPROACH)

# 12

The Y-shaped incision gives excellent exposure of the operative field but in a previously irradiated case the anterior limb should either be shortened or avoided to preserve the blood supply to the pinna.

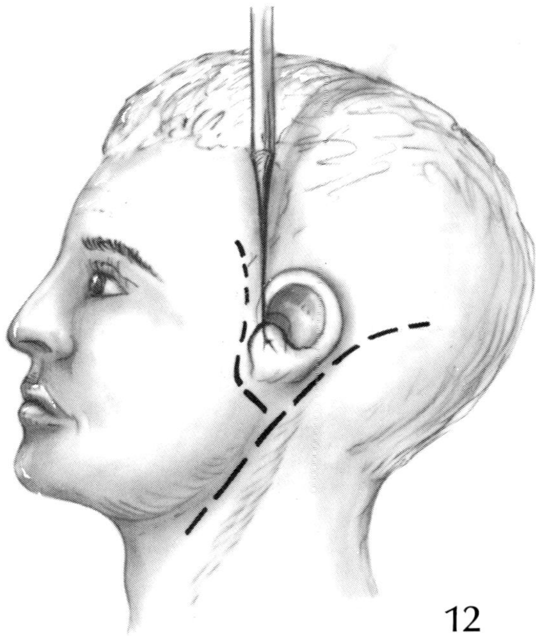

12

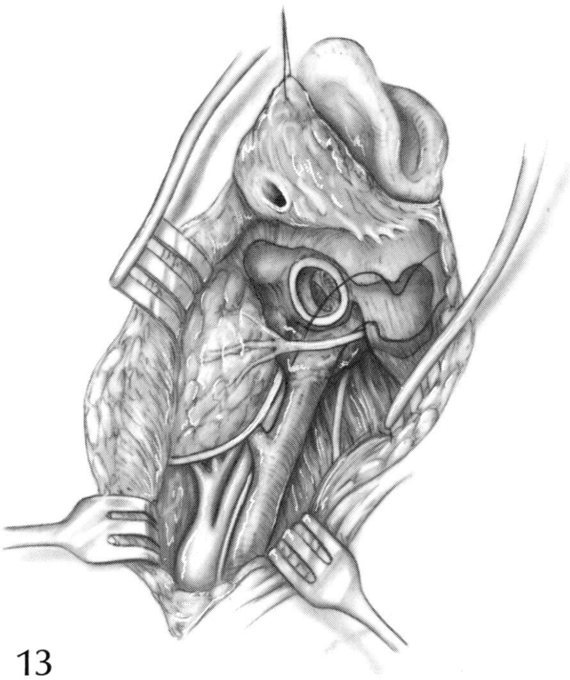

13

# 13

The meatus is transected at the junction of the bony and cartilaginous meatus and reflected superiorly. The anterior skin flap is reflected forward and a parotid dissection performed to display and mobilize the facial nerve up to its first major division. The upper neck is explored, and the nerves and vessels of the jugular foramen and adjacent skull base are carefully freed and mobilized up to their entry into the skull. The internal jugular vein is ligated and divided below the tumour. The external carotid artery may be ligated if previous embolization has not been used, and a tape is placed around the internal carotid artery to provide immediate control if necessary in an emergency.

The mastoid is exposed and a total clearance of all the cells performed with the drill to display the facial canal, sigmoid sinus and tumour.

# 14

The meatal wall and drum are removed with the ossicles, and the facial nerve decompressed in both its horizontal and vertical portions. A new bony groove is made anterosuperiorly and the facial nerve is dissected free from its normal canal and then transposed anteriorly into its new groove, thus completely displaying the tumour. The bone around the upper end of the sigmoid sinus is removed and the sinus ligated with either a ligature or Scoville clip. The tumour is then mobilized in preparation for its removal. In many cases the tumour is localized to the lateral wall of the sinus and can be removed by opening the sinus lumen and excising the tumour; in such cases the operation is straightforward, with preservation of both the dura and the neural compartment of the jugular foramen. With more extensive tumours the posterior fossa may be explored by continuing the exposure posteriorly as a formal suboccipital approach. For relatively small tumours this can be accomplished with the patient in the supine position, but if the posterior fossa component is large better exposure is obtained by repositioning the patient in the 'park-bench' position. Anteromedial extension of the tumour around the carotid canal towards the petrous apex is easily demonstrated by the anterior transposition of the facial nerve. Tumour clearance from the carotid artery and neural compartment may lead to increased neurological deficit and consideration should be given to the use of adjunctive radiotherapy, either with intraoperative implants of Iodine-125 seeds or with a postoperative external beam.

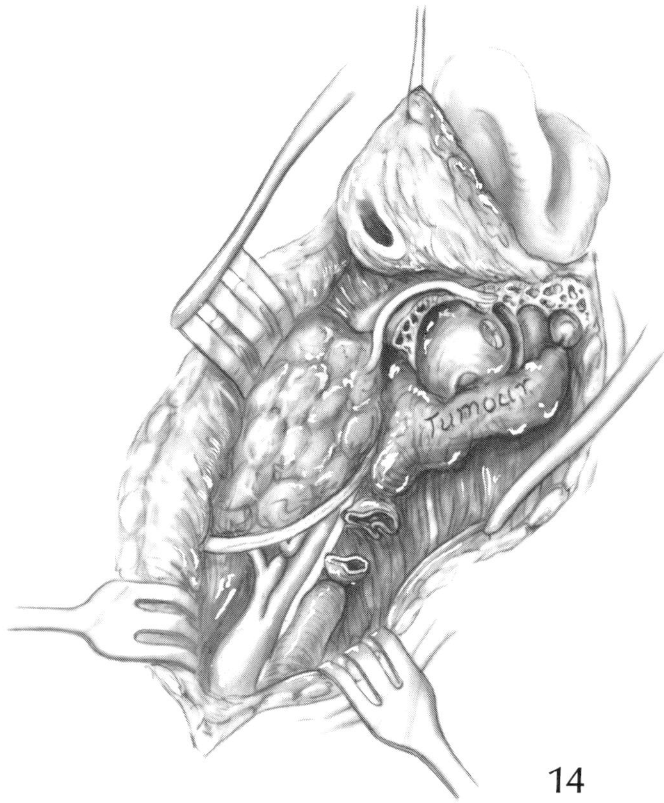


14

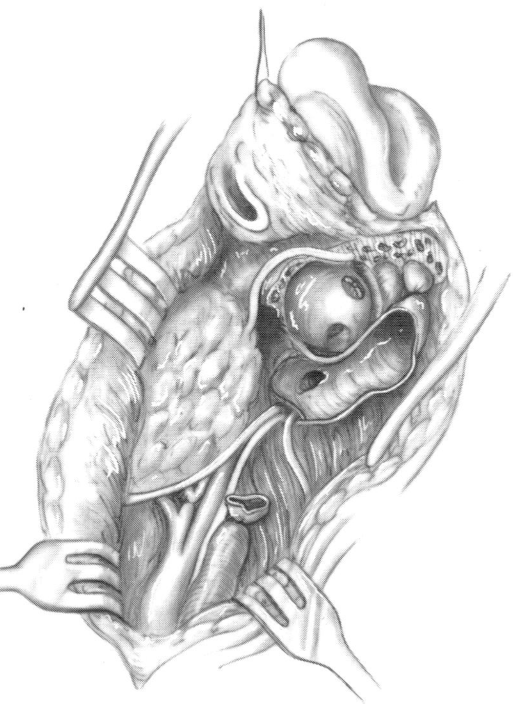

15

# 15

Following tumour removal, bleeding from the inferior petrosal sinus (which may have multiple openings) is controlled with Surgicel packing. Any dural defect is closed with either temporalis fascia or fascia lata. The facial nerve is left transposed and the Eustachian tube is closed with bone wax and free fat graft. The external auditory canal is closed off as a blind-ending sac with everting sutures to the meatal skin.

# 16

The tumour bed and the mastoid cavity are then filled with a free graft of dermal fat taken from the left abdominal wall or thigh.

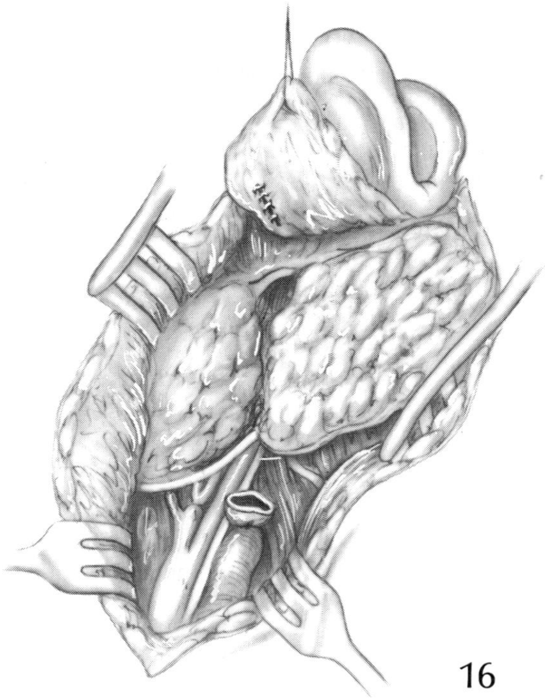

16

# 17

The wound is closed in layers with suction drainage. The suction drain is placed away from any dural repair and suction stopped if it drains cerebrospinal fluid.

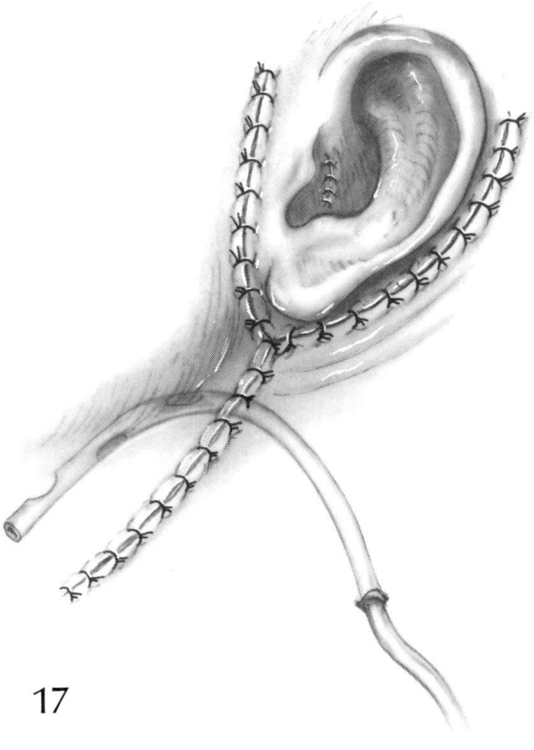

17

## POSTEROLATERAL APPROACH

This approach has been developed over the years from the infratemporal fossa approach devised by Fisch. The main advantage is the ability to develop the exposure depending on the extent of the tumour. Most type B and many type C tumours can be excised without the need to transpose the facial nerve.

Additionally, large type D tumours extending into the posterior fossa can be readily excised at a single operation. The main disadvantage of the operation is the restricted exposure of the petrous apex which results from not transposing the facial nerve, and in such cases the nerve can easily be transposed as described previously.

The patient's position on the operating table depends on the extent of the tumour. If the tumour has a large posterior fossa component, exposure is facilitated by placing the patient in the 'park-bench' position. However, this position is not ideal for the neck or skull base part of the operation; consequently with smaller tumours the patient is placed in the supine position with the head rotated away from the tumour.

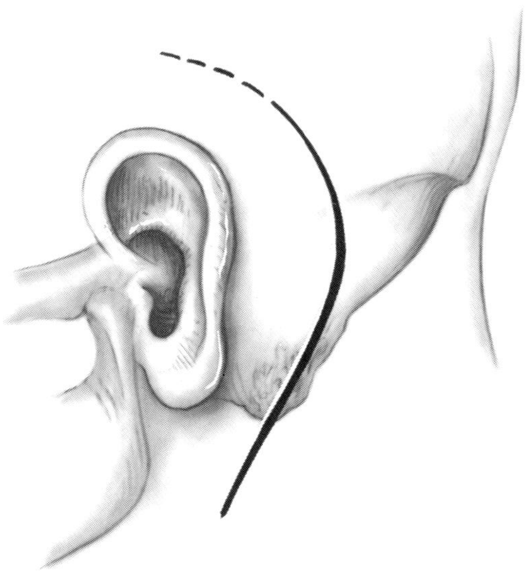

18

# 18

A single incision extending from the inferior temporal line behind the mastoid tip into the upper neck is used to ensure adequate vascularization of the pinna. It may be extended superiorly or a posterior limb made to increase exposure.

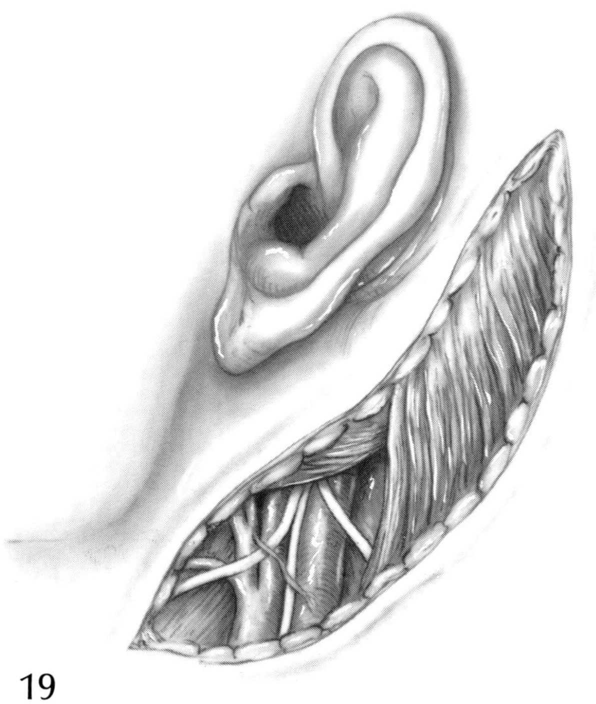

19

# 19

The incision is opened superficial to the origin of the sternomastoid and deeply into the neck to expose the carotid sheath and associated nerves.

# 20

The origin of the sternomastoid is dissected off the skull to show the underlying splenius muscle with the occipital artery on its surface. The lateral process of the atlas is displayed with its attached suboccipital muscles. The splenius and the superior suboccipital muscles must also be dissected off the occipital bone to fully expose the bone posterolateral to the jugular foramen. Care must be taken to avoid damage to the mastoid emissary vein and more deeply, superomedial to the lateral process of the atlas, the vertebral artery, as it passes superomedially to enter the skull.

The upper neck is explored and the nerves of the jugular foramen carefully freed to the skull base; the internal jugular vein is similarly freed, looking carefully for the inferior petrosal sinus which may enter the vein in the neck inferior to the skull base. The carotid arteries are identified and a tape is passed around the internal carotid to act as an emergency ligature if needed subsequently. The branches of the external carotid which supply the tumour may be ligated if not previously embolized. The internal jugular vein is ligated inferior to any neck extension of the tumour.

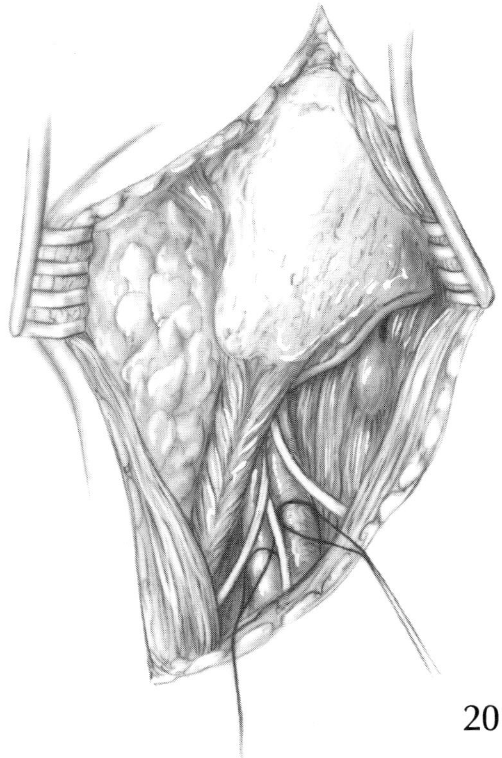

20

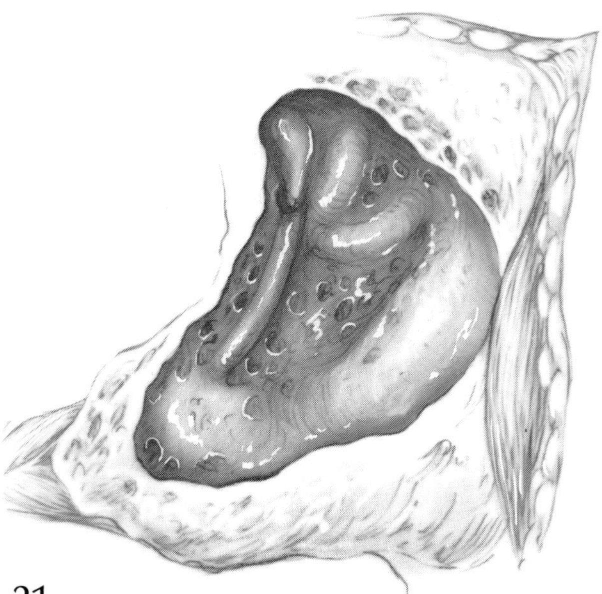

21

# 21

Using a high-speed cutting burr an extensive cortical mastoidectomy is performed. The following structures are then skeletonized using a diamond burr: the fallopian canal down to the digastric ridge, the bony labyrinth, the dural plates of both the middle and posterior fossae, and the sigmoid sinus. If tumour is known to be present in the hypotympanum, access to this region is obtained by deepening the fossa incudis into the facial recess, creating a large posterior tympanotomy. Bleeding from the tumour at this stage can be controlled with bone wax or by dry drilling with the diamond burr.

# 22

The bone removal is then continued posterior to the sigmoid sinus to expose the posterior fossa dura widely. Bone removal is continued round onto the base of the skull, the occipital bone is removed with rongeurs down to the jugular foramen, giving a small suboccipital craniectomy. The mastoid tip is removed with rongeurs and the digastric muscle sutured anteriorly to protect the facial nerve as it leaves the stylomastoid foramen. The dural plate lying over the sigmoid sinus and associated tumour is elevated and removed using gauze dissection. (Ribbon gauze (1 cm) soaked in topical adrenaline solution 1:1000 is used to separate the soft tissues from the overlying bone.) When the upper end of the sigmoid sinus is displayed it is occluded with a Scoville clip passed across the sinus via a small dural puncture.

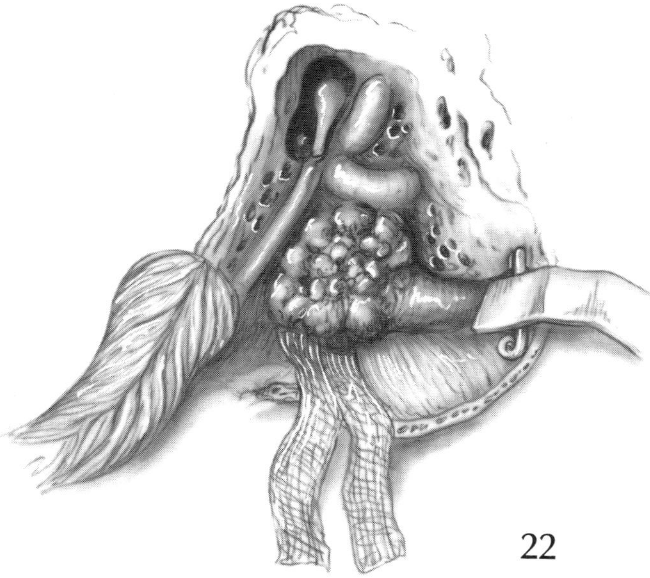

22

# 23

The tumour is further mobilized by gauze dissection and, using a diamond burr, the overlying bone is removed until the jugular bulb and tumour are clearly demonstrated. After the removal of the posterolateral wall of the jugular foramen, the skull base dissection is joined to the neck dissection and the divided internal jugular vein is freed by passing it deep to the accessory nerve. It may then be dissected up into the foramen and in many cases the tumour can be separated from the medially placed neural compartment. The tumour usually involves the lateral wall of the jugular bulb which must be excised in continuity with the tumour. This manoeuvre results in bleeding from the inferior petrosal sinus which may be controlled by packing the sinus off with Surgicel. The upper end of the sigmoid sinus is closed by suturing the anterior and posterior walls together and the Scoville clip is removed.

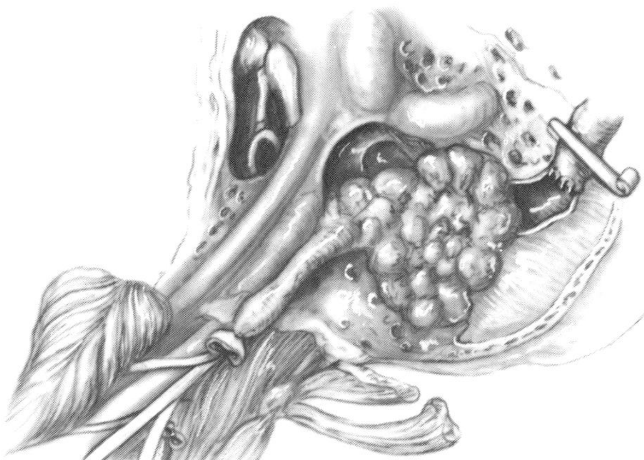

23

# 24

The tumour bed is seen with the neural compartment intact. If the tumour involves the nerves, the dissection is continued medially into the neural compartment. However, if the nerves of the jugular foramen are not clinically involved such a dissection will result in an increased neural deficit postoperatively and consideration should be given to treating such cases with adjunctive radiotherapy, either with intraoperative implantation of Iodine-125 seeds or with a postoperative external beam.

Similarly, if the tumour extends towards the petrous apex along the carotid beneath the labyrinth, a decision should be made whether radiation is to be used or surgical excision performed. In the latter situation better exposure may be obtained by transposing the facial nerve as described previously, although in our experience this is not often necessary.

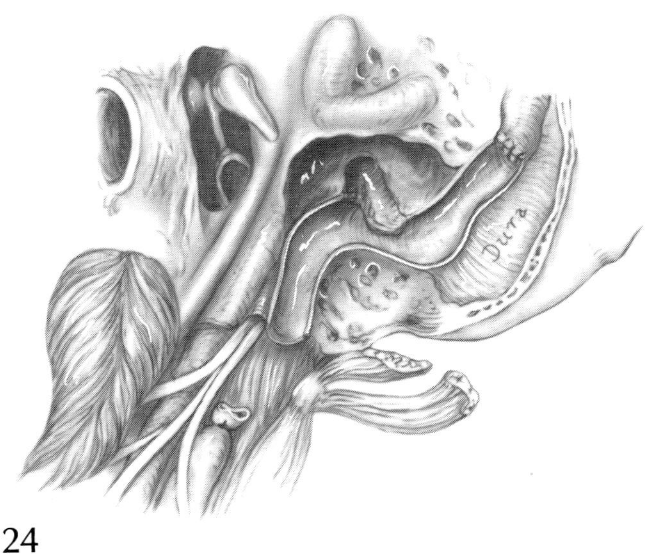


24

# 25a & b & 26

If the tumour involves the posterior fossa dura or extends into the posterior fossa it will become necessary to open the posterior fossa dura to determine the extent of the intracranial mass. The aim should be to excise the tumour as far as possible in continuity with the extracranial portion. Glomus tumours usually carry with them a covering of dura, and from the neurosurgical point of view the intracranial extension, even though massive, usually provides less technical difficulty than, for example, a posterior fossa meningioma of comparable size. After preoperative embolization and reduction in vascularity by coagulation of dural vessels entering from the vertebral artery and visible at the time of surgery, it is usually possible to separate the posterior fossa extension from cerebellum with relative ease. The tumour is often multinodular and highly vascular but it can be compressed forward into the petrous cavity already established. Thus, although these tumours were extremely formidable when tackled from the posterior fossa alone, the presence of preoperative embolization with devascularization, and an already established cavity into which the intracranial extension may be displaced, increases the relative ease of the neurosurgical portion. It is the authors' view that a one-stage operation is preferable.

When there is considerable intracranial extension, preservation of the nerves of the jugular foramen may be impossible. The intracranial portion of these thin delicate nerves will not stand dissection from a firm mass of tumour and thus preservation of the nerves of the jugular foramen in types C and D depends entirely on the tumour remaining separate from the anterior compartment of the jugular foramen, and this is relatively rare.

During the dissection of the intracranial portion it may be necessary to carry the dural excision anterior to the jugular foramen along the posterior aspect of the petrous bone. Preservation of the seventh and eighth nerves depends on the degree of involvement of the labyrinth within the bone as they are not usually involved intracranially. The inferior petrosal sinus can be occluded with Surgicel and the surgeon is then left with completion of the extracranial dissection into the petrous bone and repair of the dural defect of varying size from the jugular foramen anteriorly and posteriorly. For this repair we have commonly used autologous fascia lata taken from the upper thigh. The graft is sutured posteriorly where the dura is intact and tacked anteriorly with fibrin glue (Tisseel) to obtain a near watertight closure.

Anterior dissection of the tumour can be pursued as high as the cavernous sinus. Certain of these very advanced and extensive lesions may require resection of the carotid, but it is probable that with extensive invasion of the cavernous sinus, the tumour should be regarded as unresectable. This is particularly the case if the nerves within the carotid sinus remain uninvolved. We have, in a number of cases, ligated the internal carotid artery after test occlusion preoperatively. However, currently our view would be that if the tumour cannot be stripped from the carotid with careful microscopic dissection and with the aid of bipolar diathermy, then, particularly if the extension extends well into the cavernous sinus through the foramen lacerum, resection should be terminated at this point and reliance placed on either postoperative radiation or the use of interstitial radioactive implants such as Iodine-125. This latter technique requires preoperative arrangement with the radiotherapist and the implanted radiation may need to be supplemented by external beam radiation.

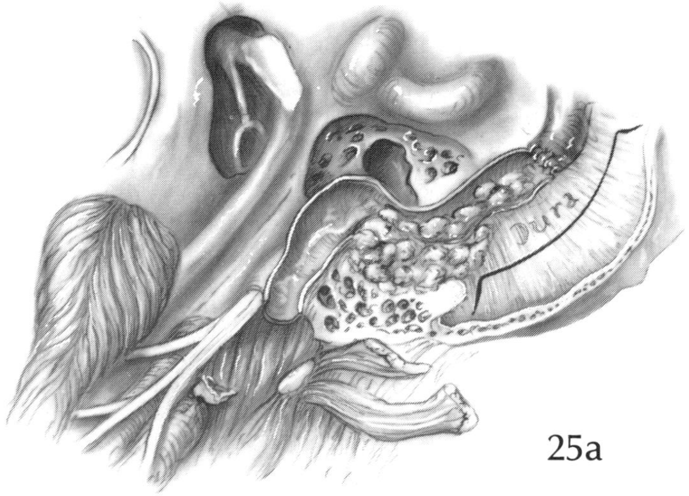


25a

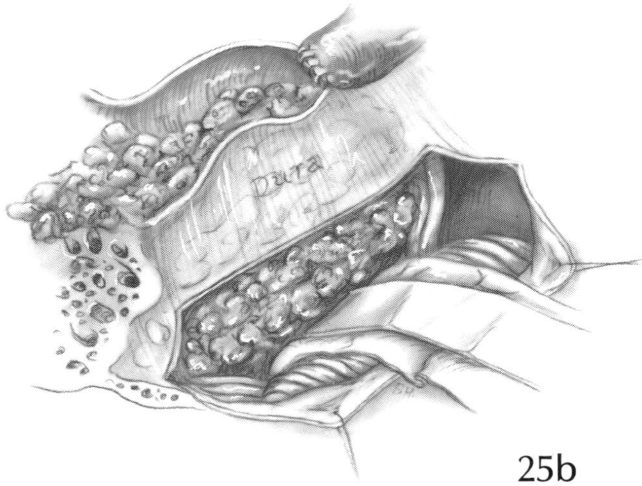


25b

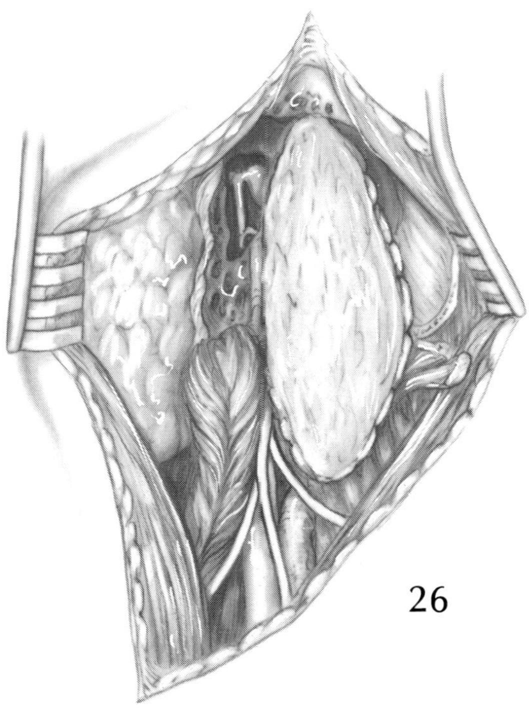

26

## Further reading

Bordi, L. T., Cheesman, A. D., Symon, L. (1989) The surgical management of glomus jugulare tumours and a description of a single staged postero-lateral combined oto-neuro-surgical approach. British Journal of Neurology (in press)

Cheesman, A. D. (1987) Glomus and other tumours of the ear. In: John B. Booth, ed. Scott-Brown's Otolaryngology, Vol. 3 Otology, pp. 546–559. London: Butterworths

Fisch, U., Fagan, P., Valvanis, A. (1984) The infratemporal fossa approach for the lateral skull base. Otolaryngological Clinics of North America, 17, 513–552

Shambaugh, G. E. (1955) Surgical approach for so-called glomus jugulare tumours of the middle ear. Laryngoscope, 65, 185–198

## Acknowledgement

Figures 3, 4, 5a–d, 9, 13, 14, 16, 20, 22, 23 and 24 are reproduced from Scott-Brown's Otolaryngology, Otology, J. B. Booth, 1987. London: Butterworths

Illustrations by Robert N. Lane

# Anterior approach to the cervical spine

**Phillip Harris** FRCS(Ed), FRCS(Glas), FRCP(Ed), FRS(Ed)
Senior Lecturer in Neurological Surgery, University of Edinburgh; Consultant Neurosurgeon, Western General Hospital, Edinburgh; The Royal Infirmary, Edinburgh; The Spinal Unit, Edenhall Hospital, Musselburgh, UK

## Introduction

Many pathological conditions involving the cervical spine that require operative treatment lie anterior to the neural and vascular elements. Attempts to treat such lesions by a posterior approach are usually hazardous, as it is unsafe to retract the spinal cord in order to gain access to the ventral aspect of the cervical spinal canal. Some lesions situated far laterally and ventrally, such as certain protruded intervertebral discs, may be safely approached by a laminectomy or facetectomy. Reliable fixation, and in particular fusion, of the cervical spine is best achieved by an anterior approach, and indeed Bailey and Badgley[1] pioneered anterior cervical spine surgery in 1952, to treat traumatic and post-surgical cervical dislocations and other lesions. Robinson and Smith[2] devised an operation to excise protruding intervertebral discs and fused the spine with iliac bone but did not excise the posterior osteophytes in patients with cervical spondylosis. Cloward[3] reported his technique in 1958, using modified Wiltberger instruments and excising posterior osteophytes. Since then, many modifications and refinements of the anterior approach have been made, e.g. in instrumentation and operative magnification, and there are several reports of cervical intervertebral disc excision operations having been carried out without any bone grafting, the first by Hirsch in 1960[4], and apparently with results comparable to those obtained by disc excision and grafting.

The operations described in this chapter are those favoured by the author, with a personal series of over 1300 patients. For the atlantoaxial area, a transoral approach is necessary, and for the second cervical to the first thoracic vertebrae the approach is transcervical. An anterior cervical operation is indicated for certain degenerative, traumatic, infective and neoplastic lesions. It is beyond the scope of this chapter to discuss in any detail the indications and contraindications for the treatment of any particular disorder. Some key references are given but no attempt has been made to provide a comprehensive bibliography for disorders and procedures which are now very extensive and varied. The main aim is to describe and depict some of the more technical aspects of the anterior cervical spinal operations.

# ANTERIOR APPROACH TO CERVICAL SPINE FROM C2 TO T1 INCLUSIVE

### Indications

Excision of a protruded intervertebral disc or of one or more degenerative discs with associated posterior osteophytes, as seen in cervical spondylosis, is best achieved by an anterior approach. In cervical spinal stenosis, depending on the pathology, the clinical syndrome and the radiological appearances, treatment may be by extensive decompressive laminectomy or by anterior decompression and bony fusion. If indicated, the latter procedure can be followed some 10 or more weeks later by a decompressive laminectomy.

A similar approach may be part of an operation required for certain patients with severe cervical spinal injury. Neoplasms and infections involving the ventral aspect of the spine also require an anterior approach.

## Preoperative

### Special equipment

This includes Gardner–Wells skull tongs (or some other form of skull caliper or a canvas occipital-chin halter), cord, pulley and weights. A firm padded rest or bridge secured to the operating table (or a very firm sandbag resting on the table) to support the patient's neck is essential.

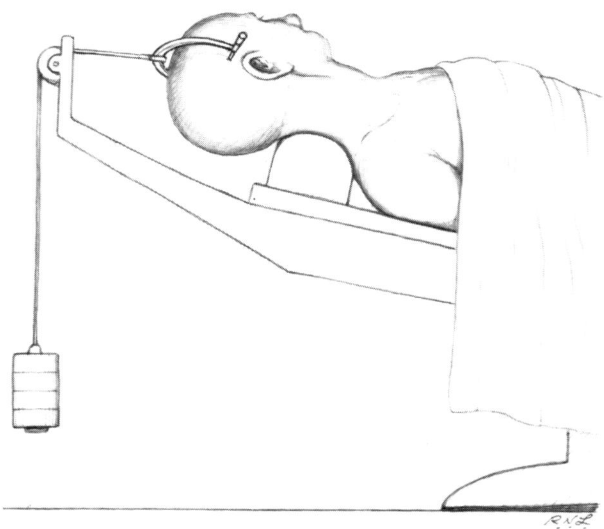

1

For anterior cervical operations, the patient should be on a Stryker turning frame, preferably with the addition of a Harris bridge to support the neck, or have had a halothoracic brace applied.

In addition to modified Wiltberger and Cloward instruments, the following are required: dowel cutter (15.5 mm); Hudson brace; two Meyerding hand retractors; two Harris hand retractors; lumbar puncture needle with guard at 10 mm from the tip; guide director and guard with handle; a flat-cutting four-fluted (12.5 mm) drill; bone curettes; obtuse-angled blunt-nosed knife (to open the posterior common ligament); up- and down-cutting sphenoidal punches (Angell James 2 mm); facing away blunt hook; dowel punch; depth gauge; operating microscope; high-speed drill. The author uses Absele (Ethicon) for bone haemostasis, and a specially designed foam plastic craniocervical support (Harris).

### Handling the patient

It should be stressed that special care is necessary in handling these patients, as sudden and/or forced movement of the neck, especially extension, may aggravate the neurological condition. Thus, the patient must be moved very gently and carefully when being transferred from bed to trolley to operating table, etc., and the neck should not be severely or suddenly extended for intubation.

### Anaesthesia

The operation is carried out under general anaesthesia. After induction with an intravenous agent, anaesthesia is maintained with nitrous oxide and oxygen. Muscular relaxants and analgesic drugs are routinely given. Intermittent positive-pressure ventilation is used and a latex-armoured orotracheal tube is preferred.

# 1

### Position of patient

The patient is placed supine on the operating table, with the neck slightly extended and firmly supported on the padded rest or bridge. Gardner–Wells traction tongs are applied to the head with about 3 kg weight over a pulley, and the table is tilted head-end upwards for countertraction. The head is turned to the left side, and a firm sandbag or bridge placed under the left buttock to facilitate access to the iliac crest. Padded crêpe bandage slings are placed around the patient's wrists so that the shoulders may be pulled down during radiography of the neck to permit visualization of all the cervical vertebrae. Surgeons who are right-handed will most likely prefer to operate on the right side of the patient's neck and on the left iliac crest. However, the recurrent laryngeal nerve is at greater risk of being inadvertently damaged if anterior operations are carried out on the right rather than the left side of the neck.

# The operation

## REMOVAL OF DOWELS FROM ILIAC BONE

## 2

### The incision

An incision is made in a skin crease just below the anterior end of the left iliac crest. Subperiosteal exposure of the crest is obtained by using cutting diathermy and a periosteal elevator. A broad, malleable spatula is placed against the inner aspect of the iliac bone and the iliac muscles are retracted.

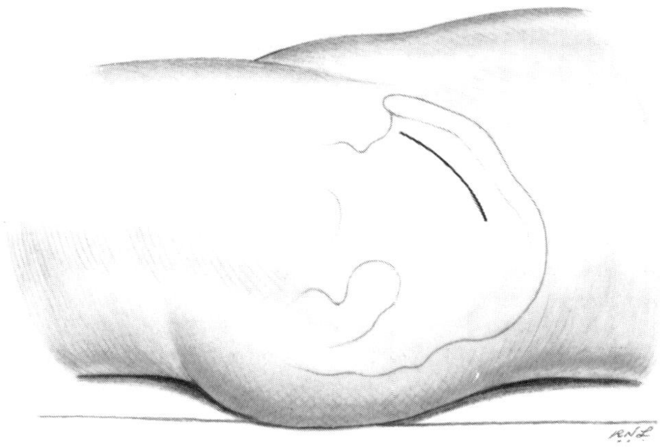

2

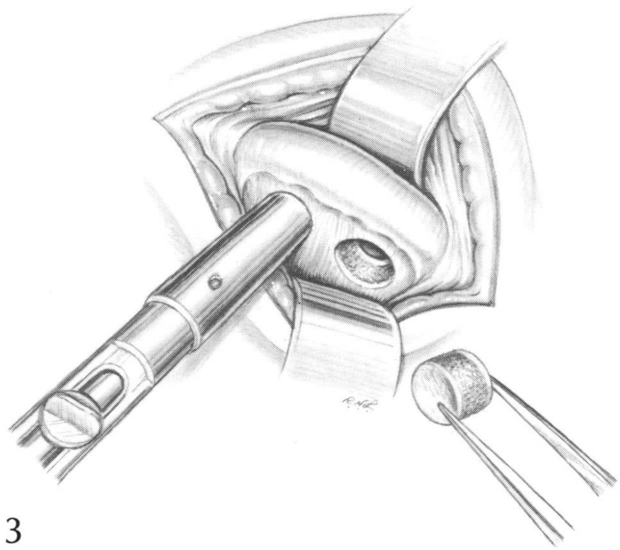

3

## 3

### Cutting the dowels

The appropriate number of full thickness dowels of iliac bone are removed from just below the iliac crest with a dowel cutter and a Hudson brace. Each dowel consists of a 'sandwich' of cancellous bone between 10 and 18 mm in thickness.

## 4a & b

### Wound closure

Bone haemostasis is obtained using Absele. The muscles on each aspect of the iliac bone are brought together with one suture or more through the drilled holes (*a*). The aponeurosis is then closed in one layer (*b*) and the skin in two layers with interrupted sutures. A closed suction drain (Davol) is left *in situ*.

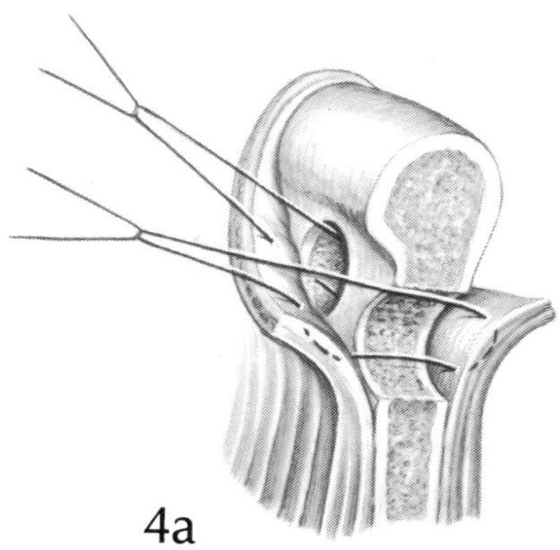

4a

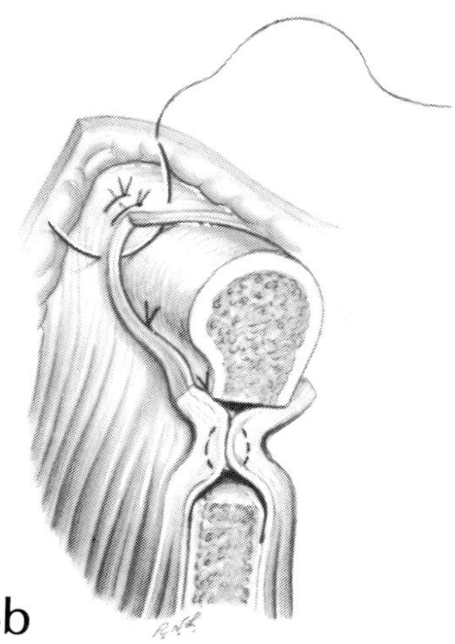

4b

## EXCISION OF INTERVERTEBRAL DISCS AND OSTEOPHYTES AND INTERBODY BONY FUSION

# 5

### The incision

A short incision is made in the line of a skin crease over the anterolateral aspect of the right side of the neck at a level appropriate to the site of the spinal disease, e.g., for the C5–C6 intervertebral disc, at the level of the cricoid cartilage. The incision extends from the anterior aspect of the sternocleidomastoid muscle to the midline of the neck. After undercutting the skin, it is held aside with a self-retaining retractor. It is possible to excise up to 4 intervertebral discs through one skin incision, and to reach as high as C2–C3 or as low as C7–T1 in any one patient by this route. The skin towels are sutured in place to facilitate the check radiological study.

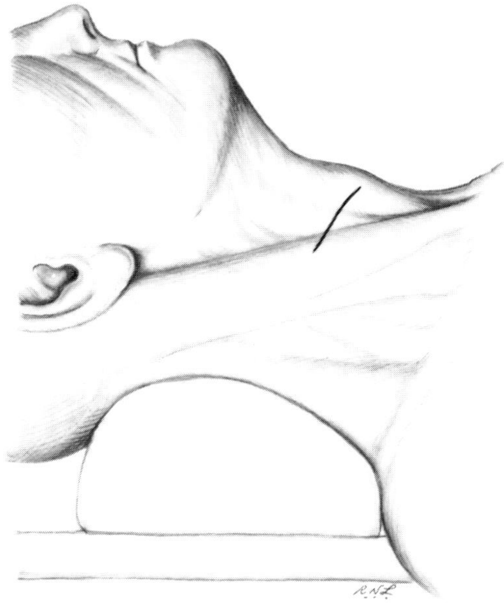

5

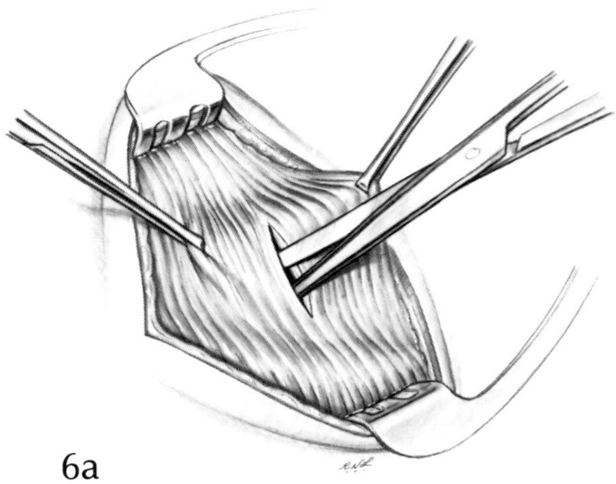

6a

# 6a & b

### Dividing the platysma

The platysma muscle is picked up with toothed forceps and divided with scissors in the line of its fibres, just medial to the sternomastoid muscle.

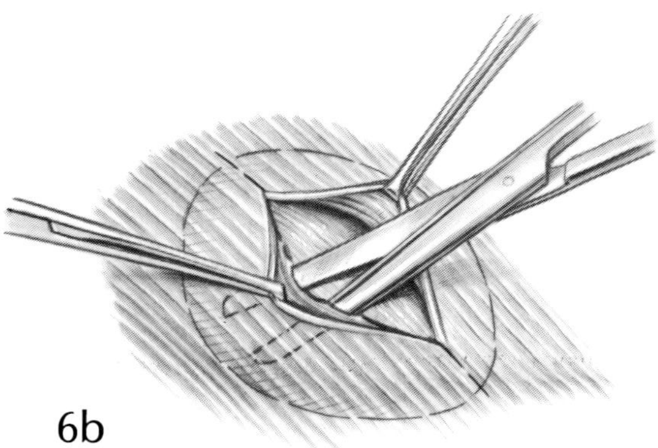

6b

## Exposure of anterior aspect of cervical spine

# 7

Blunt dissection is now carried out between the sternomastoid muscle and the carotid sheath and its contents laterally, and the oesophagus, pharynx, larynx and trachea medially. The recurrent laryngeal nerve on the right side of the neck lies between the oesophagus and the trachea, accompanied by the inferior thyroid artery. The prevertebral fascia is separated off the vertebral bodies and intervertebral discs, exposing these structures and longus colli muscles. In the lower cervical region, the omohyoid muscle is defined and retracted medially and inferiorly. It is not usually necessary to divide it. However, some tributaries of the internal jugular vein may require ligation and division.

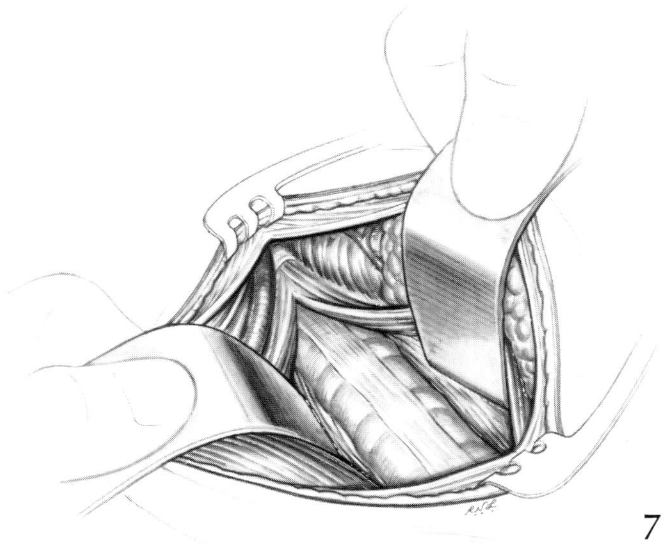

7

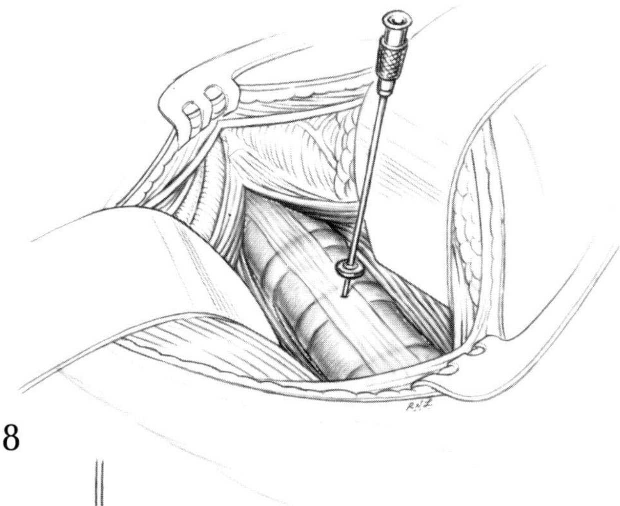

8

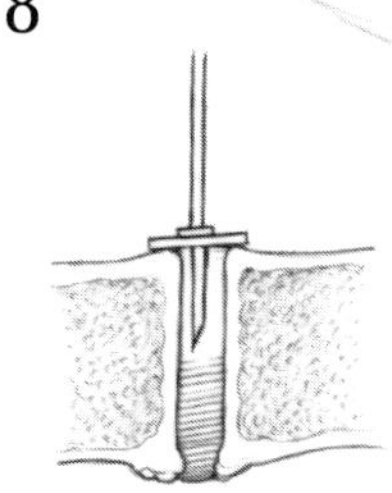

# 8

Prominent anterior osteophytes may permit precise anatomical localization of the lesion. Otherwise, after the patient's shoulders have been firmly pulled down by the crêpe bandages previously applied to the wrists, a lumbar puncture needle with a guard at 10 mm is inserted into the centre of an intervertebral disc and a lateral radiograph taken. Immediately the needle is removed, its site of entry is marked by making a surgical diathermy lesion. If desired, discography can be performed.

# 9

The author prefers to drill to about 10 mm initially, because, if for some technical reason the hole is not found to be in the ideal position, it is still possible to change the direction and even the site of the hole.

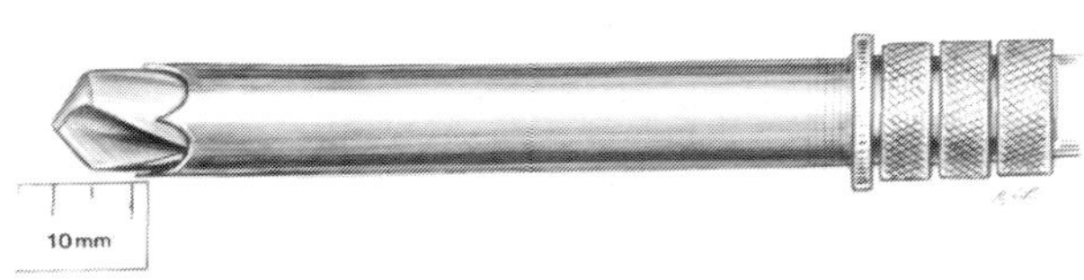


9

# 10a & b

Prominent anterior osteophytes are removed with bone rongeurs. To ensure that the drill hole will be made in the centre of the disc, a guide director is inserted firmly into the disc (*a*), and the guard (secured in the handle, which is firmly held by two assistants) is passed down over this and firmly tapped into place with a surgical hammer so that the spikes at its end are embedded in the vertebral bodies caudal and cranial to the disc being operated on (*b*). The guide director is now removed.

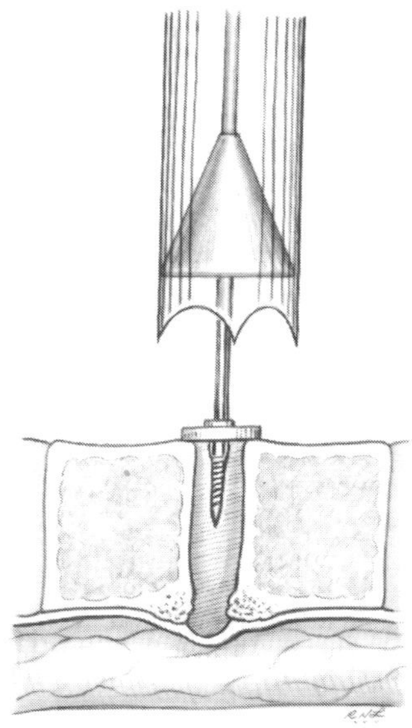

10a

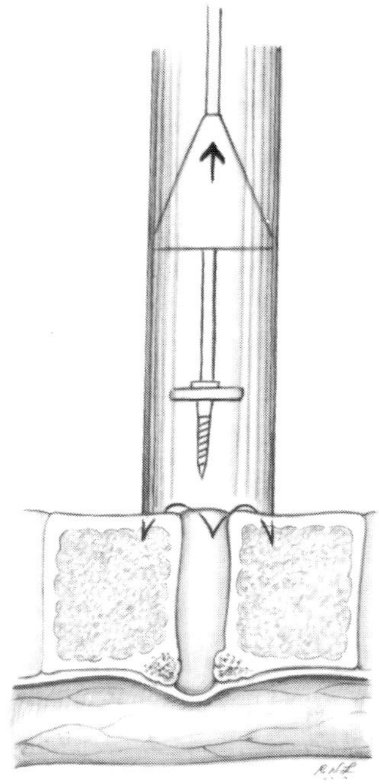

10b

## Drilling the hole

# 11

A flat-cutting four-fluted drill (12.5 mm in diameter) attached to a Hudson brace is passed down the guard, and the hole is drilled in stages, adjusting the length of drill protruding beyond the end of the guard. The hole is made through the disc and the adjacent aspects of the vertebral bodies until only a thin plaque of cortical bone remains. This plaque is now removed with bone curettes. Bone haemostasis is secured with Absele.

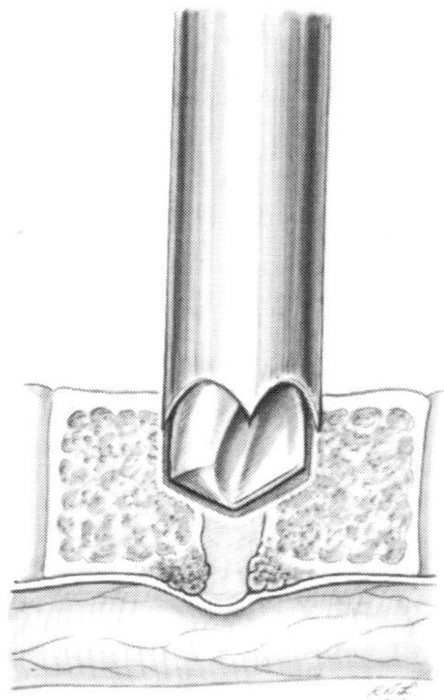

11

# 12

Gentle but firm use of small, slightly angled bone curettes allows further removal of any more laterally situated intervertebral disc tissue and posterior osteophytes on each side. By using a high-speed bone drill and magnification with a loupe or an operating microscope, very thorough decompression of the neural and vascular elements in the neural foramina can be achieved. This latter procedure is of particular importance in patients with an intervertebral disc or spondylotic radicular syndrome if interbody bony fusion is not going to be part of the operation. It is necessary to open up narrowed neural foramina and to ensure that they do not become narrow and constrict nerve roots. This is one reason why the author always prefers to do a combined decompression and interbody bony fusion procedure.

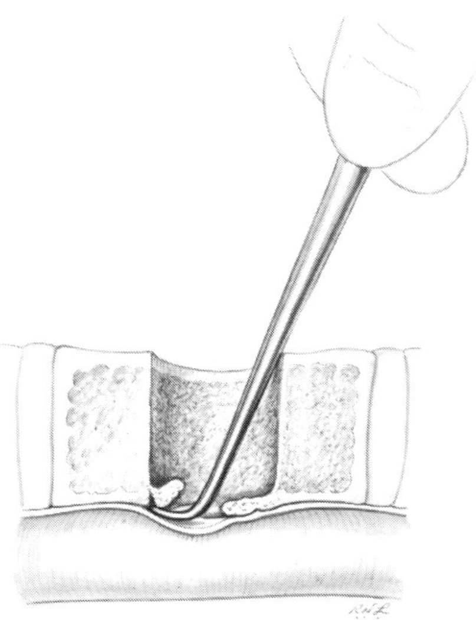

12

## Removal of posterior common ligament

# 13

The exposed posterior common ligament is split in the midline with a Harris obtuse-angled blunt-nosed knife and then removed with small up- and down-cutting sphenoidal punches, disclosing the dura. The punches and curettes can be used to remove more disc tissue and osteophytes, and excising the posterior common ligament will prevent it from buckling and acting as a nerve root compressing factor.

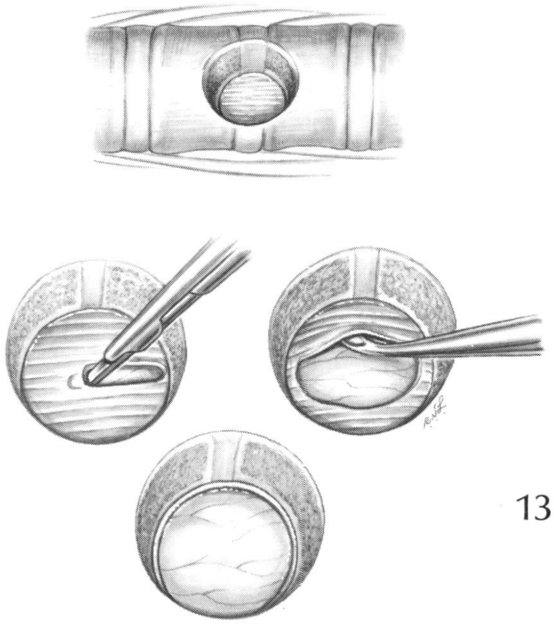

13

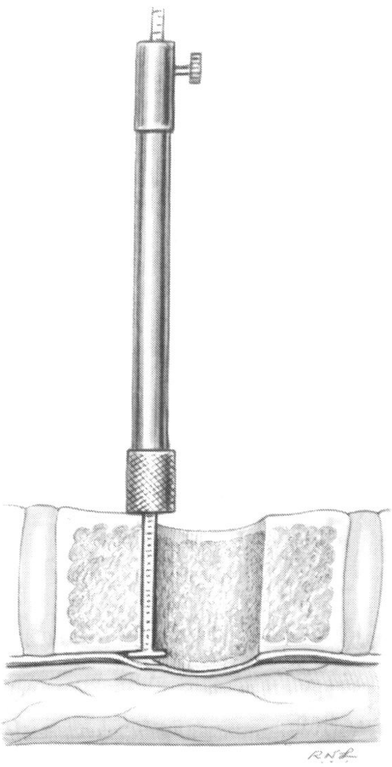

14

# 14

A depth gauge is used to measure the depth of the hole from the dura to the anterior aspect of the adjacent vertebral bodies to ensure in particular that there is no risk of inserting too long a dowel of bone, which could compress the spinal cord.

# 15a & b

## Insertion of bone dowel

The traction weight is now increased to about 16 kg (ensuring that the patient's head and neck are free to move up the table) in order to widen the space between the vertebral bodies that have been drilled. After its thickness has been measured, the dowel of iliac bone is fitted on to the end of the punch (*a*) and tapped home in the hole so that its ventral surface is flush with those of the adjacent vertebral bodies (*b*). If indicated, two or more diseased intervertebral discs may be similarly excised and the vertebrae fused. The traction weight is reduced to 3 kg.

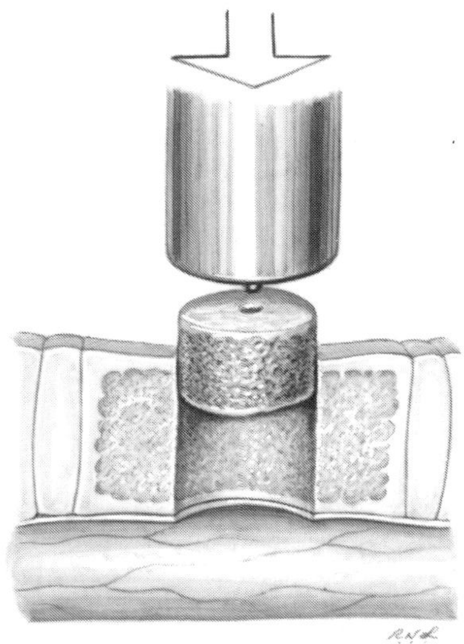

15a

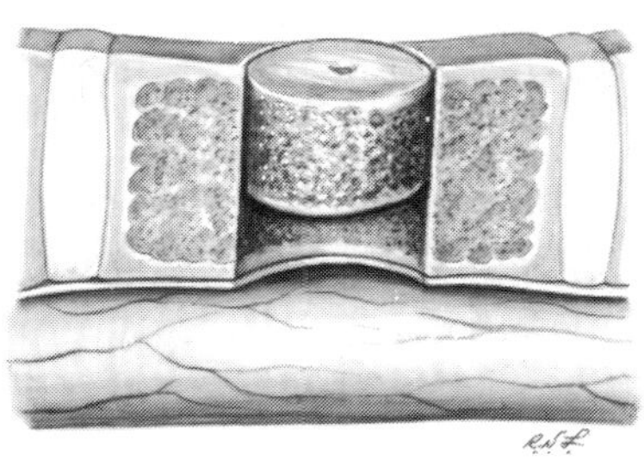

15b

# 16

### Wound closure

The platysma is closed in one layer and the subcutaneous tissues in a second layer of interrupted sutures, after a closed suction drain (Miniflap Drain; McGhan Medical Corporation) has been placed in the wound. The skin is closed with metallic clips. The Gardner–Wells tongs are removed and the small puncture wounds in the scalp are sprayed with an antibiotic.

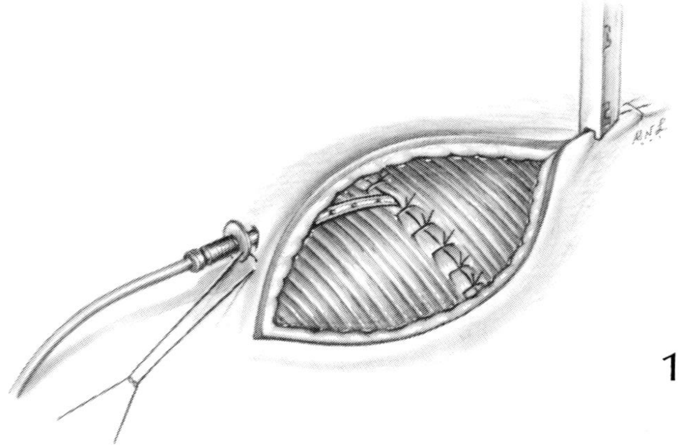

16

## Postoperative care

# 17

After the anaesthetic and drugs have been discontinued and the relaxant drugs reversed, and once the patient's clinical state is seen to be satisfactory, he is very gently transferred from the operating table to a firm bed, lying supine, with the head and neck immobilized in a foam plastic head–neck support.

A lateral radiograph of the patient's cervical spine is taken on the morning after the operation to ensure that the decompression–fusion site is satisfactory. The patient is then allowed up for increasingly frequent and longer periods. For 6 weeks a firm plastic collar with foam plastic edging is worn during the day.

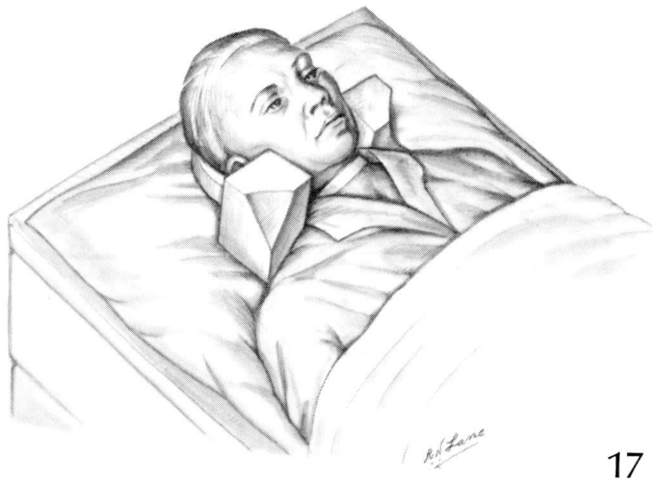

17

## Complications

Neurological complications are prevented by good patient selection, careful handling of the patient, and meticulous attention to surgical technique. In the author's experience, collapse or extrusion of a bone dowel is extremely unlikely, and indeed this should never occur. Gentle intermittent retraction in the neck and complete haemostasis should prevent postoperative dysphagia and dyspnoea. A rare complication is partial, temporary (right-sided) Horner's syndrome resulting from too vigorous lateral retraction of the cervical tissues. Another is recurrent laryngeal nerve paresis, which usually recovers fully.

In a few patients, infection of the left iliac wound has occurred, but this can be avoided by careful preparation and shaving of the pubic region. At operation, only gentle retraction should be used, and complete haemostasis must be obtained before closure.

## Results

With brachialgia (nerve root) syndromes, neck pain and/or pain in one or both upper limbs is usually absent from the time the patient wakes up from the anaesthetic. Weakness of the upper limb begins to improve in the immediate postoperative period and, if not worse than about grade 3, should recover over the next 2–3 months. Upper limb sensory changes begin to improve immediately after operation, and the prognosis is good.

With myelopathic syndromes, improvement depends in part on the acuteness of onset, the severity, the type of syndrome and the length of history. Best results are obtained in patients with anterior cord, lateral cord or subtotal cord syndromes.

# DISLOCATIONS AND FRACTURES OF THE CERVICAL SPINE FROM C2 TO T1 INCLUSIVE

## Indications

Operative treatment may be required in the following situations.

1. After reduction of cervical spine dislocations
2. In certain patients with an acute anterior cord syndrome with severe deformity of the cervical spine, and/or severe compression of the intraspinal neural and vascular elements by portions of damaged vertebral body and intervertebral disc
3. After closed reduction by traction and counter-pressure. (Full reduction should be attempted but with care being taken not to cause distraction.)

## Special equipment

In addition to the equipment described on p. 000, the following items are required: stainless steel 20 s.w.g., wire cutters, orthopaedic bone chisels, and methylmethacrylate. The substance now used is Palacos R. with gentamicin, which is radio-opaque (Kirby-Warrick, Mildenhall, UK).

For this operation and for the transoral atlantoaxial operation, halo fixation is one method of immobilizing the patient's head and neck before, during and after operation. The author has modified this apparatus so that, for a patient requiring a posterior cervical operation, the left posterior support can be removed for the duration of the operation, and for an anterior operation, the right anterior support can be removed to allow the surgeon full access to the patient.

Initially, Gardner–Wells skull tongs should be applied and a (Harris) bridge or sandbag placed under the affected portion of cervical spine. With the patient on a Stryker turning frame or other special bed, traction and expert manipulation are used to reduce the dislocation or fracture. The halo apparatus may then be applied, but more often the operation is carried out with the patient on the frame.

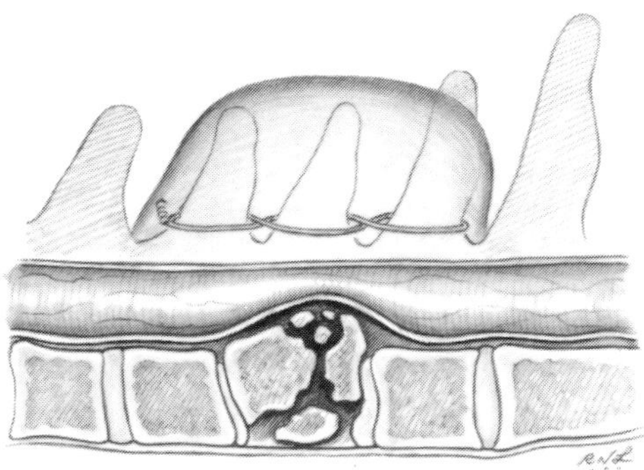

18

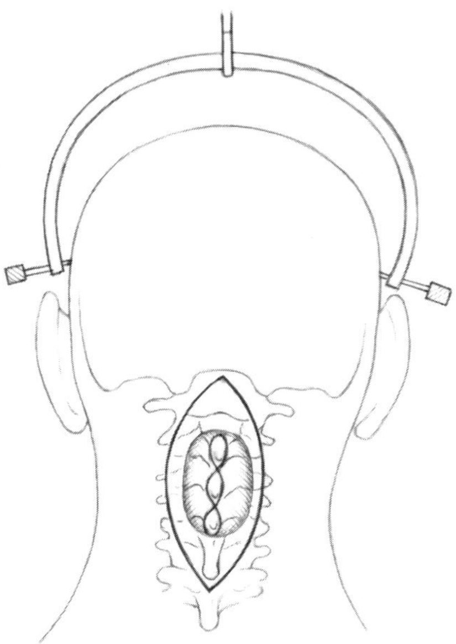

19

# The operation

This may consist of an anterior operation only, but the author usually prefers to fix the spine posteriorly before carrying out the anterior operation.

# 18 & 19

## Posterior fixation of cervical spine

The patient is placed prone. A lateral radiograph should be taken to ensure that positioning of the patient has not altered the anatomical appearance of the traumatized cervical spine. A midline cervical spine skin incision is now made. This reveals rupture of the supraspinous and interspinous ligaments commonly, and of the apophyseal ligaments and joint capsules. The spinous process and the laminae of the cervical vertebra below the point of dislocation or fracture (or traumatic disc protrusion or rupture) are exposed, as are those of the two vertebrae above this point. The three spinous processes are wired together. Methylmethacrylate of the consistency of paste is then poured onto the spinous processes, over the laminae and under their edges so that, when the material has set (in about 8 minutes), the affected portion of the spine is strongly bonded together. The wound is now closed, the cervical aponeurosis in one layer and the skin in two layers, with interrupted sutures. It is preferable to drain the wound by a closed vacuum system.

# 20

**Removal of damaged intervertebral disc or vertebral body and interbody bony fusion**

Under the same anaesthetic, the patient is now turned supine, and a further lateral radiograph is taken.

The initial procedure is similar to that described for the excision of a protruded cervical disc. As a portion of sequestrated intervertebral disc may have strayed up or down the spinal canal, away from the normal anatomical site of the disc, removal of a larger part of vertebral body may be necessary so that this free piece of disc can be located and removed. If there is a comminuted fracture with associated intervertebral disc rupture, the pieces are removed with pituitary rongeurs, and further anterior decompression of the neural and vascular elements is obtained using a high-speed bone drill. Sometimes there is a tear in the dura and arachnoid allowing cerebrospinal fluid to well out through the damaged vertebra and disc, possibly forming a pool under the anterior common ligament. The dural tear may be sutured or covered with a portion of crushed muscle.

Through an incision over the anterior part of the left iliac crest, an appropriately sized wedge of bone is removed with chisels and mallet, and this wedge, which includes part of the upper surface of the iliac crest, is trimmed so that it will fit tightly into the gap in the cervical spine left after excision of the vertebral bodies and disc. Instead of iliac bone, a portion of fibula may be used. To help retain the bone graft in place, a pinning/methylmethacrylate technique may be used as an additional measure.

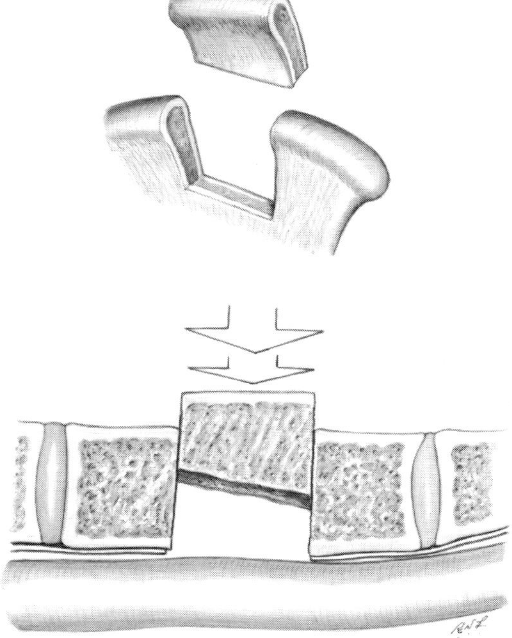

20

## Postoperative care

Depending on his neurological state and any associated injuries, the patient is mobilized and allowed up from the first postoperative day. With secure posterior cervical fixation, the halo apparatus or skull tongs may then be removed.

If the patient has a serious high cervical spinal cord lesion and or serious associated injuries, a longer period of immobilization in a halo or with skull tongs may be necessary. Further discussion is outside the scope of this chapter.

## Complications

These are similar to those mentioned on p. 388 for the anterior cervical operation. It is important that patients with a serious spinal injury are transferred, as soon as possible after the injury, to a specialized spinal paralysis unit, as their management demands special facilities and expertise.

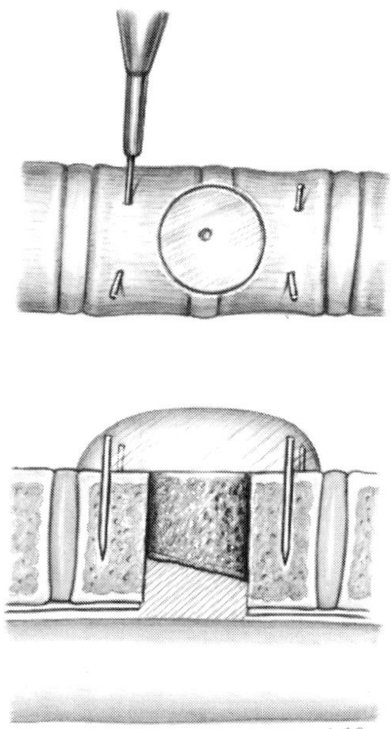

21

# TRANSORAL ATLANTO-AXIAL OPERATION

## Indications

The transoral approach may be required for certain patients with traumatic atlantoaxial dislocation or fracture–dislocation, and for infective conditions, including those causing weakness of the atlantoaxial ligaments and consequent dislocation, such as rheumatoid arthritis, in which there may also be a mass of nodular granulation tissue compressing the anterior aspect of the uppermost part of the cervical spinal cord. Tuberculosis, neoplasms and craniocervical dysplasia are other conditions where this operation may be required. In some patients with type 1 or 3 dens fracture, simple wiring of the posterior arch and tubercle of the atlas to the spinous process and laminae of the axis, with a covering of methylmethacrylate, may suffice. However, surgical access may be difficult if reduction of a dislocation or fracture–dislocation is to be maintained, and the wire may in time either cut through the bone, especially the thin posterior arch of the atlas, or break.

To remove a displaced dens, e.g. an os odontoideum, or the dens in a patient with basilar impression, and to remove rheumatoid or other pathological tissue that may be compressing the anterior aspect of the spinal cord, an anterior approach is necessary. It is also necessary if the posterior bony elements have been removed at a previous operation. A fracture through the base of the dens is most likely to heal securely if the patient's head and neck are firmly immobilized for 10–12 weeks in a halo apparatus or, as a second choice, with skull tongs and a Stryker turning frame, but posterior wiring is just as effective and very early mobilization of the patient is possible.

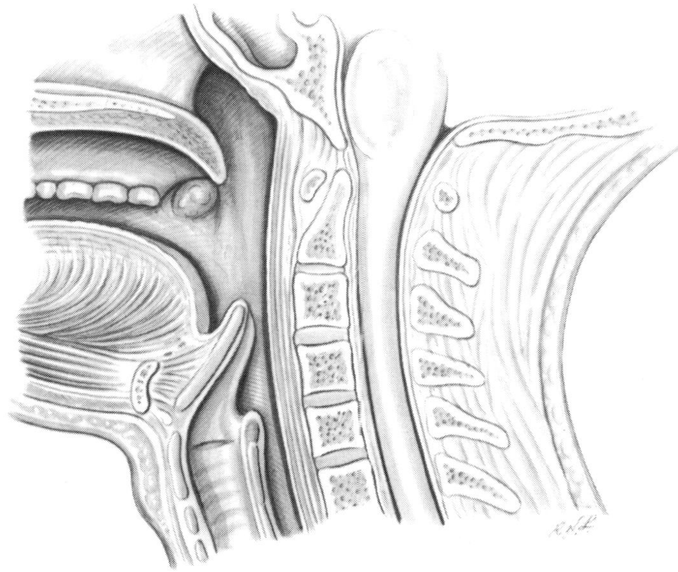

# 22

## Anatomy

It is essential that the surgeon makes himself fully familiar with the anatomy of the area, and studies in the anatomy department and autopsy room are recommended.

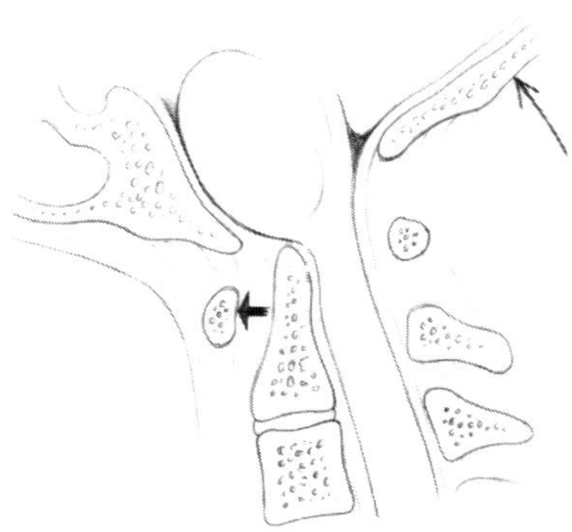

22

## Special equipment

In addition to Gardner–Wells skull tongs and a Stryker turning frame (or halo trunk traction apparatus), a Davis–Boyle mouth gag is required.

The instruments, specially modified, are similar to those used for the anterior cervical (C2–T1) operation (see p. 382): iliac bone dowel cutter (10.5 mm in diameter); two Harris hand retractors; guide director with guard and handle; four-fluted drill (8 mm); depth gauge; dowel punch; stainless steel pins and punch; methylmethacrylate; boomerang needle; 2/0 chromic catgut.

# Preoperative

## Preparation of patient

It is essential to ensure that reduction of the dislocation or fracture–dislocation has been obtained, and is being maintained, using skull tongs and a Stryker turning frame, or a halo apparatus. (The special management of infective conditions and of neoplasms will not be discussed here.) The patient should be isolated, and throat and nasal swabs taken for bacteriological study. A wide-spectrum antibiotic is given, beginning 48 hours before the operation.

## Anaesthesia

This is as for the anterior cervical operation (*see* p. 382), except that after induction a tracheostomy is performed and the anaesthetic is given through a cuffed tracheal tube. The lower pharynx is packed off with gauze, which must be removed at the end of the operation.

## Position of patient

The patient is placed supine, with the right anterior rod of the halo apparatus removed. If skull tongs and a Stryker turning frame are being used, it is important to ensure that the patient's head and neck are firmly supported posteriorly, e.g. on a Harris bridge. A check lateral radiograph of the cervical spine is then taken to outline the lesion in the atlantoaxial region.

# The operation

A standard tracheostomy is made after induction and the anaesthetic given through a cuffed tracheostomy tube. Two dowels of iliac bone are then removed from the anterior aspect of an iliac crest, as described earlier.

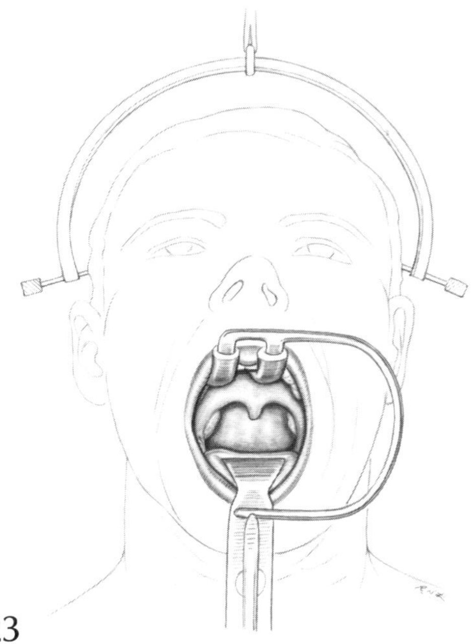

23

# 23

## Insertion of Davis-Boyle mouth gag

The gag is inserted fully. The best exposure is obtained in patients who are edentulous. The lower pharynx is packed off, and the soft palate and pillars of the fauces are stitched to the adjacent wall of the oropharynx (*see Illustration 23*). At intervals during the operation, the mouth and throat should be sprayed with an antibiotic. In patients with rheumatoid arthritis, the temporomandibular joints may be involved, limiting access to the posterior pharynx. This can be overcome by splitting the mandible to allow greater depression of the tongue.

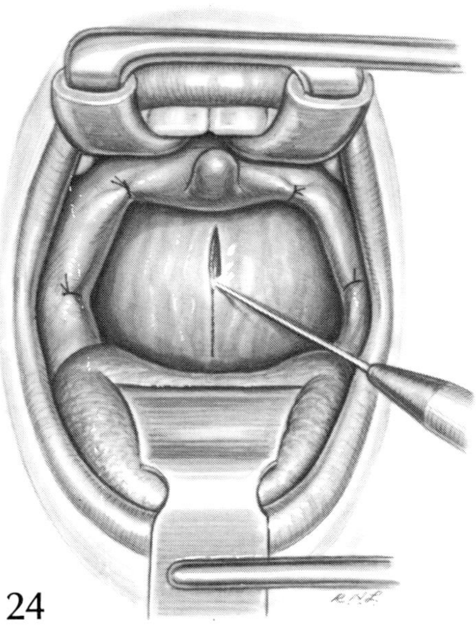

24

# 24

## Incision of posterior pharyngeal wall

The anterior tubercle and arch of the atlas, the body of the axis and the C1–C2 apophyseal joints just lateral to these are palpated and then exposed by dividing the posterior wall of the pharynx with cutting diathermy, keeping to the midline.

# 25

## Exposure of atlantoaxial region

A pair of Harris or other hand retractors is used to hold the pharyngeal soft tissues aside. Haemostasis is secured with diathermy and Absele.

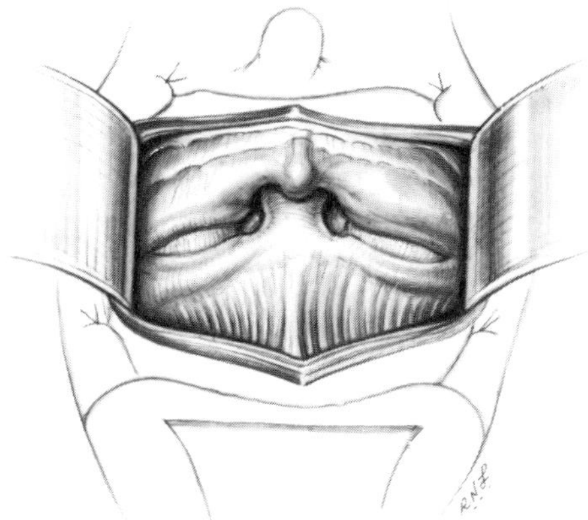

25

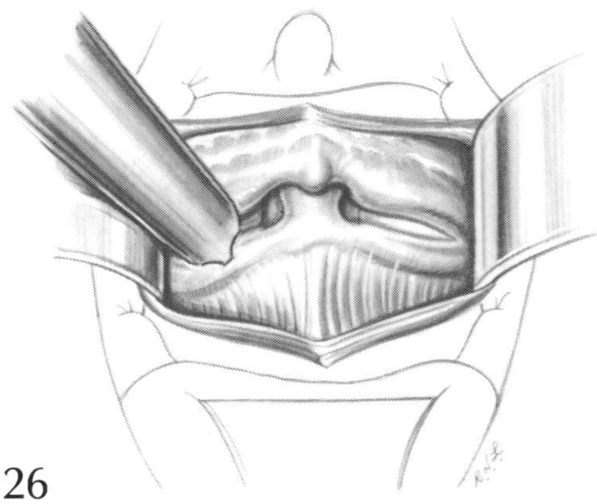

26

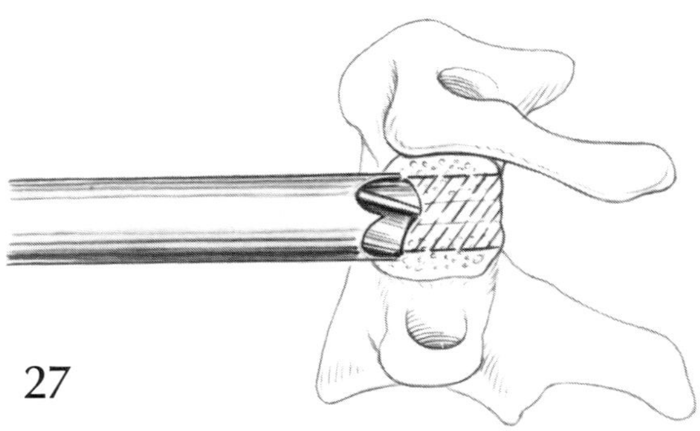

27

# 26 & 27

## Drilling the holes

The guide is inserted into the centre of one of the atlantoaxial apophyseal joints, and the guard is then passed over this and gently tapped into place so that the spikes on its end enter the bone above and below the apophyseal joint. The handle is used to steady the guard, and a hole is drilled to about 6 mm depth through the joint and adjacent aspects of the articular masses of C1 and C2. It is important not to drill beyond the confines of the joint. The procedure is then repeated on the other C1–C2 joint. The depth of the holes is then measured and the length of the iliac bone dowels is trimmed if necessary with a bone rongeur.

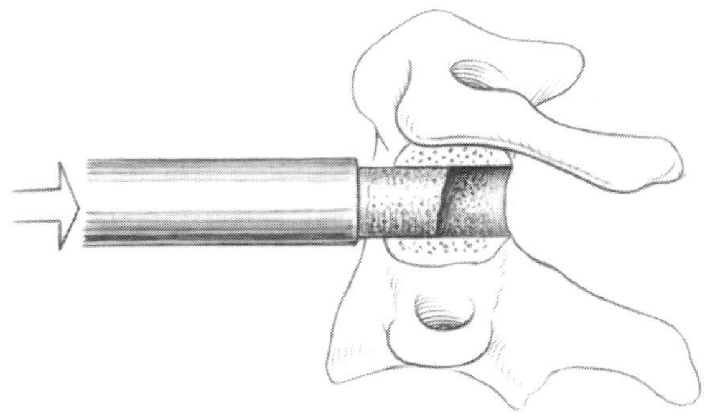

28

# 28, 29 & 30

## Insertion and fixation of bone dowels

The iliac bone dowels are now inserted into the drill holes and tapped into place. However, unlike those inserted as grafts in the lower part of the cervical spine, they do not fit snugly, and therefore a pinning/methylmethacrylate technique is used additionally. Two stainless steel pins are inserted into the anterior arch of the atlas, and two into the body of the axis, and over these and the bone dowels, methylmethacrylate is applied to bond the atlas and axis vertebrae together and to retain the bone dowels in place.

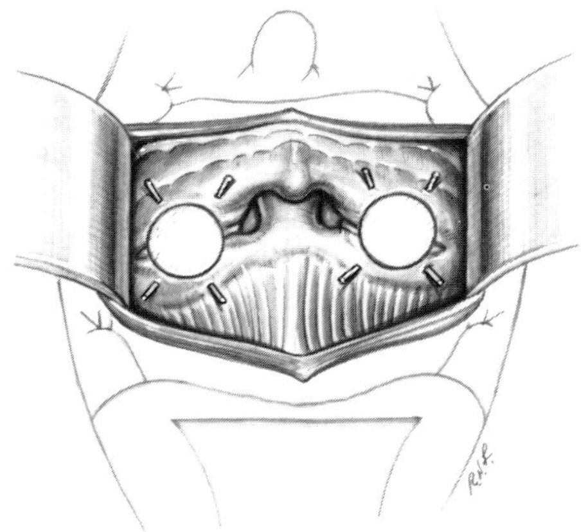

29

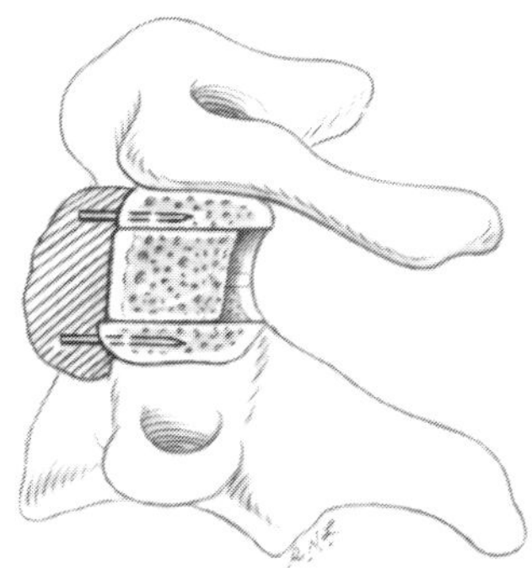

30

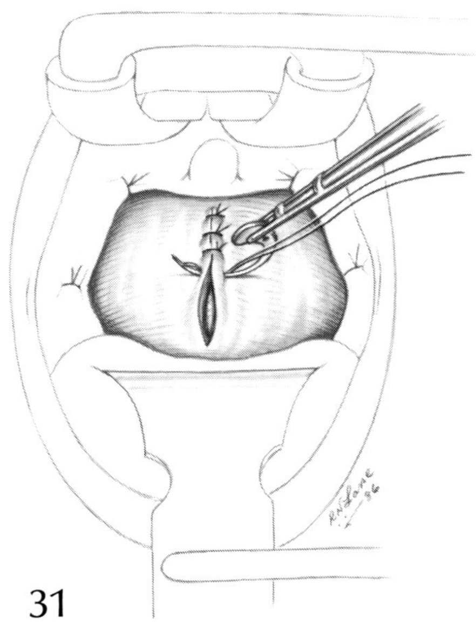

31

## Closure of posterior pharyngeal wall

# 31

The posterior pharyngeal wall is closed with a single layer of 2/0 chromic catgut sutures, using a boomerang needle. The stay sutures are then divided.

If the operation is being performed for some disorder other than to fuse the atlas and axis, then that condition is dealt with appropriately. For example, a displaced dens may be removed, and it may be necessary to excise part of the anterior arch of the atlas. Infective or neoplastic lesions may require fusion of C1 and C2, as described, in addition to their appropriate treatment.

## Postoperative care

After the pharyngeal pack and Davis–Boyle mouth gag have been removed, the anaesthetic and relaxant drugs are reversed. The patient is then placed prone initially.

During the first 48 hours, parenteral feeding is used, and for the next 3–4 days, food is given through a soft nasogastric tube, which is left *in situ*. The pharyngeal wound is inspected twice daily. With these precautions, there should be no problem with wound healing.

The tracheostomy tube is removed on the fifth or sixth postoperative day. The patient is allowed up within a few days of the operation, depending on the severity of any neurological disabilities that may be present. Check radiographs are taken.

## Complications

If the above instructions are strictly adhered to, there should not be any complications. If the hole through the C1–C2 apophyseal joint has been drilled too deeply and laterally, a vertebral artery may have been damaged. In this case it should be possible to obtain haemostasis by inserting a portion of crushed muscle or/and some Oxycel gauze (Associated Hospital Supply, UK) into the hole.

### *References*

1. Bailey, R. W., Badgley, C. E. (1960) Stabilization of the cervical spine by anterior fusion. Journal of Bone and Joint Surgery, 42A, 565

2. Robinson, R. A., Smith, G. W. (1955) Anterolateral disc removal and interbody fusion for cervical disc syndrome. Bulletin of the Johns Hopkins Hospital, 96, 223

3. Cloward, R. B. (1958) The anterior approach for removal of ruptured cervical discs. Journal of Neurosurgery, 15, 602

4. Hirsch, C. (1960) Cervical disc rupture: diagnosis and therapy. Acta Orthopaedica Scandinavica, 30, 172

# Posterior midline approach for cervical disc disease

**Kemp Clark** MD, FACS
Professor of Neurosurgery, Division of Neurological Surgery, Southwestern Medical School, Dallas, Texas, USA

The posterior midline approach for cervical disc disease is indicated for the surgical treatment of laterally placed soft cervical discs at one level. Occasionally it may prove useful for the laterally placed hard disc but this is generally best managed by an anterior approach.

## Positioning the patient

The patient may be positioned in the prone, lateral or sitting position. Skeletal fixation of the skull is a desirable adjunct as it prevents motion after the patient has been placed in the appropriate position. It is the author's preference to use the sitting position.

# The operation

A Doppler probe should be placed in the right heart for detection should air embolism occur. The patient's neck should be moderately flexed. After appropriate draping, a midline incision extending two spinous processes above and two spinous processes below the known site of disc herniation is made. This is carried down through the deep fascia of the neck and the intraspinous ligament. Using a sharp periosteal elevator the paraspinous muscles are elevated from the spinous process and lamina on the appropriate side. It may prove necessary to divide some of the attachments of the short segmental muscles which attach to the lamina sharply. It is important that the dissection be carried well laterally as the facet joint must be exposed.

An interesting modification of the skin incision has been proposed by Hunt and Miller in which they make an oblique incision. It is begun at the spinous process of the lamina involved in the pathology, and is extended laterally on the appropriate side. The trapezius muscle is then divided by a muscle splitting incision. The rest of the procedure is carried out in the manner herein described. The advantages claimed for this procedure are elimination of some neck pain and the ease of closure. The disadvantage is that it limits exposure to one, or perhaps, two interspaces. This makes the placing of the incision critical.

Once the muscles have been elevated from the lamina, an appropriate self-retaining retractor is applied. Using a fine, sharp curette, the ligamentum flavum is freed from the edge of the superior lamina. A small, angled Kerison punch is then used to remove approximately one-third to one-half of the laminar arch on the appropriate side. An alternative to using a rongeur to remove the bone is to use a high-speed air drill. This is somewhat slower, but may have an added margin of safety. As nothing is passed under the lamina, damage to the underlying root is less likely. The bony removal should include the medial part of the superior facet at the facet joint. The ligamentum flavum is then excised.

If the operating microscope is to be used, it should be introduced into the operative field at this point. The microscope provides superior illumination and vision for the operating surgeon. It also provides an observation tube for instruction of house officers or other physicians. It is not imperative that the microscope be used; cervical disc surgery was performed successfully for a long period of time before its introduction. However, it is useful for the reasons given, and the author suggests its use.

Bleeding in the epidural space should be controlled with bipolar cautery, or by packing with fine pieces of absorbable gelatin sponge soaked in thrombin. The cervical nerve root has a very short course inside the spinal canal and is rather firmly attached at both ends of that course. It is imperative, therefore, that retraction of the nerve root is gentle to prevent damage. It should also be borne in mind that the sensory and motor roots may not have fused, so the possibility exists that it is still a double root. The surgeon must be careful to be sure that the root has been totally mobilized and retracted before proceeding to the next step.

The nerve root may be retracted upward or downward depending on the location of the disc fragment under it. Once the root has been retracted the posterior longitudinal ligament should be incised in a cruciate fashion, gaining access to the offending fragment. A fine pituitary rongeur should be used to move the fragments of herniated discs. There is not a lot of disc material extruded in cervical disc disease. Because of the anatomy, much smaller extrusion is likely to produce root pain and dysfunction. It is unusual to be able to enter the disc space for removal of additional material and no attempt should be made to do so.

Once the offending fragments have been removed, a dental tool should be passed out through the neural foramen to ensure that the root is completely free and that no laterally placed fragment has been missed.

Following this the wound is irrigated and all cottonoid and gelatin sponge are removed. Closure in layers is accomplished with fine non-absorbable interrupted sutures. A soft cervical collar is applied for approximately 6 weeks. Ambulation should begin the evening of surgery and the patient should rapidly progress to full activity.

## Complications

The complications of this procedure are those of any major operative procedure, plus those unique to this particular operation. Obviously anaesthetic complications can occur intraoperatively. Haemorrhage intraoperatively usually means that the dissection has been carried too far laterally and the vertebral artery lacerated. If this occurs, exposure of the vertebral artery and the foramen transversarium should be carried out. The vessel should be repaired if possible: ligation should be used as a last resort. Postoperative wound infection may occur but this should certainly be less than 1 per cent of patients operated upon by an individual surgeon. Meticulous attention to aseptic technique will reduce the instance of this complication.

Wound haematoma is quite unusual if careful haemostasis is performed before closure. Deep vein thrombosis may occur in any postoperative patient not ambulatory in the immediate postoperative period.

Neurological complications include damage to the nerve root and to the spinal cord itself. These are the results of rough handling of tissue and lack of gentleness in retraction. It should not be necessary to retract the dura mater. If the offending disc or osteophyte lies in a paracentral location, the surgery should be performed anteriorly rather than posteriorly. Originally, even midline cervical discs were approached through a laminectomy, proceeding transdurally to remove the fragment. This is no longer appropriate to the greater efficacy and safety of the anterior approach.

The most common neurological complication is damage to the nerve root with resulting fibrosis and persistent pain or numbness, paraesthesia, and weakness. This can be avoided by careful and gentle retraction of the nerve root and by using an appropriate direction to retract the nerve root. If the disc presents largely below the root, the root should be retracted upward. If the reverse is true, the root should be retracted downward.

Illustrations by Ludwig Kempe and Robert Lane

# Transthoracic removal of thoracic disc protrusions

**Phanor L. Perot Jr** MD, PhD
Professor and Chairman, Department of Neurological Surgery, Medical University of South Carolina, Charleston, South Carolina, USA

## Introduction

Thoracic disc protrusions were first described by Key in 1838[1] and then by Middleton and Teacher in 1911[2]. They are relatively rare lesions, with an estimated incidence of one patient per year per one million population[3]. There is no stereotyped clinical presentation, but most thoracic discs present with radicular pain if they are located laterally or centrolaterally, or with signs and symptoms of myelopathy if they are located centrally. Earlier efforts at treatment of these difficult lesions through a standard posterior laminectomy approach resulted in a relatively high incidence of morbidity and mortality, particularly with central disc protrusions causing myelopathy[4]. The best results were obtained with lateral disc protrusions producing radicular symptoms only. Alternative approaches were proposed, such as a lateral costotransversectomy[5], far lateral laminectomy and partial fascetectomy[6], and a posterolateral approach through the facet joint and pedicle[7]. In 1969, the author described a transthoracic approach that is particularly applicable to central thoracic disc protrusions causing spinal cord compression[4]. Improved results have been obtained with all of these alternative approaches when compared with a standard posterior laminectomy.

# 1a & b

## Radiological evaluation

At the present time, in the author's experience, the preferred imaging technique for these lesions is computerized tomographic metrizamide myelography. This technique demonstrates these lesions clearly and accurately delineates their anatomical relationship to the spinal cord. Laterally placed lesions causing radicular pain (*a*) may be dealt with adequately through posterolateral approaches. The more centrolateral or centrally placed lesions (*b*) are best approached by a more anterior route, and in the author's experience the transthoracic approach has proved most satisfactory[8].

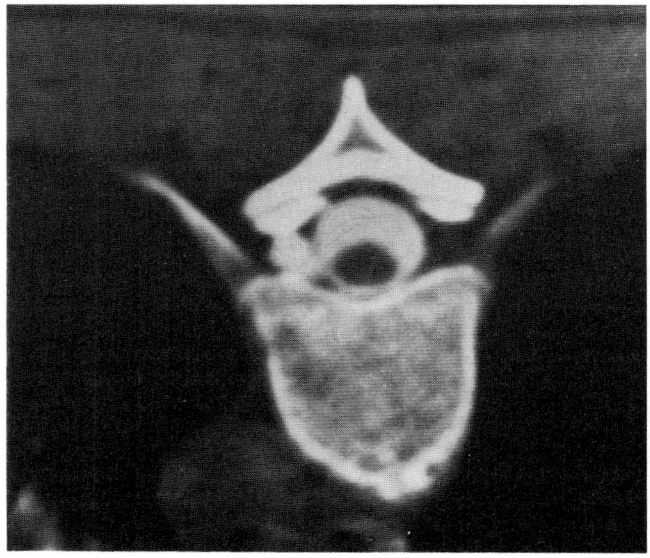

1a

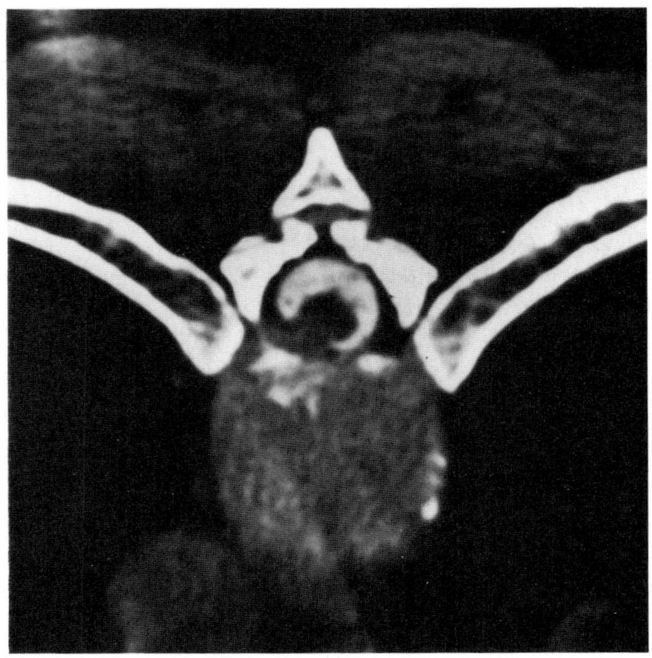

1b

# Preoperative

Great care must be taken to locate the involved disc space accurately; good scout films on the CT scanner, allowing one to count from above or below, are essential. Preoperative intercostal angiography has been advocated by some authors. The author uses it for laterally situated disc protrusions that are to be approached posterolaterally, because it is good to be forewarned of the presence of a significant radicular artery entering the spinal canal along the nerve root at the operative level. It is probably not necessary to perform preoperative intercostal angiography when approaching these lesions transthoracically, because the dissection is carried out at a fairly safe distance from the usual site of entry of any significant radicular vessels into the spinal canal.

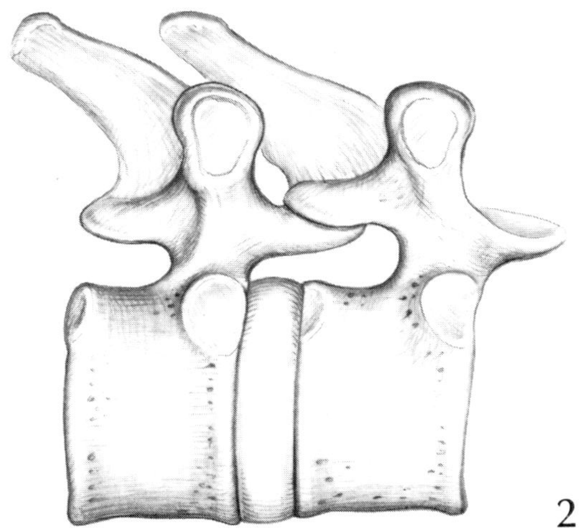

2

## Anatomical considerations

### 2

It is important to appreciate that the intervertebral disc lies at the most caudal and ventral aspect of the intervertebral foramen. The disc lies very close to the pedicle of the vertebra below it and at some distance from the pedicle of the vertebra above it.

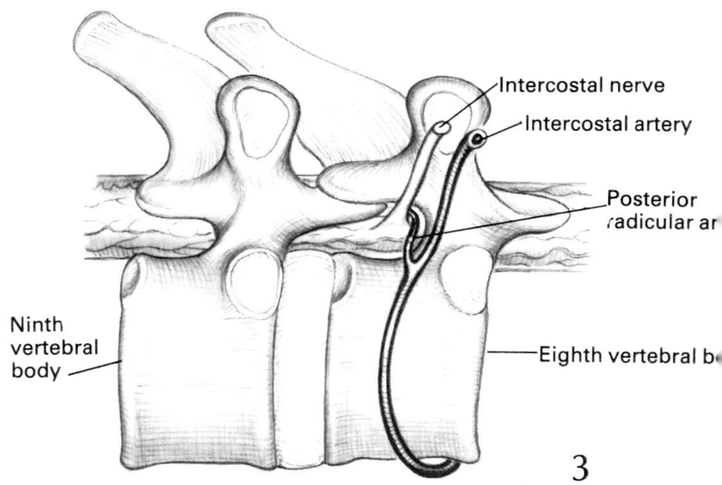


3

### 3

The spinal nerve root exits the foramen at its cranial end. The intercostal artery courses dorsally over the midportion of the vertebral body, halfway between adjacent intervertebral discs. As it passes the cranial end of the intervertebral foramen it may or may not give off small epidural arteries, or a significant radicular artery inside the spinal canal, before joining the intercostal nerve to course beneath the rib edge. Since the disc lies at the caudal end of the foramen, one operates at a little distance from the intercostal artery and also away from any significant vessels that might supply the anterior spinal artery.

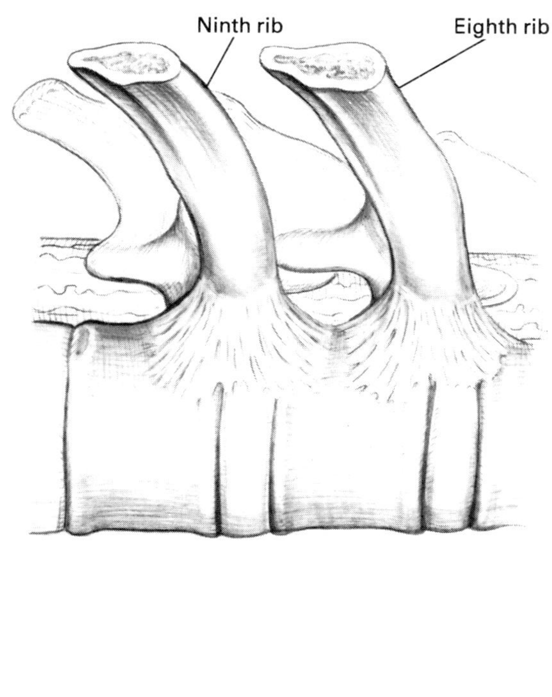


4

### 4

The rib head articulates with the vertebral body above and below the disc space. The head is firmly attached to the adjacent vertebrae over the disc by the radiate ligament. It is apparent that to reach the disc protrusion the head of the rib has to be removed along with its ligamentous attachments to the vertebral bodies.

# The operation

## Position of patient

### 5

For midline thoracic disc protrusions causing myelopathy the author prefers a right-sided approach. The heart and great vessels are less in the way, and significant radicular arteries tend to enter the spinal canal more often from the left side than from the right. More centrolaterally placed lesions can be safely approached from whichever side allows the most direct access.

The patient is postured in a standard right-side-up thoracotomy position. Careful attention is given to padding of the dependent limbs, and the upper arm is brought up and away from the operative site. Anaesthesia is given through a double-lumen endotracheal tube so that the patient may be ventilated using the dependent lung, and the upper lung is deflated and packed off during the operation. It is convenient to open the chest between the ribs just above the involved interspace, as this will allow more direct lateral exposure of the appropriate thoracic disc through the thoracotomy. The surgeon stands facing the front of the patient, and the operating microscope is normally used.

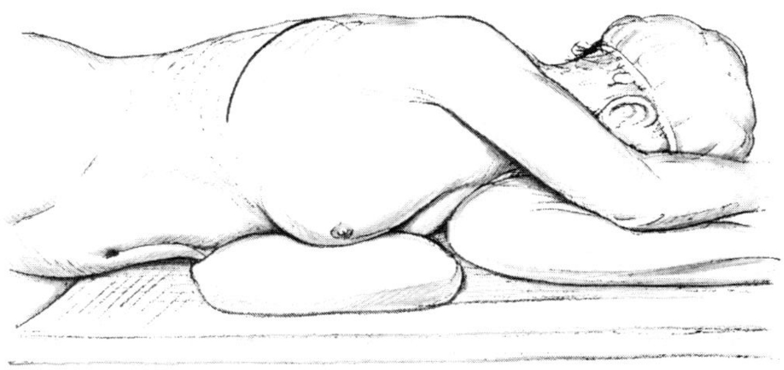

5

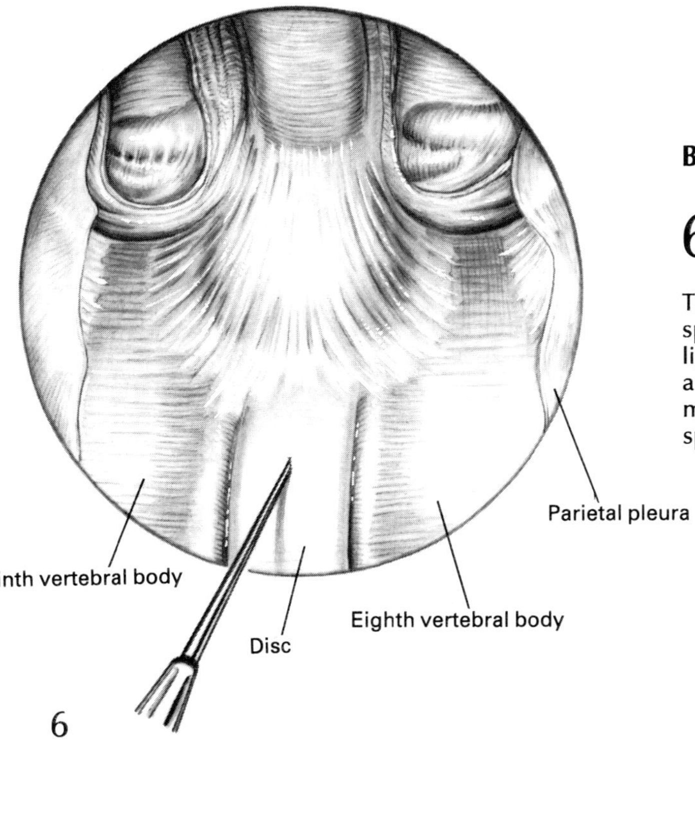


6

## Beginning the dissection

### 6

The parietal pleura is opened over the appropriate disc space, exposing the head of the rib and its radiate ligament. A needle is inserted in the disc space and anteroposterior and/or lateral thoracic spine films are made to confirm identification of the appropriate disc space.

# 7

## Removal of the rib head

The disc space is entered with a sharp knife and some disc tissue is removed laterally. Following this, a high-speed nitrogen-driven drill is used to remove the head of the rib as it articulates with the vertebral bodies above and below the affected disc space. The fibrocartilaginous attachments of the rib to the vertebral bodies will be removed and more disc will be curetted away as the dissection proceeds more medially. Note that the bone removal will extend into the pedicle of the vertebra caudal to the affected disc space, but not into the pedicle of the vertebra cranial to the disc space.

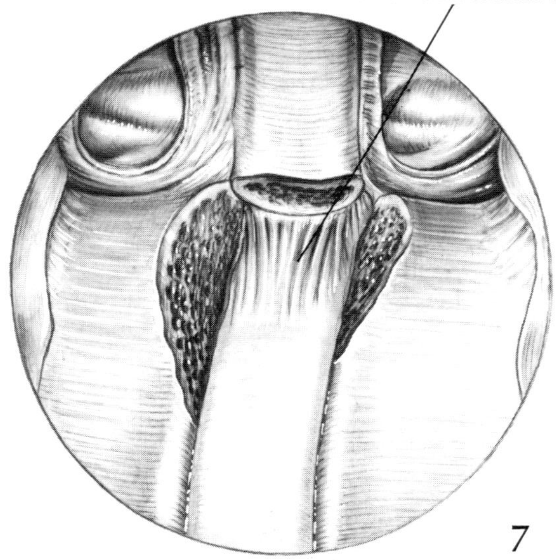

7

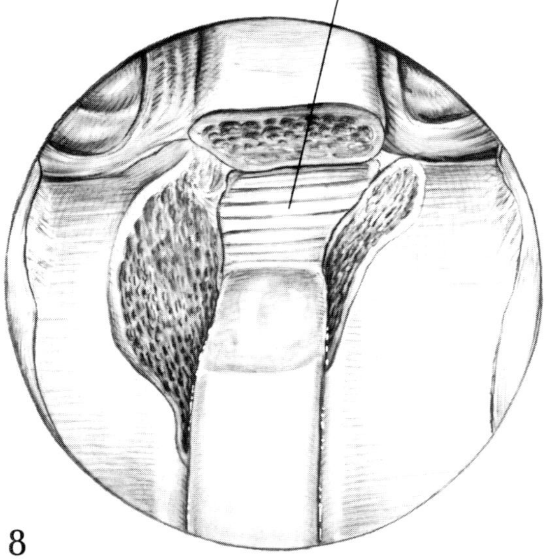

8

# 8

## Exposure of the posterior longitudinal ligament

When the fibrocartilaginous attachment of the rib head to the adjacent vertebral bodies is penetrated, the dense fibres of the posterior longitudinal ligament are encountered running transversely across the exposure and covering the epidural space.

# 9

## Removal of the posterior longitudinal ligament

Using an elevator and sharp dissection, the posterior longitudinal ligament is excised laterally and anteriorly, exposing the epidural space. Bleeding from the epidural venous plexus is usually encountered at this stage and is controlled by bipolar coagulation or small amounts of absorbable gelatin sponge. The ligament is excised from the most cranial to the most caudal extent of the exposure anterolaterally.

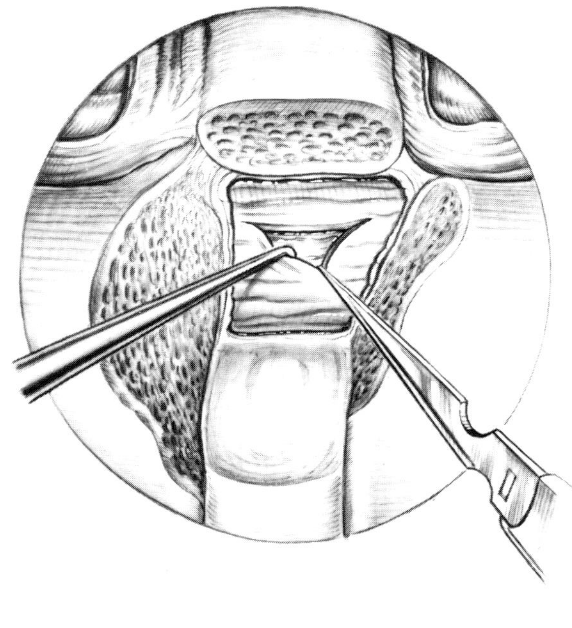
9

# 10

## Relation of dura to disc protrusion

With central protrusions, the disc may be completely covered laterally by the dura that caps the protrusion. It is important not to retract or manipulate the dura and the compressed spinal cord.

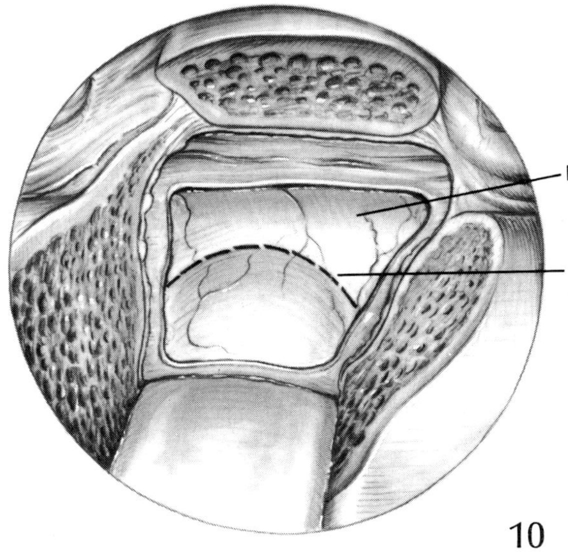


10

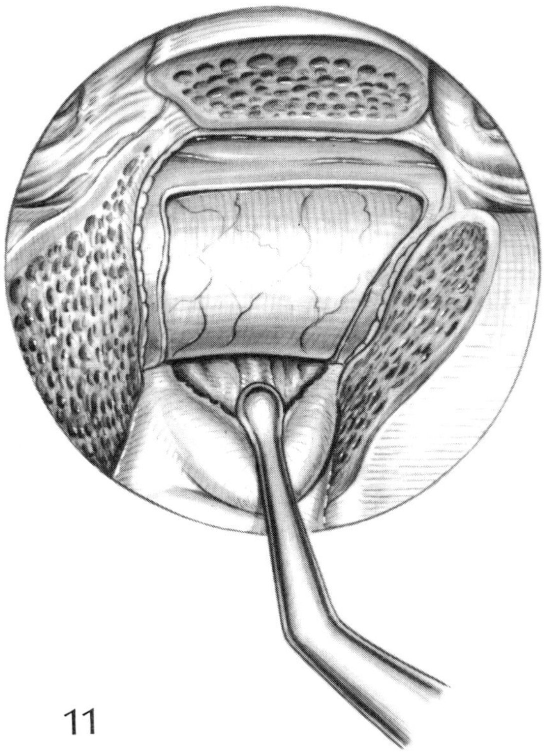

11

# 11 & 12

## Disc removal

Using angled backward-cutting curettes the disc tissue can be pulled away from the anterior surface of the dural tube without any manipulation of the spinal cord. Disc material is curetted away from the spinal cord into the trough created by the removal of bone and disc anteriorly. Posteriorly projecting osteophytes from the opposing posterior surfaces of the vertebral bodies may have to be broken away with the curette or removed with the high-speed drill. Care must be taken to identify those rare situations where disc tissue may have actually penetrated the dura and may be adherent to the overlying spinal cord.

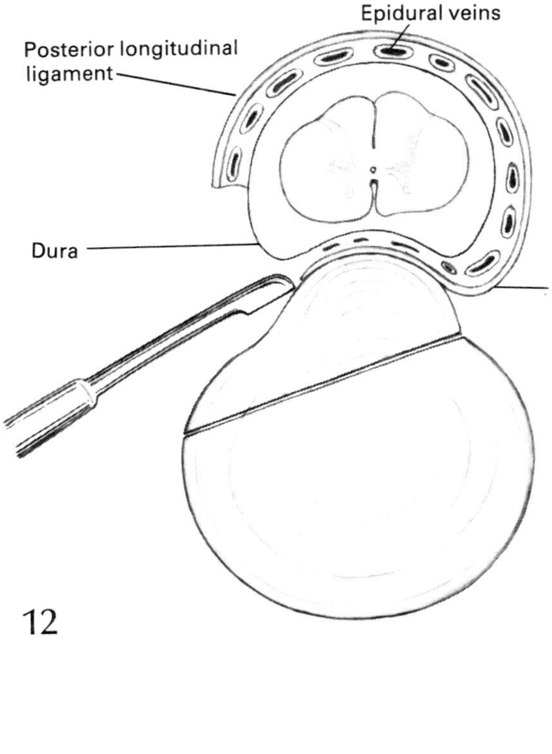


12

## Postoperative care and complications

The thoracotomy wound is closed in the usual fashion, and two large-bore chest tubes are brought out through separate stab wounds. The chest tubes are removed on the second or third postoperative day. The sutures are removed after 7 days and Steri-Strips (3M, UK) applied to the wound. The patient is mobilized as soon as the chest tubes are removed. No internal stabilization or external bracing is required. Extrapleural effusions or haematomas can occur, but these are rare.

### *References*

1. Key, C. A. (1838) On paraplegia depending on disease of the ligaments of the spine. Guy's Hospital Reports, 3, 17–34

2. Middleton, G. S., Teacher, J. H. (1911) Injury of the spinal cord due to rupture of an intervertebral disc during muscular effort. Glasgow Medical Journal, 76, 1–6

3. Hawk, W. A. (1936) Spinal compression caused by ecchondrosis of the intervertebral fibrocartilage: with a review of the recent literature. Brain, 59, 204–224

4. Perot, P. L. Jr., Munro, D. D. (1969) Transthoracic removal of midline thoracic disc protrusions causing spinal cord compression. Journal of Neurosurgery, 31, 452–458

5. Hulme, A. (1960) The surgical approach to thoracic intervertebral disc protrusions. Journal of Neurology, Neurosurgery and Psychiatry, 23, 133–137

6. Carson, J., Gumpert, J., Jefferson, A. (1971) Diagnosis and treatment of thoracic intervertebral disc protrusions. Journal of Neurology, Neurosurgery and Psychiatry, 34, 68–77

7. Patterson, R. H. Jr., Arbit, E. (1978) A surgical approach through the pedicle to protruded thoracic discs. Journal of Neurosurgery, 48, 768–772

8. Perot, P. L. Jr. (1985) Thoracic disc disease. In: Neurosurgery, Vol. 3, Wilkins, R. H., Rengachary, S. S. (eds), pp. 2245–2250. New York: McGraw-Hill

Illustrations by Anne S. Greene

# Surgery of the lumbar spine

**Charles A. Fager** MD
Chairman Emeritus, Department of Neurosurgery, Lahey Clinic Medical Center, Burlington, Massachusetts, USA

The success of any lumbar spinal operation depends on proper selection of patients and on appropriateness of operation for the disc or spondylotic disorder. Although no cure exists for a so-called 'bad back', few operations are more gratifying than removal of an extruded disc. The patient is dramatically relieved of the intense pain and immobility due to nerve root compression, can leave the hospital in 2–3 days, and in most instances may return to work within 3 weeks.

Conversely, nothing is more damaging than spinal operation for back or lower limb pain *without* neural compression because this adds further trauma to the underlying irremediable problem. Patients with recurring acute back syndrome, musculoligamentous pain after operation, and degenerative or arthritic changes without nerve root involvement are advised to pursue a programme of exercises, physiotherapy and analgesics when necessary.

The decision to operate demands a clear history and symptoms, if not signs, of nerve root or cauda equina compression confirmed by lumbar myelography, which is still the definitive diagnostic procedure before surgical intervention. Computerized tomography (CT) may be helpful, especially in patients with far lateral disc rupture, and may even be used as the sole procedure in those with a definite history and certain findings of disc extrusion. However, CT may be misleading and usually does not show the size and location of the lesion as well as myelography. Electromyography, thermography, discography and epidural venography have no additional value in diagnosis.

The surgeon must interpret the myelographic or CT findings in the light of the patient's symptoms and should never rely on a radiological report of a bulging disc (often at two levels), as this is common in patients with and without back pain and is not in itself an indication for operation, especially in those who have had an industrial or vehicular accident. There is also no indication for removing more than one disc because intervertebral discs seldom, if ever, actually rupture and produce neural compression at more than one level simultaneously.

Search for improved methods of treatment thus far has yielded nothing better than the natural progression of disc disease and spondylosis. The so-called failed back syndrome results from either operating on the wrong patient or performing the wrong operation. Similarly, alternative methods such as chemonucleolysis, microdiscectomy and percutaneous discectomy are almost certain to produce the same iatrogenic disasters.

# LUMBAR DISC RUPTURE

Most patients with disc protrusion and some with frank rupture recover spontaneously. The sciatic pain gradually decreases over a period varying from 1 to 4 months; minor weakness and sensory symptoms clear completely. The patient requiring operation tends to have persistent sciatic or femoral pain, usually attended by clear neurological signs of nerve root compression. Severe neurological deficit due to a massive extruded disc may require early or urgent operative intervention, especially if the patient has acute midline rupture with cauda equina compression.

When operation is necessary, the surgeon invariably finds a fragment of disc that has either extruded completely from its space or has erupted through the annulus fibrosus and is incarcerated beneath the distended, thinned or partially torn posterior longitudinal ligament. In the latter instance, a large fragment has been thrust mushroom-like through a small opening and may be constricted by annulus and ligament at its neck, sequestered beneath nerve root and dura mater.

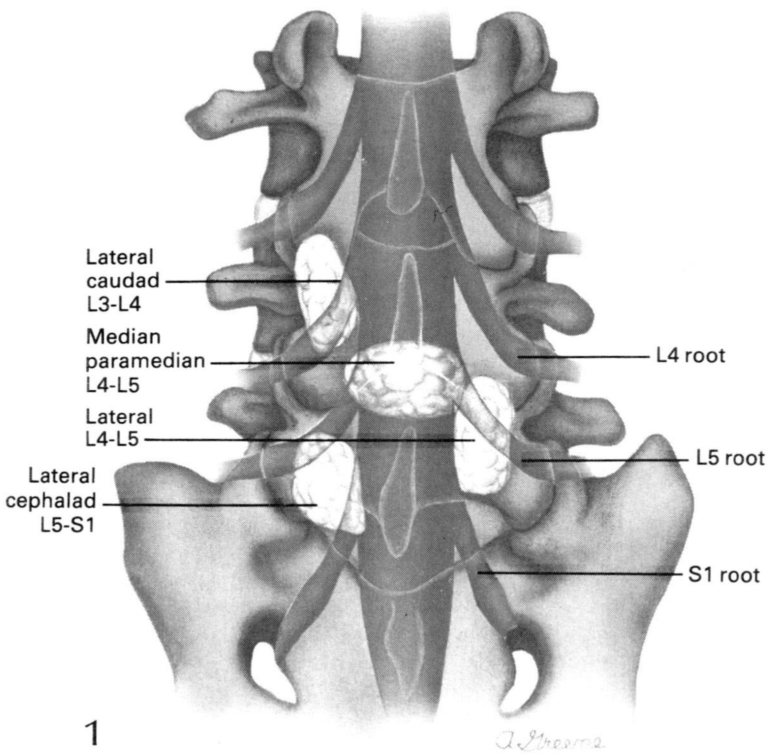


1

## 1 & 2

The common path for extrusion of ruptured lumbar disc fragments is posterolateral so that they present immediately anterior or anterior and lateral to the nerve root coursing over the disc space.

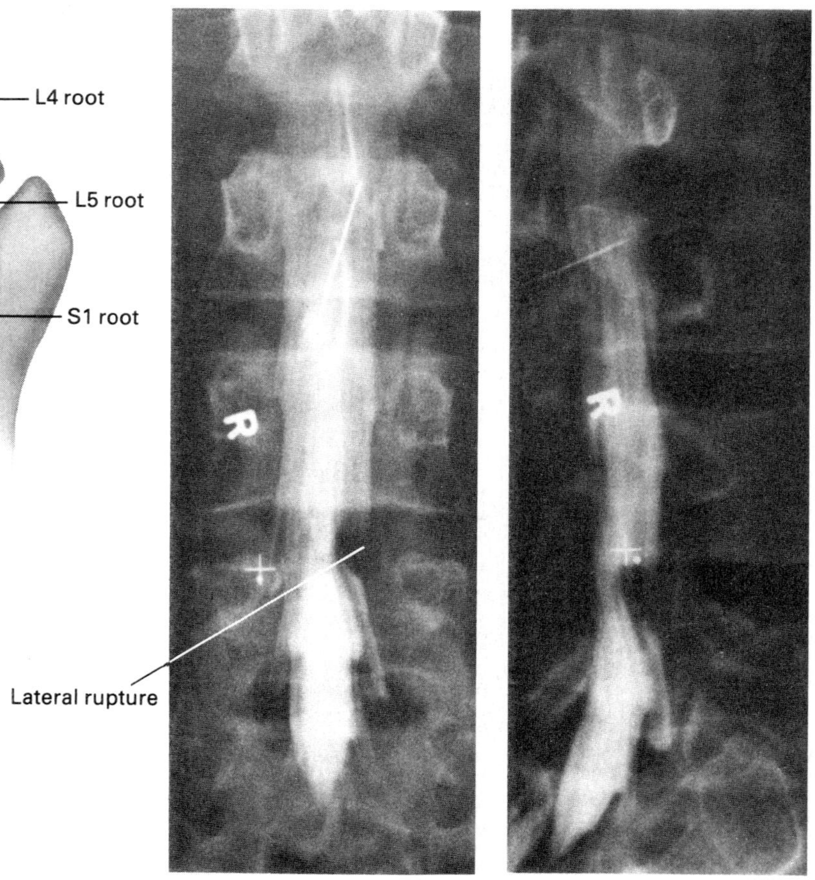


2

## 3

Larger fragments extruding more laterally and superiorly may also compress the root above at its foramen. This escape route probably develops most often because of the midline tenacity and thickness of the posterior longitudinal ligament. Nevertheless, attenuation of this ligament occurs, permitting fragments to extrude and occupy a median or paramedian position, or to extend above or below the disc space once in the open spinal canal. Such median or paramedian ruptures commonly produce complete or partial myelographic block and occur in about 15 per cent of patients with ruptured lumbar disc.

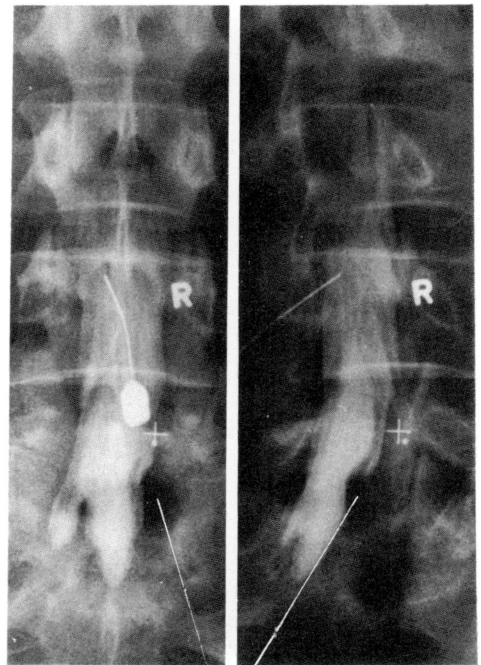


3

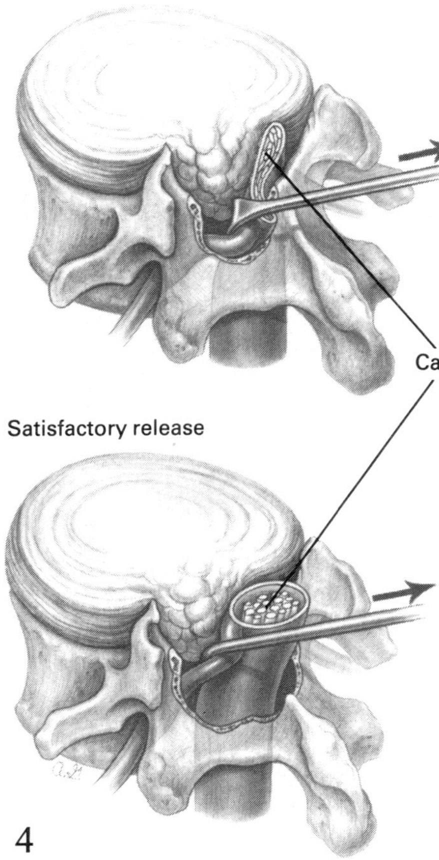


4

## 4

A fundamental surgical doctrine is that a routine operation for ruptured lumbar disc does not exist. Although the procedure for common lateral disc rupture may be standard, it must often be modified to the size and location of the lesion. Perhaps the commonest surgical error is the habitual use of a small bony opening or laminotomy, a term lacking definition, regardless of the pathological condition (*top*). The abiding principle in lumbar and all other spinal operations remains adequate bony removal above, below and lateral to the lesion to allow a posterolateral approach with minimal traction or surgical compression of neural elements (*bottom*).

Unfortunately, spondylotic constriction or so-called annular or waist-like myelographic deformity has often been misinterpreted as midline disc protrusion and has led to disc removal through bilateral limited exposures. This kind of operation, rather than relieving nerve root or cauda equina compression, intensifies constriction because of contusion, early root oedema in a confined canal followed later by epidural fibrosis, and cohesion of nerve roots often referred to as adhesive arachnoiditis.

## The operation

### 5

Special equipment and positions are not necessary as long as the patient's abdomen is free, with padded lifts beneath the chest and each iliac crest. Flexion of the operating table reduces or eliminates lumbar lordosis. With the myelogram or CT film in the operating room the surgeon can visualize the size and location of the ruptured disc fragment. The patient's lumbar spine radiographs should also be available not only for localization of associated pathological conditions but to clarify the appropriate level in patients with transitional vertebrae.

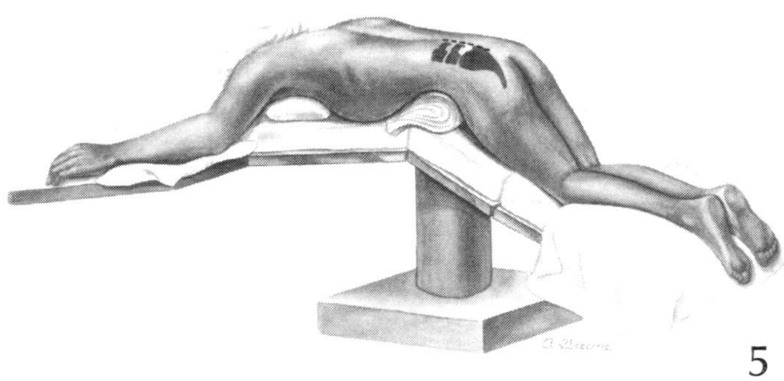

5

### 6

Incision of the deep paravertebral fascia just lateral to the spinous processes and retraction medially over the spine permits dissection of paravertebral muscles, beginning precisely at the midline. By use of fine cutting electrocautery and sharp dissection, the muscles are separated cleanly from laminal margins and laminae. Paralytic agents such as suxamethonium (succinylcholine) are given by the anaesthetist to allow easy retraction of the muscle mass.

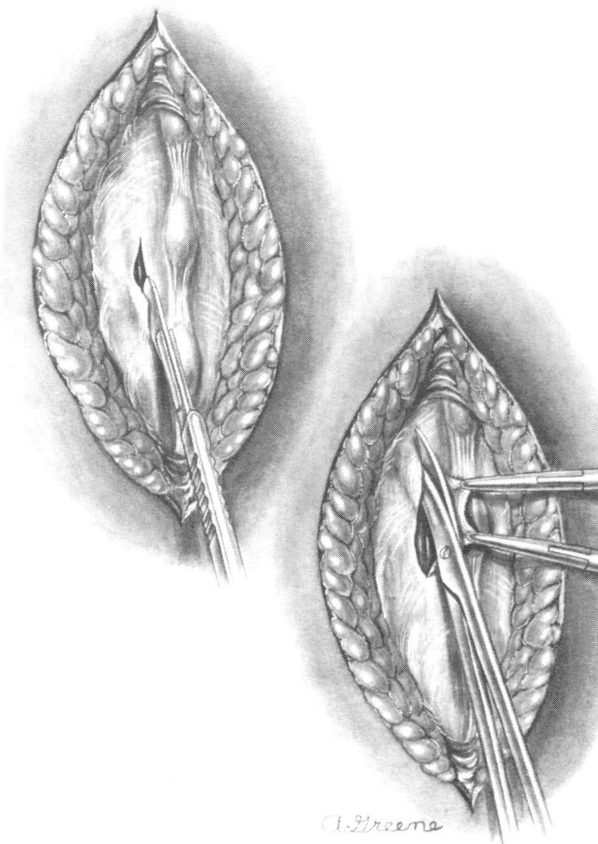

6

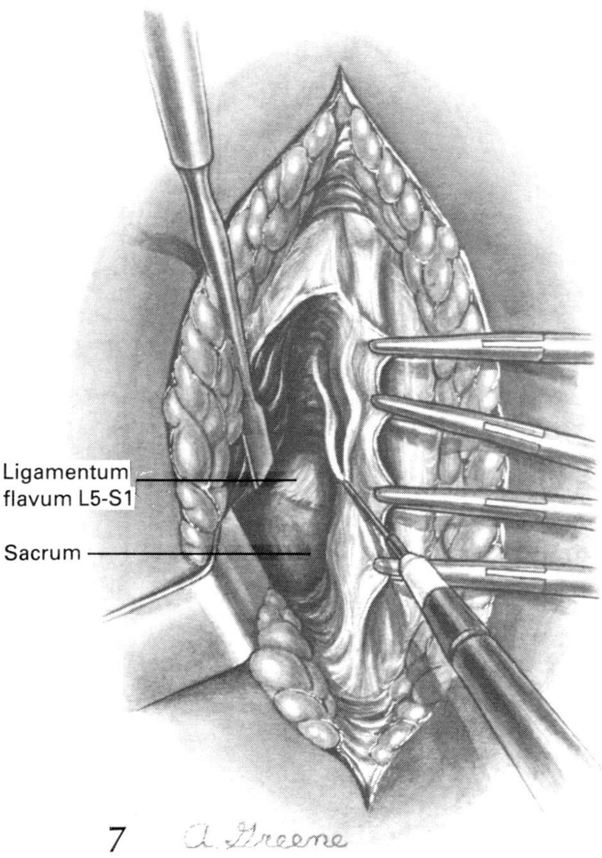


7

### 7

A skin and fascial incision long enough to provide longitudinal release and atraumatic retraction without contusion or bleeding within muscle is essential. This is the most important factor in preventing postoperative muscle spasm and allowing ambulation on the same day. Satisfactory longitudinal release is also mandatory because muscle must be retracted to the lateral margin of the facet for adequate posterolateral exposure.

# 8

The common lateral disc rupture at L5–S1 requires exposure of the upper sacrum and all of the L5 hemilamina. The ligamentum flavum should be exposed above the L5 lamina and at L5–S1. The lower margin of the lamina of L4 is visualized in heavy or muscular patients. Fat is extracted to give a clear view of bony margins.

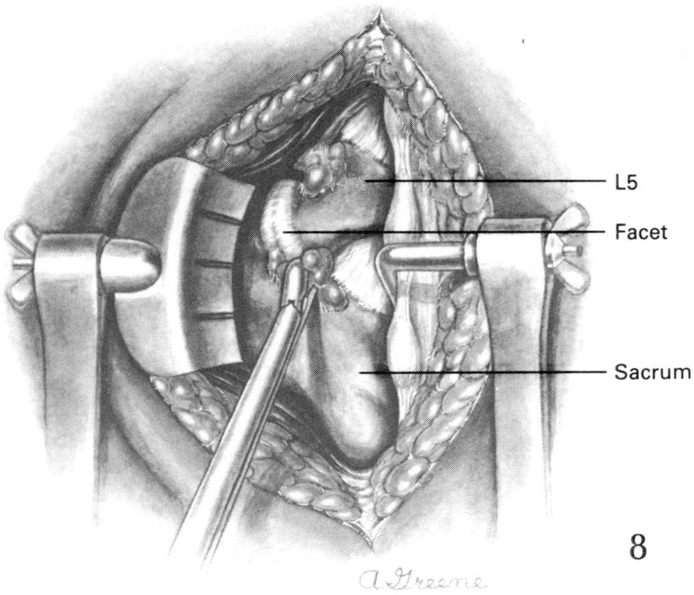


8

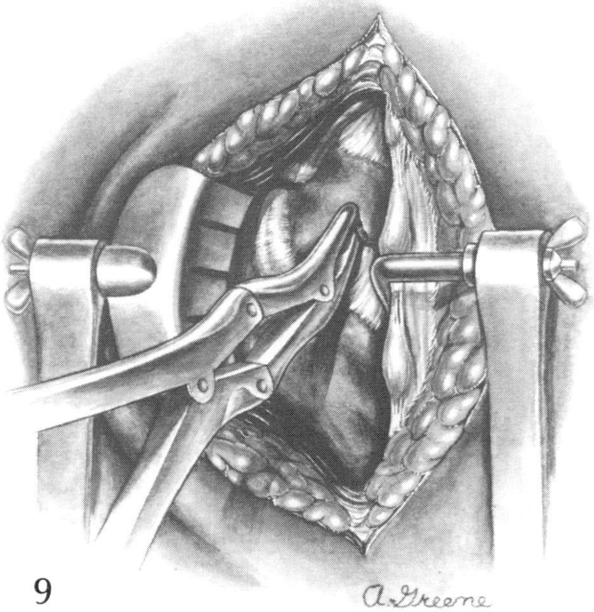


9

# 9

The hemilamina of L5 is removed with Leksell rongeurs above the superior margin of the ligamentum flavum to expose the dura mater and overlying epidural veins. This usually, although not always, ensures epidural exposure cephalad to the disc space.

# 10

Once the ligamentum flavum has been excised away from its attachment to the sacrum, and as far laterally as possible, bone excision for full exposure of nerve root and lesion can be completed.

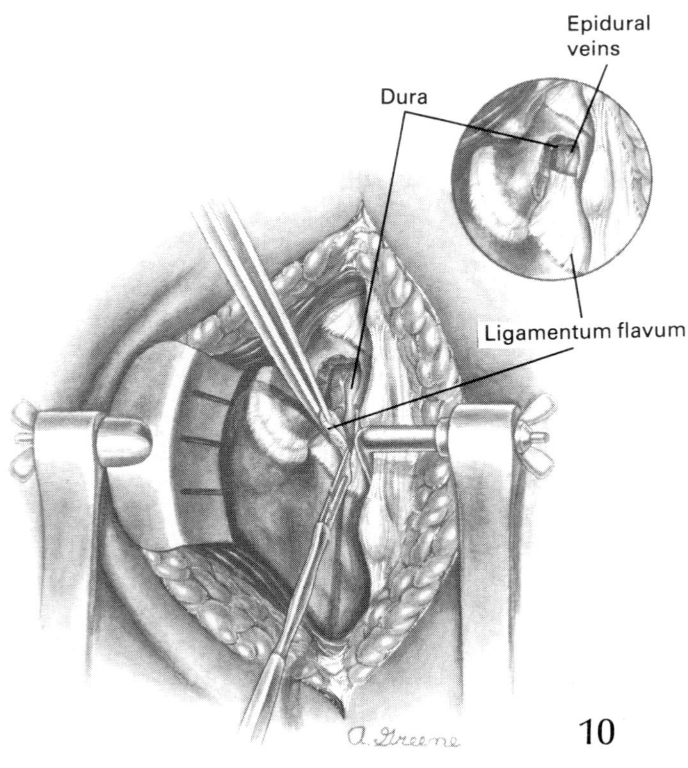


10

# 11

This is best accomplished with angled thin-plated Kerison rongeurs, starting from above. It is important to excise bone with any residual lateral ligamentum beyond the lateral margin of dura mater. A lateral ruptured fragment usually compresses the nerve root tightly against the sacral rim so that the upper sacrum and medial margins of the facet are excised by first working alternately medially and laterally to the nerve root rather than directly over the root itself.

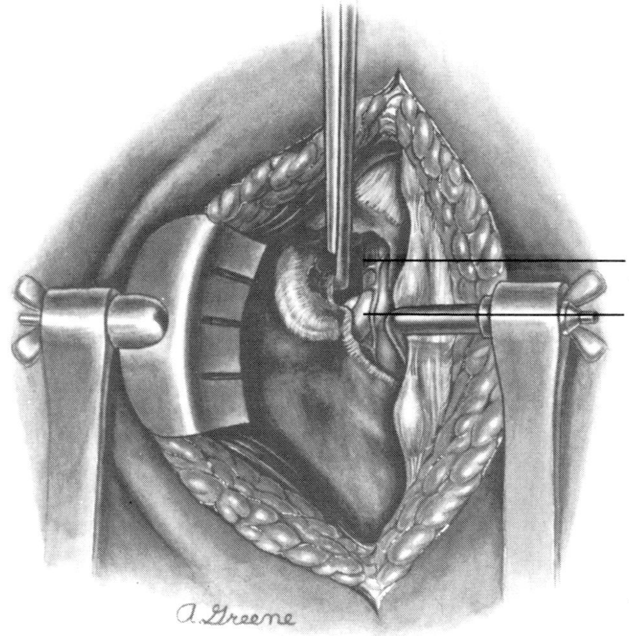


11

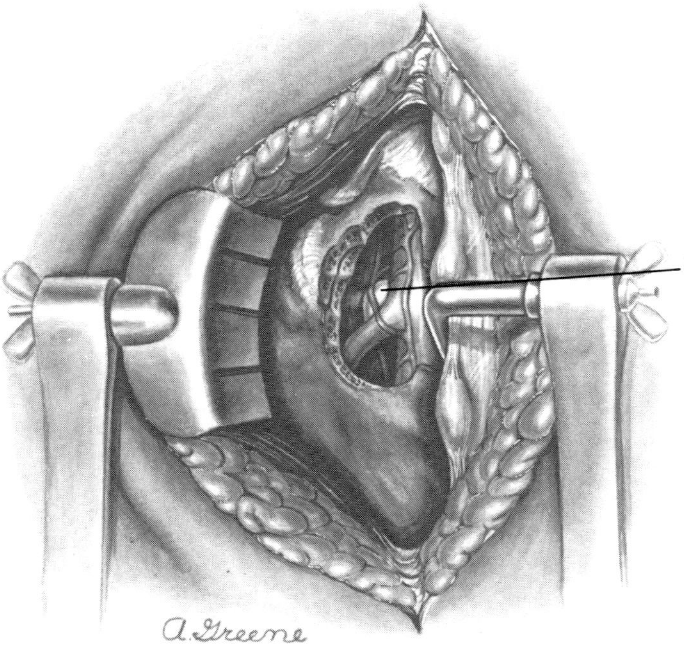


12

# 12

Bone is removed caudad to the disc space, usually to the foraminal level, to provide mobility for the nerve root so that its directly overlying bone can be excised without compression. The ruptured fragment of disc then comes into view. Overlying stretched epidural veins are coagulated and divided well away from the nerve root or, after slight retraction of the nerve root as the fragment is dissected free, liberated from the surrounding ligamentum and annulus and excised.

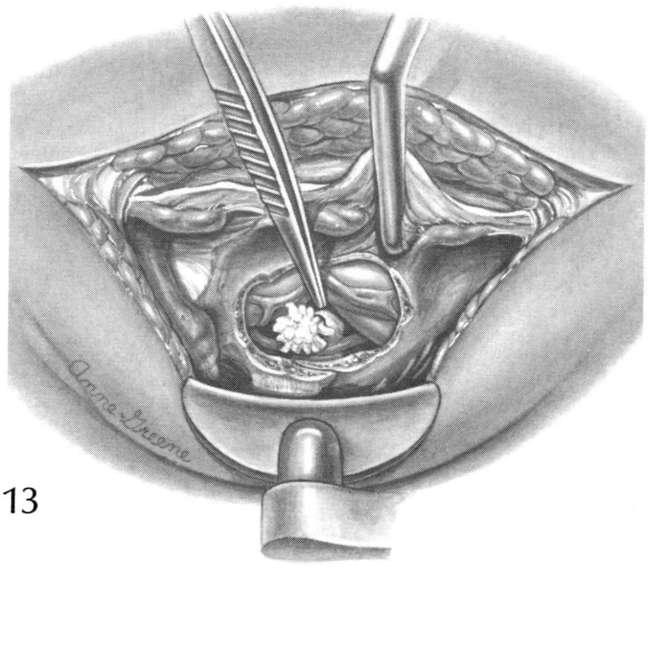

13

# 13

The posterolateral approach requires little retraction of the nerve root or lateral cauda equina. A small blunt nerve hook may occasionally be necessary during the dissection, but nerve root retractors, especially those held by an assistant, are inadvisable. Nothing more than a forceps displaces and protects the nerve root and lateral dura mater. Small cottonoid pledgets may be placed, not packed, into the lateral epidural recess above and below the disc space because additional epidural bleeding may be encountered as the nerve root is visualized. (*Illustration 13* shows the surgeon's view.)

# 14

Frequently, a tight constriction at the neck of the disc fragment requires piecemeal removal, and the small opening in the annulus and ligament must then be extended medially and laterally or in cruciate or circular fashion. This is not necessary when the disc has been expelled through a large tear.

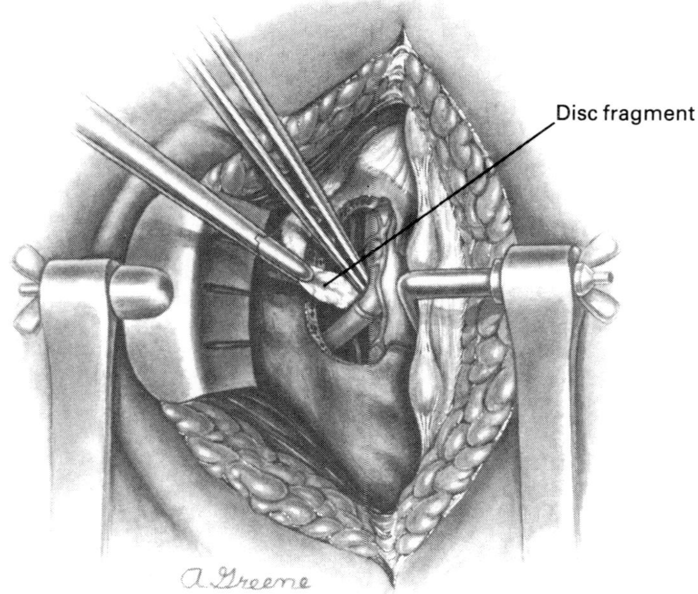


14

# 15

The disc space is entered and cleared of remaining degenerated material with straight and angled pituitary rongeurs. Adherent portions of degenerated disc may be loosened with a curette if necessary, but there is no evidence that curettage of cartilaginous plates provides any additional benefit or reduces the rate of recurrence, which is about 7–10 per cent. The only certain method of preventing injury to iliac vessels or the ureter is to maintain direct vision of the tip of the rongeur at all times. Because this is not always possible, the surgeon must estimate its position and project its location, being constantly mindful of the depth of the disc space, and avoid penetration of the anterior ligament. The same approach is used for lateral disc rupture at L4–L5 and L3–L4, including exposure of the upper sacrum.

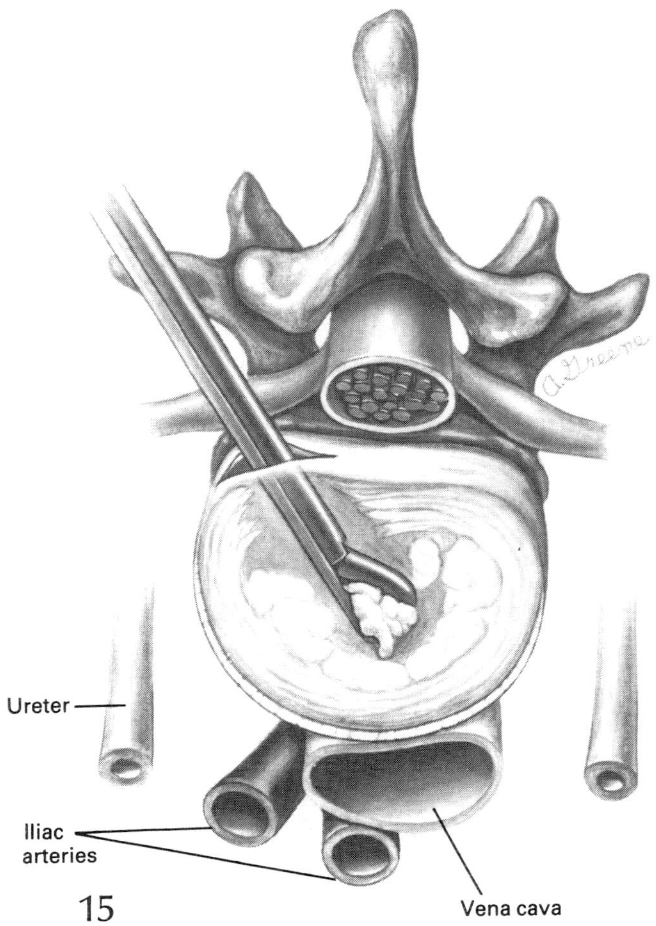


15

## Medial rupture

# 16, 17 & 18

The approach to fragments of disc that have ruptured medial to the nerve root demands more extensive hemilaminectomy, and sometimes even complete hemilaminectomy above and below the disc space or extension of the laminectomy across the midline, depending mainly on the size of the fragment. Lateral excision of bone is equally important and allows a lateral passage to the lesion. No harm is caused by excision of additional bone, but removal of a large fragment through limited exposure may cause considerable neurological damage or a dural tear, and bleeding from epidural veins is difficult to control. Postoperative relief of radicular pain is most complete when adequate decompression has been provided.

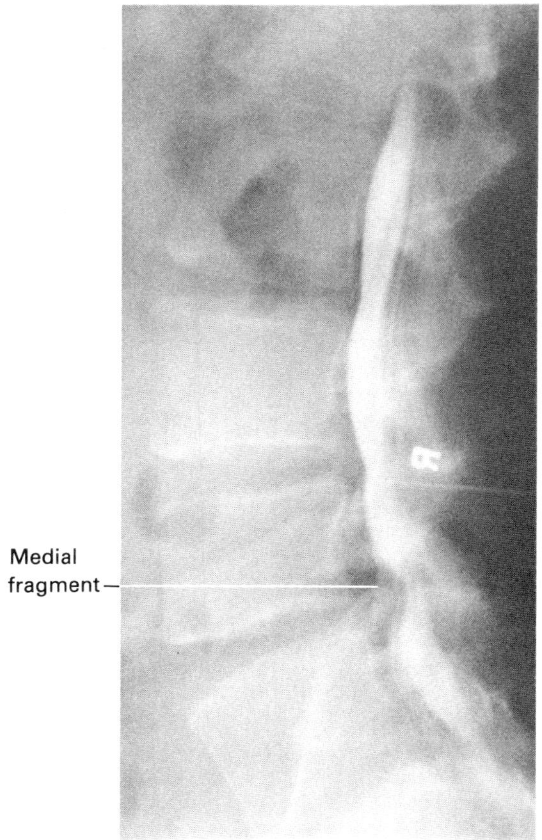


16

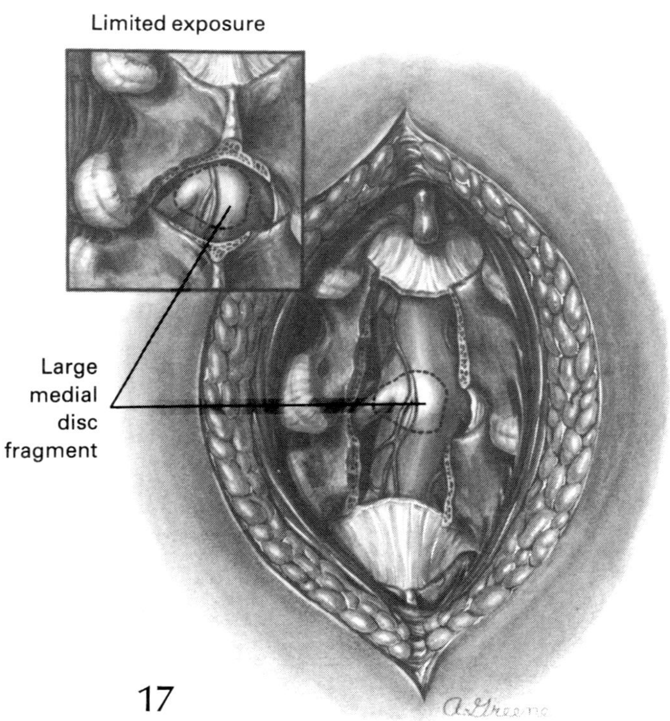


17

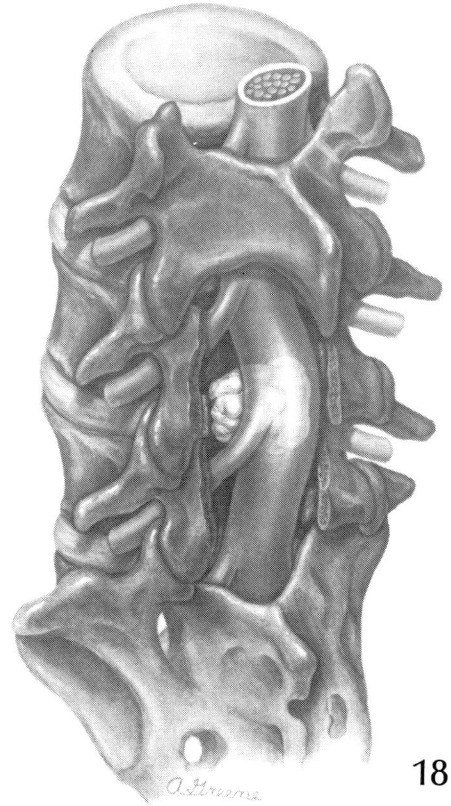

18

# 19, 20 & 21

A medial rent in the annulus is likely to be particularly small at the fragment's neck so that even with adequate release of overlying neural structures it may not come away easily. Rather than attempt to retract the nerve root over its apex, it is sometimes expedient to incise the posterior longitudinal ligament and annulus laterally from the lateral margin of the aperture, and draw the fragment first anteriorly into the disc space and then laterally as its peak is dissected away from the anterior dura mater.

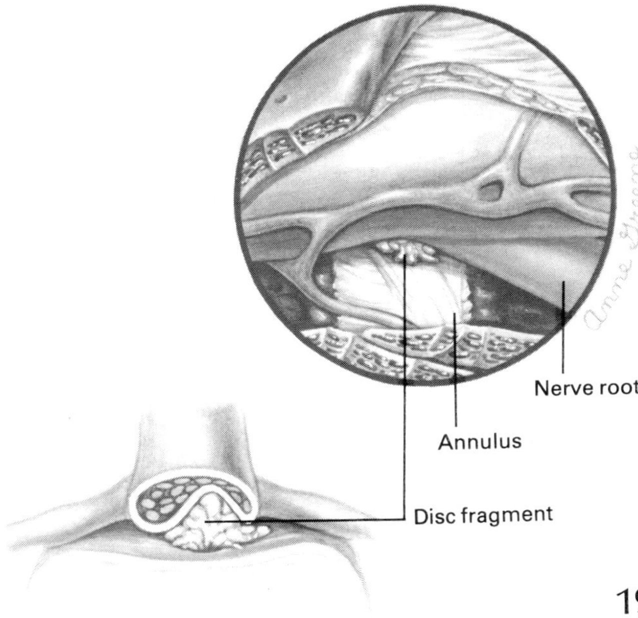


19

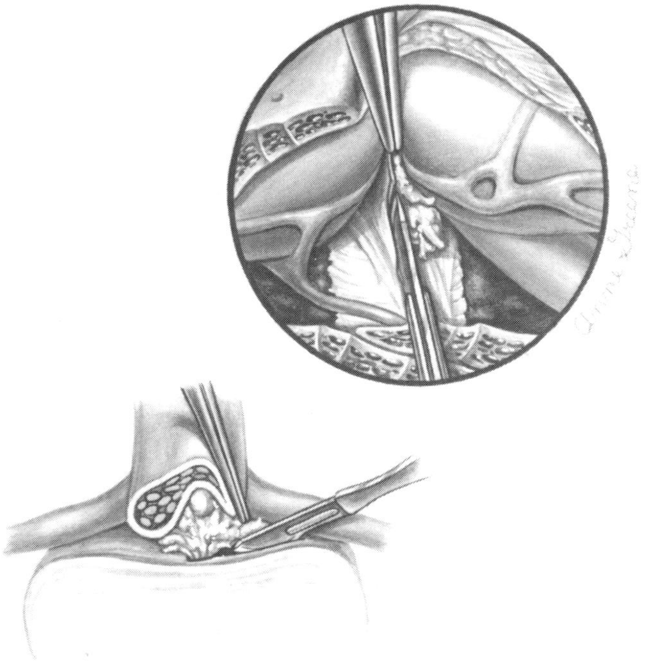

20

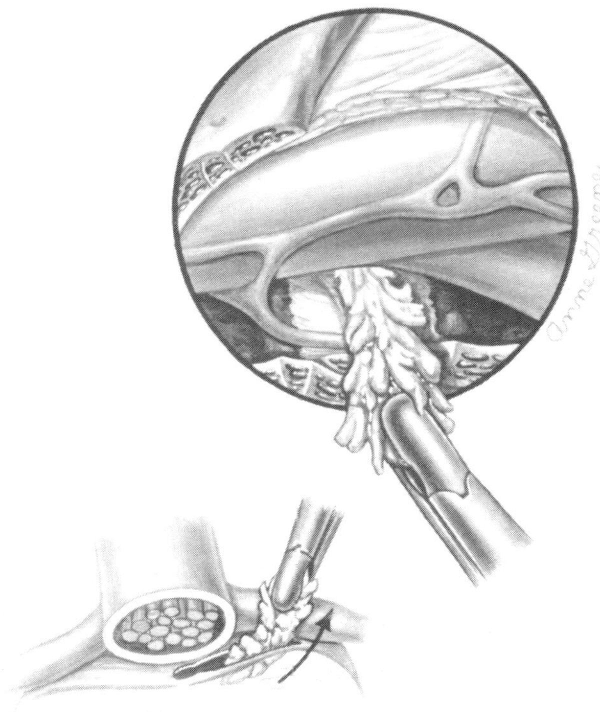

21

## Cephalad and caudad rupture

# 22–26

Access to fragments that extend above or below the disc space and may compress two nerve roots requires extensive bony removal and often wide foraminal exposure rather than limited exposure because their migration is most frequently lateral. Disc fragments that have erupted from either L4–L5 or L5–S1 may straddle the L5 nerve root and commonly erode the posterior L5 body, leaving a saucer-like excavation after removal. It is not unusual to have signs of L5 and S1 root compression and to see both roots affected during operation.

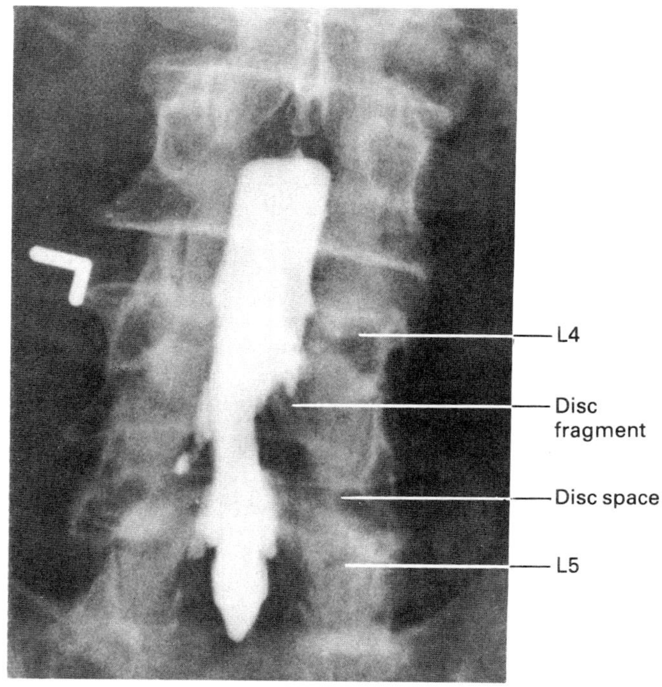


22

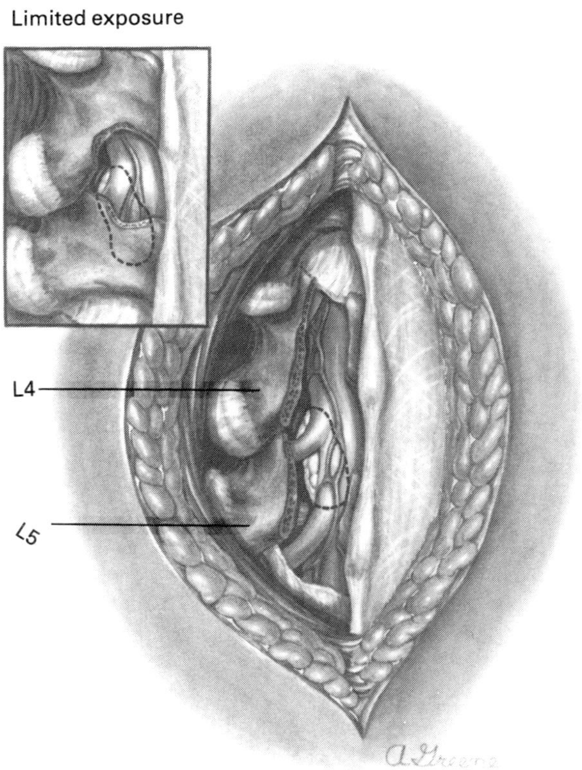
Limited exposure
L4
L5

23

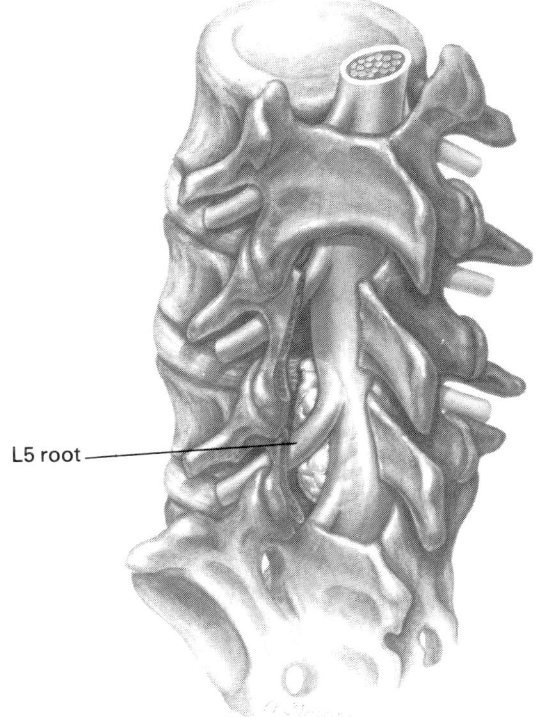
L5 root

24

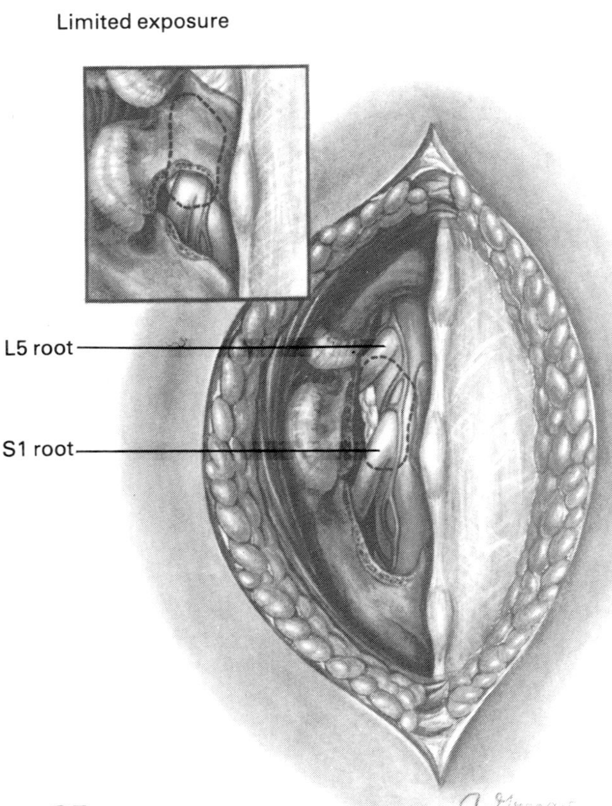
Limited exposure
L5 root
S1 root

25

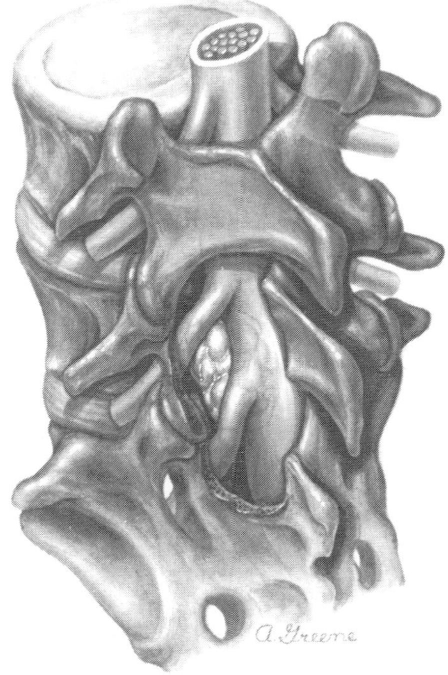

26

# 27

Medial fragments of disc lying within the sacral canal must be dissected away cautiously from the sacral nerve roots with which they become interlaced.

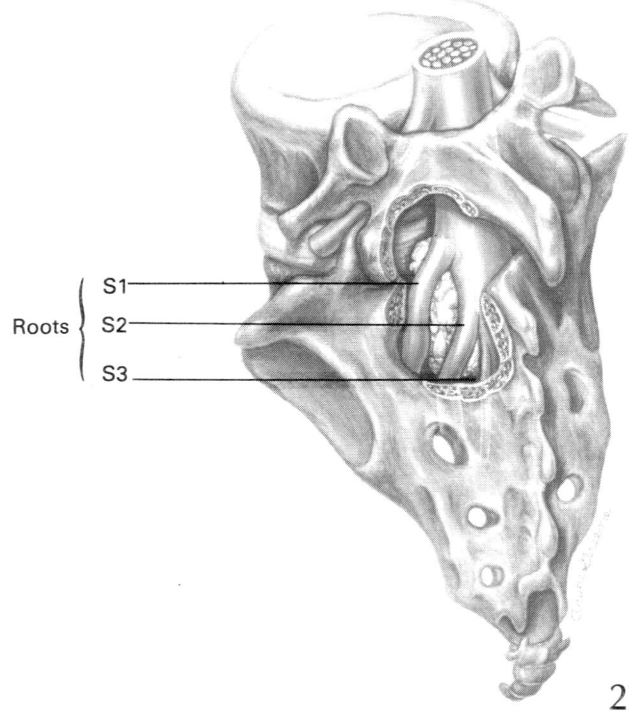


27

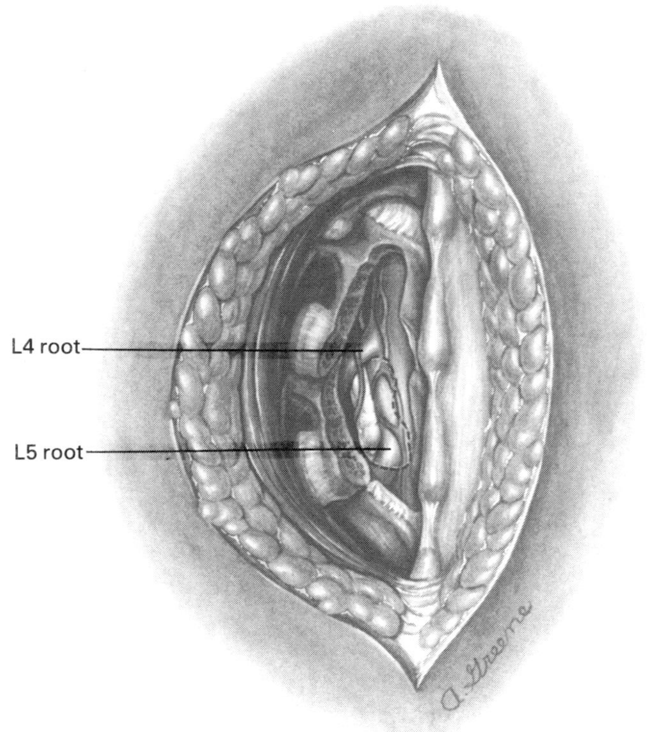


28

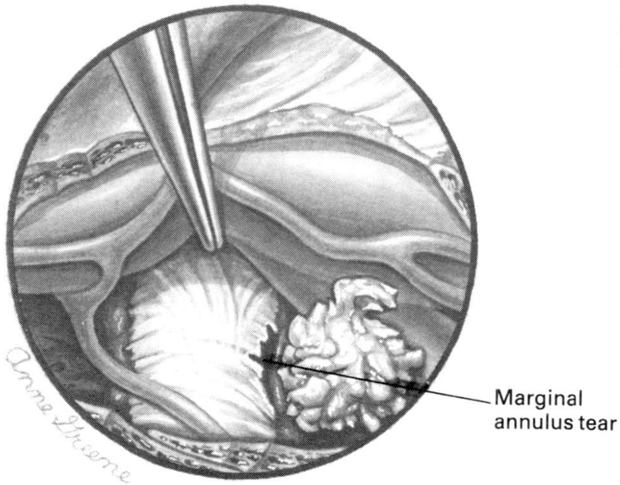


29

# 28 & 29

A disc ruptured at the L3–L4 level may likewise erupt laterally and downward and impinge on L4 and L5 nerve roots. When such caudad or cephalad migration occurs, the annulus tear is often found at its upper or lower margin.

These possibilities can be predicted from neurological evaluation and myelography and must be anticipated and dealt with operatively according to the axiom that excision of laminal and facet elements proceeds from areas where most space is available towards the crown of the ruptured fragment. Complete lateral hemilaminectomy of two segments may be necessary.

## Median and paramedian rupture

# 30, 31 & 32

Median and paramedian disc rupture produces partial or complete myelographic block in more than 70 per cent of patients with this type of lesion, yet most of these present either with unilateral pain and neurological deficit or a preponderance of symptoms on one side. This is important in determining the appropriate surgical approach.

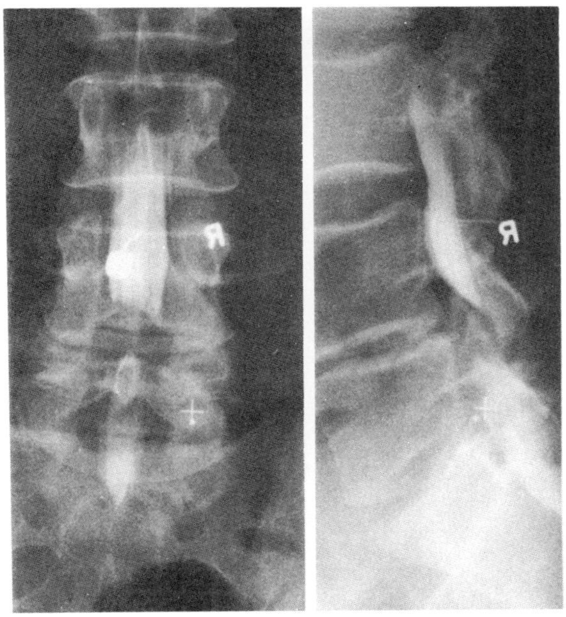

30

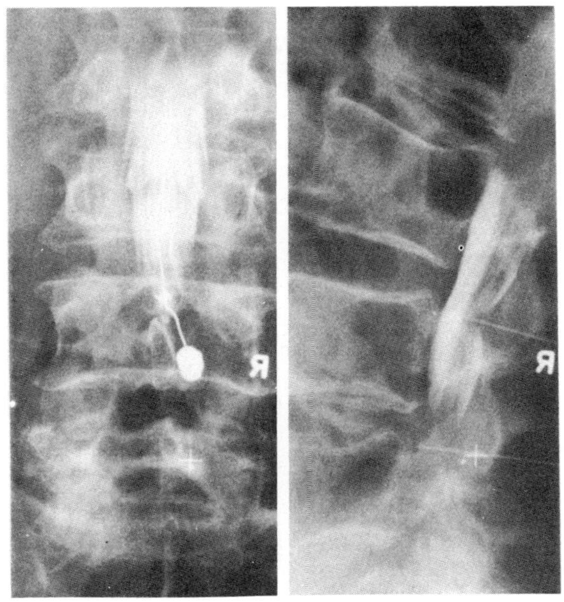

31

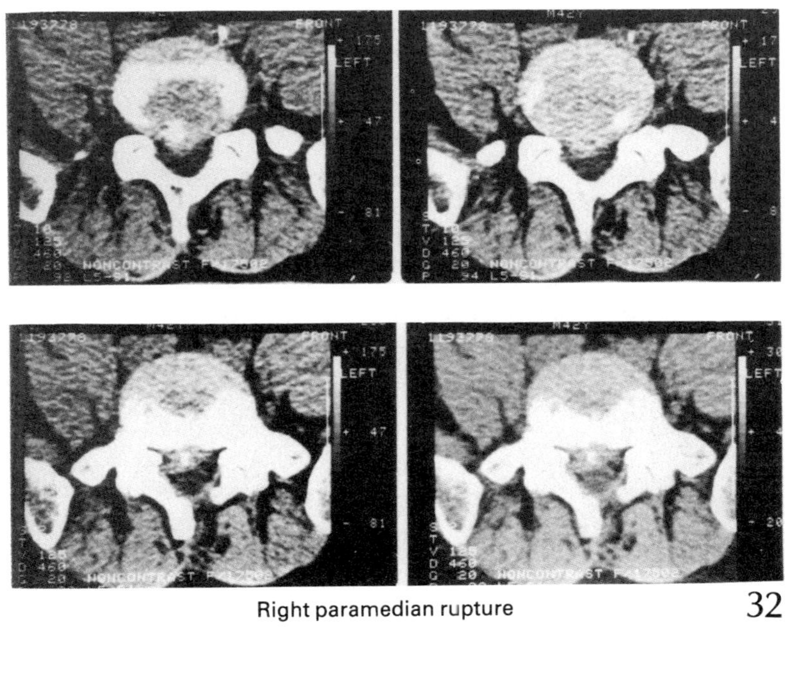


Right paramedian rupture

32

## 33

If a large fragment of disc has extruded into the midline, usually more to one side, retraction of the nerve root or cauda equina over its crest is impossible without adequate removal of bone. Therefore, no satisfactory alternative to complete laminectomy exists. As in operations for obstructive intraspinal tumours, laminectomy begins where space is abundant, for example in patients with L4–L5 block, at the lower margin of L5, and must include the full caudocephalad length of L5 and L4 laminae.

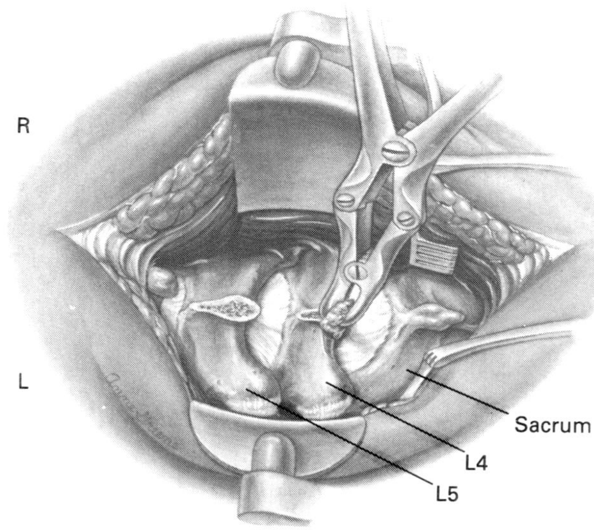


Unilateral facet exposure

33

## 34

The ligamentum flavum is excised, beginning in the midline and as far laterally as possible.

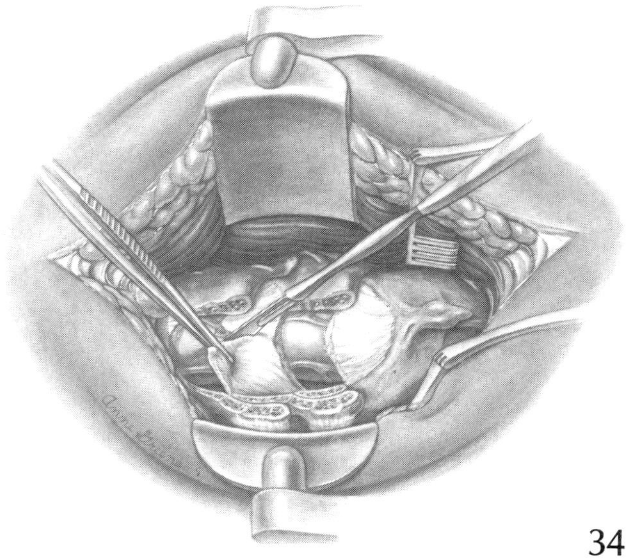

34

## 35

Bone is then removed beyond the lateral margin of dura mater on one side (that of greater pain or deficit), starting above the level of the ligamentum flavum and continuing this lateral excision with removal of medial facet elements to the segment below.

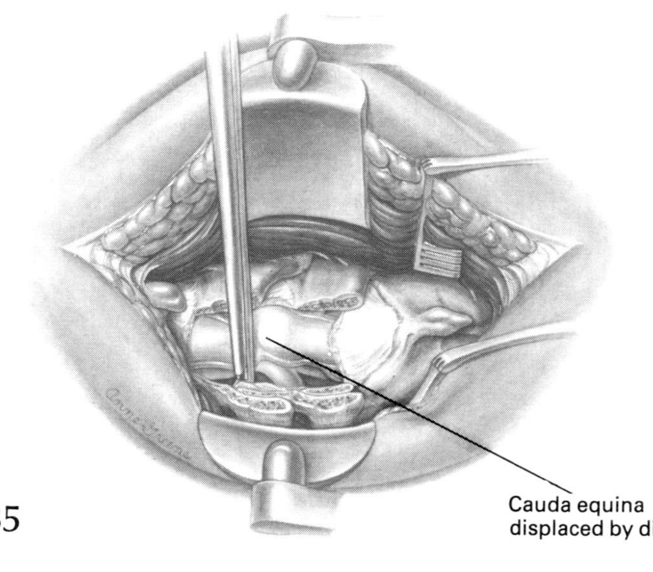


35

# 36

Posterolateral exposure allows access from one side initially and requires minimal retraction of dura mater and cauda equina over the ruptured fragment of disc.

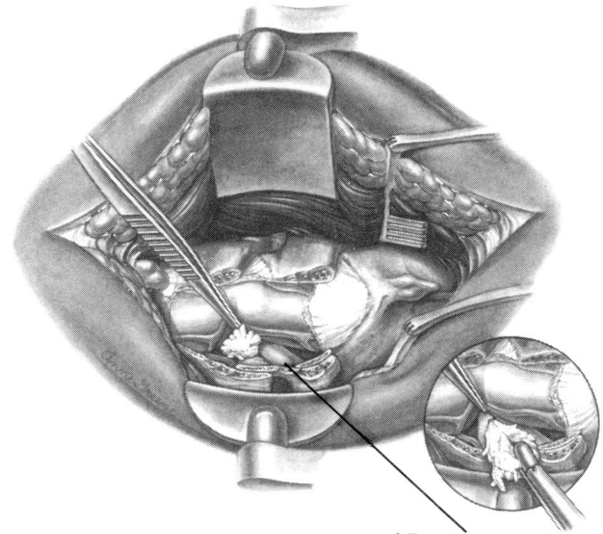


36

# 37

Once the extruded or incarcerated portion of disc has been removed, adequate space is available for epidural exposure of the anterior canal well across the midline, and for additional bony removal and secondary approach from the opposite side should any doubt exist about retained fragments on that side. Bilateral exposure of this type, however, is seldom necessary. The medial tear in the annulus and posterior longitudinal ligament, which is often quite small in relation to the ruptured disc material, is easily extended laterally so that the disc space can be cleared of residual degenerative material.

At the lumbosacral level, after laminectomy of L5 and excision of the ligamentum flavum, the upper sacrum is carefully excised from laterally to medially, in contradistinction to the medial-to-lateral removal of bone for a lateral disc extrusion beneath the S1 nerve root. Leaving the facets intact on one side permits the same early mobilization as in patients with a simple lateral ruptured disc.

Opening the dura mater is not necessary because exposed root and the dura mater with its enclosed cauda equina are adequately released by the extent of the laminectomy. The only indication for opening the dura mater during excision of a lumbar disc is the presence of a conjoined root sleeve that prohibits nerve root mobilization.

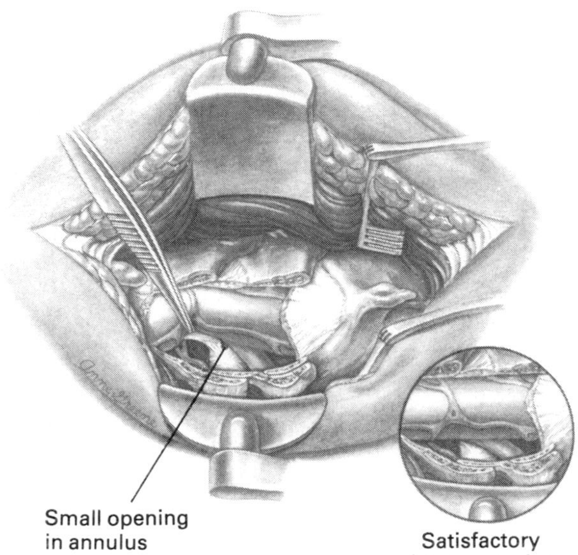


37

# RUPTURED DISC WITH LUMBAR SPONDYLOSIS

## 38 & 39

In patients with severe lumbar spondylosis, who may also have extensive degenerative disc disease and spondyloarthrosis, a sciatic syndrome develops in which nerve root compression may be caused by disc rupture or chronic disc protrusion at one level, associated with extensive hypertrophic changes evident radiographically.

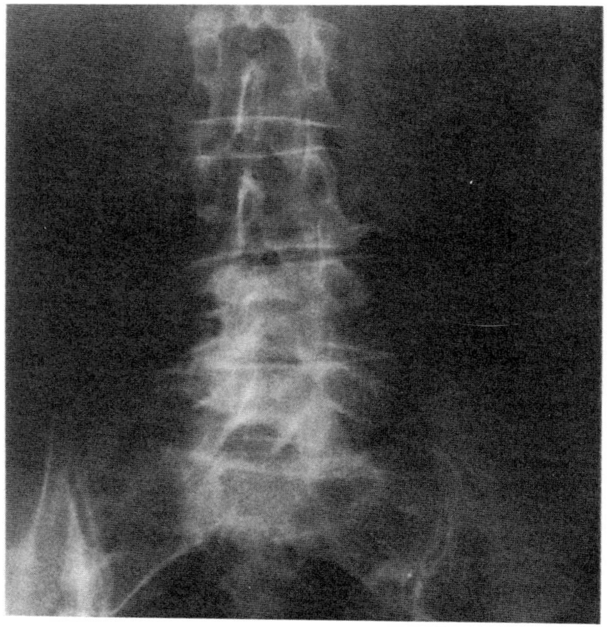

38

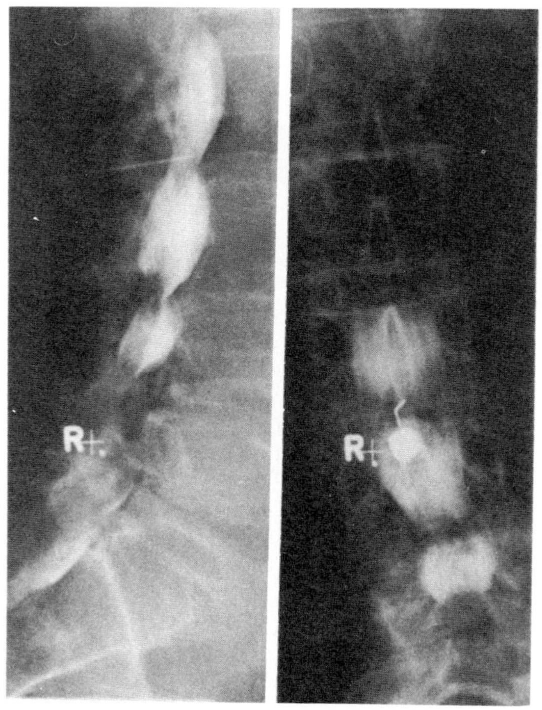

39

## The operation

# 40, 41 & 42

This creates a problem in diagnosis requiring reliance on acuteness of onset, distribution of pain, and signs of specific nerve root compression. CT may be helpful in determining the exact nature of radicular pain because it can demonstrate a soft or semi-soft erupted fragment in association with osseous occlusions of foramina or spinal canal. However, in the presence of multiple areas of obstruction caused by spondylosis, the choice of surgical approach becomes critical. Judicious extensive laminectomy releases the cauda equina, provides adequate decompression and avoids postoperative complications from worsening spinal stenosis, which is intensified by the postoperative oedema associated with limited operation.

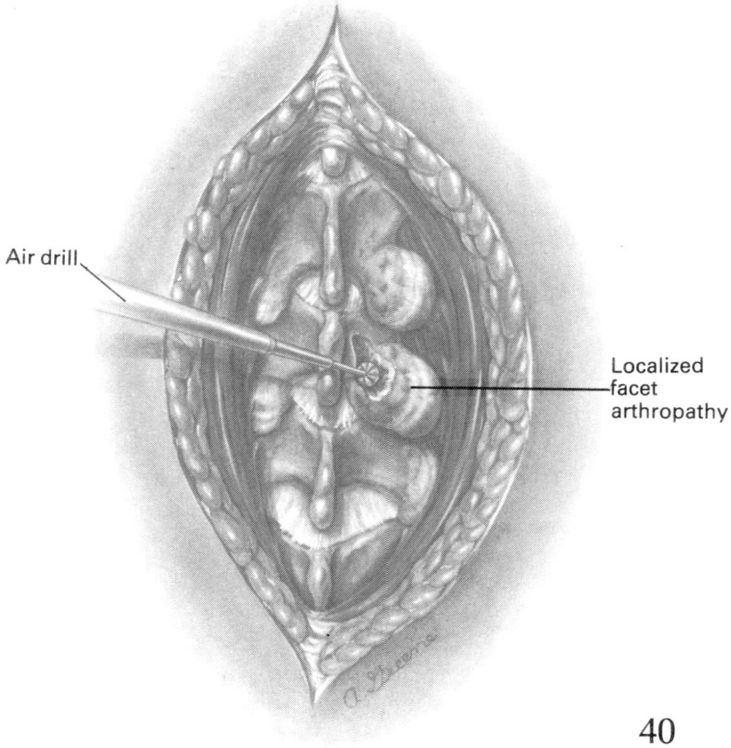


40

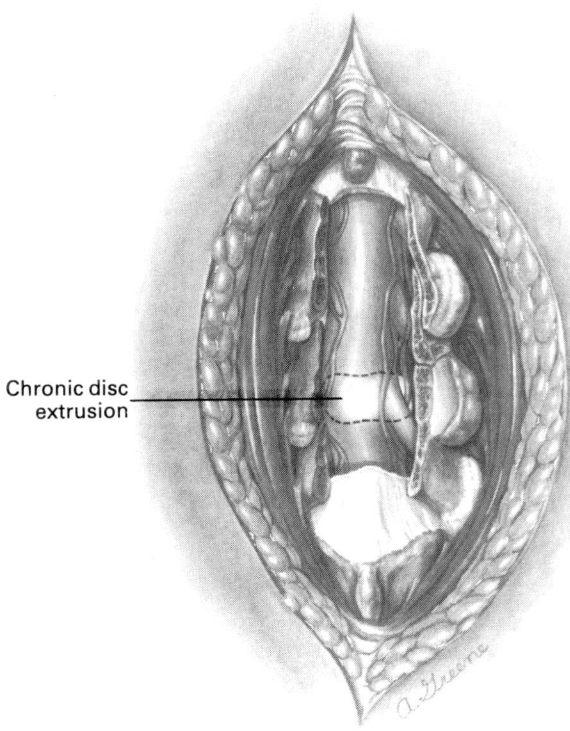


41

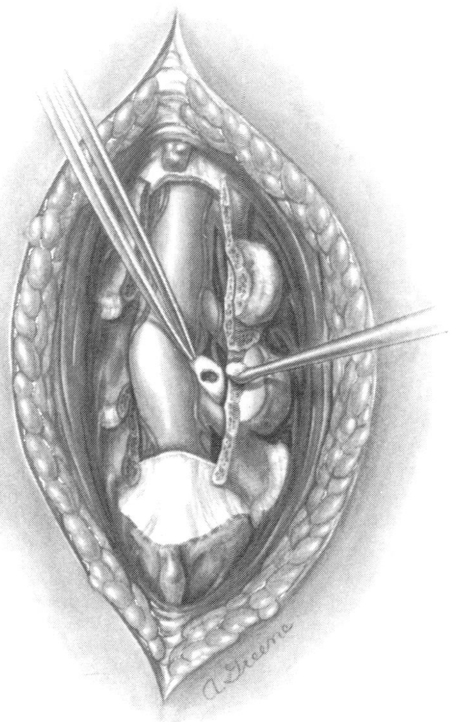

42

# LUMBAR SPONDYLOSIS

## 43 & 44

The conspicuous element of cauda equina compression in patients with severe lumbar spondylosis is encroachment on the spinal canal from posterolateral expansion of facets and compression from ventral ridges.

This may occur at only one level, especially in elderly women who have secondary spondylolisthesis related to severe facet arthropathy without congenital abnormality.

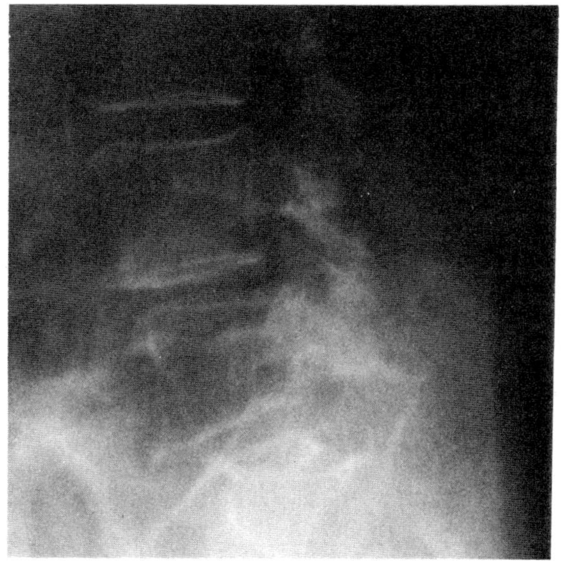

43

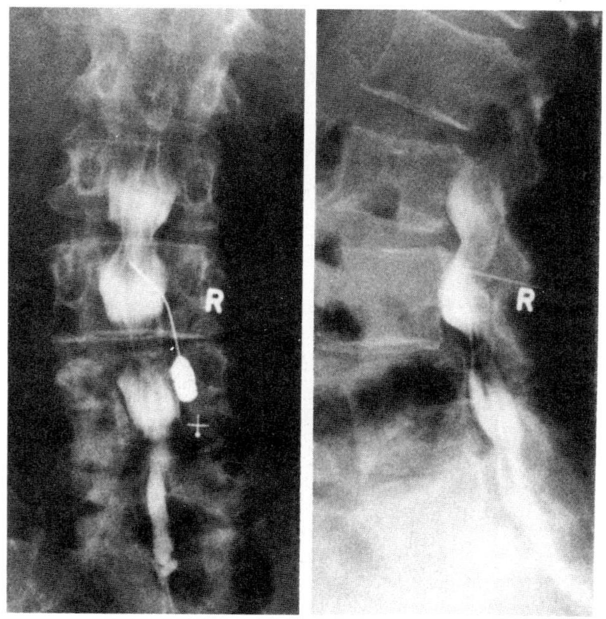


44

# 45, 46 & 47

However, it commonly involves multiple segments throughout the lower lumbar spine, at times extending upward to include even L1 and L2 segments. A typical syndrome is that of neurogenic claudication and radicular pain, often with paraesthesia extending to one or both lower limbs. Relief is obtained by bending forward, sitting, or lying at rest. Despite the symptoms of cauda equina compression these patients show surprisingly little neurological deficit except at an advanced stage after many years of neural compression. Usually no neurological signs are found (other than absence of Achilles tendon reflexes) despite the severe radicular pain extending to both lower legs.

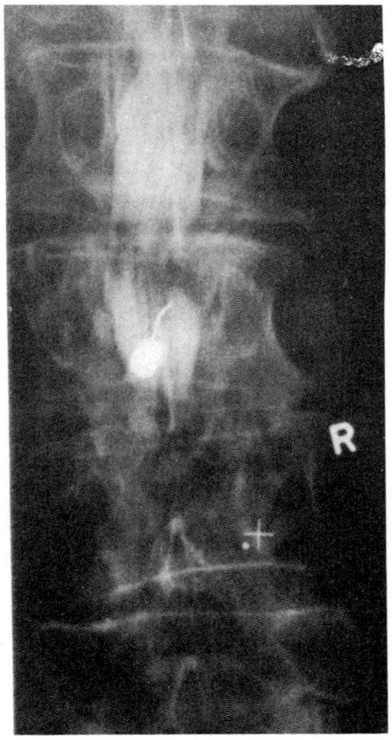

45

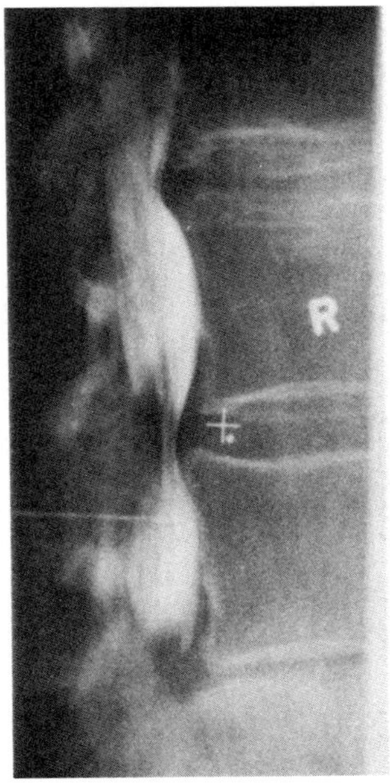

46

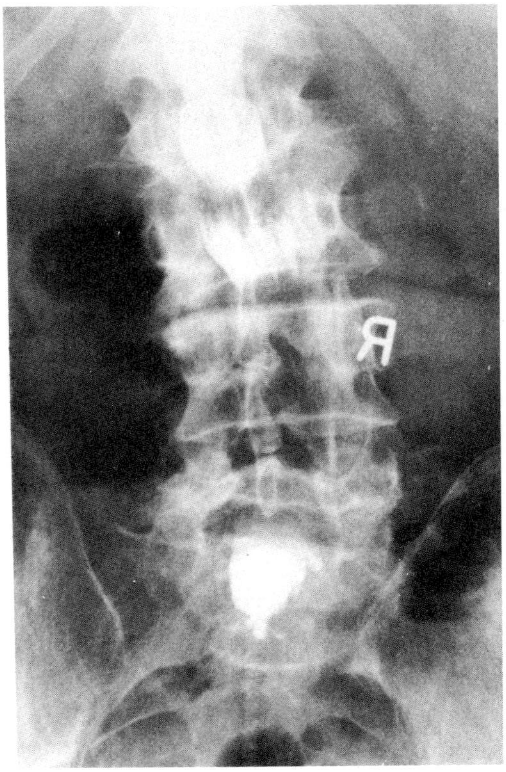

47

# The operation

## 48

Surgical technique is difficult and tedious and requires painstaking attention to detail. From the beginning, the operation is fraught with problems, not least of which is the unwrapping the facets that have often expanded into the midline of the overlying paravertebral muscles. To avoid excessive bleeding and muscle trauma, this must be accomplished by methodical and meticulous dissection at each level from above downward. The fine cutting electrocautery tip is used to dissect towards the facet from the uppermost part of the spinous process and lamina, and then laterally around each facet, keeping the muscle intact as much as possible, to provide bilateral exposure of the full joint at each involved segment.

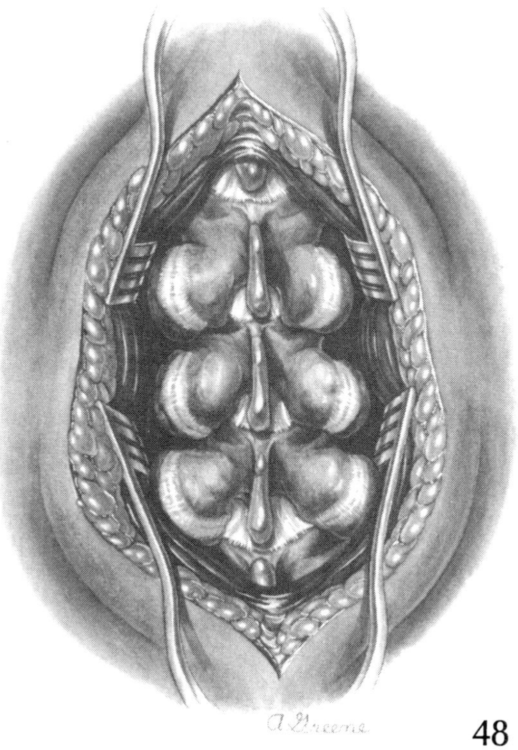

48

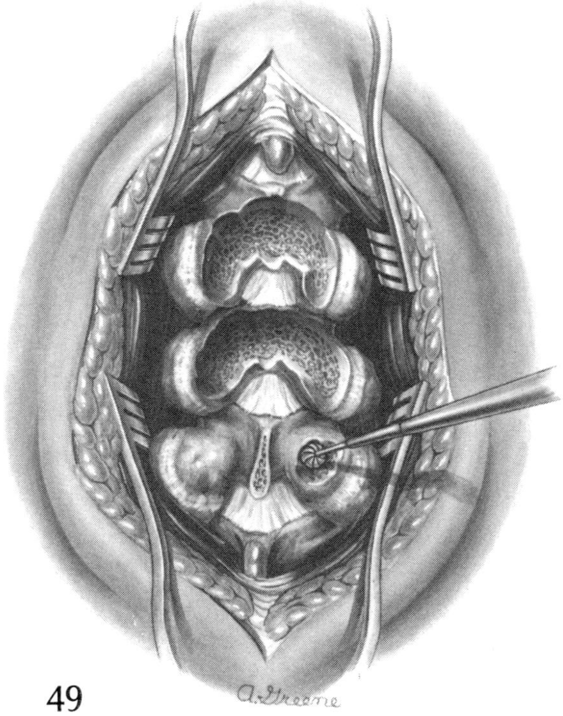

49

## 49

Generous facets increased in amplitude and breadth are associated with considerable thickening of laminae. Posterolateral elements are best excised by first thinning the dense bone with an air drill in a crescent shape. This must be done carefully in the midline, although the thick enfolded ligamentum flavum usually provides protection to the dura mater. However, particular caution must be exercised with the drill and subsequently with rongeurs over the dura mater between each ligamentum flavum where it may easily be torn.

## 50 & 51

Once the epidural space is exposed in the midline at each level and the ligamentum bulges posteriorly, it is excised, and bone and lateral ligament are taken away to the lateral margin of dura mater on each side. Foraminotomy may be performed for additional decompression if one particular nerve root is believed to be compressed at the foraminal level. Such radiculopathy is difficult to evaluate and probably accounts for persistence of root pain in some patients despite extensive decompression.

In patients with secondary spondylolisthesis, full laminectomy and bimedial facetectomy may be undertaken without danger of further vertebral displacement as long as the annulus fibrosus is left intact and the disc is not excised. This problem almost always occurs at L4–L5, but laminectomy of L3, L4 and L5 should be accomplished to achieve adequate posterior decompression and longitudinal release of the cauda equina.

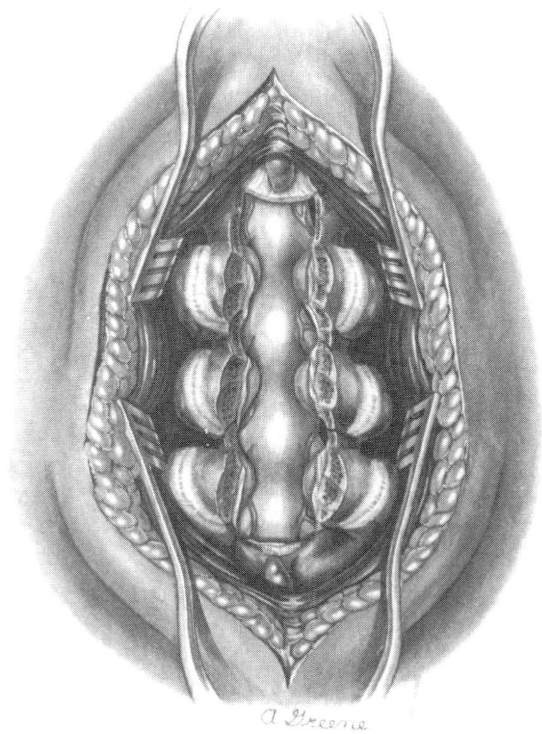

50

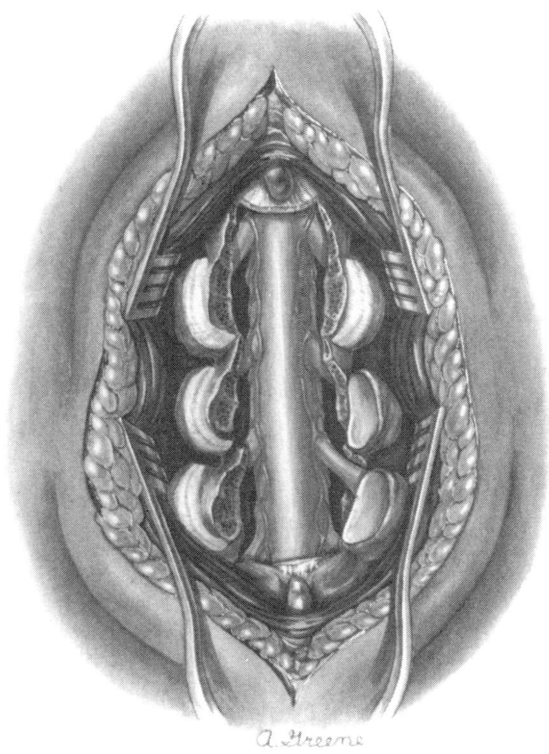

51

## Acknowledgments

*Illustration 17* has been reproduced by courtesy of C. A. Fager and the publisher; *18, 31–37, 40* and *46*[1] have been adapted or reproduced by courtesy of C. A. Fager and Elsevier Science Publishing Co[2]. *Illustrations 9–12, 14, 47, 48, 50* and *51* have been adapted or reproduced by courtesy of C. A. Fager and Raven Press[3]. *Illustration 22* has been reproduced by courtesy of W. B. Saunders Company[4].

## References

1. Fager, C. A. (1984) Facts and fallacies of spinal disorders: a neurosurgeon's viewpoint. In: Evaluation and treatment of chronic pain. Aronoff, G. M. (ed.), pp. 351–357. Baltimore: Urban and Schwartzenberg
2. Fager, C. A. (1985) Ruptured median and paramedian lumbar disc: a review of 243 cases. Surgical Neurology 23, 309–323
3. Fager, C. A. (1982) Lumbar disc disease – surgical treatment. In: Lumbar disc disease, Hardy, R. W. (ed.), pp. 119–145. New York: Raven Press
4. Fager, C. A. (1980) Surgical approaches to lumbar disc lesions and spondylosis. Surgical Clinics of North America, 60, 649–663

## Further reading

Alexander, E., Jr. (1969) Significance of the small lumbar spinal canal: cauda equina compression syndromes due to spondylosis. Part V: Achondroplasia. Journal of Neurosurgery, 31, 513–519

Clark, K. (1969) Significance of the small lumbar spinal canal: cauda equina compression syndromes due to spondylosis. Part II: Clinical and surgical significance. Journal of Neurosurgery, 31, 495–498

Ehni, G. (1969) Significance of the small lumbar spinal canal: cauda equina compression syndromes due to spondylosis. Part I: Introduction; Part IV: Acute compression artificially-induced during operation. Journal of Neurosurgery, 31, 490–494; 507–512

Fager, C. A., Freidberg, S. R. (1980) Analysis of failures and poor results of lumbar spine surgery. Spine, 5, 87–94

Gindin, R. A., Volcan, I. J. (1978) Rupture of the intervertebral disc producing cauda equina syndrome. American Surgeon, 44, 585–593

Shephard, R. H. (1959) Diagnosis and prognosis of cauda equina syndrome produced by protrusion of lumbar disc. British Medical Journal, 2, 1434–1439

Shephard, R. H. (1960) Compression of cauda equina by lumbar disc. Modern Medicine, 28, 133–134

Illustrations by Barbara Hyams and Ludwig G. Kempe

# Surgery of epilepsy

**Sidney Goldring** MD
Head of Neurological Surgery, Washington University School of Medicine, St Louis, Missouri, USA

**Erik M. Gregorie** MD
Chief, Neurosurgery Service, Brooke Army Medical Center, Fort Sam Houston, Texas, USA

**Rene Tempelhoff** MD
Chief of Neuroanesthesia, Washington University School of Medicine, St Louis, Missouri, USA

## Introduction

Conservative estimates indicate that about 60 000 individuals in the United States of America have focal epilepsy that would benefit from surgery, yet only several hundred operations for epilepsy are carried out annually. Similar underutilization of surgical management occurs uniformly throughout the world, including Canada where epilepsy surgery gained most popularity through the efforts of the late Wilder Penfield and colleagues[1].

The main reason for the underutilization of surgery is that most of the medical community are not aware that surgery safely abolishes seizures in about two-thirds of patients who undergo excision of an epileptogenic focus. Even more important is that most physicians have not had the personal experience of witnessing the unemployed and socially stigmatized epileptic, incapacitated for years, undergo surgery, which at once abolishes the seizures. This is an event which not only offers a new life for the patient, but also the family who have shared the burden. For the surgeon, the result is one of the most gratifying experiences that can be encountered, because in all surgery there is no more grateful patient or family.

In operations for focal epilepsy, excision of brain that does not harbour a progressively growing lesion and that frequently appears normal on visual inspection may seem to be a drastic step. In reality, however, one is careful to remove tissue that serves no important purpose and only exerts an adverse effect expressed in repeated convulsions. Furthermore, histological examination of the focus will usually show pathological features. It may seem paradoxical that operative excision, which in itself produces focal brain damage and glial scarring, should act to prevent the development of convulsions, but fortunately this is the case. In patients in whom the epileptogenic cicatrix is a residuum of a previous open head injury or brain abscess, the paradox may be explained by the histological features of the scars. They frequently harbour both mesenchymal and glial elements. The former are thought by some to be more epileptogenic, although data in support of this thesis are not compelling. In any case, we lack a full explanation of the epileptogenicity of pathological scars and other lesions, compared with the relatively weak epileptogenic effect of an operative cicatrix.

This chapter deals with current procedures used most commonly in the surgery of epilepsy, these being cortical excision of an epileptogenic focus giving rise to simple partial seizures, anterior temporal lobectomy for complex partial seizures, and section of the corpus callosum for generalized seizures, especially drop attacks.

## Preoperative evaluation for surgery

The most critical and specialized aspect of surgical management of epilepsy is the accumulation of evidence establishing that the clinical seizure arises from a single focus in a functionally silent area of the brain. The evidence for a focal origin comes from a variety of sources: (*1*) clinical history; (*2*) physical examination; (*3*) routine EEG; (*4*) simultaneous EEG and video monitoring to determine whether the onset of the clinical seizure is preceded by a focal electrical seizure discharge; (*5*) nasopharyngeal and/or sphenoidal electrodes to capture seizure discharges emanating from the hippocampal region in patients with complex partial seizures; (*6*) psychological testing; (*7*) radiological imaging procedures, i.e. computerized tomography (CT scans), magnetic resonance imaging (MRI scans), cerebral angiography and positron emission tomography (PET scans).

The main value of CT and MRI scans is to evaluate the possibility of a mass lesion, or other focal structural pathology as a cause of the seizures. Both also provide information regarding asymmetries in ventricular size indicating focal atrophy and chronic incisural herniation of the medial temporal lobe, which may be associated with mesial temporal sclerosis. PET scanning is being used with increasing frequency in patients with complex partial seizures. In those who prove to have mesial temporal sclerosis, the PET scan may show decreased metabolic activity in the affected temporal lobe[2]. Arteriography, of course, provides important information regarding the distribution of the normal vasculature and the possibility of a vascular malformation as a cause of the seizure disorder.

In addition, during arteriography, the Wada test[3] may be carried out to determine which hemisphere is concerned with language function. This test is used whenever an anterior temporal lobectomy is planned for complex partial seizures, or a cortical excision is anticipated in the vicinity of the sylvian fissure. The test utilizes intracarotid injection of sodium amylobarbitone. Dominant-side injections produce aphasia in addition to paresis of the contralateral limbs. In conjunction with the injection of sodium amylobarbitone, the ability of either temporal lobe to subserve the function of recent recall is also tested[4]. Immediately preceding the injection, the patient is shown three items, e.g. pictures of two objects and the first line of a nursery rhyme, and asked to remember them. After the injection, failure to recall the items suggests that the temporal lobe on the uninjected side is incapable of storing the items. Such a result would suggest that anterior temporal lobectomy on the injected side might risk impairment of recent recall. When injecting the dominant hemisphere, the testing for recall is delayed until the aphasia has cleared.

# Cortical excisions for simple partial seizures

Given that one study, or a combination of the above studies, suggests the general site (e.g. right frontal lobe) of the epileptogenic focus, one then proceeds to obtain data which more precisely map the boundaries of the focus which is to be excised. The procedure used most commonly requires that a craniotomy be performed under local anaesthesia[5]. General anaesthesia is avoided because it suppresses electrocorticographic seizure activity used to identify the focus. It also suppresses the motor responses to electrical stimulation of the cortical surface which are used to identify the sensorimotor region.

Not all patients, however, can undergo surgery under local anaesthesia with the necessary degree of cooperation, and this is especially true of children. We have also encountered patients in whom interictal electrical discharges observed during surgery were unreliable for localizing the focus, whether they occurred spontaneously or were induced by electrical stimulation (afterdischarge). Even an afterdischarge associated with the development of the clinical seizure may be misleading[6]. We, along with others[6–8], have become increasingly convinced that the most reliable evidence for localizing an epileptogenic focus is the change in the electrocorticogram made during the spontaneous development of the patient's symptomatic seizures, an undesirable event during craniotomy. It was these observations and our demonstration that somatosensory evoked responses could be used to localize the sensorimotor region under general anaesthesia[9,10] that led us to develop the method of extraoperative electrocorticography using epidural electrode arrays for the localization of the epileptogenic focus[6].

The main features of the procedure are: (*1*) all surgical manipulation is carried out under general, rather than local anaesthesia; (*2*) the sensorimotor region is readily identified in the anaesthetized patient by recording cortical sensory evoked responses in conjunction with cortical electrostimulation to produce movement; (*3*) the epileptogenic focus is localized by extraoperative electrocorticography via indwelling surface epidural electrode arrays, localization being derived predominantly from recordings made during spontaneously occurring seizures.

## Anaesthesia

Craniotomy is performed under general anaesthesia. It permits both the recording of somatosensory evoked responses and the elicitation of motor responses to cortical stimulation. The method currently in use was developed by Dr Rene Tempelhoff and differs somewhat from that described previously[11–13]. Patients, both children and adult, are premedicated with metoclopramide 0.2 mg/kg and cimetidine 5 mg/kg to decrease the risk of aspiration pneumonitis during induction. In adults, an intravenous line is started and incremental doses of fentanyl (8–20 μg/kg) and droperidol (0.08–0.2 mg/kg) are introduced progressively. Induction is carried out following administration of a short-acting muscle relaxant, vecuronium 0.1 mg/kg, and anaesthesia is maintained with a fentanyl drip, 3–6 μg/kg per hour, $N_2O/O_2$ (65/35 per cent) and end-tidal isoflurane 0.25 per cent to obtain complete amnesia. When functional localization is completed, muscle relaxation is reintroduced and the patient is maintained on $N_2O/O_2$ (65/35 per cent) and fentanyl for the remainder of the procedure.

In children, if there is an intravenous catheter in place, or if one can be readily introduced, the protocol is the same as in adults. If the child is uncooperative or has poor venous access, induction is started with progressive introduction of halothane up to 3 per cent with $N_2O/O_2$ (65/35 per cent) and an intravenous line is set up as soon as possible. The child is then given vecuronium 0.1 mg/kg, intubated, and the halothane is discontinued. Thereafter the method is the same as that described for adults.

## CRANIOTOMY FOR LOCALIZATION AND INSERTION OF THE EPIDURAL ELECTRODE ARRAY[12,13]

### Incisions

# 1

A large question-mark type scalp flap is turned. The flap may encompass the frontal, parietal, occipital and temporal regions; the specific size and position of the flap depends on the suspected size and location of the focus. The medial limb of the incision is placed 2 cm from the midline, except for the anterior 2–3 cm which are directed to end just behind the apex of the hairline. The posterior limb is extended laterally from the medial limb to just behind and above the pinna. It is carried over the ear and downward 1.5 cm anterior to the tragus to end at the zygoma.

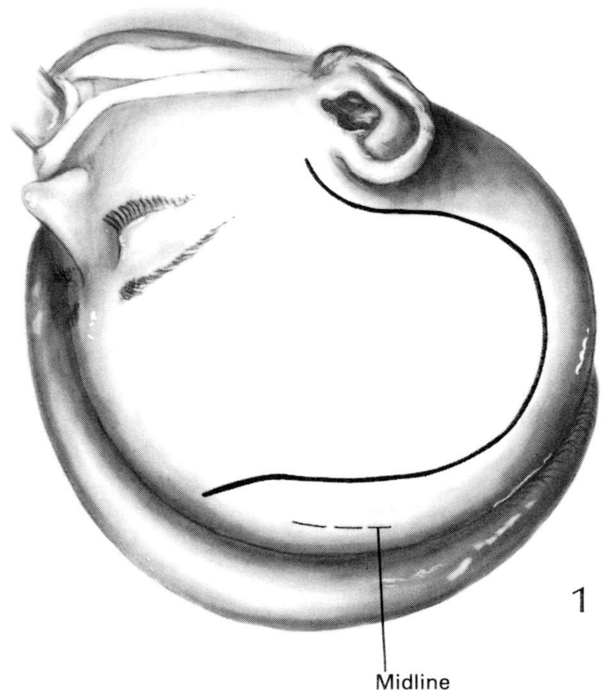


1

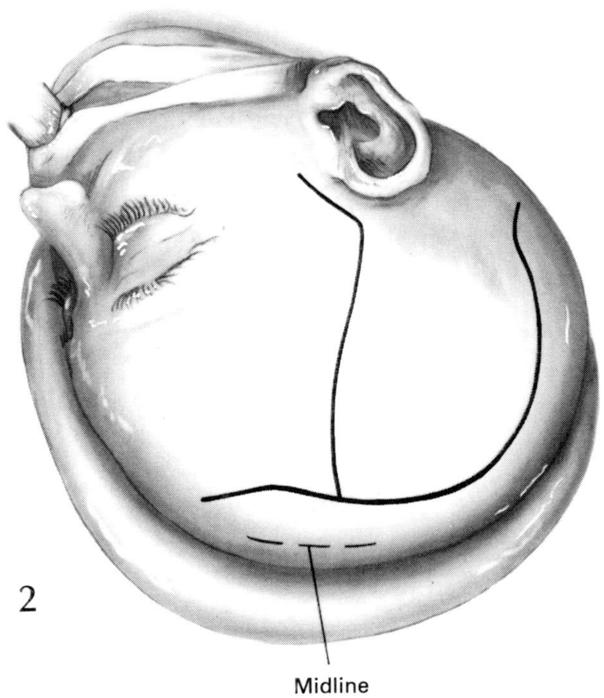


2

# 2

If an unusually large flap is required (e.g. to carry out subtotal hemispherectomy), the incision is modified. The posterior limb ends behind the ear and a vertical incision is made from about the middle of the medial limb to the zygoma, about 1.5 cm anterior to the tragus. This creates two scalp flaps, each with an adequate blood supply.

## Opening of dura

# 3

The pericranium and temporalis fascia and muscle are stripped from the underlying bone and a free bone flap is removed. The dural incision is made around the *entire* periphery of the exposed dura, the dural edges along the midline (toward the bottom in *Illustration 3*) are sutured, and the dural flap reflected out of the field on the sutured medial hinge. This is done to produce a free dural graft, which minimizes the development of epidural clot that could attenuate the extraoperative recorded electrical activity.

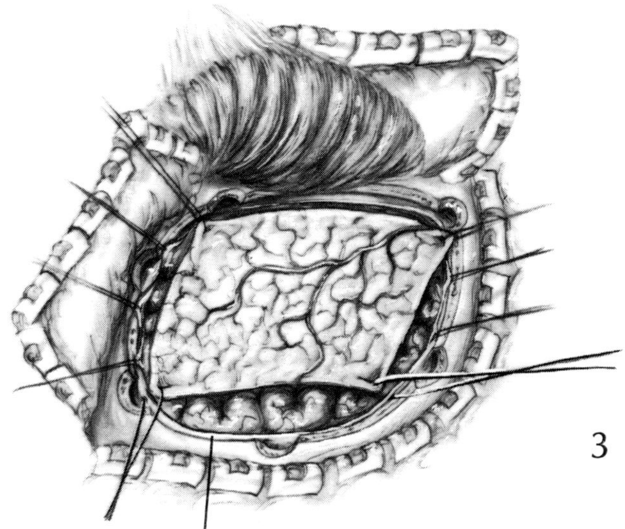


3

## Recording evoked responses

# 4

Cortical sensory evoked responses are then recorded to identify the sensorimotor region. A Silastic (Dow Corning, UK) template holding three rows of eight linearly orientated electrodes is placed on the cortical surface in a plane parallel to the midline and spanning the presumed location of the sensorimotor region. The interelectrode distance is 1 cm and each row is separated by 1.5 cm. In *Illustration 4*, the midline is shown toward the bottom. An elliptical 1 × 2 mm platinum disc underlies each numbered ticket. The lead wires from each of the electrodes are collected in a bundle and exit at the top.

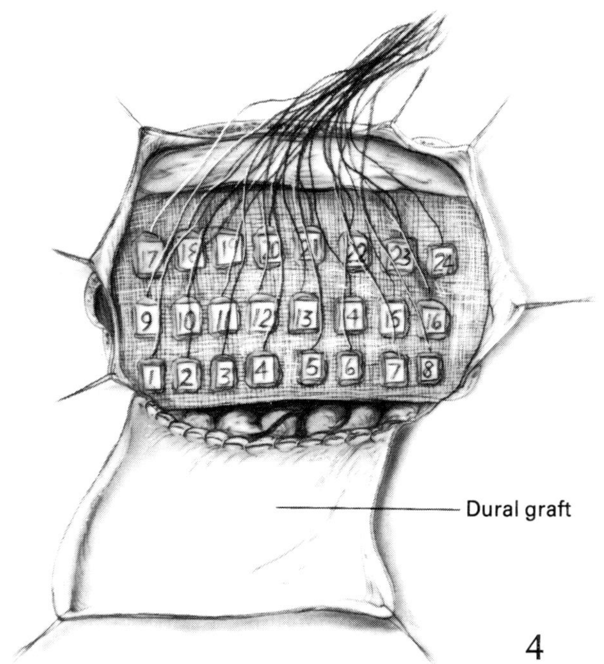


4

Simultaneous records are made from each adjacent pair of electrodes in the first row (that is, 1–2, 2–3, 3–4) while the contralateral median nerve is electrically pulsed transcutaneously (1 per second) at the wrist. Stimulus strength is adjusted to just above the threshold for eliciting movement of the thumb. If an evoked response is not obtained, then recordings are made from the second row of electrodes, etc. A switching matrix controlled by a microprocessor under keyboard command can select any row of recording sites in the brief time it takes to type in the command (e.g. 'Matrix A'). A special purpose computer is used to expose the sensory evoked response quickly by averaging 25–50 post-stimulus epochs (100 milliseconds in duration) of electrical activity. The face area is similarly identified. The facial nerve is electrically pulsed transcutaneously by a pair of disc electrodes, with one placed over the parotid gland just anterior to the tragus and the other just beneath the angle of the mandible.

5

When a response is evoked only in the somatosensory area, the tracings from the row of linearly orientated electrode sites usually show responses from only two adjacent pairs of electrode combinations, and these responses are reversed in polarity. For example, simultaneous recordings made from a row of electrodes 1–2, 2–3, etc. show a response only from 5–6 and 6–7(*A*). Tracings from all other electrode sites show either no response or inconsequential deflections. Since electrode sites 5 and 7 show a response only when they are paired with electrode 6, and not when they are paired with the other electrodes to which they are adjacent, electrode site 6 is identified as overlying the somatosensory area. In some cases, smaller responses are recorded from the areas immediately adjacent to the two sites which yield responses showing phase reversal. These are not locally generated; they reflect, instead, distant pick-up of the response generated in the somatosensory area. It is the phase reversal between two responses recorded from two adjacent electrode pairs sharing a common electrode that establishes the site of somatosensory representation. When a response is evoked in the motor cortex in addition to the somatosensory area, responses are recorded from four adjacent pairs of electrode sites, rather than two, and there is a double phase reversal (*B*).

*Illustration 5* shows somatosensory evoked responses identifying the somatosensory and motor hand areas. Vertical lines between traces indicate phase reversal of responses recorded bipolarly from adjacent areas. Deflections at the beginning of each trace are shock artefacts; time calibration is at the bottom. Recordings in a patient in whom only the somatosensory area yielded a response are shown in *A*: numbers to the left of each trace are electrode combinations. Recordings in a patient in whom both the somatosensory and motor hand areas yielded responses are depicted in *B*.

In a small number of cases, phase reversal is not seen and only responses of varying amplitude from several adjacent electrode combinations occur. In these instances, the largest amplitude response usually occurs in the somatosensory area. It is these patients and the patients who show a response in the motor cortex as well as in the somatosensory area in whom it is especially important to verify the location of the motor cortex with cortical stimulation. This can be accomplished by stimulating through the pair of recording electrodes just anterior to those overlying the sensory area. For carrying out more detailed cortical stimulation, the electrode array is replaced with a mock array that consists of numbered tickets which are fused to a matrix of narrow Silastic stripping. The position of each ticket corresponds precisely to the electrode positions in the electrode array, and the grid is orientated in the exact position that had been occupied by the electrode array to identify the somatosensory hand area. Since the matrix is not embedded in a solid sheet of Silastic, it permits more extensive exploration with a hand-held bipolar electrode (interelectrode distance 0.5 mm).

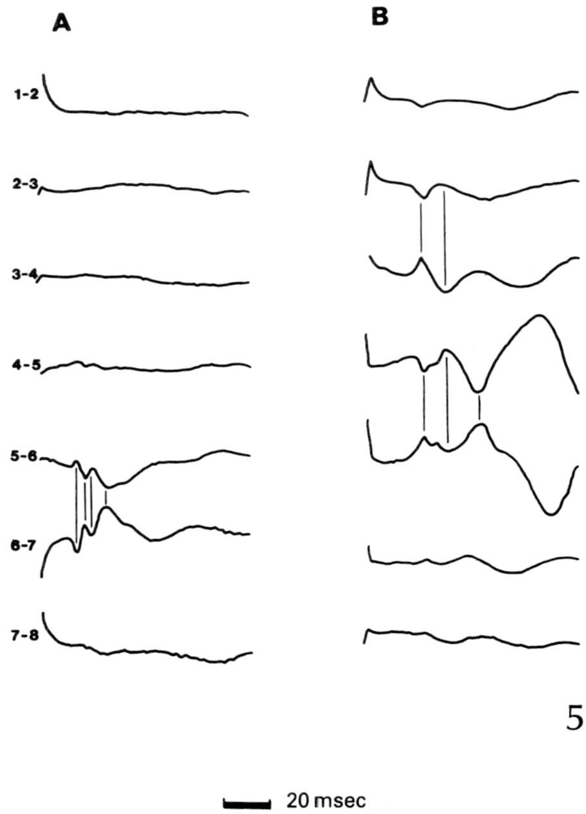


5

Since it is possible to localize the sensorimotor region with cortical stimulation under general anaesthesia without neuromuscular paralysis, the use of somatosensory evoked response for functional localization may appear redundant and unnecessary. However, during general anaesthesia the threshold for producing movement is raised; much time is spent varying stimulus intensities and exploring the cortical surface with the stimulating electrode. Also, depending on the level of general anaesthesia, the extent of the electrically excitable cortex may be constricted. By using somatosensory evoked responses prior to cortical stimulation, the time spent and frustration frequently experienced in searching blindly for the domain of sensorimotor cortex are avoided.

## 6

After the central fissure is identified, it is overlaid with a thread. Then a square grid is draped over the exposed brain, and a photograph is made. In *Illustration 6*, anterior is to the left, midline is toward the bottom, and the meandering broken line is the central fissure. Measurements between several peripheral points on the grid lines and the adjacent cranial sites are made, the grid is removed and the dura is closed.

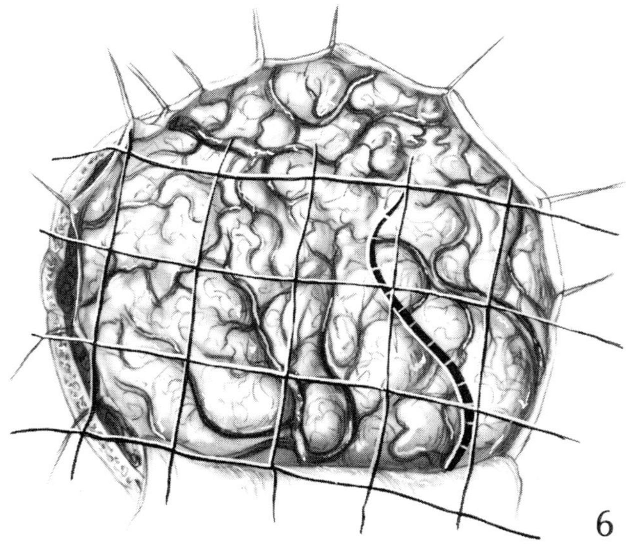

6

## 7

A quasirectangular template of medical grade Silastic holding 48 electrodes is sewn in epidurally. In *Illustration 7*, anterior is to the left and midline is toward the bottom. An elliptical 1 ×2 mm platinum electrode underlies each numbered ticket. The lead wires from each electrode are collected in a bundle and exit at the bottom. The meandering broken line is the central fissure. The electrodes are arranged in rows with interelectrode distances of 1.0 and 1.5 cm in the sagittal and coronal planes, respectively. The electrode array is placed so that it spans the suspected area of epileptogenicity, its surround and the sensorimotor region. The previously made measurements are used to place the grid of rectangular squares over the electrode array in an identical position to that previously occupied when draped over the exposed brain. By referring to the photograph of the exposed brain, the grid lines are used to locate approximately the central fissure epidurally. The sylvian fissure is identified similarly.

Knowledge of these important landmarks during the extraoperative monitoring expedites the retrieval of information that demonstrates the relationship of the epileptogenic focus to the sensorimotor area, and language cortex if the focus is in the dominant hemisphere. Motor responses and speech arrest are readily obtained by transdural cortical stimulation.

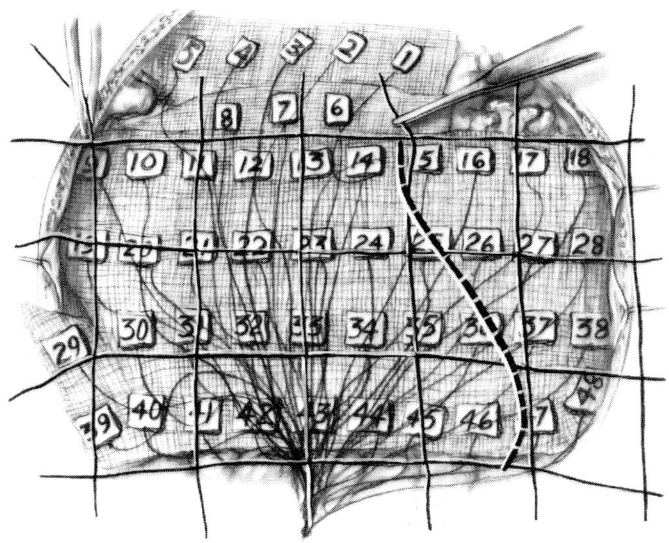


7

8

The remainder of the closure is completed and recordings are usually begun on the same day. *Illustration 8* shows the distribution of epidural electrodes. In patients in whom the medial surface of a hemisphere is suspected of harbouring the focus, a subdural electrode array is inserted[14].

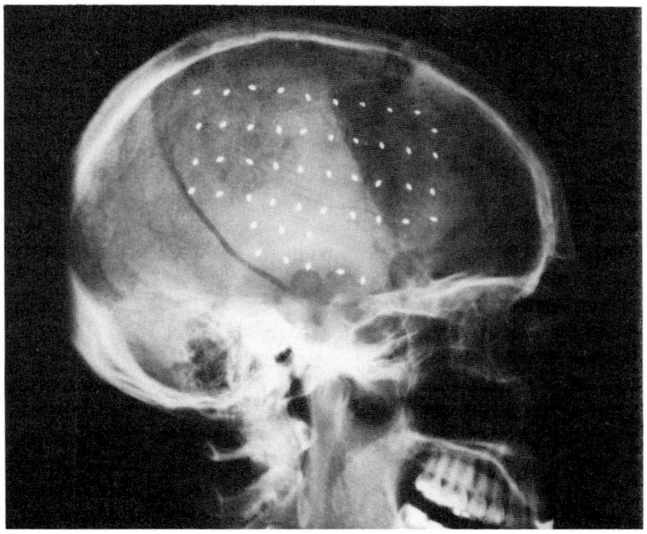

8

Both the patient's behaviour and the electrocorticogram (ECG) are recorded continuously and displayed side by side on the split screen of a television monitor. The taping of these recordings permits the additional opportunity for replays of any seizure that might occur. This is necessary to determine accurately which cortical area shows the first sign of abnormal activity in the moments preceding the onset of a clinical convulsion – essential information for localizing the focus. Because the patient is awake, it is possible to record motor responses to transdural cortical stimulation in addition to sensory evoked responses, and to identify the relationship between the sensorimotor region and the focus. If the recordings are from the dominant hemisphere, speech arrest produced by electrical stimulation is used to determine the boundaries of the speech area. Furthermore, in young children who are unable to undergo the Wada test, this technique may be the only method for determining whether the hemisphere being evaluated is concerned with language function. Thus, all the techniques used in localizing an epileptogenic focus during the usual surgical procedure under local anaesthesia can be performed by recording and stimulating epidurally with indwelling epidural electrode arrays. The recordings are performed in a leisurely manner, free from the usual stresses of the operating room, and the opportunity for recording the ECG during a spontaneous clinical seizure, or if necessary an activated one, is markedly enhanced.

Recording with the epidural electrode array usually continues for 1–6 days, since most patients have daily-to-weekly seizures. Anticonvulsant medication is frequently reduced to increase the probability that seizures will occur during the period of monitoring. If the observations identify the boundaries of a single epileptogenic focus, then brain tissue within the epileptogenic zone is excised at a second craniotomy; if not, the epidural electrode array is removed and the operative wound is closed.

## FOCAL CORTICAL RESECTION

Under general endotracheal anaesthesia the wound is opened to expose the epidural recording electrode array. Measurements are made of the distance between several peripherally situated electrode sites in the array and adjacent points on the calvarium. The electrode array is removed, the dura is opened and the brain exposed.

# 9 & 10

Using the measurements previously taken, a mock electrode array is orientated on the brain to correspond precisely to the position of the electrode array. The epileptogenic focus is mapped, based on the information obtained during the extraoperative recordings. The cortical resection is carried out using bipolar cautery, suction, and blunt and sharp dissection, wherever possible respecting gyral boundaries by subpial resection.

*Illustrations 9* and *10* show the mock electrode array of numbered tickets embedded in a matrix of medical grade Silastic stripping, and the manner in which it is draped over the cerebral cortex of the right hemisphere. Anterior is to the left and midline is toward the bottom. Tickets 1–5 overlie the temporal lobe; tickets 6–8 are just medial to the sylvian fissure. The meandering broken line is the central fissure.

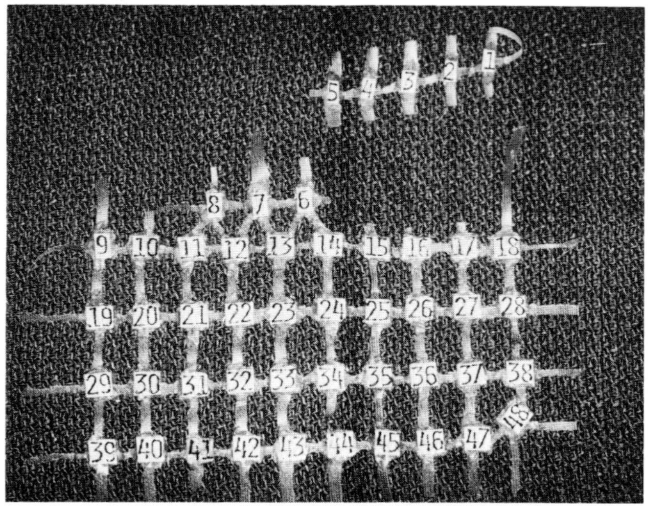

9

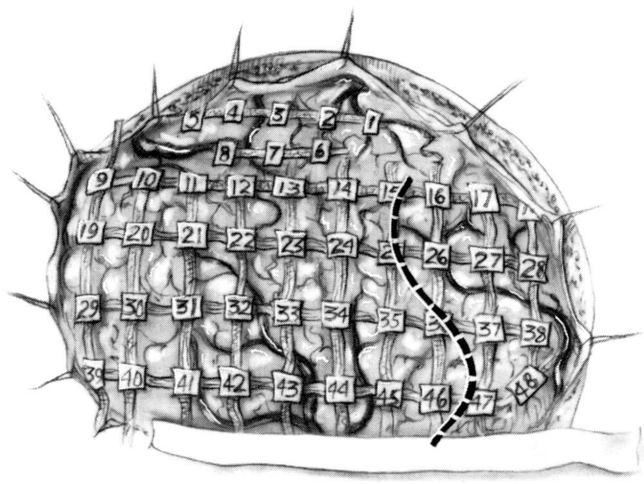

10

Anticonvulsant medication is begun immediately postoperatively. Usually the same medication that the patient was taking at the time of admission is prescribed. The prophylactic antibiotic vancomycin, which was begun at the time of insertion of the epidural electrode array and continued during the extraoperative recordings, is given for 24 hours. Dexamethasone, which was also started at the time of the first procedure, is reduced and discontinued over a 7-day period.

## Results

Seventy-two of one hundred patients evaluated with epidural arrays underwent resection of an epileptogenic focus[11]. The remainder either exhibited a diffuse or multifocal epileptogenic focus, failed to show an electrographic focus in association with the clinical seizure, or failed either to have a seizure during the monitoring, or to show in the interictal record conclusive changes for identifying a focus. Fifty-seven of the seventy-two patients who had a resection have been followed-up for 1 year or more. Of these, 29 were children and 18 (62 per cent) have had a good result. Of the 28 adults, 18 (64 per cent) show a good result. A 'good result' is defined as either complete cessation of all seizures or a reduction in seizure frequency, permitting employment or education, neither of which was possible before surgery, or a reduction in seizure frequency, avoiding institutionalization; in other words, a good result is one which unambiguously produced an improvement in the quality of life.

## Limitations and complications

One disadvantage of the procedure is the necessity of a secondary craniotomy. We believe, however, that this disadvantage is outweighed by the following considerations: (*1*) a long and arduous operation under local anaesthesia is avoided; (*2*) the procedure permits management of both children and those adults who cannot undergo surgery under local anaesthesia; and (*3*) localization of the epileptogenic focus is frequently more precise.

One patient developed a subgaleal wound infection which responded to drainage and antibiotic therapy and another developed aseptic necrosis of the bone flap, which had to be replaced by cranioplasty.

Since reporting in 1984 on the 100 cases summarized here[11], another patient developed a subgaleal wound infection. This occurred in a child who scratched his wound and caused a dehiscence. This infection also responded to drainage and antibiotics. Also two intracranial haematomas have occurred. One patient developed an epidural haematoma, which was evacuated and left no neurological deficit. The other developed a temporal lobe clot which was evacuated. The patient was left with a superior quadrantic hemianopia. It is not clear, however, whether this deficit was the result of the haematoma, or the anterior temporal lobectomy which the patient underwent 1 week after removal of the haematoma. Prior to the lobectomy, the field cut was diminishing progressively in size.

# Anterior temporal lobectomy for complex partial seizures

In some of those patients in whom the various preoperative examinations fail to identify the symptomatic temporal lobe, it is possible to do so by extraoperative electrocorticography with implanted recording electrodes. This is usually carried out with depth electrodes, stereotactically implanted in the medial temporal lobe[7,8]. However, we no longer use depth recordings. Since 1980, patients who were considered to be candidates for depth electrode recording for localization of their focus have been evaluated instead with epidural recording arrays[11].

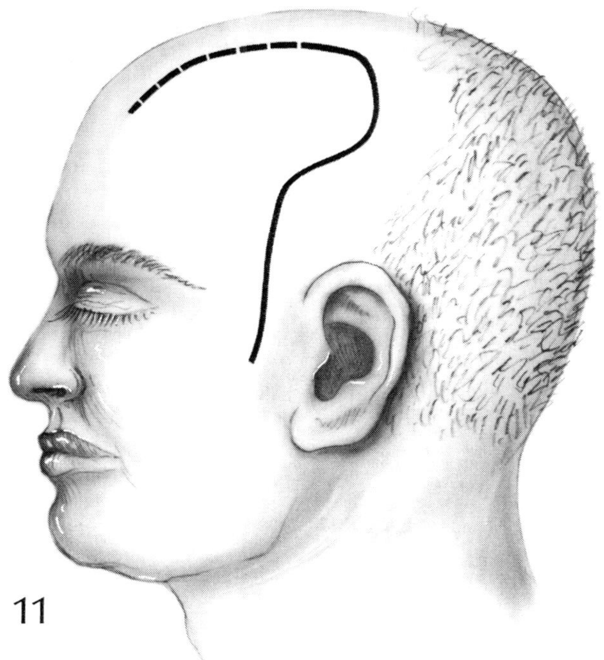

11

## LOCALIZATION OF THE EPILEPTOGENIC FOCUS

### 11

Under general anaesthesia, an abbreviated question-mark skin incision is made for inserting the temporal lobe epidural electrode array (solid line) with an extension (broken line) for anterior temporal lobectomy. The incision begins at the zygoma, 1.5 cm anterior to the tragus, and extends vertically for 4 cm. From this point it courses rostrally in the shape of a C. The most rostral point in the C ends 3 cm directly above the rostral end of the vertical segment of the incision. The apex of the convexity in the C is 2 cm posterior to the plane of the vertical segment. The temporalis muscle is incised along the same plane as the scalp incision and is stripped from the underlying bone, which is exposed with self-retaining retractors.

A burr hole is made just above the root of the zygoma. Using the burr hole as the point of entry, a craniotome is used to cut out a 2.5 × 2 cm rectangle of bone. Additional temporal bone is rongeured away on either side of the burr hole.

# 12a, b & c

An electrode array for epidural monitoring of temporal lobe seizures is used. Platinum discs ($1 \times 2$ mm) are embedded in a medical grade Silastic. Wires are led to an Amphonol connector.

The dura is stripped from the floor of the temporal fossa to reach the foramen ovale. It is not necessary to divide the middle meningeal artery. The electrode array, fashioned as a quasistrip and containing the seven electrode contacts (*a*) is inserted extradurally until the most medially situated electrode lies adjacent to the foramen ovale. The other six electrode contacts are located in the strip as three separate, horizontally orientated pairs, the interelectrode distance in each pair being 1 cm. It is estimated that the most medially situated electrodes, 1, 2 and 3, lie adjacent to the hippocampal and fusiform gyri. The other two pairs lie approximately over the inferior and middle temporal gyri respectively. The lead wires are anchored to the temporalis muscle, the rectangular bone button is replaced and the wound is closed in layers. The procedure is carried out bilaterally. Recordings are made from 1–2, 1–3, 2–3, 4–5 and 6–7.

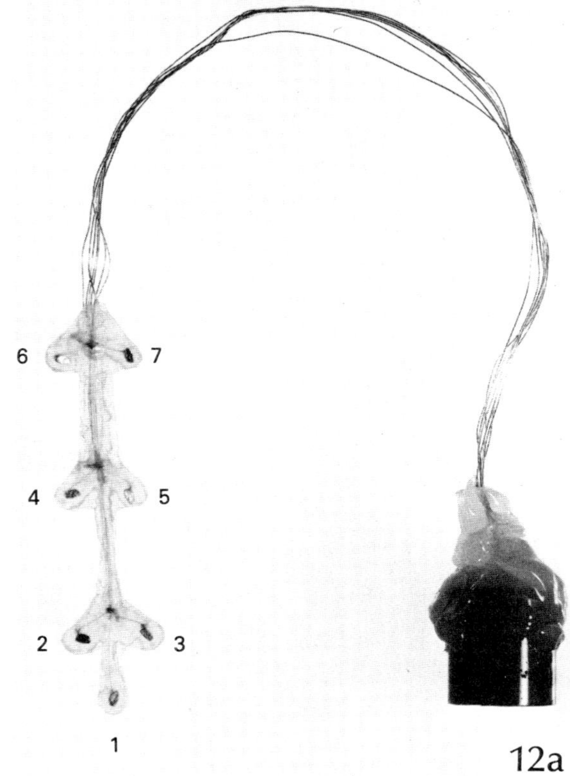


12a

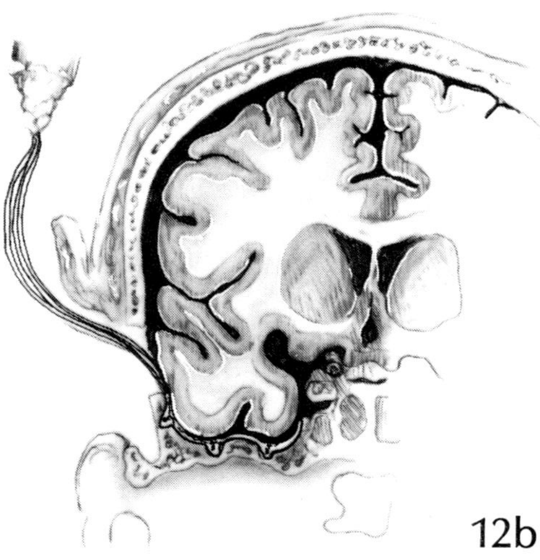

12b

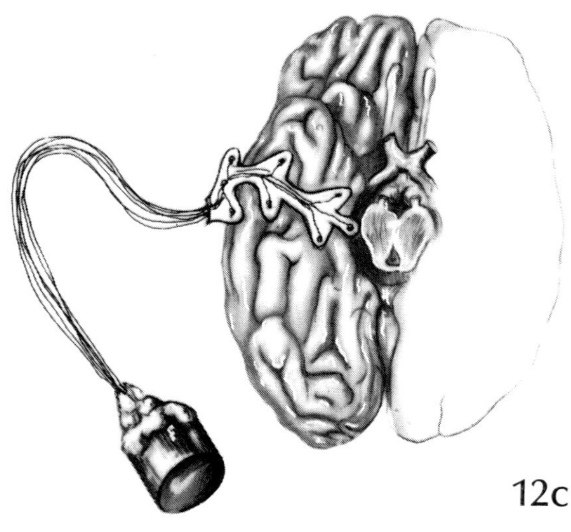

12c

## Extraoperative monitoring and management

# 13

X-rays are obtained postoperatively to check orientation of the electrode arrays. Extraoperative monitoring, identical to that described for patients with hemispheric recording arrays, is carried out. In those patients in whom a unilateral focus can be demonstrated, anterior temporal lobectomy is carried out when the epidural arrays are removed.

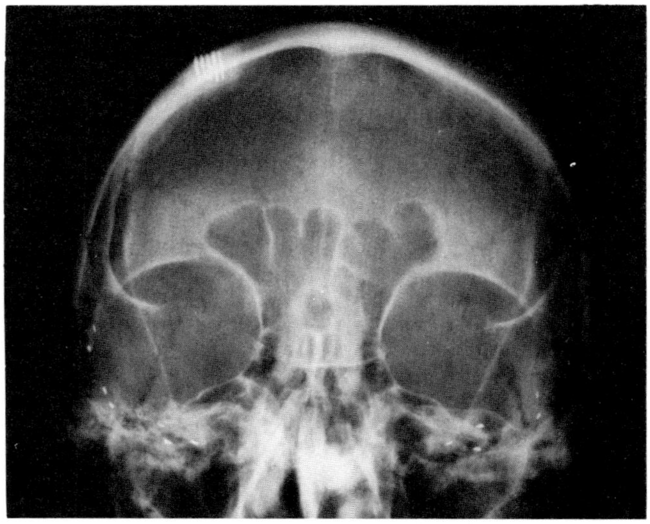

13

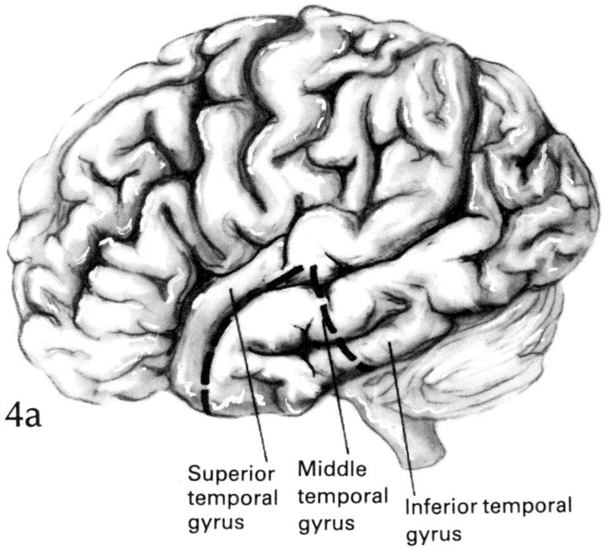


14a

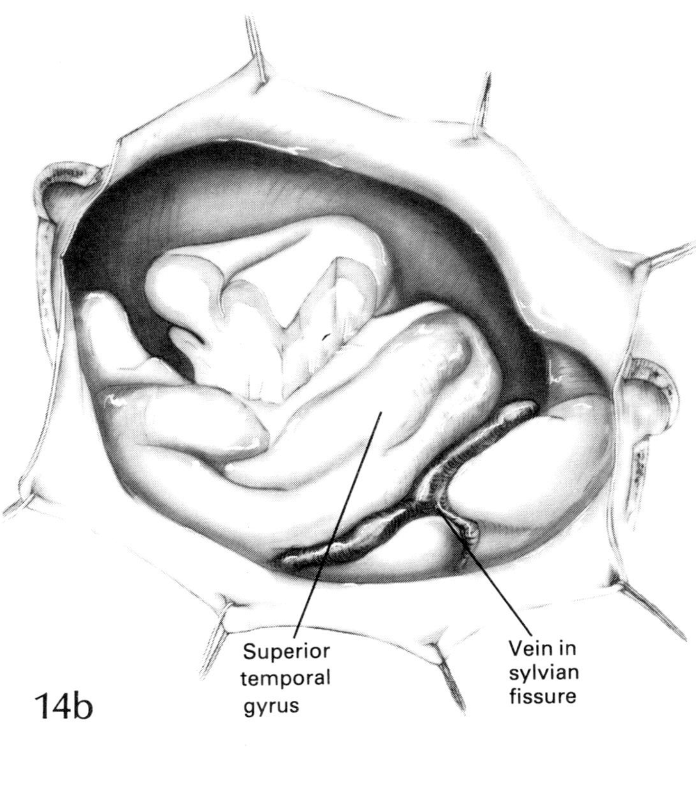


14b

## ANTERIOR TEMPORAL LOBECTOMY

On the side planned for lobectomy, exposure is obtained by extending the rostral end of the scalp incision anteriorly to the hairline in a curvilinear fashion (*see Illustration 11*). The incision in the temporalis fascia and muscle is extended to fashion a flap of temporalis muscle which is retracted laterally on a hinge of temporalis muscle. The rectangular plug of bone is removed and saved for later replacement. A free bone flap which will permit exposure of the anterior 6 cm of the temporal lobe, sylvian fissure and inferior frontal gyrus is removed, and additional inferior temporal bone is also removed to provide easy access to the floor of the anterior temporal fossa. The dura is opened inferiorly along the edge of the craniotomy and reflected on a medial hinge to expose the anterior temporal lobe and sylvian fissure.

# 14a & b

The middle temporal gyrus is incised vertically 4–4.5 cm posterior to the anterior temporal tip, keeping the incision closer to 4 cm on the side concerned with language function. Using bipolar cautery, sharp dissection and suction, this cortical incision is extended obliquely in a posterior direction through the fusiform and inferior temporal gyri and the lateral aspect of the parahippocampal gyrus. The incision through these gyri is carried to the white matter. Next, the bottom of the sulcus between the superior and middle temporal gyri is exposed and divided to reveal the white matter from the transverse incision in the middle temporal gyrus to the anterior tip of the temporal lobe. Then, working from posterior to anterior and medial to lateral, the white matter is divided. There remains only the parahippocampal gyrus and its arachnoid holding the mobilized lateral temporal cortex. This attachment is divided longitudinally and the lateral temporal cortex and associated white matter is delivered *en bloc*.

# 15

The white matter is incised to reveal the anterior temporal horn and the incision is extended horizontally to expose the anterior 2.4–3 cm of the hippocampus. In *Illustration 15* the parahippocampal gyrus has been removed and included in the resected block of lateral temporal cortex.

# 16

The parahippocampal gyrus and hippocampus are divided transversely approximately 2.5 cm posterior to the anterior tip of the hippocampus. The choroid plexus is exposed and gently retracted to reveal the choroidal fissure. The inset of *Illustration 16* is a magnified view showing hippocampus, choroid plexus and choroidal fissure. The fissure has been opened by retracting the hippocampus laterally to expose the arachnoid covering the brain stem.

# 17

The transverse incision in the hippocampus is carried down to the arachnoid overlying the basis pedunculi and the fissure is opened along its entire extent. Then, beginning at the previously made transverse cut in the hippocampus and hippocampal gyrus, these structures are gently swept off of the arachnoid which protects the cerebral peduncle, the third and fourth cranial nerves, and the posterior cerebral artery. The hippocampal tissue is removed *en bloc* to permit adequate pathological examination, especially for the presence of mesial temporal sclerosis. The amygdala is not included in the resection, but a biopsy of the medial portion is obtained in most of our cases. Histological examination of this tissue has usually been normal or shown only gliosis. This finding, however, may only be a matter of sampling. Haemostasis is secured and a routine closure is performed.

## Results

Eighty patients have been evaluated using temporal epidural recording electrode arrays. In 65, a unilateral focus was identified and the patients underwent an anterior temporal lobectomy. Forty-eight of these patients have been followed-up for 1–8 years. Of these, 34 (71 per cent) have had a good result. These results compare very favourably with those reported in the literature for temporal lobe epilepsy[15].

Thirty-one of the 34 patients who had a good result showed mesial temporal sclerosis (neuronal drop-out and astrocytosis of the hippocampus) in the resected tissue. Lateral temporal sclerosis, focal cortical dysplasia and gliosis were found in the remaining three. Of the 14 who failed to respond to surgery, seven showed only gliosis, one showed lateral and mesial temporal sclerosis and six showed mesial temporal sclerosis.

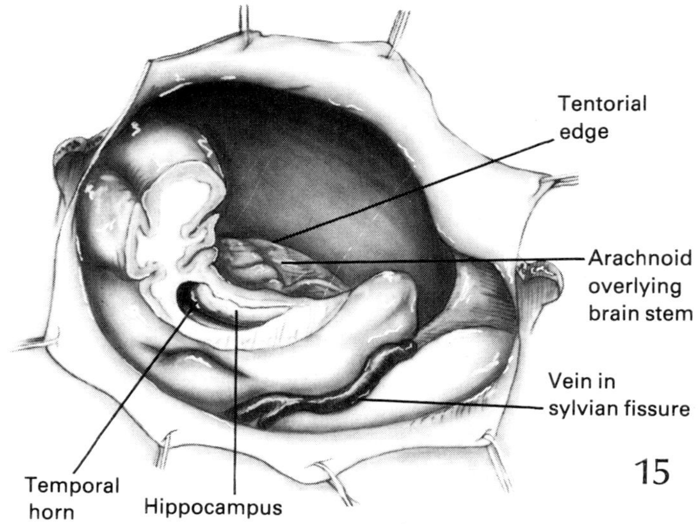

15

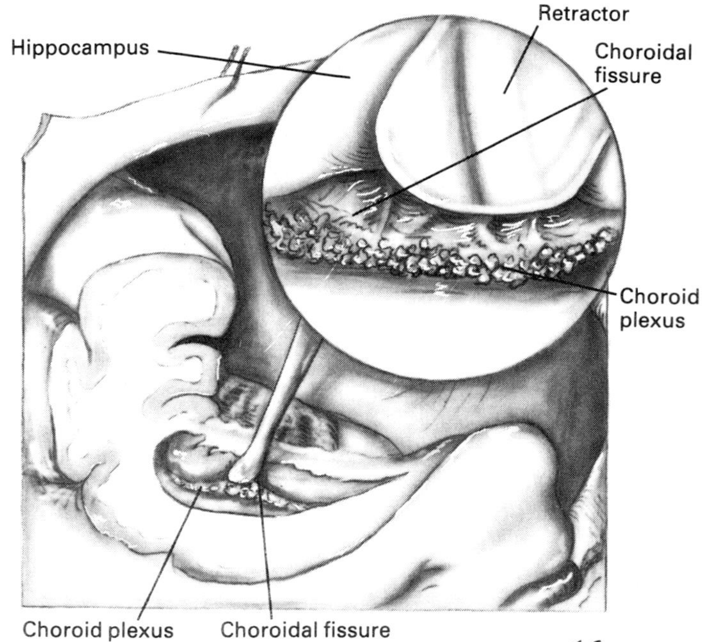

16

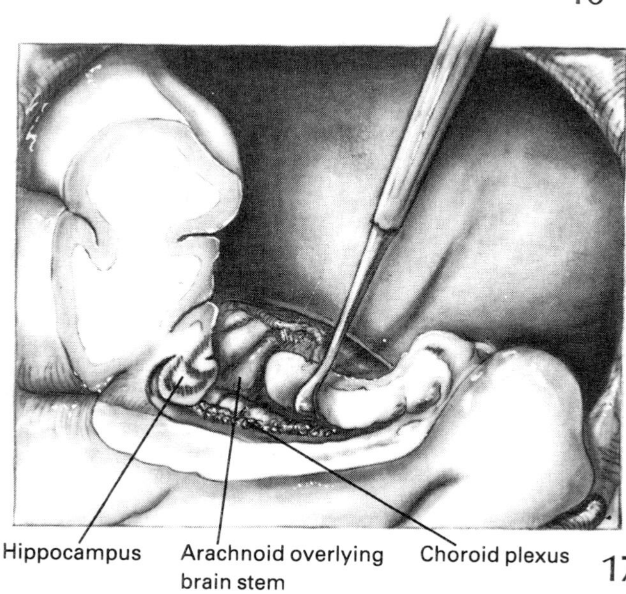

17

# Section of the corpus callosum for generalized seizures

Those who have studied human epilepsy with indwelling recording electrodes have observed localized electrical seizure discharges unaccompanied by clinical manifestations. Such abnormal discharges occur in presumably functionally silent areas of the brain, and a clinical seizure only becomes manifest if the electrical discharge invades a critical region (e.g. motor cortex or language area). The finding suggests that an alternative method of dealing with drug-resistant epilepsies might be the interruption of paths of preferential spread of seizure discharge. Such an approach is especially useful in those patients with intractable generalized seizures in whom an epileptogenic focus cannot be demonstrated or is ill-defined, or in in-patients with focal seizures that become generalized, but in whom the focus is located in a vital area where an operative resection risks the production of an unacceptable neurological deficit.

This is the rationale that prompted Van Wagenen and Heren in 1940[16] and later others[17-20] to carry out various degrees and combinations of sections of the cerebral commissures (i.e. corpus callosum, fornix, anterior commissure) for generalized convulsions. The early results suggested that commissurotomy produced a significant reduction in seizure frequency in some patients. Also important was that the ultimate neurological impairment produced by the procedures was relatively minor[21]. The deficits were usually revealed only by psychological testing and did not affect routine daily living. An example is the inability of blindfolded, right-handed subjects to name objects placed in the left hand. Information regarding size, shape and texture of the object felt with that hand is registered in the right hemisphere. The commissurotomy prevents such information from being transferred to the dominant hemisphere, a prerequisite for verbal recognition of the object held. Nevertheless, until the last decade commissurotomy was performed infrequently. Generally, it was not accepted that commissurotomy was a practical therapeutic alternative for the surgical treatment of epilepsy, and although patients could ultimately make a good neurological recovery, the early postoperative morbidity was substantial, and the time of convalescence long. Hemiparesis or ataxia of the left limbs, mutism, confusion and apathy were common findings in the postoperative period.

It was the observations of Wilson and collaborators[20,22] that sparked the current increased usage of commissurotomy. His results and those accumulating from others[23] demonstrate that only the corpus callosum needs to be divided and, in many, an anterior section sparing the splenium is just as effective as is a total section in controlling generalized seizures. Of particular importance is the demonstration that the procedure was especially effective in controlling drop attacks. Also, the early postoperative morbidity is significantly reduced and the convalescence shortened, although the transient postoperative neurological deficits mentioned above still occur in lesser and varying degrees. Wilson attributed the smoother postoperative course following limited callosal section to the use of microsurgical technique, and to not entering the lateral ventricle by leaving its ependymal lining intact. The relative importance of these latter methods in affecting the postoperative course, however, is questionable.

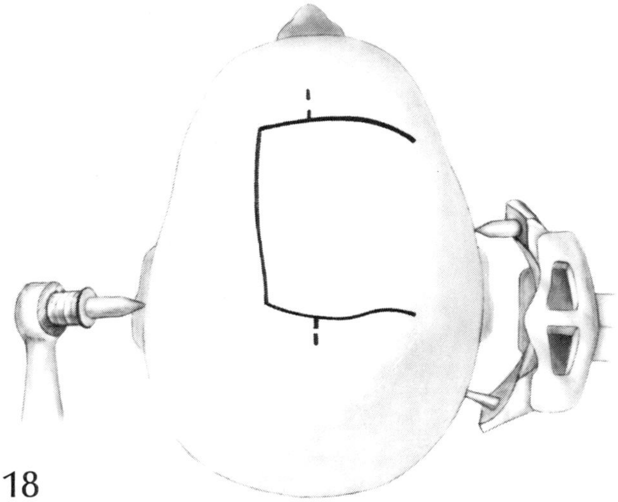

18

## ANTERIOR CALLOSTOMY

We stage our callosal section, not to reduce postoperative morbidity, but because in most patients anterior callostomy sparing the splenium has controlled the seizures. Also, there is evidence that preservation of the splenium prevents the disconnection symptoms seen after total callosal section[24]. Only if anterior callostomy fails to control the seizures do we divide the splenium at a second stage.

## 18

The procedure is performed under general endotracheal anaesthesia. The patient is placed in the supine position with the back elevated 30°, and the head straight, moderately flexed and secured with skeletal fixation in a Mayfield head holder. A U-shaped scalp flap is fashioned high in the right frontoparietal area. It extends about 3 cm across the midline with its base on the right side about 6 cm from the midline. The anterior limb is just behind the hairline and about 9 cm anterior to the posterior limb.

# 19

The pericranium is stripped from the cranium and a free bone flap elevated. This is accomplished usually with four burr holes – one at each corner of the exposure. Prior to using the craniotome to remove the bone flap, the dura is carefully separated from the cranium overlying the sagittal sinus. This is accomplished by inserting a staphylorrhaphy or similar instrument through the left-sided burr holes.

If the dura cannot be readily separated, then two additional burr holes are made about 1 cm to the right of the midline, opposite the left-sided burr holes, and the separation of the dura and sinus is completed from the right side. The dura is opened as a U-shaped flap and reflected on a medial hinge at the falx. Adhesions between the arachnoid and dura are coagulated and divided to permit access to the callosum through the longitudinal fissure. Usually an anterior bridging vein has to be coagulated and divided. Posterior bridging veins are preserved and access to the corpus callosum is gained by working on either side of them. Loupe magnification is used to expose the callosum. The medial surface of the hemisphere is easily separated from the falx down to the cingulate gyri. Separating these gyri presents varying degrees of difficulty due to adhesions. In some cases there are areas where the gyri are inseparable, and in these situations we perform a subpial dissection of the right cingulate gyrus to separate the gyri and expose the callosum.

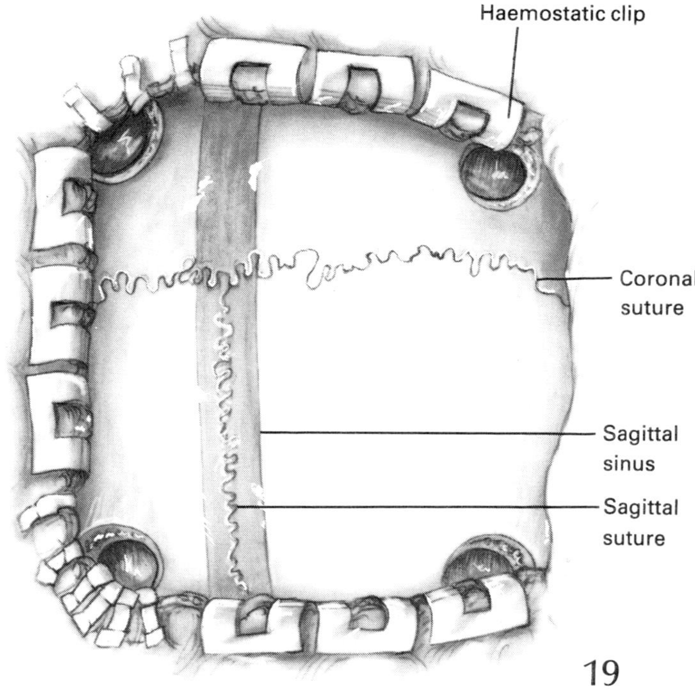


19

# 20

The pericallosal vessels are identified. Their courses meander to differing extents; in some cases the right pericallosal vessel runs for varying distances on the left and vice versa. From this point on we use about 10 × magnification. The vessels are freed up and mobilized out of the way.

Using bipolar coagulation and suction through a small tip (No. 5) the corpus callosum is divided back to the splenium. The callosal vessels are trivial and present no problem.

20

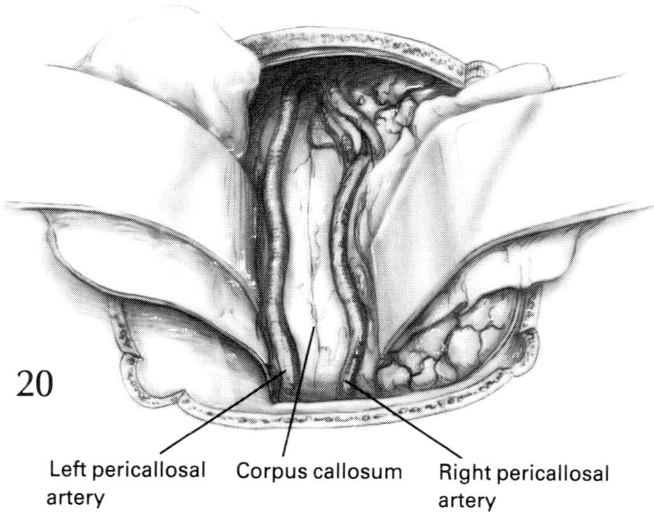

21

Complete section of the genu is accomplished by exposing and following the anterior bend of the pericallosal vessels around the genu.

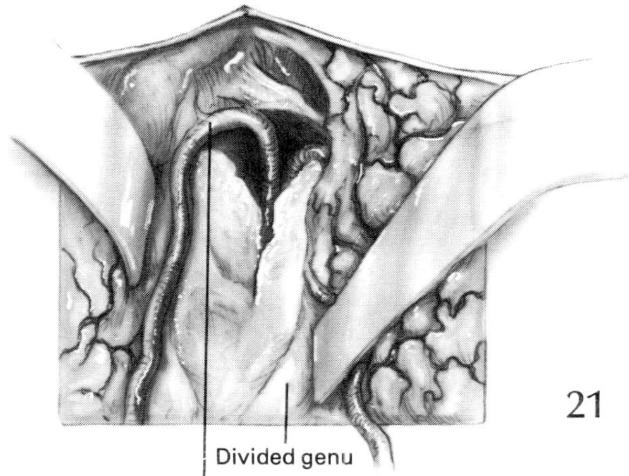


21

We make some effort to preserve the ependyma and try to avoid opening the ventricle, but are not compulsive about this. We are not convinced that just opening the ventricle adds any more morbidity than opening the temporal horn when performing an anterior temporal lobectomy. We believe that the morbidity which has been attributed to opening the ventricle[22] was in some cases related to the intraventricular manipulation which occurred in gaining access to the fornix and anterior commissure. It is undesirable, however, to open the ventricle when these are enlarged. In such cases the ventricular enlargement may represent arrested hydrocephalus, and a subdural hygroma may occur if the ventricle is opened.

Following section of the anterior corpus callosum, routine closure is carried out. Postoperative management with anticonvulsant medication, antibiotics and steroids is similar to that for patients undergoing craniotomy for simple and complex partial seizures.

## Results

In a multicentre review of callosal section[23], it was concluded that the procedure eliminates drop attacks and generalized tonic–clonic seizures in the majority of patients. The patients continue to have partial seizures, with the frequency being reduced in many although increased in some.

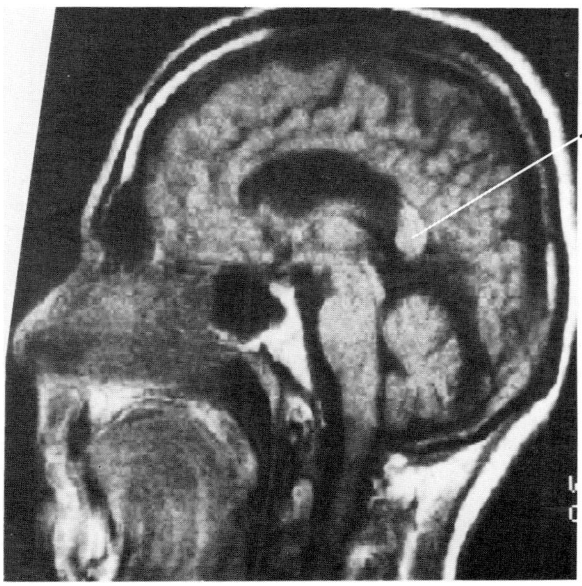


22

22

We have carried out callosal section in eleven patients (anterior section in nine, total section in two). Nine of these patients, who suffered from drop attacks, have been followed-up for 1 year or more. Seven have had good results. The drop attacks have been eliminated in six and markedly reduced in the seventh patient, but all continue to have partial seizures. None has incurred any permanent neurological complication.

## Acknowledgements

Illustrations 4–10 have been modified with permission from Surgical Treatment of the Epilepsies, ed. Jerome Engel, Jr, Raven Press, New York.

I am grateful to Ludwig Kempe MD for drawings of Illustrations 14–17 depicting the procedure of anterior temporal lobectomy. The technical help of Isaac Edwards, Gary Harding and Karl Probst is also gratefully acknowledged.

This work was supported in part by NINCDS Grant 2 P01 NS 1483407.


## References


1. Ward, A. A. Jr. (1983) In: Ward, A. A., Penry, J. K., Purpura, D. P. (eds.) Epilepsy. Research Publications: Association for Research in Nervous and Mental Disease, 61, 371–390. New York: Raven Press
2. Engel, J. Jr., Brown, W. J., Kuhl, D. E., Phelps, M. E., Mazziotta, J. C., Crandall, P. H. (1982) Pathological findings underlying focal temporal lobe hypometabolism in partial epilepsy. Annals of Neurology, 12, 518–528
3. Branch, C., Milner, B., Rasmussen, T. (1964) Intracarotid sodium amytal for the lateralization of cerebral speech dominance: observations in 123 patients. Journal of Neurosurgery, 21, 399–405
4. Milner, B. (1975) Psychological aspects of focal epilepsy and its neurosurgical management. In: Purpura, D. P., Penry, J. K., Walter, R. D. (eds.) Neurosurgical management of the epilepsies. Advances in Neurology, 8, 299–321. New York: Raven Press
5. Penfield, W., Jasper, H. H. (1954) Epilepsy and the functional anatomy of the human brain. Boston: Little, Brown & Co.
6. Goldring, S. (1978) A method for surgical management of focal epilepsy, especially as it relates to children. Journal of Neurosurgery, 49, 344–356
7. Crandall, P. H. (1973) Developments in direct recordings from epileptogenic regions in the surgical treatment of partial epilepsies. In: Epilepsy: Its Phenomena in Man, Brazier, M. A. B. (ed.), pp. 287–310. New York, London: Academic Press
8. Talairach, J., Bancaud, J. (1966) Lesion, 'irritative' zone and epileptogenic focus. Confinia Neurologica, 27, 91–94
9. Stohr, P. E., Goldring, S. (1969) Origin of somatosensory evoked scalp responses in man. Journal of Neurosurgery, 31, 117–127
10. Goldring, S., Aras, E., Weber, P. C. (1970) Comparative study of sensory input to motor cortex in animals and man. Electroencephalography and Clinical Neurophysiology, 29, 537–550
11. Goldring, S., Gregorie, E. M. (1984) Surgical management of epilepsy using epidural recordings to localize the seizure focus: a review of 100 cases. Journal of Neurosurgery, 60, 457–466
12. Goldring, S. (1987) Surgical management of epilepsy in children. In: Surgical Treatment of the Epilepsies, Engel, J. Jr, (ed.), pp. 445–464. New York: Raven Press
13. Goldring, S., Gregorie, E. M., Picker, S. (1987) Placement of epidural grid electrodes at Washington University Medical Center, St. Louis. In: Surgical Treatment of the Epilepsies, Engel, J. Jr, (ed.), pp. 629–634. New York: Raven Press
14. Lueders, H., Lesser, R. P., Hahn, J., Dinner, D. S., Klem, G. (1983) Cortical somatosensory evoked potentials in response to hand stimulation. Journal of Neurosurgery, 58, 885–894
15. Jasper, H. (1983) Epilogue. In: Ward, A. A., Penry, J. K., Purpura, D. P. (eds.). Epilepsy. Research Publications: Association for Research in Nervous and Mental Disease, 61, 391–393. New York: Raven Press
16. Van Wagenen, W. P., Heren, R. Y. (1940) Surgical division of commissural pathways in the corpus callosum: relationship to spread of an epileptic attack. Archives of Neurology and Psychiatry, 44, 740–759
17. Bogen, J. E., Vogel, P. J. (1962) Cerebral commissurotomy in man: preliminary case report. Bulletin of the Los Angeles Neurological Society, 27, 169–172
18. Bogen, J. E., Vogel, P. J. (1975) Neurologic status in the long term following complete cerebral commissurotomy. In: Les Syndromes de Disconnexion Calleuse ches l'Homme, Michel, F., Schott, B. (ed.), p. 227. Lyon: Hôpital Neurologique
19. Luessenhop, A. J., dela Cruz, T. C., Fenichel, G. M. (1970) Surgical disconnection of the cerebral hemispheres for intractable seizures. Journal of the American Medical Association, 213, 1630–1636
20. Wilson, D. H., Reeves, A., Gazzaniga, M., Culver, C. (1977) Cerebral commissurotomy for control of intractable seizures. Neurology, 27, 708–715
21. Akelaitis, A. J. (1944) A study of gnosis, praxis and language following section of the corpus callosum and anterior commissure. Journal of Neurosurgery, 1, 94–102
22. Wilson, D. H., Reeves, A. G., Gazzaniga, M. S. (1982) 'Central' commissurotomy for intractable generalized epilepsy: Series two. Neurology, 32, 687–697
23. Spencer, S. S., Gates, J. R., Reeves, A. R., Spencer, D. D., Maxwell, R. E., Roberts, D. (1987) Corpus callosum section. In: Surgical Treatment of the Epilepsies, Engel, J. Jr, (ed.), pp. 425–444. New York: Raven Press
24. Gordon, H. W., Bogen, J. E., Sperry, R. W. (1971) Absence of deconnexion syndrome in two patients with partial section of the neocommissures. Brain, 94, 327–336

Illustrations by Barbara Hyams

# Posterior fossa approach for trigeminal neuralgia

**R. D. Illingworth** FRCS
Consultant Neurosurgeon, Regional Neurosciences Centre, Charing Cross Hospital, London;
Honorary Consultant Neurosurgeon, Westminster and Central Middlesex Hospitals, London, UK

## Introduction

In the last 20 years there have been three major advances in the management of trigeminal neuralgia. The first was the introduction of carbamazepine, which provided for the first time an effective medical treatment; the second was the refinement of the technique of percutaneous radiofrequency thermocoagulation which allowed localized differential lesions to be produced in the posterior trigeminal root without significant risk; and the third was the development of a surgical operation, microvascular decompression, from Dandy's posterior fossa approach[1] which now treats what appears to be a major factor in the cause of most cases of trigeminal neuralgia.

Dandy's original operation was a fractional prepontine section, which he believed would avoid dysaesthesiae and keratitis[1]. Later, in 1934, he described anatomical and pathological structures which he found impinging on the posterior trigeminal root in 60 per cent of 215 patients with trigeminal neuralgia, and suggested that these were the cause of the condition[2]. He never attempted to treat trigeminal neuralgia by relieving the nerve of this compression and this appears to have been performed first by Gardner and Miklos in 1959[3]. Since 1967 the operation of posterior fossa microvascular decompression has been developed and documented in a number of series, notably by Jannetta[4] and Apfelbaum[5].

The operative findings in these large series (totalling over 600 patients) are remarkably consistent, and similar compression of the trigeminal nerve has only rarely been found in cadavers without a prior history of trigeminal neuralgia[6]. The evidence, which is discussed in detail elsewhere[7], supports the view that a local lesion affects the posterior root in virtually all cases of apparently idiopathic trigeminal neuralgia.

## Indications for operation and choice of procedure

Carbamazepine is so effective that most patients will choose medical management initially. Surgery tends to be considered only if carbamazepine causes unacceptable side-effects or fails to provide adequate relief.

Percutaneous radiofrequency thermocoagulation is so safe and so controllable that it should replace the open middle fossa and posterior fossa section operations. Peripheral procedures including cryosurgery usually give only temporary relief but may still be useful in the elderly and in the rare patients with ophthalmic pain. Despite the safety of radiofrequency thermocoagulation there are significant drawbacks to the procedure since, in common with all destructive methods, there is a risk of causing unpleasant sensory symptoms, and occasionally anaesthesia dolorosa or keratitis. Between 15 and 37 per cent of patients develop unpleasant numbness or paraesthesia[8,9], and anaesthesia dolorosa can occur in up to 3 per cent[10]. If the risk of these problems is minimized by producing less sensory loss, the penalty is an increased relapse rate[11].

Microvascular decompression offers the prospect of permanent relief of symptoms, with a relapse rate of 10–20 per cent. It should produce no sensory loss and hence avoid dysaesthesiae and keratitis, but is a major procedure which carries some risk and may result in damage to other cranial nerves. The choice patients face when medical management fails is therefore between a safe, destructive method with risk of dysaesthesiae and relapse, and a major surgical operation with some risk of morbidity and mortality. Many patients with trigeminal neuralgia are elderly and often unfit, and for these, and those who are not worried about sensory loss and its possible consequences, radiofrequency thermocoagulation is the procedure of choice. In general, microvascular decompression is suitable for younger, fit patients who are not fearful of operation and who wish to avoid sensory loss. No upper age limit for the operation is suggested, but 70 years in a fit normotensive patient is not too old. Clearly, one procedure will not suit everyone and patients should be able, with medical advice, to choose what is appropriate. The author has therefore prepared a leaflet which explains in simple terms the condition of trigeminal neuralgia, and describes the operations of radiofrequency thermocoagulation and microvascular decompression, and their advantages and disadvantages. All patients considering operation are given this leaflet to take home and are asked to read it at leisure before deciding which operation to have.

It should be emphasized that the operation of microvascular decompression requires some expertise in microsurgical technique in the posterior cranial fossa.

# Preoperative

Careful evaluation of the presenting symptoms is essential since the procedure to be described is only suitable for patients with trigeminal neuralgia. The characteristics and distribution of the pain should be typical and, although many patients will have no clinical signs of impairment of trigeminal nerve function, careful testing may disclose minor subjective differences in sensation or in the corneal reflex between the two sides.

Preoperative investigation includes computerized tomography with enhancement to reduce the risk of unexpected discovery of a tumour, large aneurysm or arteriovenous malformation. Vertebral angiography is not performed routinely. It will always show arteries in the region of the trigeminal nerve but only at operation can the precise anatomical relationships be identified, and the investigation does not provide sufficient useful information to influence the choice of procedure or to justify the slight risk involved.

The patient's general medical state, and in particular the cardiovascular state, should be assessed to detect myocardial ischaemia or arterial hypertension, which may be contraindications to this procedure. Other preparation is as performed routinely for major surgery, but cross-matched blood is not required.

Dexamethasone 4 mg 6-hourly is started 24 hours before operation and continued in reducing dose for several days after. Anaesthesia with moderate hyperventilation to produce an arterial $P_{CO_2}$ of about 30 mmHg (4.0 kPa) is used, but hypotension is not required and should be avoided in older patients.

## Instrumentation

The operating microscope with a 300 mm objective lens and inclined eye pieces is used. A self-retaining cerebellar retractor with a narrow blade is essential to allow the surgeon to use both hands for dissection. Fine suckers operating with gentle suction, bayonet-handled microscissors, and a set of fine dissecting instruments are needed. The set of instruments devised by Jannetta (American V. Mueller) is ideal. The most useful of these is a fine blunt hook with the hook end at 135° to the line of the shaft, which is slightly bent. To avoid snagging important structures during the deeper part of the dissection, right-angled blunt hooks should not be used.

## Position of patient

The lateral position is preferred for this procedure. It allows easy access to the cerebellopontine angle and is free of the risk of air embolism. In the lateral position the cerebellum tends to be rather full, but once CSF has been drained, the fifth nerve can be exposed with minimal cerebellar retraction. Apfelbaum[5] prefers the semi-sitting position, arguing that this gives the best access and allows CSF and blood to drain, and that the risk of air embolism can be minimized by ventilating the patient and using the Doppler detector. In practice, when the lateral position is used, sufficient CSF is easily drained by lumbar puncture, and intradural bleeding in any case should be minimal. Patients, particularly older ones, appear to have a smoother postoperative course when operated on in the lateral rather than the sitting position. The transtentorial approach seems to have no surgical advantages and carries the risk of producing neurological disturbance or epilepsy from retraction of the cerebral hemisphere.

# 1

The patient is placed on the operating table with the side to be operated on uppermost and the lateral popliteal and circumflex nerves protected by padding. A small, firm pad under the upper chest lifts the weight of the trunk off the lower arm. The trunk is stabilized on the table with two strips of adhesive tape passed across the shoulder and across the pelvis, and the upper shoulder is drawn slightly downwards by a further strip of tape. The operating table is tipped about 5° head-up. A lumbar puncture is now performed and a drainage system is set up but left closed.

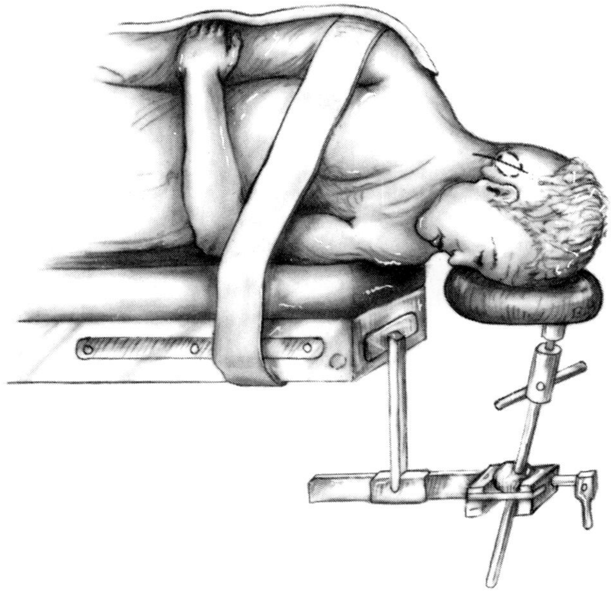

1

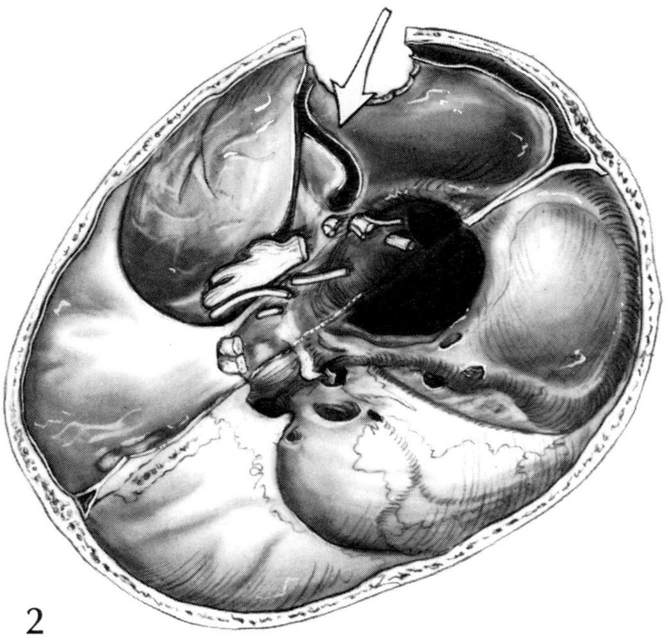

2

# 2

The position of the patient's head in relation to the trunk and the surgeon's line of vision is critical. The line of exposure is through a narrow triangular tunnel formed by the posterior surface of the petrous bone on one side, the retracted cerebellum on the other, and the inferior surface of the tentorium towards the surgeon. This tunnel should run approximately vertically, and certainly not be inclined at all towards the patient's feet. Turning the patient's head so that it faces approximately 45° towards the floor will bring the posterior surface of the petrous bone into the vertical. The neck must be flexed laterally about 15° to make the inferior surface of the tentorium vertical. When the microscope with angled eye pieces is used, this position allows the fifth nerve to be exposed easily, with little cerebellar retraction, and the surgeon to work in a comfortable posture.

# The operation

## The incision

### 3

After routine skin preparation the incision is marked and the head towelled. A straight incision about 8 cm long is marked one-third above and two-thirds below the superior nuchal line (or one-third below and two-thirds above the tip of the mastoid process) and about 1–2 cm behind the posterior margin of the mastoid process. (This and all subsequent illustrations are as seen by the surgeon exposing the right fifth nerve.) Accurate placement of the incision is important to allow the craniectomy to be precisely sited.

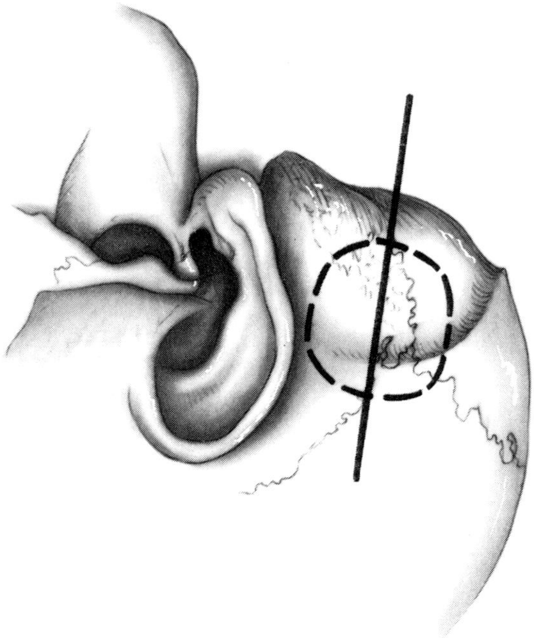

3

### 4

The incision is made, and the muscles are divided in the line of their fibres down to the occipital bone, freed from the bone and retracted. Some sharp dissection or use of cutting diathermy will be needed to free the muscles from the superior nuchal line. The muscles must be freed and retracted anteriorly up to the back of the mastoid process. The muscle incision need not be carried down to the arch of the atlas and care should be taken that this is not done inadvertently in case the vertebral artery is damaged. A suitable muscle retractor is placed at this point: the Apfelbaum self-retaining cerebellar retractor (Codman) is ideal. The retractor blades are opened widely and its handles fixed to the towels with a length of cotton gauze and a towel clip to ensure stable fixation and allow a cerebellar retractor to be safely attached.

A burr hole is made on the asterion where the temporal, occipital and parietal bones meet. Ideally the burr hole will expose the transverse sinus and thus define the upper limit of the craniectomy. Bone is rongeured away to produce a defect 3.5–4.0 cm in diameter which must expose the transverse sinus superiorly and the sigmoid sinus anteriorly. This is essential to allow the exposure to be made with minimal cerebellar retraction. Mastoid air cells are usually opened when the craniectomy is made, and these must be carefully sealed with bone wax to prevent CSF leakage into the middle ear. The bone is usually thin over the cerebellum but much thicker over the sinuses and at the back of the mastoid. Occasionally the bone may be so thick anteriorly that it cannot be removed with rongeurs and a high-speed drill will be required. Failure to remove bone to expose the junction of transverse and sigmoid sinuses will severely impair access, and if it is found when the dura is opened that the sinus has not been exposed, it is worth going back and removing more bone. Once bone removal has been completed, all extradural bleeding is meticulously stopped. Failure to carry out this simple step may result in the deeper part of the dissection, which should be bloodless, being obscured by blood trickling in.

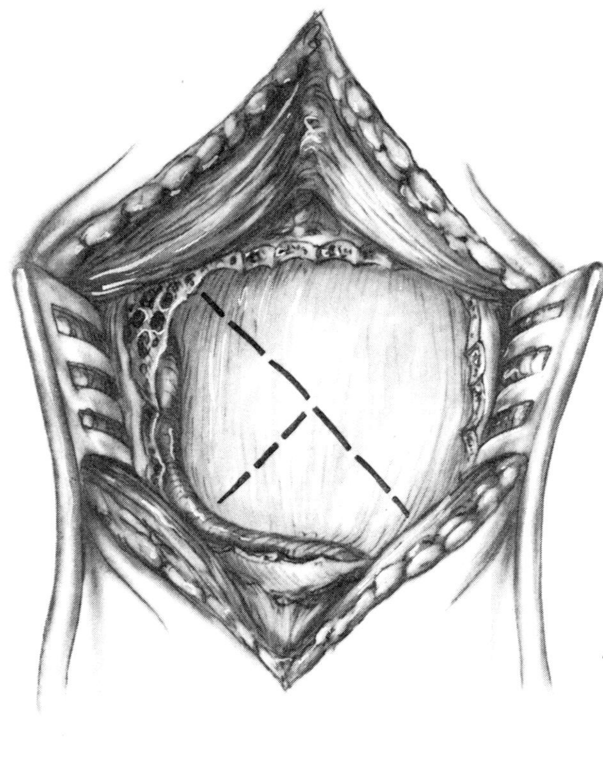

4

At this point the dura is usually fairly full, and the lumbar CSF drain should be opened. The release of approximately 20–30 ml of CSF will relax the dura, which is now opened with an inverted Y-shaped incision and retracted with sutures to allow maximal exposure in the upper anterior part.

# 5

The microscope is now brought into use and the cerebellum lightly retracted with a 6 mm wide, slightly curved retractor blade. The tension in the Apfelbaum flexible arm is adjusted so that the retractor will maintain its position but can be easily moved by hand without re-tensioning being needed. The retractor blade is placed on the upper anterior corner of the cerebellum, which is protected by cottonoid strips. This opens the triangular tunnel between the back of the petrous bone, the undersurface of the tentorium and the retracted cerebellum. If the retractor is placed lower down on the cerebellum it will be nearer to the seventh and eighth cranial nerves and can produce traction on these nerves and cause permanent damage. The eighth nerve appears to be particularly vulnerable from axial traction. If the head has been correctly positioned with some lateral flexion of the neck, the seventh and eighth nerves will not be in the line of the exposure. A short length of these nerves will usually be visible as they pass between the internal auditory meatus and the cerebellum, but they need not be exposed or dissected any further.

The cerebellum is gently retracted and further CSF aspirated as the triangular tunnel is opened deeper. Usually a few small veins or arachnoid strands will be found passing across the space and these should be coagulated with bipolar diathermy and divided. Occasionally a small vein running from the top of the cerebellum to the tentorium may be detached, and any venous bleeding at this point must be controlled before the dissection proceeds further. In the depths of the wound the petropontine vein is now usually seen surrounded by arachnoid.

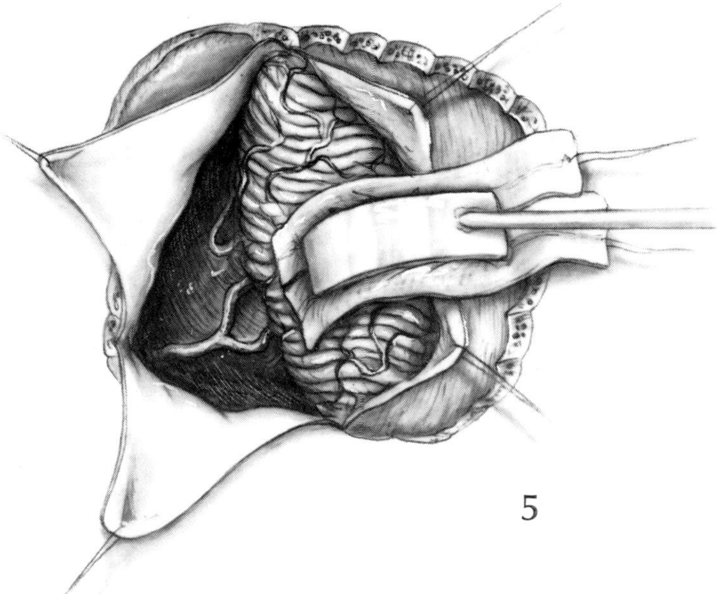

5

## Division of petropontine vein (petrosal vein)

This usually passes from the cerebellum to the tentorium just behind the point where the tentorium meets the petrous bone. Two limbs from the cerebellum, sometimes three, join to make a trunk just a few millimetres long. The vein is usually found a few millimetres superficial to the fifth nerve but may be right on the nerve and compressing it, or may not be present at all. The vein must be coagulated and divided to allow the nerve to be exposed and this manoeuvre occasionally gives rise to problems. The vein is surrounded by arachnoid, which must be opened to allow the vein and its branches to be seen fully. The arachnoid is usually thin but may be thick and require sharp dissection. Once defined, the vein is coagulated with bipolar diathermy and divided with fine scissors. Even if it appears to be occluded by the diathermy, it is best to divide it partially at first and only complete the section if no bleeding occurs. Once divided, the cerebellar end of the vein tends to retract and if not completely sealed may be difficult to pick up again. A more serious problem may occur if the main stem of the vein becomes detached from the tentorium before it has been coagulated and divided. This can happen fairly easily since the vein is thin-walled and runs a very short course. Either cerebellar retraction or closing the diathermy forceps on the vein may result in a little bleeding from the junction with the tentorium. As the coagulation shrinks the vein, the bleeding will increase and a fairly brisk venous haemorrhage can result. The problem is best handled by using a fine sucker over the bleeding to keep the field clear while the vein is dissected and divided. Bipolar diathermy will stop the bleeding from the cerebellar end, and bleeding from the tentorial end is usually easily controlled with bipolar diathermy once the vein has been divided if there is a little stump, or by monopolar diathermy if this is not the case. Care must be taken that any monopolar diathermy is applied very precisely, to avoid damage to the fourth and fifth nerves. Once the petropontine vein has been divided, the cerebellar retractor blade can be advanced and the fifth nerve exposed.

## Dissection of fifth cranial nerve

The nerve is surrounded by arachnoid and this needs to be opened before the nerve can be fully seen. If thin, the arachnoid can be opened by gentle dissection with fine hooks but no tugging should be used, as this can cause bleeding or damage to the fourth cranial nerve. This nerve runs just above, medial and parallel to the upper border of the fifth nerve and is usually close to the edge of the tentorium and a little distance from the fifth nerve. Sometimes it is very close, held by arachnoid bands or displaced by blood vessels, and great care must be taken to avoid damage. Sharp dissection should be with fine scissors, the points of which must always be kept in view to avoid injury to the structures present in this area. Further CSF is aspirated as dissection proceeds, and every effort should be made to avoid bleeding, since even minor bleeding at this stage will stain the arachnoid and render recognition of the detail more difficult.

## 6

The fifth nerve must be exposed up to its point of entry into the pons since this is the area where the significant findings lie. The nerve reaches the side of the pons obliquely and the lateral side of the nerve follows almost the same line as the lateral side of the pons. The precise point of entry may therefore not be clear initially, but by observing the upper and lower margins of the nerve the point can be defined. Once the arachnoid has been opened up to the root entry zone and the cerebellum retracted sufficiently, the relevant anatomical findings are seen. The commonest is that the superior cerebellar artery makes a downward loop as it comes around the brainstem from deeply. The loop passes from above the nerve downwards, medial to the nerve, and then loops back upwards again to pass above the nerve as it enters the side of the pons. The nerve may be widened or kinked laterally at this point, as it is compressed from the medial side. The downward loop may be quite shallow and pass almost along the upper border of the nerve, or loop down as low as the seventh and eighth nerves.

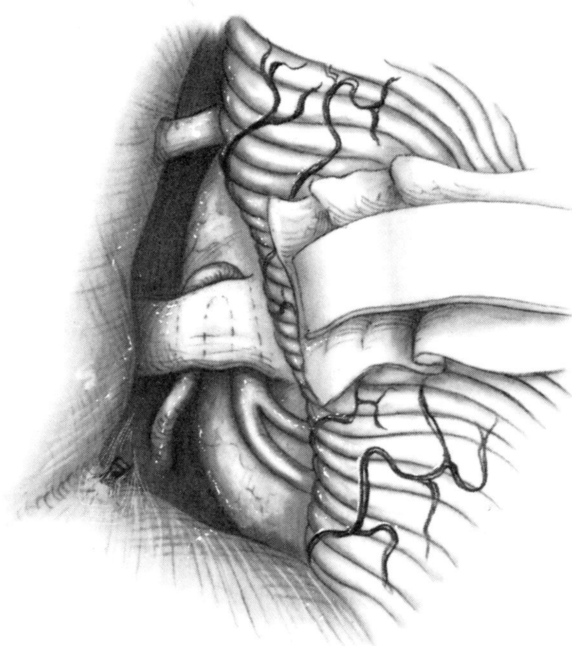

6

The findings may not be immediately apparent since the proximal part of the artery may lie entirely medial to the nerve in the exposure, or may lie so deeply in the field that it is covered by CSF or outside the depth of field of the microscope. The artery may also not be seen at the distal end if the nerve is not exposed right up to the pons. It is emphasized that the relevant findings are only those at the point where the nerve enters the pons and that this area must be adequately exposed. The superior cerebellar artery often divides into two branches which run together backwards at this point, and cross-compression of the nerve may occur from one or both of these branches, which are occasionally widely separated. It is important to look carefully for such double compression. Occasionally the nerve is cross-compressed by an arterial loop from below or from laterally. A vein may pass across the nerve, grooving it at the pons, or pass through the nerve, and combined compression from an artery and a vein may also be present. Compression may occur from medially or inferiorly by grossly ectatic vertebral or basilar arteries. The point of compression on the nerve does not appear to be related to the distribution of trigeminal neuralgia on the face.

Arterial compression has been found in 59 per cent of patients, combined arterial and venous compression in 23 per cent[4], and arterial compression with or without venous compression in 80 per cent[5]. Compression by veins alone is found in about 12–14 per cent and by clinically unsuspected tumours in about 3–3.6 per cent[4,5]. If nothing is found, the surgeon should consider whether the exposure and dissection are adequate or whether retraction of the cerebellum may have altered the anatomical relationships in the exposure.

## Decompression

# 7 & 8

If the nerve has been compressed by the superior cerebellar artery from medially, decompression is achieved by lifting the downward loop out from medial to the nerve and placing it above and lateral. The artery may loop deeply medial to the nerve but can be displaced upwards and laterally by gentle dissection with two angled blunt hooks around the convex side of the loop. No branches should run off on this side but arachnoid strands and small veins may be encountered and these may need to be divided.

Great care should be taken that no artery, however small, is damaged or coagulated with diathermy, and that the artery in its new position is not kinked. Some adjustment may be necessary to achieve this.

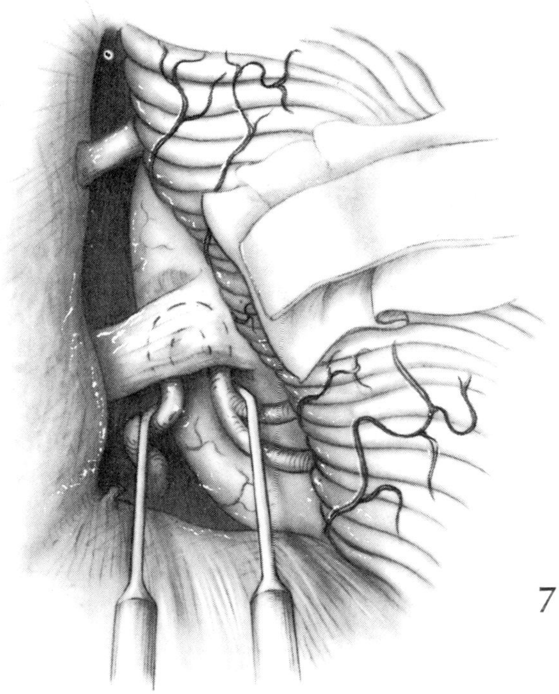

7

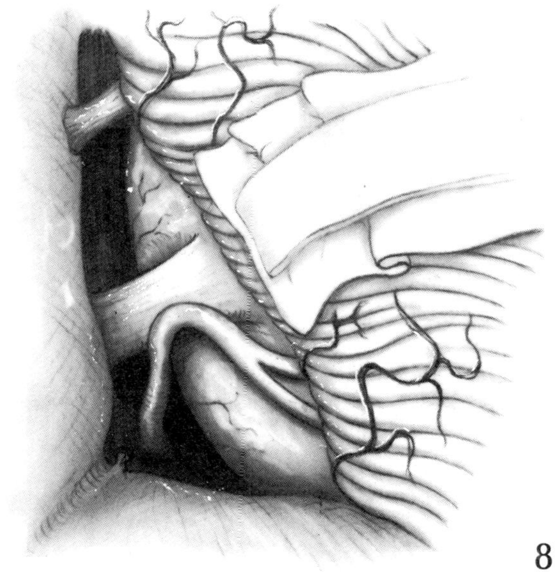

8

# 9 & 10

Once the artery has been displaced laterally or above the nerve, a small permanent implant needs to be inserted to prevent renewed contact with the nerve at the root entry zone. Non-absorbable material must be used for this, and gel sponge and muscle are not adequate. Shredded PTFE[4], or Ivalon sponge (Unipoint Laboratories, Highpoint, North Carolina, USA) carved to fit between the artery and nerve[5] have been recommended to hold the artery away from the nerve. The author uses cotton ribbon gauze or cottonoid. A single piece 10 mm × 5 mm, often folded double and placed between the artery and nerve or between the artery and the brainstem is usually sufficient. Cotton gauze is soft and pliant when wet and conforms well to the surfaces of contact, and adheres sufficiently not to be easily displaced. Alternatively, the artery can be held up against the tentorium and away from the nerve with a small piece of gauze or cottonoid looped around the artery. The ends are then placed up against the tentorium. Pieces of oxidized cellulose (Surgicel, Ethicon, UK) are placed over the gauze to hold it in place until it adheres, and to keep the artery away from the nerve until this occurs. This method is now preferred. Veins compressing the nerve are coagulated with bipolar diathermy and divided.

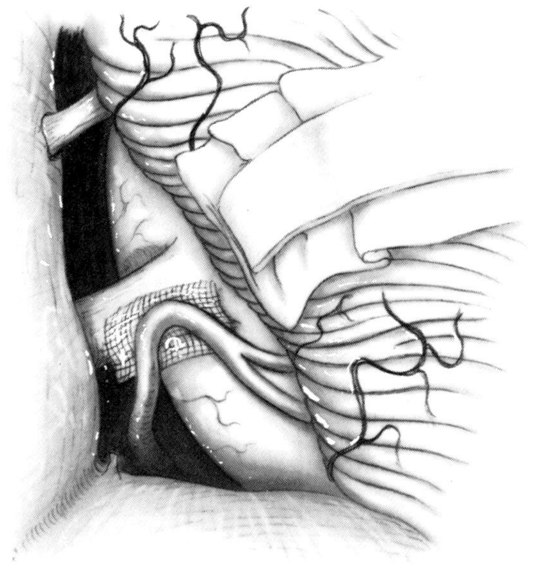

9

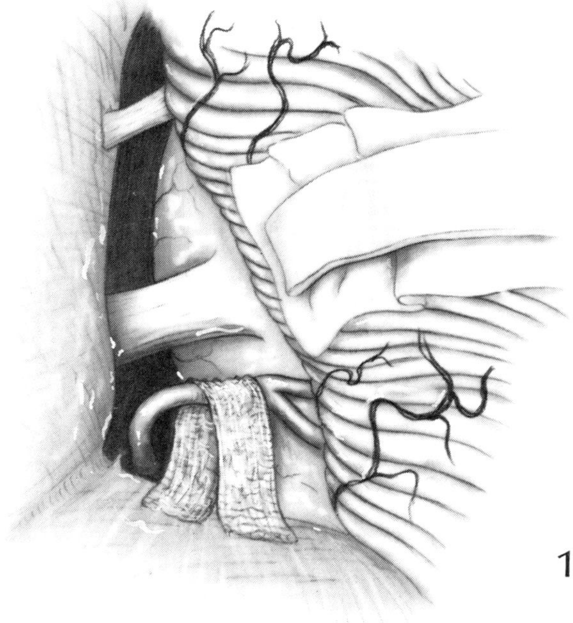

10

## Nerve section

When operating on earlier cases, the author did not always find compression of the nerve and was in any case initially uncertain of its significance. Because of this, a number of patients underwent fractional fifth nerve section with preservation of the intermediate fibres and the motor root which lie medially. All 25 of these patients obtained satisfactory relief of trigeminal neuralgia from this operation and in 15 there was marked dissociation of sensory loss with preservation of light touch sensation[12]. Some patients with larger sections and more sensory loss have been troubled by unpleasant dysaesthesiae. The author now feels that elective posterior fossa fifth nerve section has been superseded by the easier and safer procedure of percutaneous radiofrequency thermocoagulation and that posterior fossa approaches for trigeminal neuralgia should be used only where microvascular decompression is the aim, or in the rare instances of bilateral trigeminal neuralgia where preservation of the motor root is important.

## Closure

Before closure the blood pressure, if it has fallen, is restored to normal and the venous pressure raised to check haemostasis. The subarachnoid space is filled with saline and the dura closed with interrupted sutures to make as water-tight a closure as possible. The muscles are closed in three layers in the deep inferior part and with one layer in the upper part. The subcutaneous tissues are closed with interrupted sutures and the skin with staples. No drain is used.

## Postoperative management

Patients are nursed lying down until the next day. The incision is painful for the first 24 hours, but codeine phosphate provides adequate relief. Patients often complain of headache and nausea, but this rarely lasts longer than 24 hours although occasionally nausea may persist for several days. The dose of dexamethasone is progressively reduced and stopped after 3 days. The day after operation patients can begin to drink and then eat unless nausea persists. Patients sit out of bed on the second postoperative day and are then progressively mobilized. Discharge from hospital depends on the patient's progress and home circumstances, but may be as early as the fifth postoperative day. Sutures are removed on the tenth postoperative day.

The pain of trigeminal neuralgia is usually relieved immediately after operation, but it may take a few days to die out and on rare occasions it persists for much longer. Carbamazepine should be continued for at least a few days and then discontinued. Patients should be warned that relief of pain is not always immediate, and it should not be assumed that the procedure has failed if pain persists.

## Results

The results of two large series have been published. In Jannetta's series[4] of 411 patients, 83.5 per cent obtained lasting relief (although 3.7 per cent required a repeat operation to achieve this), 9.3 per cent continued to have pain which could be controlled by carbamazepine, 4.1 per cent required a radiofrequency lesion for pain relief, and 1.2 per cent continued to have severe pain. The period of follow-up is not given.

In Apfelbaum's series[5] of 200 patients, initial pain relief was achieved in 93.4 per cent. Thereafter 71.2 per cent remained free of pain without medication, 20.1 per cent had pain controlled by carbamazepine, and 8.7 per cent had pain which could not be controlled by medical treatment. The follow-up in this series was 5 months to 5 years (mean 3 years). Most relapses occurred within 6 months of operation, and the pain in many patients could then be controlled by a smaller dose of carbamazepine than before operation.

No sensory symptoms are reported from either series, but the incidence of permanent disturbances of other cranial nerves was 5.6 per cent[4] and 4.5 per cent[5] respectively. The nerve usually involved is the eighth, but transient fourth and seventh nerve palsies have also been reported. Some major morbidity can occur from cerebral or cerebellar haemorrhage or infarction, and in one series[5] the incidence of transient cerebellar symptoms was 7 per cent. The reported mortality was 1.2 per cent[4] and 1.5 per cent[5] respectively. Not all results have been as good. For example, in a series of 52 patients, the incidence of permanent postoperative cranial nerve palsies was 27 per cent, and of transient palsies 31 per cent[13].

The author's published series of 39 patients with trigeminal neuralgia and glossopharyngeal neuralgia treated by microvascular decompression[14] has now increased to 59 (up to December 1985). Of these, 48 (81 per cent) have remained pain free and off all medication. There have been eight relapses (14 per cent) occurring at intervals between 2 months and 5 years (mean 25 months) after operation: two of these were very minor and no medication or other treatment was required; three remain pain free on a smaller dose of carbamazepine than previously; and the other three have had more serious pain requiring radiofrequency lesions for relief. In three patients (5 per cent) the operation failed to give relief of pain. One of these has been treated with a radiofrequency lesion and two remain on carbamazepine. As in other series, there have been some cranial nerve complications. Two patients have minor facial paraesthesiae which are not disturbing, and one is aware of some sensory loss. There has been one transient facial palsy, one transient fourth nerve palsy, and one delayed but permanent ipsilateral deafness. There have been no such complications in the last 20 patients, but one patient with glossopharyngeal neuralgia developed a purulent but sterile granuloma around the implanted cotton gauze. Reoperation to remove the gauze was followed by rapid neurological improvement without relapse of the neuralgia. There was no other morbidity and no mortality in this series. Follow-up is complete and extends from 9 years to 2 months (mean 32 months). Of the 19 patients followed for more than 4 years, 17 (89 per cent) have remained off medication and free from all pain.

When a relapse does not respond to medical treatment, radiofrequency thermocoagulation appears to be the treatment of choice. No information on the operative findings in patients who relapse and are re-explored appears to be available. It should be remembered that there is very little information on the long-term follow-up of patients treated by microvascular decompression. It appears that some may develop recurrent trigeminal neuralgia despite relief of vascular cross-compression and the reason for this is not clear. Surgeons performing the operation are encouraged to maintain all patients on long-term follow-up and report the results.

## *References*


1. Dandy, W. E. (1929) An operation for the cure of tic douloureux; partial section of the sensory root at the pons. Archives of Surgery, 18, 687–734

2. Dandy, W. E. (1934) Concerning the cause of trigeminal neuralgia. American Journal of Surgery, 24, 447–455

3. Gardner, W. J., Miklos, M. V. (1959) Response of trigeminal neuralgia to 'decompression' of sensory root: discussion of cause of trigeminal neuralgia. Journal of the American Medical Association, 170, 1773–1776

4. Jannetta, P. J. (1981) Vascular decompression in trigeminal neuralgia. In: The Cranial Nerves: anatomy, pathology, pathophysiology, diagnosis and treatment, M. Samii, P. J. Jannetta (eds), pp. 331–340. Berlin, Heidelberg, New York: Springer-Verlag

5. Apfelbaum, R. I. (1982) Microvascular decompression for tic douloureux: results. In: Neurological Surgery of the Ear and Skull Base, D. E. Brackmann (ed.), pp. 175–180. New York: Raven Press

6. Sunderland, S. (1948) Neurovascular relations and anomalies at the base of the brain. Journal of Neurology, Neurosurgery and Psychiatry, 11, 243–257

7. Illingworth, R. (1986) Trigeminal neuralgia: surgical aspects. In: Headache, F. Clifford Rose (ed.) Handbook of Clinical Neurology, review series 4, vol. 48, 449–458. Amsterdam, Elsevier Science Publishers

8. Tew, J. M. Jr, Keller, J. P. (1977) The treatment of trigeminal neuralgia by percutaneous radiofrequency technique. Clinical Neurology, 24, 557–578

9. Sweet, W. M. (1976) Treatment of facial pain by percutaneous differential thermal trigeminal rhizotomy. In: Progress in Neurological Surgery, H. Krayenbuhl, P. E. Mosper, W. H. Sweet (eds) 7, 153–179. Basel: S Kager

10. Siegfried, J. (1981) Percutaneous controlled thermocoagulation of Gasserian ganglion in trigeminal neuralgia. Experience with 1000 cases. In: The Cranial Nerves: anatomy, pathology, pathophysiology, diagnosis and treatment, M. Samii, P. J. Jannetta (eds) pp. 322–330. Berlin, Heidelberg, New York: Springer-Verlag

11. Latcham, J. P., Hardy, R. W., Forsythe, S. B., Cook, A. F. (1983) Trigeminal neuralgia treated by radiofrequency coagulation. Journal of Neurosurgery, 59, 479–484

12. Hussein, M., Wilson, L. A., Illingworth, R. (1982) Patterns of sensory loss following fractional posterior fossa Vth nerve section for trigeminal neuralgia. Journal of Neurology, Neurosurgery and Psychiatry, 45, 786–790

13. Breeze, R., Ignelzi, R. J. (1982) Microsurgical decompression for trigeminal neuralgia. Results with special reference to the late recurrence rate. Journal of Neurosurgery, 57, 487–490

14. Illingworth, R., Richards, P. (1984) Microvascular decompression: definitive surgical treatment without nerve section for trigeminal and glossopharyngeal neuralgias. Journal of Neurology, Neurosurgery and Psychiatry, 47, 1053–1054

Illustrations by R. N. Lane

# Percutaneous radiofrequency cordotomy

**Edward Hitchcock** ChM, FRCS
Professor and Head of Department of Neurosurgery, University of Birmingham, Birmingham, UK

In 1963 Mullan *et al.*[1] used a lateral percutaneous technique to place a strontium needle close to the anterior quadrant of the spinal cord between C1 and C2. This was soon replaced, in 1965, by electrolytic coagulation because of the unpredictable effects of the strontium needle method, which produced lesions of less controllable size.

Rosomoff[2] reported his experience with the radiofrequency method in 177 patients, in whom 268 procedures had been performed. The introduction of this relatively simple technique resulted in the open cordotomy procedure being virtually supplanted in many centres.

It is now realized, however, that percutaneous radiofrequency cordotomy is less benign than previously supposed. Lipton[3] noted that 10 per cent of his patients had severe postoperative weakness preventing weightbearing, although 80 per cent of these recovered after one month. Additional problems that many patients, particularly the aged, are unlikely to cooperate with procedures under local anaesthesia, and that cervical spine spondylosis or neoplasia may prevent ready passage of the needle. Nonetheless, because of its advantages over the open procedure, percutaneous cordotomy continues to enjoy a well deserved popularity. Mullan has outlined these advantages, which include the ability to localize a lesion precisely by stimulation in the alert patient and the possibility of avoiding complications by repeated assessment during increments of the current and thus the lesion size.

## Indications

The indications for open cordotomy apply equally to the percutaneous procedure. The chief indication is malignant disease, especially if it is unilateral. Its use for lumbosacral plexus invasion has the same drawbacks as open cordotomy, namely that the disease is frequently bilateral and that a staged bilateral procedure may be necessary. There are fewer indications for its use in benign pain, although it has been recommended for brachial plexus avulsion, postoperative lumbar disc pain, amputation pain, coccydynia, incisional pain and postherpetic neuralgia[4,5]. It has also been recommended for non-phantom paraplegic pain but experience does not support its use for deafferentation pain. It is not always easy to achieve a high level of analgesia, e.g. with supraclavicular pain, although most authors suggest that in general percutaneous cordotomy is suitable for somatic pain below the mandible. In summary then, it is a useful and generally safe simple procedure for unilateral cancer pain, which is its chief indication.

Rosomoff[2] has had extensive experience with the procedure and his technique or modifications of it is the one generally used. Taren *et al.*[6] listed four important steps: (*1*) definition of the radiological coordinates of the target; (*2*) use of a precision apparatus; (*3*) physiological confirmation of the target; and (*4*) precise target destruction.

*Note: it is essential to confirm the correct position of the electrode tip before making a lesion.*

## Anatomy of cervical vertebrae and cord

# 1

The percutaneous procedure is possible at cervical level because there is little laminal overlap and because the interarticular joints of C1–C2 are more anterior than at lower levels. This allows penetration of the anterior cord by the passage of a needle immediately behind the facet. This is not possible at the atlanto-occipital interval because of the presence of the vertebral artery as it emerges from the foramen transversarium and enters the foramen magnum.

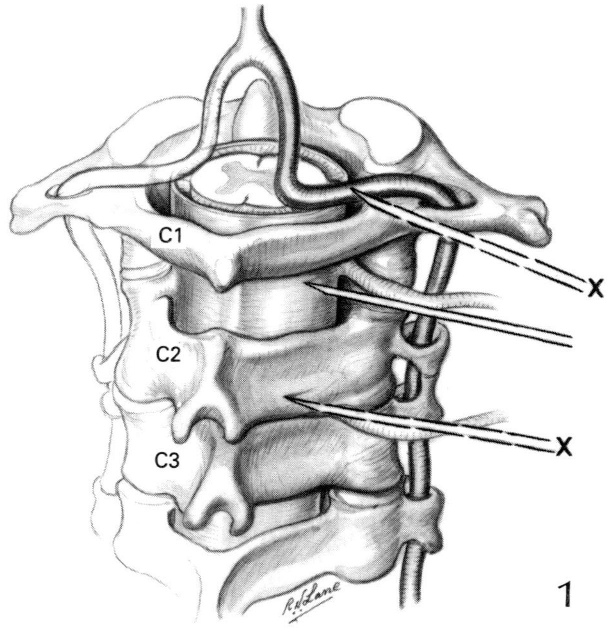


1

# 2

There are several representations of the arrangement of fibres within the spinothalamic tract. The traditional view of the spinothalamic fibres being arranged in an onion skin pattern with the cervical fibres being deep and the lumbosacral fibres on the periphery is incomplete, for the overlap is only partial and there is a gradual movement of the fibres from the lower part of the body more posteriorly as newer fibres from higher areas enter. This displacement results in the lumbosacral fibres being located close to the dentate ligament near the equatorial line of the cord and the cervicothoracic fibres being located more anteriorly. There is also some modality organization, with superficial pain and temperature being located in the periphery and deep pain more centrally.

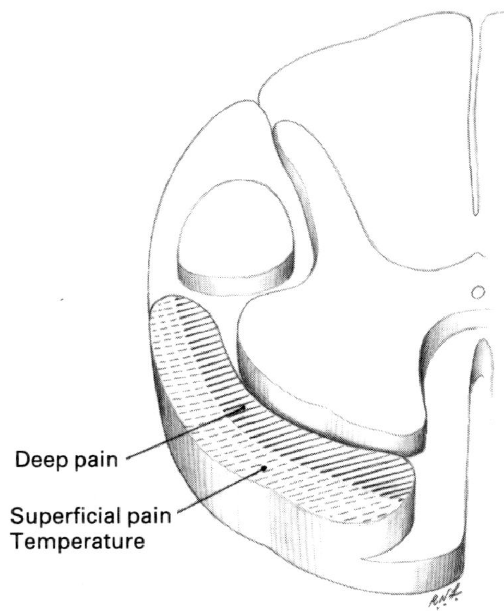


2

# 3

The ventrolateral reticulospinal tract contains the descending respiratory pathway (R) which lies deep to the spinothalamic tract (S) but with some mixture of fibres in the anterior part of the tract. This pathway lies close to the cervicothoracic portion of the tract and a similar somatotopic relationship exists between descending micturition pathways, which lie close to the lumbosacral segments[7, 8]. Fibres from both respiratory pathway and corticospinal tract synapse with the anterior horn cells (A). The diaphragmatic fibres lie anteriorly (D). If the descending respiratory pathway is destroyed, automatic respiration is impaired, which makes bilateral cordotomy particularly hazardous. Sleep-induced apnoea is a major complication of bilateral cordotomy: at the onset of sleep voluntary respiratory efforts cease and, with the loss of automatic respiration, the patient's respiratory efforts become less although on arousal he is able to breathe voluntarily again. Even with unilateral lesions, however, severe respiratory impairment will result if the ipsilateral descending respiratory pathway to an intact apparatus is damaged during a procedure designed to relieve contralateral pain in a damaged respiratory apparatus, for example in a patient who has had a thoracotomy and pneumonectomy[7,9]. Respiratory complications after percutaneous cordotomy have been reported in as many as 9 per cent of patients. These findings support the thesis that visceral functions are associated with appropriate somatic representatives within the cervical cord of man. Micturition pathways also bear a somatotopic relationship to the lumbosacral portion of the spinothalamic tract[7].

The proximity of these and other important tracts to the target zone makes accurate confirmation of correct electrode position mandatory.

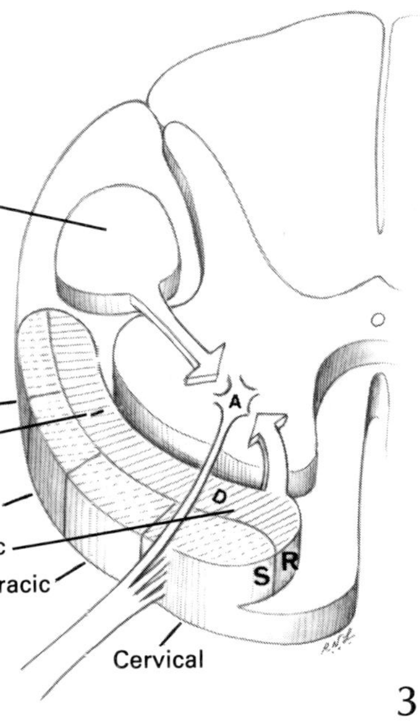


3

# 4

The corticospinal tracts decussate from the obex to C1 or C2 to lie in the posterolateral portion of the cord, the arm fibres crossing before the leg fibres. The decussation may extend beyond C1 to C2 and the later crossing leg fibres may then be damaged. As Taren *et al.*[6] have pointed out, there is considerable variation in the proportion of decussated fibres within the corticospinal tract. Despite these variations it is convenient to have a simple concept of fibre arrangement within the cord. There appears to be a 'spinothalamic homunculus' and a 'posterior column homunculus' and this somatomal arrangement within the cord[10] has been confirmed by others[11, 12]. At the C1–C2 region the cord is oval in cross section, approximately 14 mm wide and 10 mm thick.

Knowledge of these arrangements explains the complications of the procedure, such as sleep-induced apnoea, urinary and rectal incontinence and extremity paresis.

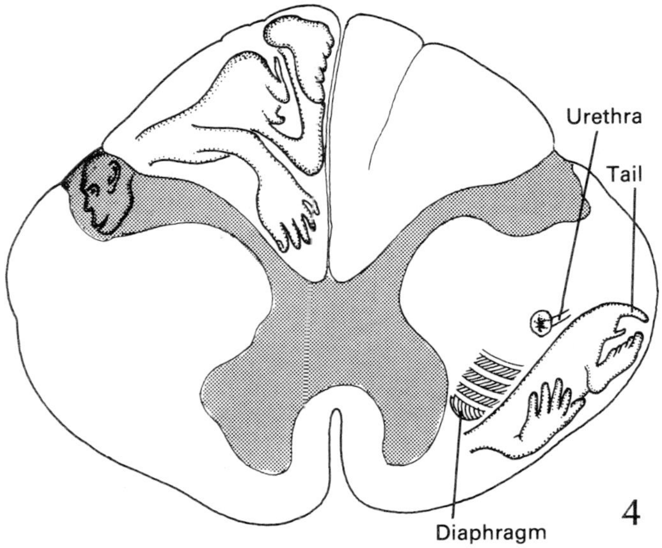


4

# Preoperative

## Preparation of patient

It is essential and indeed extremely helpful to discuss the procedure in some detail with the patient, explaining in a simple manner the sensations that may be experienced and the importance of reporting these to the operator. Most patients take an intelligent interest in this treatment in which their cooperation is vital. If there is any doubt about the ability of the patient to comprehend simple instructions and report sensations accurately, it might be wiser to consider an alternative procedure. The chance of success, which is high, and the relatively low risks should be explained although for most patients with terminal malignant disease even high risks may be acceptable. The particular hazards of micturition difficulties and the possibility of catheterization should be mentioned and also that a transient ipsilateral weakness may occur. Finally, the patient should be warned that headache is common following the procedure. Bilateral procedures are inadvisable because of the imprecise nature of the procedure and the great risk of respiratory disorder.

The cervical spine should be X-rayed to ensure that there is no mechanical obstruction to the passage of the needle and blood should be collected for haematology and electrolyte determination.

Estimation of respiratory function is particularly important. Flow rate and minute volume should be measured but in practice simple vitalograph measurements of forced vital capacity (FVC) and forced expiratory volume ($FEV_1$) are usually adequate. There is a substantial risk of respiratory disorder if the $FEV_1$ is less than 1.5 litres. If values less than 50 per cent of the predicted value are obtained, there is a high risk of 'sleep apnoea' and some other analgesic procedure should be considered.

The patient is starved for at least 4 hours before the procedure and opiate analgesics are discontinued 24 hours before operation by substitution with a non-opiate preparation. This is not always possible in patients with high opiate dosages and in such cases the undoubted higher risks may need to be accepted.

Immediately before operation a simple tranquillizer or sedative such as diazepam can be prescribed but preparations which have a respiratory depressive effect should be avoided.

## Instrumentation

5

A number of commercial kits are available which include a Teflon-coated 0.5 mm steel electrode with a 2–3 mm uninsulated tip which passes through an 18-gauge short bevelled lumbar puncture needle. Units which include arrangements for measurement of impedance, stimulation and electrode coagulation are also available, the best of which is the Radionics RFG-2A (Radionics Corporation, Burlington, Mass., USA). The commercial kits include micromanipulators to permit simple needle adjustments and special head holders which are helpful but not essential. The Rosomoff kit provides all the necessary equipment.

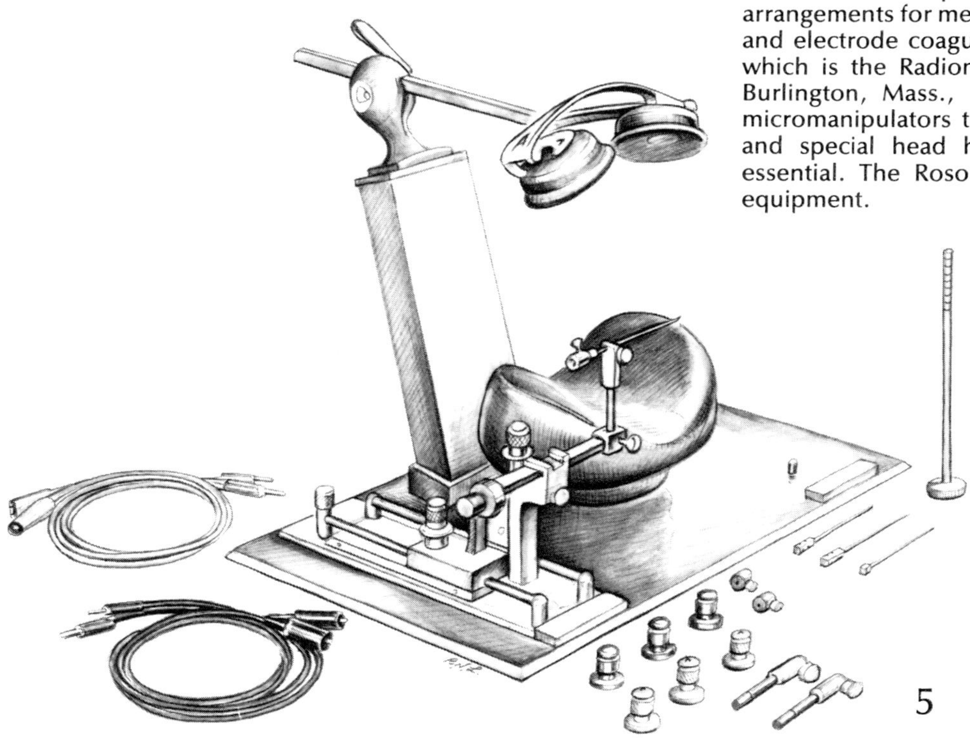

5

6

Biplane radiography with image intensification using a C-arm facilitates the procedure but the temptation to use fluoroscopy extensively should be resisted because of the danger of radiation. If facilities for fluoroscopy biplane radiography are not available, a portable X-ray unit can be used with a wooden or plastic cassette box beneath the head and a lateral cassette holder to allow films to be placed and removed without disturbing the patient's head and neck pillows.

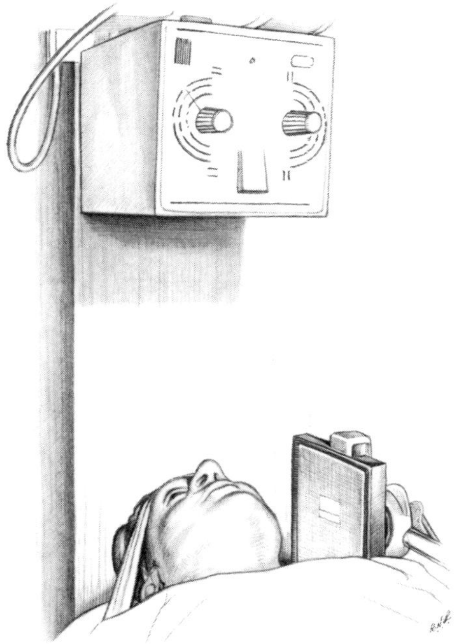

6

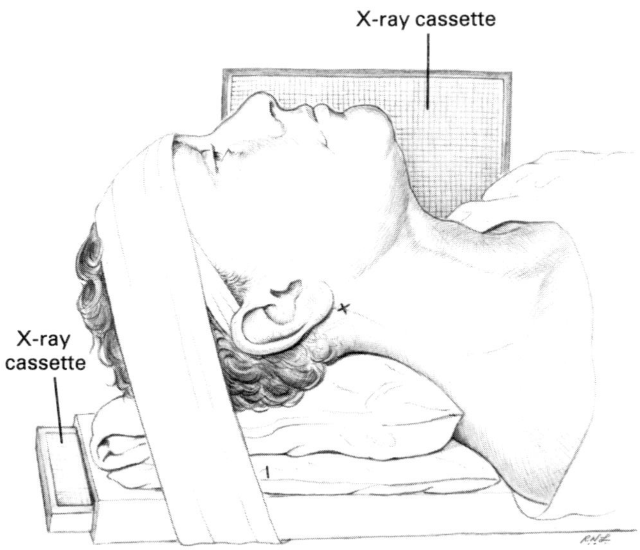


7

## The operations

### LATERAL PERCUTANEOUS CORDOTOMY

7

The patient lies supine with the head resting on a plastic sponge so that the dentate ligament is horizontal. The head is then clamped in place or secured by a U-shaped plastic plate with sponges on either side of the head; alternatively, it can be secured by a strap. Cassette holders are arranged beneath the neck and laterally. A large earth plate is placed on the shoulder; alternatively, a lumbar puncture needle in the scalp or the hub of the outer cordotomy needle can serve as the earth.

The skin is cleansed below and behind the tip of the mastoid and the ear, and sterile towels are draped around the neck. The commercially available plastic films to cover operation sites are convenient to keep hair out of the operative field and give secure coverage of a wide area.

The electrode is passed through the needle and beyond the selected depth, and a stop is placed on the electrode. An alternative method, more accurate but also rather more tedious, is to measure the total length of the electrode protruding from the hub of the needle with the electrode tip at the needle tip.

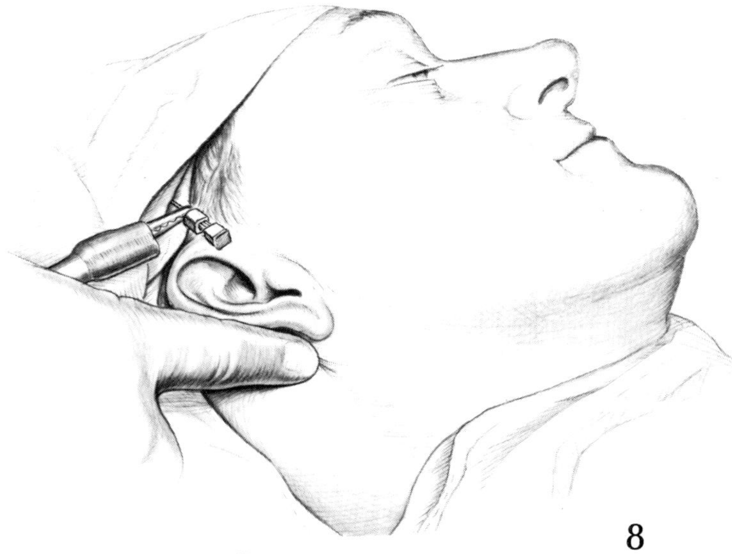

8

# 8 & 9

The tip of the mastoid is palpated and a point chosen 1 cm below and behind it. At this level, the target is approximately 10–12 mm behind the posterior body of the C2 vertebra and should be closer to C2 than to C1 because of the risk of making a high insertion and the added hazard of injury to the corticospinal tract.

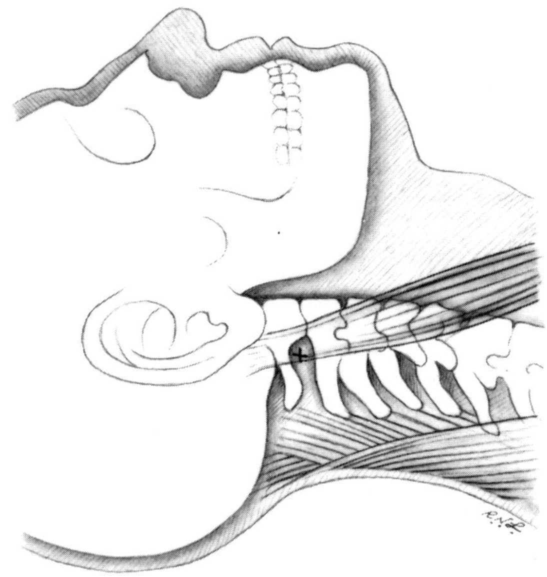

9

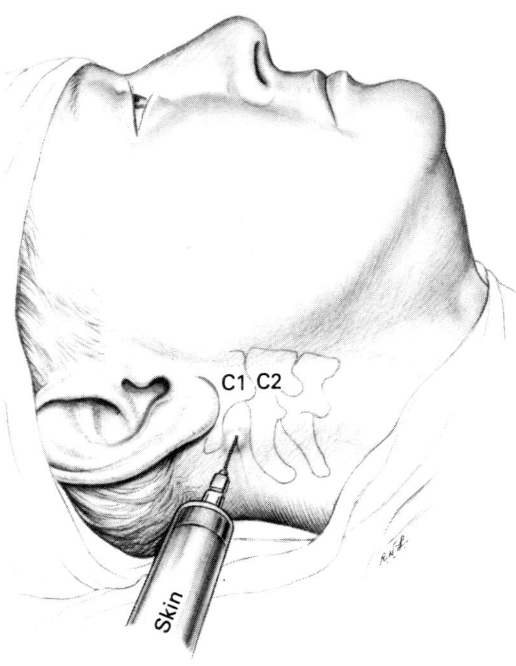


10

## Local anaesthesia

# 10

The puncture area is then infiltrated with 1 per cent lignocaine, using a 25-gauge needle for the skin and a 22-gauge needle for the subcutaneous tissue and muscles. A total of 5–10 ml of local anaesthetic should be injected approximately 3 cm deep, almost up to the vertebra. The depth can be checked radiologically but with experience this becomes unnecessary. The needle is directed about 10 mm behind the posterior border of C2 and advanced horizontally. The passage of the needle may be painful and provoke unilateral headache when the C2 root is touched. This can usually be relieved by the injection of up to 2 ml of local anaesthetic. The operator should avoid injecting large amounts of local anaesthetic because of the risk of leakage into the subarachnoid space and the production of temporary respiratory failure.

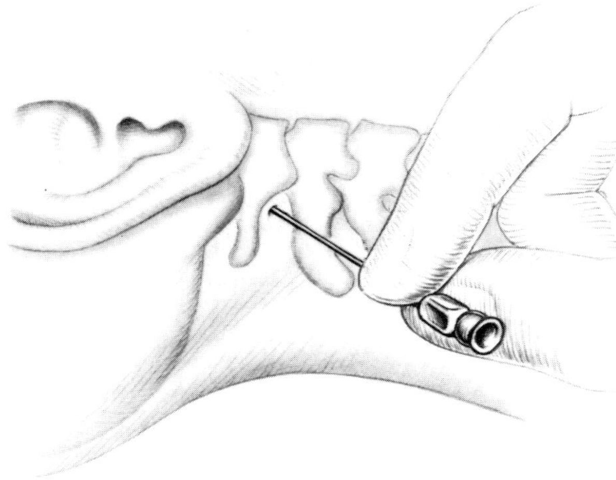

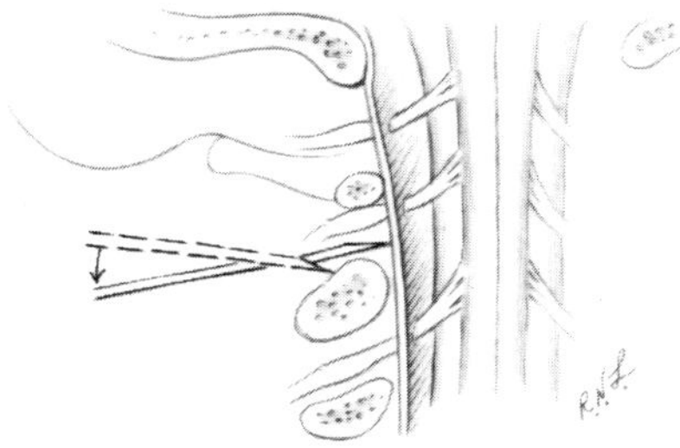

11

## 11 & 12

A lumbar puncture needle is then slowly advanced through the puncture site between C1 and C2 to penetrate the dura. If the needle's passage is obstructed, it is usually by lamina. If after readjustment the obstruction persists, an X-ray should be taken and the angle readjusted so that the needle point lies in the interlaminal space.

The dura gives a slight resistance and then a characteristic relaxation sensation as the needle tip penetrates it and enters the subarachnoid space. Usually cerebrospinal fluid escapes through the needle but, if not, a small quantity should be cautiously aspirated to confirm placement within the subarachnoid space. If blood is aspirated, the needle is usually too anterior and in the extradural space, very often having passed anterior to the dura. The needle should be retracted to the subcutaneous level and reinserted at a different angle.

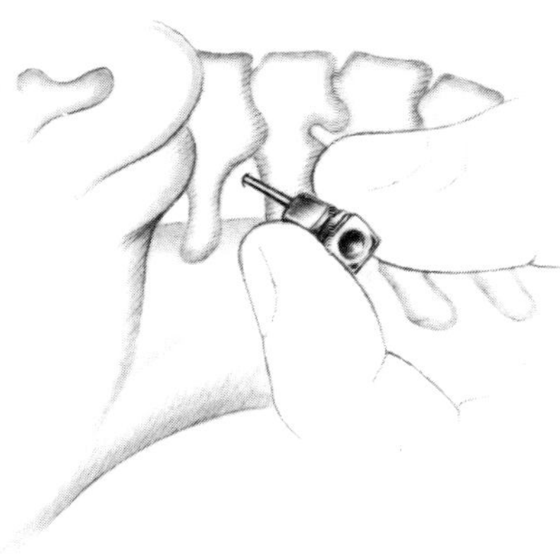

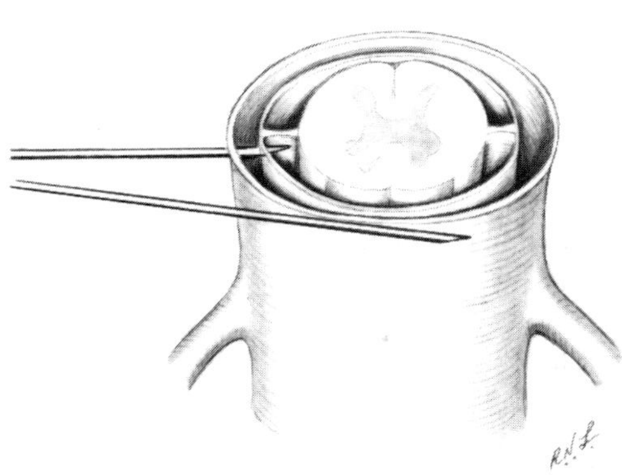

12

# 13

After subarachnoid puncture has been confirmed, the needle may be attached to the micromanipulator or held by hand or taped to a support. A plastic stopcock is attached to the needle and approximately 2 ml of a water-soluble radio-opaque dye is injected; alternatively an injection of 10 ml air may be used. Myodil was previously used to outline the dentate ligament but because of its well known tendency to produce arachnoiditis its use is now contraindicated.

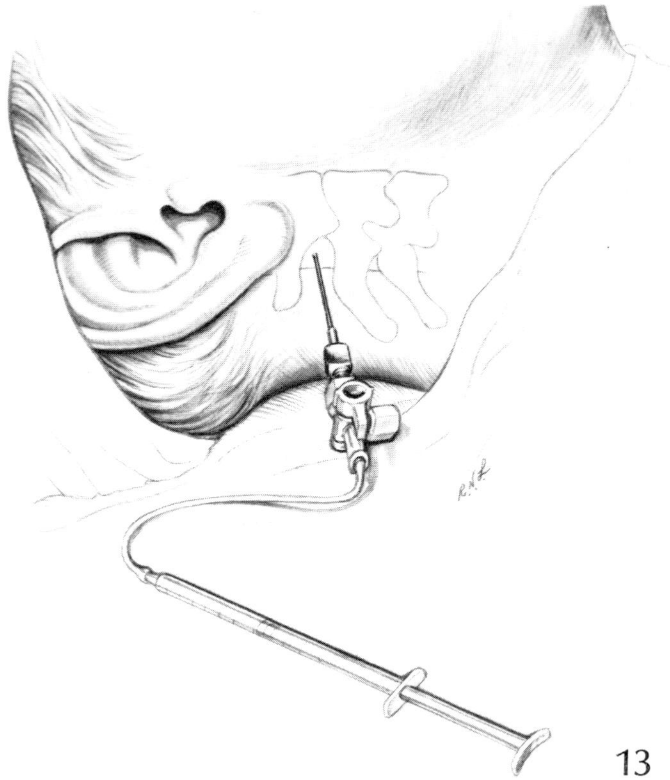

13

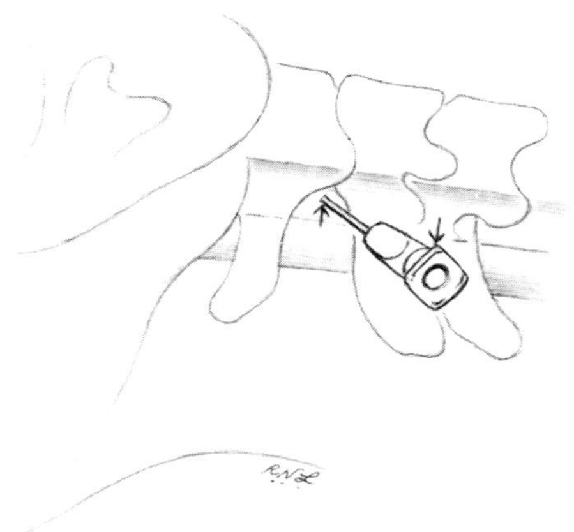

14

# 14 & 15

Lateral and anteroposterior views through the open mouth are then taken, using either conventional X-ray or a fluoroscopic technique. The lateral radiograph is inspected first. The anterior border of the cord is outlined approximately 8 mm behind the posterior border of C2. The needle should be directed to a point halfway between the middle of the cord and its anterior margin by raising or lowering the needle hub. On the anteroposterior film the needle tip should lie close to, but not past, the lateral edge of the odontoid.

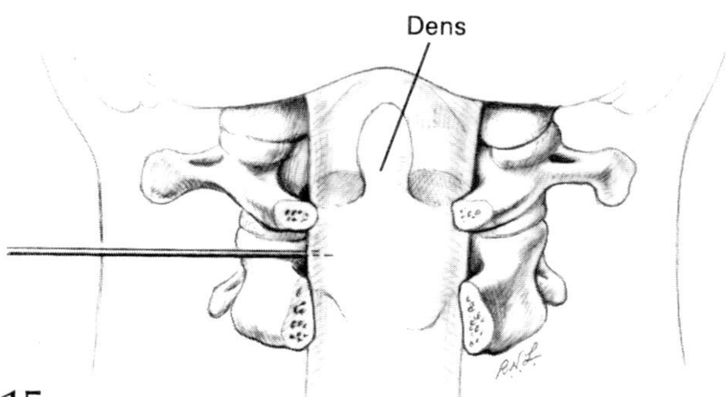


15

# 16

For relief of arm pain the needle point should be directed approximately 2 mm posterior to the anterior cord shadow, for leg pain about 3 mm. It must be appreciated that such apparently fine adjustments are only part of a simple aiming technique. There is little opportunity for accurate selective lesion-making.

The position of the needle tip can be secured by fixing the needle in a micromanipulator which permits fine adjustments. The same effect can be achieved less elegantly but equally effectively by taping the needle to a support bar attached to the head holder or table or, even more simply, by holding the needle hub by hand while the electrode is inserted. Adjustments are permitted by the mobile skin and muscle but there is relatively little movement at the dural level, which can be regarded as the fulcrum. Large hub movements are therefore necessary to produce small anterior or posterior adjustments of the needle. Radiological confirmation of correct position is then obtained.

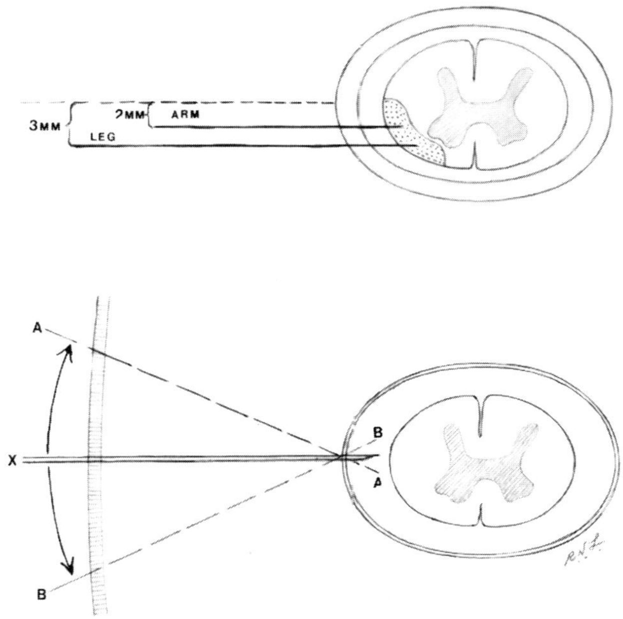


16

# 17 & 18

## Electrode insertion

The point of the electrode should be carefully examined and protected before insertion. The arachnoid is tough and, unless the electrode is very sharp, the cord will be displaced rather than penetrated. The electrical cables are now clipped to the earth (which can be the outer needle) and the electrode. The electrode is then advanced through the needle until it touches the cord. This often produces a distinctive sensation and the patient may complain of pain. The pia may be very tough so that the cord is sometimes displaced rather than penetrated. In this case the electrode should be withdrawn and advanced with a quick thrust.

During the passage of the electrode the impedance is measured to determine the depth of penetration. It is approximately 200 ohm within cerebrospinal fluid, rises on contact with the spinal cord and increases to more than 400–750 ohm as the cord is penetrated. If the electrode is advanced any further, there is another slight increase in resistance and some pain as the insulated portion of the needle is reached.

X-rays are taken to show the electrode tip, which is sometimes so fine that it is difficult to see.

The electrical cables are connected appropriately: active cable to electrode and inactive cable to earth.

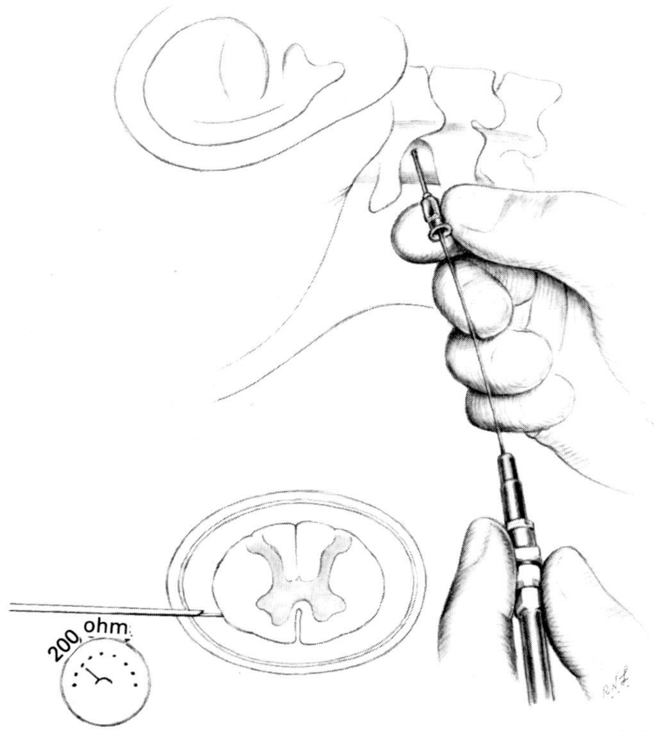


17

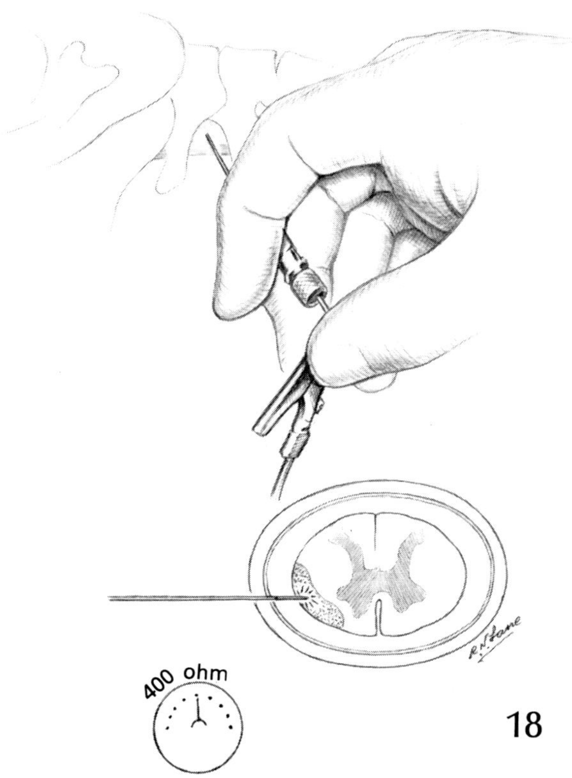


18

# 19

## Stimulation

Electrical stimulation is now used first at 5 Hz with stimuli of 1 ms duration. At around 0.5–1.5 V there should be contraction of the ipsilateral neck muscles and trapezius. The higher the voltage required to produce this response, the further away is the electrode tip from the anterior cord. To this extent, therefore, the response is a useful confirmation of correct positioning. However, there should be no contraction of the arm or leg. Such contractions below 1.5 V indicate that the electrode is in or close to the corticospinal tract. In this case, the electrode should be withdrawn and reinserted more anteriorly to avoid the corticospinal tract. If the electrode is properly sited, stimulation at 50 Hz will usually produce sensory responses at less than 0.3 V. The patient then complains of paraesthesiae in the contralateral body in the form of numbness, cold or warm or an electric-shock-like sensation. Lower limb sensations indicate more dorsal placement than for the arm. Ipsilateral responses are probably due to posterior placement within posterior columns. Occasionally bilateral sensations are produced; they usually occur when the tip lies in the centre of the cord. To some extent the voltage required to produce responses correlates with the proximity of the tip to the spinothalamic fibres. Thus low voltages imply good placement. A stimulus of more than 0.5 V implies that the tip is close to but not within the tract and larger voltages imply a position farther away. If sensations cannot be obtained at less than 0.5 V the electrode should be reinserted and the outer needle readjusted. The electrode is then introduced and stimulation repeated. The paraesthesia experienced in, for example, the leg gradually spreads up or down the body.

If appropriate sensations are produced, then a lesion can be made.

## Making the lesion

There are two methods of making a radiofrequency lesion: (*1*) by keeping the current constant and increasing the time and (*2*) by using a standard time and increasing the current.

19

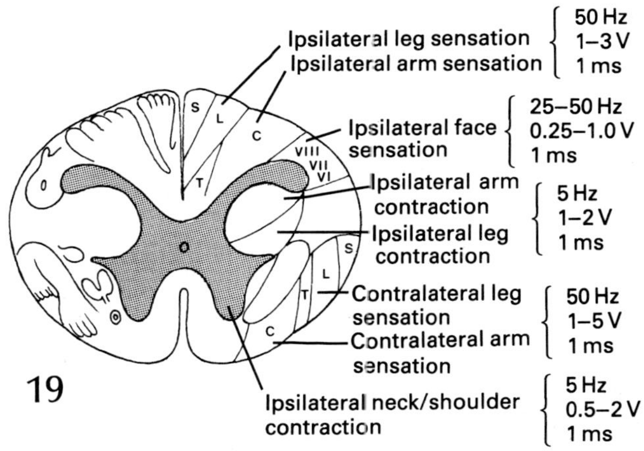


C, cervical; T, thoracic; L, lumbar; S, sacral; VIII, VII, VI, trigeminal nucleus

For the constant current method not more than 50 mA should be used. Lesions are made at 2.5 s increments.

The constant time method uses a standard time of 30 s and 5–10 mA increments of current from 20 mA to 50 mA. The latter method is preferable but the introduction of a fine temperature monitoring electrode permits better control than either of these two so that lesions can be made by producing a selected temperature.

The patient's reactions should be tested after each increment or lesion stage. Sensation to pin prick should be tested with a safety pin. Grip strength of both hands should be tested and the power of hip flexion and ankle dorsiflexion. Arm and knee reflexes should also be noted. Lesion-making should continue until the area of confirmed analgesia extends at least two dermatomes beyond the area of pain. Usually analgesia begins at lower dermatomes and rises as the lesion enlarges. If a high analgesic level cannot be obtained, the electrode should be advanced by 1 mm steps and the process repeated.

## Postoperative care and complications

The patient should remain in bed overnight and be carefully monitored. Headache is a frequent complaint and can be treated by simple analgesics. Severe neck rigidity usually indicates a subarachnoid haemorrhage but if it develops several hours after the operation a lumbar puncture should be performed to exclude the possibility of meningitis. If it has been impossible to wean the patient off opiate analgesics preoperatively, they should now be gradually reduced over the succeeding 36 hours. The danger of continued administration of opiates is the enhancement of any respiratory depression produced by injury to the respiratory pathways. This is indeed a major postoperative complication and nursing observations should be frequent. Respiratory disorders occur in approximately 2 per cent of these patients and if respiratory function is poor oxygen should be administered. Grossly inadequate respiratory efforts may require artificial ventilation for some days, after which the oedema surrounding the lesion will have diminished and respiratory function may improve.

Ipsilateral weakness, usually in the legs, may be due to hypotonia associated with injury to extrapyramidal pathways. Injury to the corticospinal tract is accompanied by increased reflexes and an abnormal plantar reflex. About 4.7 per cent of patients develop postoperative paresis, which is permanent in 1 per cent.

Micturition disorders (incontinence or, more frequently, retention) have been reported in 2 per cent. The patient should be catheterized for a few days before attempting to restore normal bladder function. Dizziness and nausea are not infrequent but usually subside within 24 hours. Postural hypotension also occurs and mobilization should be carefully supervised. Before discharge the patient should be warned of the danger of analgesia and especially of the danger of thermanaesthesia to avoid burns. Patients should also be advised to inspect analgesic areas for ulceration, especially their feet if they are ambulant. Bed-ridden patients should have a relative or nurse inspect the prominence of sacrum and calcaneum.

### BILATERAL CORDOTOMY

High cervical bilateral cordotomy is not recommended because of the high risk of respiratory failure[13, 14], although Rosomoff[15], who has performed staged bilateral cordotomy on one-third of his patients, believes that pain relief may require such treatment despite a mortality rate of 12 per cent. He points out that in only 2 per cent was there a clear relationship between the cause of death and the procedure. The other hazard of unilateral cordotomy, bladder dysfunction, increases from 5 to 15 per cent. In patients with bilateral arm pain, other procedures, such as myelotomy or a low cervical cordotomy by the anterior approach, should be considered (*see* below).

## Results

Despite the large number of reported cases, there are only relatively few and short follow-up reports after percutaneous cordotomy.

Lorenz[16] quoted an initial success rate of 86 per cent in 3742 cases collected from the literature. In a more detailed study of a smaller number of cases (2840), the initial success rate was 85 per cent but at 'late' follow-up this had fallen to 59 per cent. In a large personal series of Rosomoff (725 patients) the initial success rate of 90 per cent fell to 86 per cent at 1 year; yet by the third year it was only 42 per cent. A later (1979) study reported loss of analgesia in 60 per cent by 2 years.

White and Sweet[17], by questionnaire, collected statistics of 3357 patients treated by percutaneous cordotomy and compared them with open cordotomy in 371 patients. Only 84 patients with percutaneous cordotomy had records for more than 6 months and, of these, 41 had lost their initial analgesia. They concluded that percutaneous cordotomy was indicated for the treatment of pain due to malignancy because of its lower morbidity and mortality but its long-term effectiveness was not proved.

Tasker[18] found that a 96 per cent immediate relief had fallen to 85 per cent at the latest (undefined) follow-up after percutaneous cordotomy. Although 68 per cent of patients obtained pain relief after bilateral cordotomy, 19 per cent had transient paresis and 21 per cent aggravated bladder dysfunction. In a subsequent review of 244 patients with percutaneous cordotomy, 88 per cent had complete relief at the time of hospital discharge and 71 per cent had complete relief after 1 month[19]. In contrast, only 33.8 per cent of patients with deafferentation pain had complete relief at follow-up.

In a recent series of 100 patients undergoing 121 lateral percutaneous cordotomies, 64 per cent had complete pain relief and 23 per cent partial relief[20]. Ten patients had bilateral procedures. Unfortunately no follow-up was included but presumably the results are similar to those of other authors. Transient ipsilateral weakness occurred in 69 per cent but permanent weakness in only 4 per cent. Bladder dysfunction was also common (19 per cent) but only 3 per cent had permanent bladder dysfunction. As in other forms of cordotomy, and in agreement with other workers, 6 per cent of patients developed dysaesthesiae. The mortality of 6 per cent was related exclusively to postoperative respiratory dysfunction.

### ANTERIOR PERCUTANEOUS LOWER CERVICAL CORDOTOMY

To reduce the risk of respiratory disorder following cordotomy, Lin *et al.*[21] devised an anterior approach in which the electrode is inserted through the cervical intervertebral disc below the phrenic nerve fibres. The procedure is particularly useful if there is a great risk of respiratory impairment or when a second bilateral lesion is required. Another advantage is the lower incidence of micturition disorders and a better chance of obtaining selective analgesia. Against this must be set the difficulty in readjustment of needle position and the rather more detailed calculations required to use the needle. High analgesic levels cannot be obtained as readily as by the lateral high cervical approach but for low analgesic levels the procedure has many advantages.

## Position of patient and equipment

The equipment is the same as for the high cervical lateral method.

The patient lies supine with the head immobilized by Rosomoff head clamps or by some other method such as adhesive tape. Cassette holders are arranged below the head and laterally in such a way that the head and neck need not be disturbed during the procedure. For the anteroposterior view the tube-to-film distance should be 90 cm, with the cervical canal about 15 cm from the film. This can be achieved by appropriate padding or pillowing. The lateral tube-to-film distance should also be 90 cm, again with the midline of the lower cervical canal 15 cm away from the film so that the film magnification is the same for both anteroposterior and lateral films. At this magnification the anteroposterior dimension of the cord is 18 mm and the lateral dimension 10 mm.

*Note*: the needle insertion is made diagonally from the opposite side to the intended lesion.

# 20

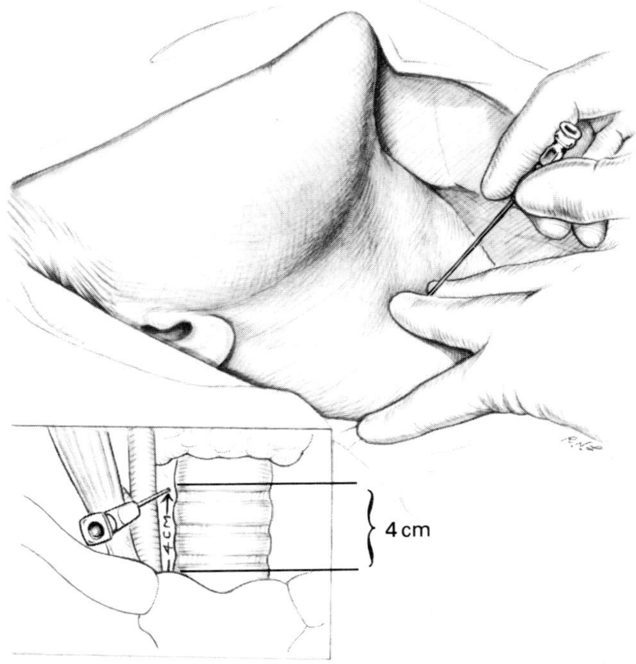


## Anaesthesia

Local anaesthetic is injected at a point 4 cm above the sternoclavicular joint between the carotid sheath and medial structure of trachea and oesophagus. The skin and subcutaneous tissues are infiltrated down to the prevertebral fascia.

# 21, 22 & 23

An 18-gauge lumbar puncture needle is then passed between the sternomastoid and trachea towards the C6–C7 or C5–C6 disc space at an angle directed towards the opposite anterolateral quadrant of the cord. The soft elastic disc space is identified by moving the needle point and the needle is then advanced through the disc for a few millimetres. Anteroposterior and lateral films are then taken so that the angle of insertion can be calculated (*see below*).

The target is chosen according to the area of desired analgesia. In the supine position the cord lies against the posterior wall of the cervical canal and is approximately 10 mm wide so that the dentate ligament lies approximately 5 mm anterior to the posterior wall of the canal. This is the lateral target point for the lumbosacral fibres; the anteroposterior target is approximately 7 mm from the midline. Cervical thoracic fibres lie more anteriorly, a few millimetres posterior to the anterior border of the cord, and about 3 mm from the midline at the same magnification.

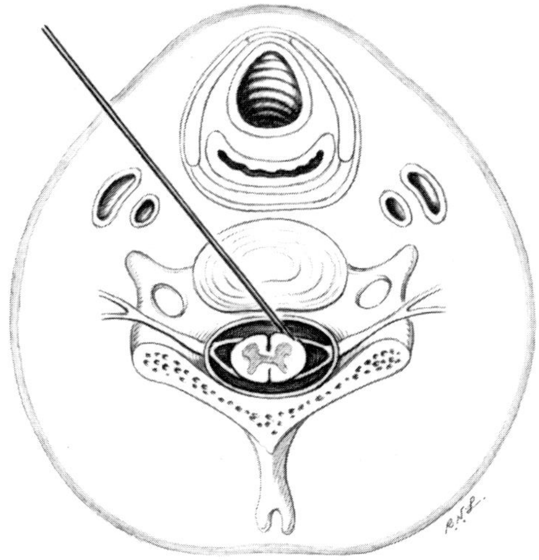

20

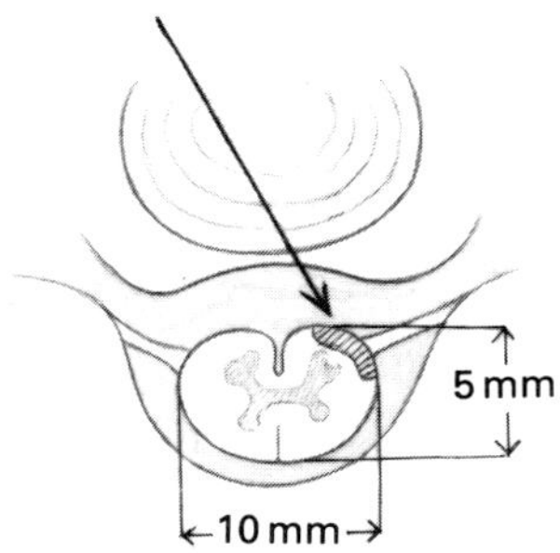


21

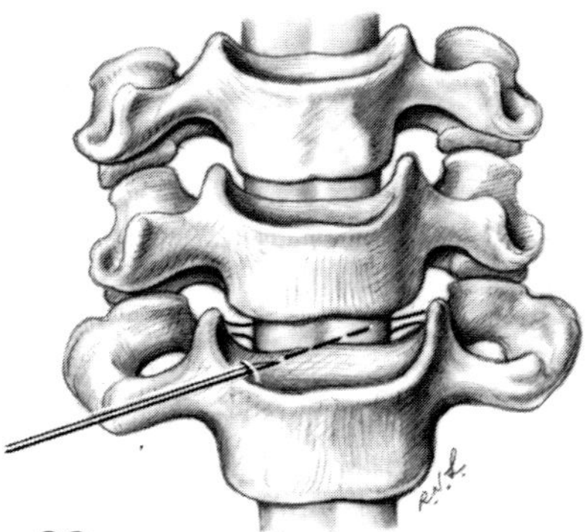

22

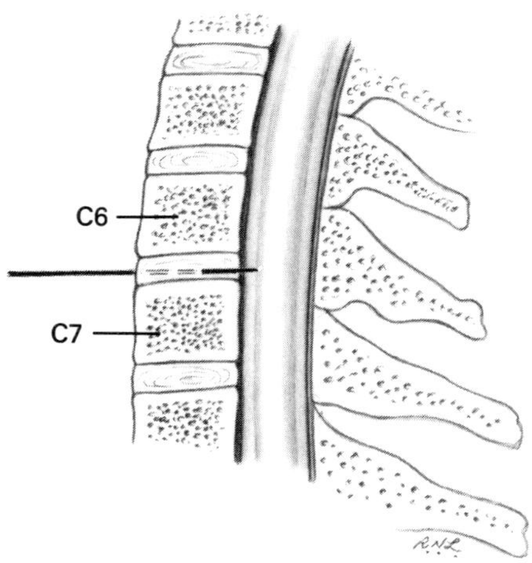


23

# 24

## Calculating the angle of insertion

The target point is marked on the lateral film and the distance from the needle point to the target (L) is measured. The target point is also marked on the anteroposterior film and its distance from the needle tip measured (A). The correct angle of insertion (X) is obtained by transferring these two measurements to the corner of a card and connecting their end points. The deviation of the resultant line from the sagittal plane gives the angle X. This card is held up below the patient's chin so that the operator can make the appropriate adjustment.

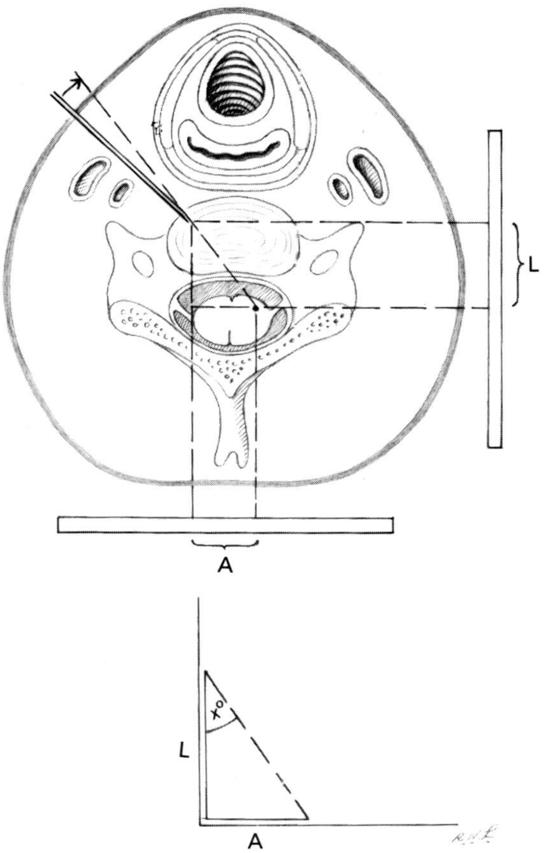


24

The needle is then advanced through the disc to its posterior part, and anteroposterior and lateral films are taken to confirm correct positioning. After any necessary readjustment, the needle is advanced through the dura into the subarachnoid space until cerebrospinal fluid flows out of the needle. At this stage 10 ml of air is injected and further X-rays are taken to outline the cord and verify that the needle is in the correct position.

The electrode is then introduced through the needle to penetrate the cord with a quick thrust and the rest of the procedure continues as for lateral percutaneous cordotomy.

## *References*


1. Mullan, S., Hekmatpanah, J., Dobbern, G. (1965) Percutaneous intramedullary cordotomy utilizing the unipolar anodal electrolytic lesion. Journal of Neurosurgery, 22, 554–583
2. Rosomoff, H. L. (1974) Percutaneous radiofrequency cervical cordotomy for relief of intractable pain. In: International Symposium on Pain, J. J. Bonica (ed.). Advances in Neurology, 4, 683–688. New York: Raven Press
3. Lipton, S. (1979) Relief of pain in clinical practice. Oxford: Blackwell Scientific Publications
4. Taren, J. A. (1977) Stereotaxic lesions for pain control. In: Pain Management, J. Fletcher-Leigh (ed.). Baltimore: Williams and Wilkins
5. Entzian, W., Linke, D. (1975) Experience with percutaneous cordotomy. In: Brain Hypoxia. Pain, H. Penzholz, M. Brock, J. Hamer, M. Klinger, D. Spoerri (eds.). Advances in Neurosurgery, 3, 190–194. Berlin, Heidelberg, New York: Springer
6. Taren, J. A., Davis, R., Crosby, E. C. (1969) Target physiologic corroboration in stereotaxic cervical cordotomy. Journal of Neurosurgery, 31, 569–584
7. Hitchcock, E., Leece, B. (1967) Somatotopic representation of the respiratory pathways in the cervical cord of man. Journal of Neurosurgery, 27, 320–329
8. Hitchcock, E., Newsome, D., Salama, M. (1974) The somatotopic representation of the micturition pathways in the cervical cord of man. British Journal of Surgery, 61, 395–401
9. Belmusto, L., Brown, E., Owens, G. (1963) Clinical observations on respiratory and vasomotor disturbances as related to cervical cordotomies. Journal of Neurosurgery, 20, 225–232
10. Hitchcock, E. (1972) Electrophysiological exploration of the cervico-medullary region. In: Neurophysiology Studied in Man, G. Somjen (ed.), pp. 237–245. Amsterdam: Excerpta Medica
11. Schvarcz, J. R. (1974) Spinal cord stereotactic surgery. In: Recent Progress in Neurological Surgery, K. Sano, S. Ishii (eds.), pp. 234–241. Amsterdam: Excerpta Medica
12. Illingworth, R. D., Molina-Negro, P. (1974) Spontaneous and electrically evoked activity in the anterolateral column of the spinal cord in dogs. Journal of Neurosurgery, 40, 58–64
13. Rosomoff, H. L., Krieger, A. J., Kuperman, A. S. (1969) Effects of percutaneous cervical cordotomy on pulmonary function. Journal of Neurosurgery 31, 620–627
14. Ganz, E., Mullen, S. (1977) Percutaneous cordotomy. In: Persistent Pain, S. Lipton (ed.), 1, 21–34. London: Academic Press

15. Rosomoff, J. L. (1985) Percutaneous spinothalamic cordotomy. In: Neurosurgery, R. H. Wilkins, R. R. Setti (eds.), 3, 2446–2451. New York: McGraw Hill

16. Lorenz, R. (1976) Methods of percutaneous spinothalamic tract section. In: Advances and Technical Standards in Neurosurgery, 3, 123–145

17. White, J. C., Sweet, W. H. (1979) Anterolateral cordotomy: open versus closed comparison of end results. Advances in Pain Research and Therapy, 3, 911–919

18. Tasker, R. R. (1976) The merits of percutaneous cordotomy over the open operation. In: Current Controversies in Neurosurgery, T. P. Morley (ed.), pp. 496–501. Philadelphia: W. B. Saunders

19. Tasker, R. R., Organ, L. W., Hawaylyshyn, P. (1982) Percutaneous cordotomy: the lateral high cervical technique. In: Current Techniques in Operative Neurosurgery, H. H. Schmidek, W. H. Sweet (eds.). New York: Grune and Stratton

20. Lahuetra, J., Lipton, S., Wells, J. C. D. (1985)[20] Percutaneous cervical cordotomy: results and complications in a recent series of 100 patients. Annals of the Royal College of Surgeons of England, 67, 41–44

21. Lin, P. M., Gildenberg, P. L., Polakoff, P. P. (1966) An anterior approach to percutaneous lower cervical cordotomy. Journal of Neurosurgery, 25, 553–560

Illustrations by Barbara Hyams

# Contemporary methods for stereotactic ventralis lateralis thalamotomy and for the stereotactic biopsy of intracranial neoplasms

**Patrick J. Kelly** MD
Department of Neurosurgery, Mayo Clinic and Mayo Medical School, Rochester, Minnesota, USA

## Introduction

In 1908, Horsley and his engineer R. H. Clarke developed the first stereotactic instrument, used initially for exploration of deep cerebellar nuclei in small animals[1]. However, human subcortical stereotactic procedures were not practical until the development of ventriculography. In 1947, Spiegel *et al.* were the first to perform a human stereotactic procedure[2]. Thereafter, others soon developed their own instrumentation, methods and indications for stereotactic procedures.

In the 1960s, the placement of subcortical lesions for the palliation of Parkinsonian tremor and rigidity was the most common application for stereotactic technique. Nevertheless, the advent of L-dopa in the late 1960s brought about a precipitous decline in the number of stereotactic procedures. Few stereotactic operations were carried out after 1968 and only then for the rare Parkinson patient unable to take, or unable to derive benefit from, L-dopa, or for patients with other types of movement disorders and chronic pain.

The availability of the precise three-dimensional database provided by computerized tomography (CT) in the 1970s prompted many neurosurgeons to re-evaluate their thinking as regards conventional versus stereotactic approaches to common intracranial tumours, and this has brought about a renaissance for stereotactic surgery[3]. Old stereotactic instruments were modified and new instruments developed which would take advantage of the CT database[4–6]. As technology continues to provide new instrumentation, new stereotactic surgical techniques emerge, and new indications are derived. However, the most common contemporary applications for stereotactic technique are neuroablative procedures for movement disorders, and the stereotactic biopsy of subcortical neoplasms. This chapter describes the technique and results for these procedures as practised at our institution.

# Stereotactic ventralis lateralis thalamotomy for movement disorder

After almost 20 years of experience with L-dopa and L-dopa/carbidopa in Parkinson's disease, it is clear that there are many individuals whose tremor is not well controlled medically. However, these patients can be helped by a stereotactic thalamotomy which will delay the onset of disability for many years before bradykinesia becomes a significant problem[7]. Incorporation of imaging technology and neurophysiological methods for localization of structures and optimal lesion sites has increased the precision of stereotactic neuroablative procedures which maximize the therapeutic benefits and reduce the surgical risk. The following will review the history for movement disorder surgery and describe our technique for stereotactic ventralis lateralis (VL) thalamotomy.

## Historical aspects

Surgeons have placed lesions in various locations within the extrapyramidal system and have noted beneficial results on the treatment of tremor and rigidity associated with Parkinson's disease. In 1909, Horsley[8] and later Bucy[9], extirpated the motor cortex and noted ablation of resting tremor. Russell Meyers lesioned the ansa lenticularis by means of craniotomy and transventricular approach in 1942[10]. He also noted cessation of tremor. He concluded that destruction of the pallidothalamic tracts was the key to the control of tremor and rigidity. In 1950, Fenelon in Paris successfully produced lesions of the ansa lenticularis by inserting a coagulating electrode utilizing a less hazardous subfrontal route[11].

Irving Cooper[12] and Guiot [13] placed stereotactic lesions in the internal segment of the globus pallidus in the late 1950s and reported beneficial results in the treatment of tremor and rigidity. Later, Cooper[14] and Hassler[15] found that lesions in the ventral lateral thalamus more effectively abolished tremor and rigidity, with acceptable levels of morbidity. This target, ventralis lateralis (VL), remains the most common contemporary lesion site for the control of many types of movement disorders.

### PROCEDURE FOR VENTRALIS LATERALIS THALAMOTOMY

There is some variation in the target localization methodology for VL thalamotomy as performed in different centres. In general, the stereotactic neuroradiological investigation establishes the *approximate position* of the subcortical target structures in reference to the stereotactic frame. The precise position of the target structure is established by microelectrode recording and/or subcortical stimulation.

We use a Todd–Wells stereotactic frame and a preoperative database consisting of stereotactic CT scanning, a computer-resident stereotactic atlas, positive contrast ventriculography, and microelectrode exploration[16]. Lesion sites are corroborated by stimulation, and lesions are made with a radiofrequency system. Stereotactic neuroablative procedures are usually done under mild sedation and local anaesthesia in order to monitor carefully the clinical effects of stimulation and lesion production. The operation is performed in two sessions: first, a data acquisition procedure and second, a microelectrode recording and lesioning procedure.

## Data acquisition

A CT-compatible stereotactic headframe is applied to the patient under local anaesthesia and mild sedation, as described in previous reports[7,17–23]. This fixes to the skull by four carbon fibre pins inserted in holes drilled in the outer table of the skull into the diploe. The depth of the pins in relation to the vertical support elements of the headframe is measured by micrometers.

# 1a & b

The patient then undergoes stereotactic CT scanning on a General Electric 8800 or 9800 CT scanning unit (General Electric Medical Systems, New Berlin, Wisconsin, USA). A CT localization system containing nine carbon fibre rods in the shape of the letter N on either side of the head and anteriorly is attached to the stereotactic head holder.

This produces nine reference marks on each CT slice, which allow calculation of stereotactic coordinates of any selected point on the CT slice. Five-millimetre CT slices overlapping at 3 mm intervals are obtained through the region of the third ventricle. The CT data is then transferred to an operating-room computer system.

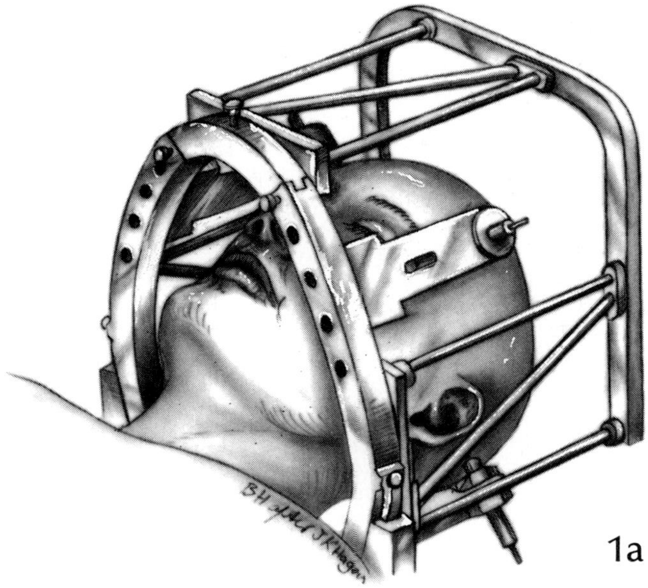

1a

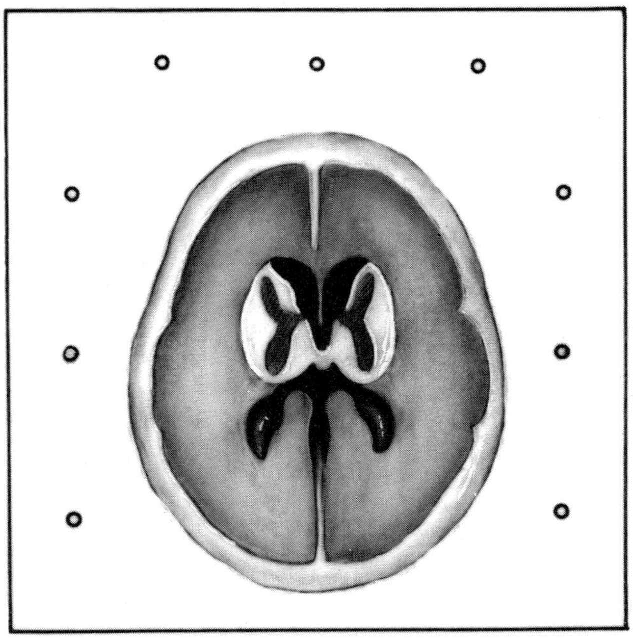

1b

2

A computer-resident digitized Shaltenbrand–Wahren stereotactic atlas is scaled by computer and superimposed on the CT slice within defined landmarks (the lateral wall of the third ventricle, pulvinar, and medial border of the internal capsule). The computer-scaled outlines of individual thalamic nuclei are then drawn in over the CT slice by the computer.

The CT slice is reformatted with respect to the anterior commissure/posterior commissure (AC/PC) line and displayed (top left). The surgeon traces around the boundaries of the thalamus, indicating the lateral wall of the third ventricle and medial extension of the internal capsule (top right). The computer adjusts the configuration of the thalamic substructures held within the computer-resident stereotactic atlas and displays each within the defined boundary (bottom left). The surgeon designates to the computer the desired substructure of interest (in this case ventralis intermedius – the ventralis intermedius). The computer then places the reformatted outline of the structure within the thalamus. The surgeon places a cursor in the desired portion of the ventralis intermedius. The computer automatically calculates stereotactic frame coordinates at this point (bottom right). Any thalamic nucleus may be selected by cursor on the display console, and stereotactic coordinates calculated as has been described previously[24].

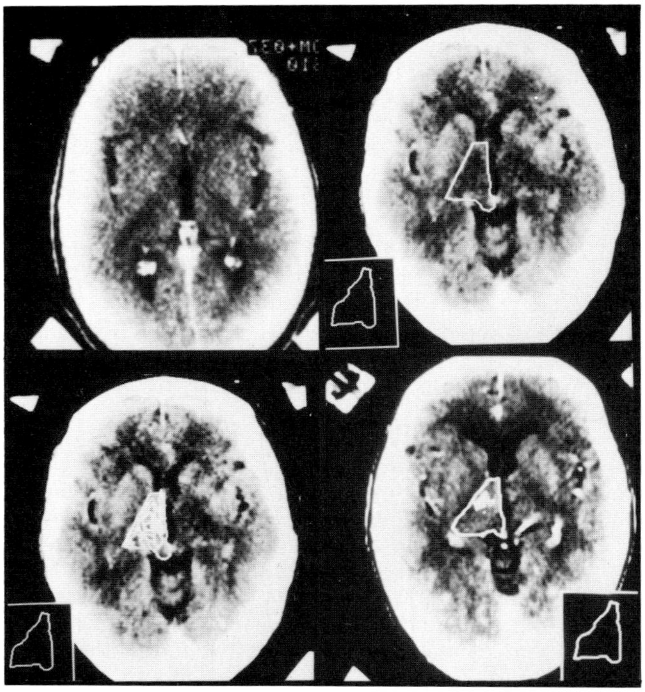

2

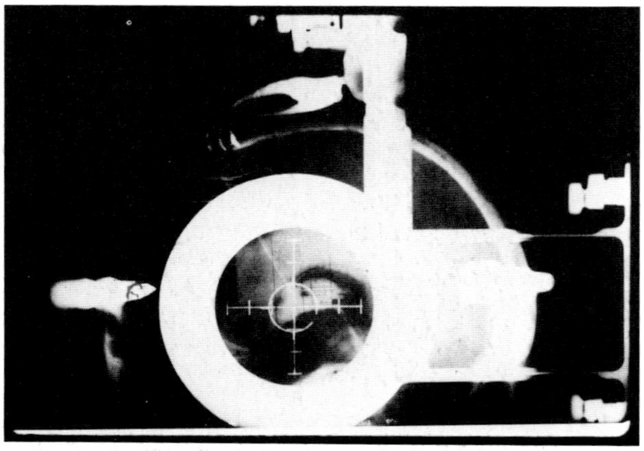

3

## Stereotactic ventriculography

3

The lateral ventricle is tapped stereotactically through a burr hole made 12 cm posterior to the nasion and 2.5 cm from the midline, and a contrast ventriculogram is performed utilizing a 220 mg per cent concentration of metrizamide. The anterior and posterior commissures are identified. The approximate location of the various thalamic subnuclei are determined utilizing a method developed by Guiot and described elsewhere[25]. Following this procedure the wound is closed and the patient removed from the stereotactic frame for that day.

## Semi-microelectrode recording

The patient is returned to the operating room on the next operating day for reapplication of the frame. Reapplication in the same frame position is assured by the fact that the headholder fixes to the patient's skull by pins inserted into holes drilled in the outer table of the skull which were made during the first application of the headholder. The headholder's position is checked by micrometer settings which measure the depth of the fixation pins relative to the vertical supports of the headholder.

Under sedation and local infiltration anaesthesia the patient is replaced in the stereotactic frame and the coronal wound opened. A bipolar concentric microelectrode with a 10–50 μm active recording tip and a 400 μm tip-to-ring distance is directed from the coronal burr hole to an intracranial target point 1 mm anterior to the posterior commissure on the AC/PC line and 11.5–13 mm lateral to the lateral wall of the third ventricle. The electrode is connected to a head-stage preamplifier and DC amplifier (DAM 5A, WPI Instruments, Westboro, Connecticut, USA). The recorded electrical activity is presented aurally and visually by audiomonitor and oscilloscope, respectively. Distinctive cellular activity is encountered at the cortex, the caudate nucleus and dorsal thalamus. Background amplitude of the cellular activity increases as the electrode enters the ventralis posterior (VP).

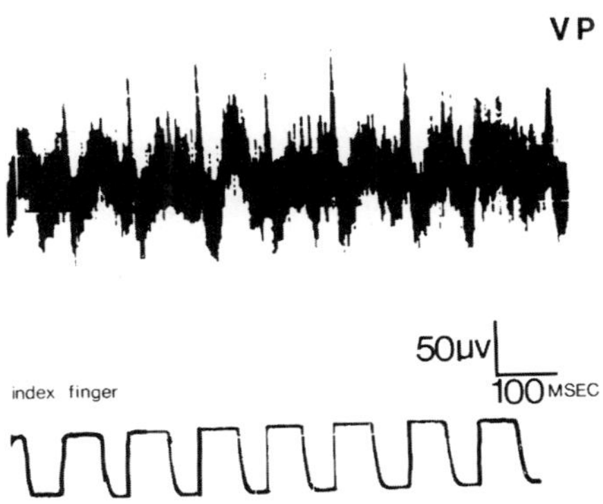


4

4

At this point the contralateral side of the patient's body is tapped or brushed. High-amplitude (150 μV) responses are obtained when touching the part of the face, trunk, arm, leg or digits represented by the part of the thalamus in which the electrode lies. Using this method, it is possible to establish the VP representation of specific body parts within an individual patient's thalamus. Somatosensory evoked responses recorded in the VP are used to define the neurophysiological laterality of the proposed lesion site.

Responses to nerve stimulation are quite focal and specific within the VP. As the electrode enters the medial lemniscus, responses become more generalized, with evoked potentials recorded at one site with stimulation of different nerves on different limbs. The inferior aspect of the thalamus frequently, but not always, corresponds to the AC/PC line. Anteroposterior and lateral radiographs which demonstrate the position of the tip of the microelectrode are obtained when the specificity of the evoked response is lost and the response becomes more generalized. These are compared with the ventriculogram and the final height coordinate for the lesion site is corrected in relationship to the actual location of the physiological inferior thalamic boundary.

## Lesioning procedure

5

The target point for the lesion site is 2.5 mm above the inferior boundary of the thalamus, 3 mm posterior to the midpoint of the AC/PC line, and at a laterality determined from the microelectrode recording. For the treatment of upper extremity tremor, lesions should be made in the VL anterior to the VP representation of the corner of the mouth, thumb or the index finger[16,25]. The lesion should be slightly more lateral for the treatment of lower-extremity tremor (anterior to the VP representation of the fifth finger). Radiofrequency lesions are made with a 1.1–1.6 mm diameter, 4 mm exposed temperature-monitored electrode. First a test lesion is made in which the electrode tip is heated to 42°C for 60 seconds. The patient is then examined to assess the neurological effects of the lesion on tremor, strength and coordination. Speech is carefully tested by a speech pathologist when the procedure is being performed on the left side. The onset or worsening of dysarthria, perseveration or disorientation, the development of aphasic verbal errors or increased verbal response latencies are particularly important signs of undesirable neurological sequelae. If no untoward effects have resulted from the test lesion, the electrode tip is then heated to 70–78°C for 60 seconds. This generates a lesion approximately 4 mm in diameter and 4–5 mm in length.

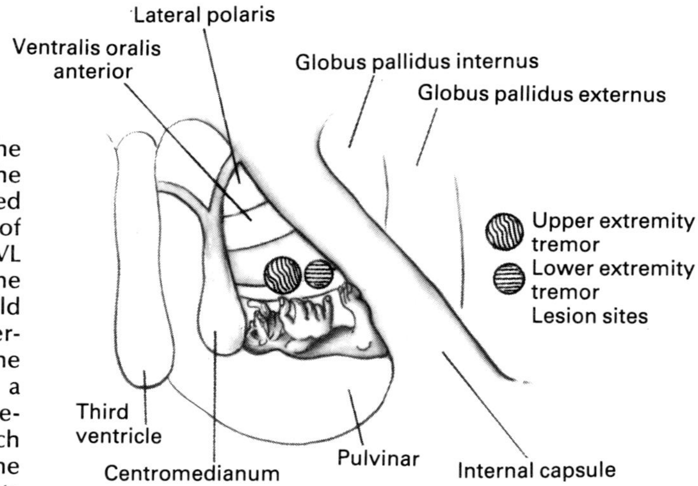


5

### Intention tremor

Selected patients with multiple sclerosis who are disabled by intention tremor derive significant benefit from VL thalamotomy[28]. Eighty to eighty-five per cent of operated patients will regain some useful function of the treated limb. Unfortunately, because of the degenerative nature of the disease, the ultimate long-term results will not be gratifying. In addition, younger patients having intention tremor related to cerebellar injuries can have good palliation by VL thalamotomy.

### Essential or familial tremor

These patients do not have a degenerative disease. Therefore they are excellent candidates for stereotactic thalamotomy when disabling tremor is refractory to medication such as anticholinergic drugs and propranolol.

# INDICATIONS FOR VENTRALIS LATERALIS THALAMOTOMY

## Parkinson's disease: tremor and rigidity

No therapy alters the relentless progression of Parkinson's disease. Therapy is symptomatic, with a goal of palliating the symptoms causing the disability[7]. Initially, tremor and rigidity are responsible for disability. Later in the course of the disease, bradykinesia results in significant disability and debilitation. Surgery is of particular benefit in patients with unilateral tremor who do not develop 'midline symptoms' (i.e. bradykinesia, mental deterioration, and speech and gait disturbances)[26]. Stereotactic surgery will abolish contralateral tremor in 90 per cent and rigidity in 88 per cent of patients[7]. In addition, in patients with bilateral tremor, bilateral VL thalamotomy staged at least 3 months apart can provide effective long-term palliation from tremor and rigidity[7,27]. Surgery is of no benefit in patients having rigidity and bradykinesia without tremor or in those who have rapidly progressive parkinsonism.

### Dystonia musculorum deformans

In some hands good results can be obtained in patients with dystonia[14,29]. The results of VL lesions are better if the patient's dystonia is confined distally to an extremity[14]. Patients having midline dystonic syndromes, including torticollis and retrocollis, do not usually derive lasting benefit from central stereotactic procedures, and they require peripheral intervention as well[30].

### Cerebral palsy

Some authors have reported favourable results with tension athetosis involving the upper extremities. It must be recognized that the basic pathological process has resulted in considerable destruction of cortex and basal ganglia. Therapeutic subcortical lesions may result in significant gait, speech or intellectual complications, even though surgery may have a beneficial effect on the tension athetosis.

# Stereotactic procedures for tumours

## STEREOTACTIC BIOPSY

With the CT- and MRI-based stereotactic biopsy procedures available, there is no excuse for not establishing the histological nature of any suspicious subcortical intracranial lesion. Stereotactic biopsies can establish the histological diagnosis of subcortical tumours with minimal morbidity. Reported mortality/morbidity rates for stereotactic biopsy procedures are low[4,19,31,32]. Apuzzo and Sabshin reported a 4 per cent morbidity in their series of 83 CT-based stereotactic biopsy procedures[4]. Lunsford and Martinez reported no permanent morbidity in 98 procedures[33]. In our experience with 422 stereotactic biopsy procedures, two patients had neurological complications and one patient died as a result of postoperative haematomas. In addition, the diagnostic yield has been very high (98 per cent)[17,19]. The stereotactic coordinates of the lesion are obtained from CT or MRI.

### Indications

Stereotactic biopsies are usually performed on intra-axial lesions. Traditionally these are usually deep-seated lesions which are not suitable for conventional craniotomy, owing to the risk of being unable to find them at an open procedure. Subcortical centrally located, basal ganglia, thalamic, brainstem, or deep cerebellar tumours can be biopsied easily and safely by computer assisted stereotactic techniques. In addition, stereotactic biopsy is the preferred method for obtaining a tissue diagnosis in hypodense lesions on CT scanning which do not enhance with contrast. These are usually infiltrating tumours which, when radically resected, are complicated by a neurological deficit if located in important brain tissue. Other possible candidates for stereotactic biopsy are patients who are too ill to undergo conventional craniotomy. Stereotactic biopsy procedures can usually be performed under local anaesthesia with little risk to the patient.

### Contraindications

In competent hands, stereotactic biopsy is a low-risk procedure. However, certain lesions pose more risk than others. Patients having lesions with significant mass effect risk cerebral herniation following stereotactic biopsy. Craniotomy with internal decompression is more advisable in these cases. In addition, lesions presenting as an intense contrast-enhancing abnormality on CT scanning, with or without vascular stain on cerebral angiography, could be cavernous or thrombosed vascular malformations. These lesions can haemorrhage when biopsied stereotactically. Pituitary-stalk lesions within the circle of Willis can be biopsied, but with considerable trepidation.

### Goals

There are three goals for most stereotactic biopsy procedures: (*1*) to establish tissue diagnosis; (*2*) to determine the extent of the neoplasm; and (*3*) to determine whether the neoplasm is composed of tumour tissue or infiltrated parenchyma. Adequate sampling of the CT or MRI defined abnormality is necessary to establish a tissue diagnosis. In addition, serial stereotactic biopsy samples obtained from perilesional CT- and MRI-normal as well as abnormal areas are required in order to establish the limits of a tumour along the biopsy trajectory[20,34]. Stereotactic sampling must also be adequate to determine whether the tumour comprises solid tumour tissue alone, parenchyma infiltrated by isolated tumour cells, or a combination of tumour tissue and infiltrated parenchyma[20,34]. Tissue diagnosis, tumour extent, and tumour composition have important ramifications on therapeutic procedures which will be offered subsequently.

### Instruments available

In order to perform stereotactic biopsies, a surgeon requires an imaging-compatible stereotactic instrument and a method for imaging (CT, MRI, digital angiography) data acquisition. In addition, instruments for the control of bleeding as well as the actual instruments for obtaining the specimens are required. The most popular appear to be the standard bronchoscopy-type forceps[4,19,31] and the side-biting window cannula[20], although other types of biopsy instruments have been described[4,35].

## PROCEDURAL ASPECTS

### Database acquisition

*Application of the stereotactic head frame*

Patients are sedated with neuroleptic analgesia. The CT/MRI-compatible headholder is fixed to the patient's head by means of four flanged carbon fibre pins which are inserted through 7/64-inch holes drilled in the outer table of the skull into the diploe.

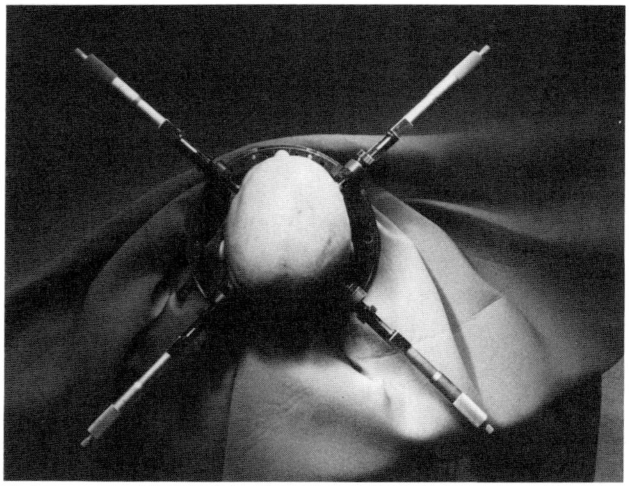

6

# 6

Micrometers are attached to the vertical supports and are advanced to the end of the carbon fibre pin. These measurements are noted in the patient's record.

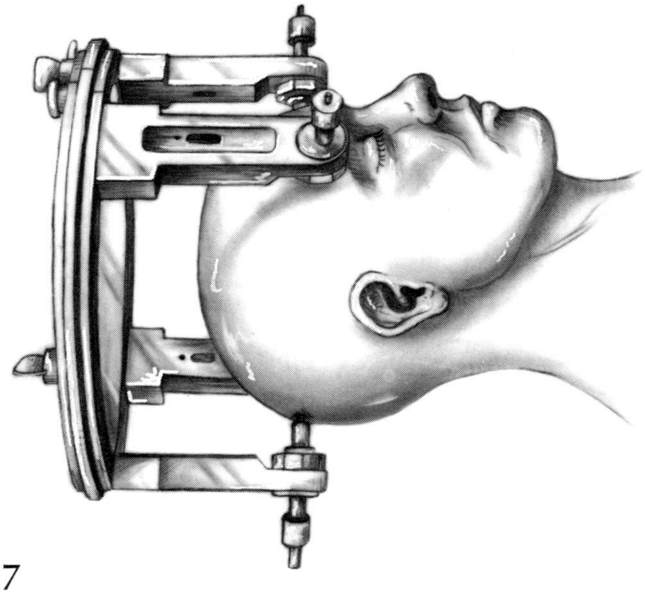

7

# 7

Posterior fossa procedures are carried out in the prone position with the round stereotactic headholder applied in the inverted position as shown. This will allow unobstructed access to the posterior fossa.

## Stereotactic CT scanning

8

The localization system described above attaches to the base ring of the stereotactic headholder in such a way that a set of three N-shaped rods is located on either side of the head and anteriorly. The localization system produces nine reference marks on each CT slice from which three vertical heights above the base ring are calculated, three points in space derived thereby, and the position and inclination of the CT slice plane above the base ring established. The zero point of the coordinate arcs defined by the localization system is related to mechanical adjustments of the stereotactic instrument by bias factors[5,19].

Following CT scanning, the stereotactic calculations may be performed by a program on the CT computer (which is identical to the computer located in the operating suite) or the archived CT data tape may be input to the operating room computer system.

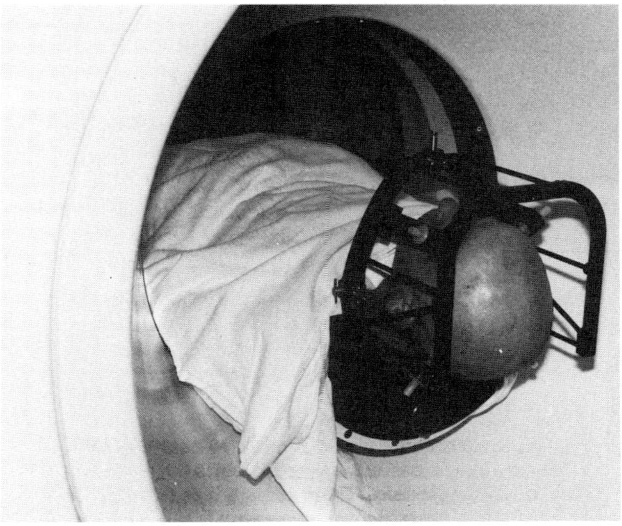

8

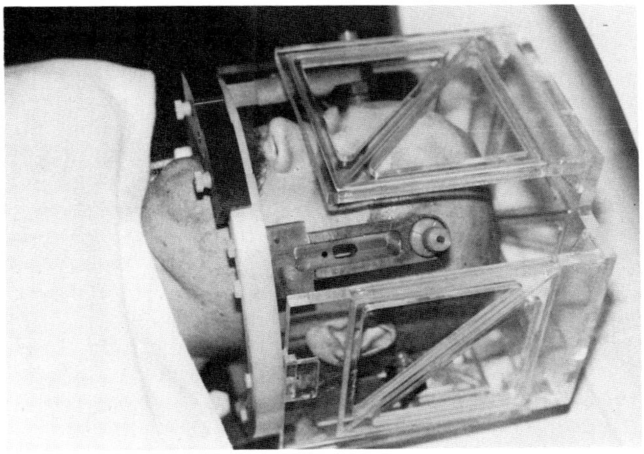

9

## Stereotactic magnetic resonance imaging (MRI)

9

Stereotactic MRI examinations are performed on a Picker (Picker International, UK) 0.15 tesla resistive unit or a General Electric Signa 1.5 tesla superconducting system. An MRI-compatible base ring constructed of carbon fibre utilizes the same vertical support and fixation system described for CT. A multiplanar localization system is used to calculate stereotactic coordinates from coronal and sagittal planes, as well as transverse images. Following the stereotactic MRI scan, the archived data tape is also input to the operating room computer system for stereotactic target calculations.

## Avoidance of vascular structures

In order to perform safe stereotactic biopsies, the precise positions of important vascular structures in relation to CT and MRI target points should be known. There are several methods currently employed at other centres. First, large vascular structures are visible on stereotactic CT and high-quality MR images and those can be avoided by the biopsy trajectory.

Secondly, an arteriogram can also be performed with the patient in the stereotactic frame utilizing a direct puncture of the carotid artery or a transfemoral catheterization technique. 'Single shot' arterial and venous phase images can then be obtained, utilizing the stereotactic teleradiographic equipment if a serialograph for stereotactic work is unavailable. Utilizing this method, magnification for the angiogram and the subsequent stereotactic radiographs will be identical, and calculations based on these will be accurate.

We believe that the most convenient method for arteriographic control involves the use of an operating-room computer system. The computer establishes a two-dimensional matrix for anteroposterior and lateral arterial and venous phases of the arteriogram which can be related by the computer to the CT and MRI databases as described below.

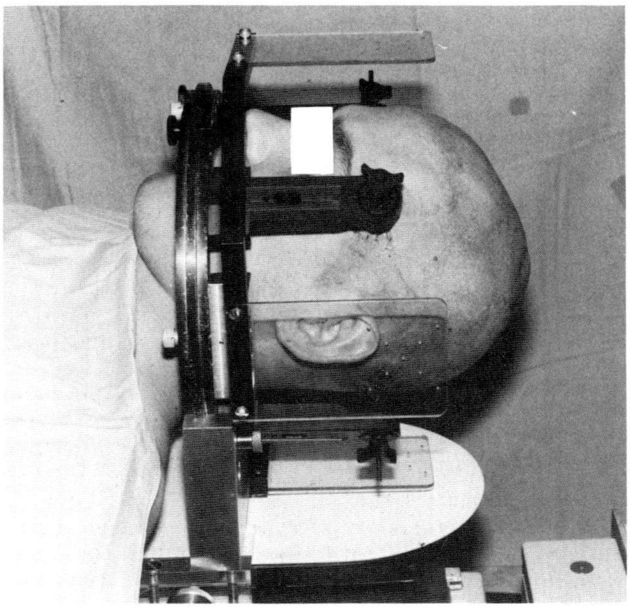

10a

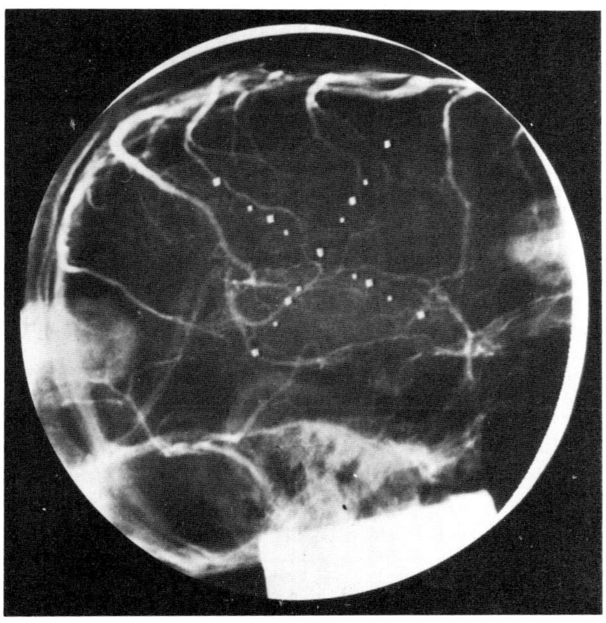

10b

## Stereotactic digital angiography

# 10a & b

Patients undergo digital angiography (DA) examination with their heads fixed in the CT/MRI-compatible stereotactic headholder as described above. A DA table adaptation system for the General Electric DF 3000 or 5000 unit receives the stereotactic headholder. An arteriographic reference system (ARS) fits onto the headholder (*a*). The ARS contains arrays of nine points suspended in radiolucent reference plates which attach to each side of the base ring of the headholder. The reference plates are positioned bilaterally, anteriorly and posteriorly. This creates 18 reference marks on each DA image (*b*). The reference marks define coordinate axes of the ARS and provide grids for the computer calculation of X-ray magnification at any three-dimensionally defined point in space. A computer program transforms X, Y, Z points in space (from stereotactic CT and MRI calculations) as a function of distances from the central X-ray beam and ARS reference plates, and interpolates the magnification factor for the correct annotation of that point on the DA images. With appropriate computer software, target points and entry points on anteroposterior and lateral views of the stereotactic arteriogram can be displayed.

## Data input

The archived data tapes from the CT, MRI and DA examinations are transferred to the operating room computer system. Decoding programs have been written for CT, MRI and DA image formats so that each CT slice, MR or DA image may be displayed on the central Ramtek (General Electric Medical Systems) console for convenient calculation of stereotactic coordinates and for treatment planning. The surgeon communicates with the operating-room computer by means of an alphanumerical keyboard, a trackball which manipulates a cursor on the display screen, and a deposit key. User-friendly programs allow rapid calculations of stereotactic targets, cross-correlation of target points between CT, MRI, DA and a computer-resident stereotactic atlas. Probe trajectory simulations[19,21], radionuclide source isodose configurations[22], tumour volume displays[20] and reconstructions can be viewed with respect to the MRI, CT and DA database[18,36].

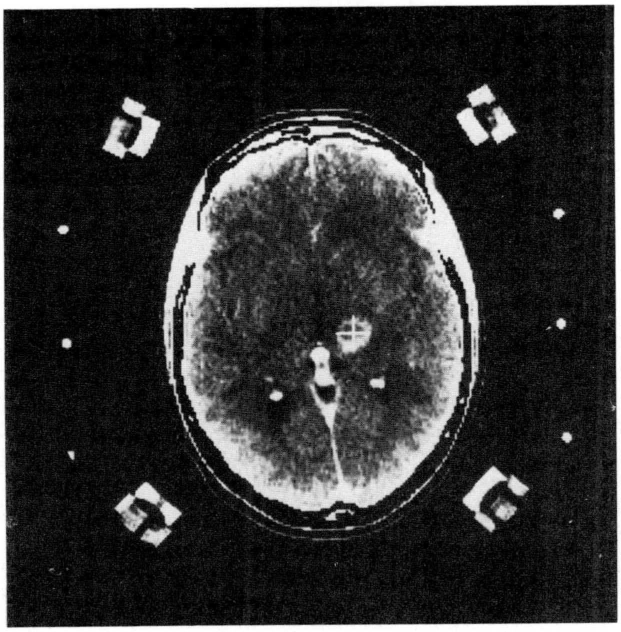

11

## 11

The surgeon selects target points from CT slices or MR images utilizing the cursor and trackball subsystems. A computer program computes screen coordinates for target points and converts these to stereotactic mechanical adjustments on the frame.

The frame adjustments are output on the computer screen or a line printer. All the calculations are done instantaneously by the computer. The numbers are then duplicated on the stereotactic instrument. These will bring the target points selected on CT or MRI into the focal point of the stereotactic arc-quadrant. The measured accuracy of this system for CT is ±500 μm in X and Y and within one-half of the CT slice thickness in Z. The tested accuracy of the MRI localization system is 1.1 mm in X and Y and within one-half of the MRI slice thickness in Z.

The DA images are displayed on the screen. First the surgeon digitizes all the 18 reference marks, utilizing the cursor and trackball subsystem. These establish reference points within a three-dimensional computer image matrix which can be related to the coordinates established for CT and MRI.

## Point in space

# 12a & b

The surgeon selects his target from displayed CT slices or MR images with the cursor and deposit key. The mathematical manipulations for the simple translation of a point selected on a CT slice to mechanical adjustments in a stereotactic frame are within the capabilities of a hand-held calculator or an inexpensive microprocessor-based computer. However, many more useful options exist if a more capacious microcomputer or minicomputer is available. The surgeon is able to simulate probe trajectories on arterial and venous phases of the arteriogram (*a*).

After the optimal trajectory has been selected, the computer outputs the arc and collar settings which represent these approach angles on the stereotactic instrument. Probe trajectories through contiguous CT or MRI slices given the calculated target coordinates and trajectory angles may also be displayed (*b*).

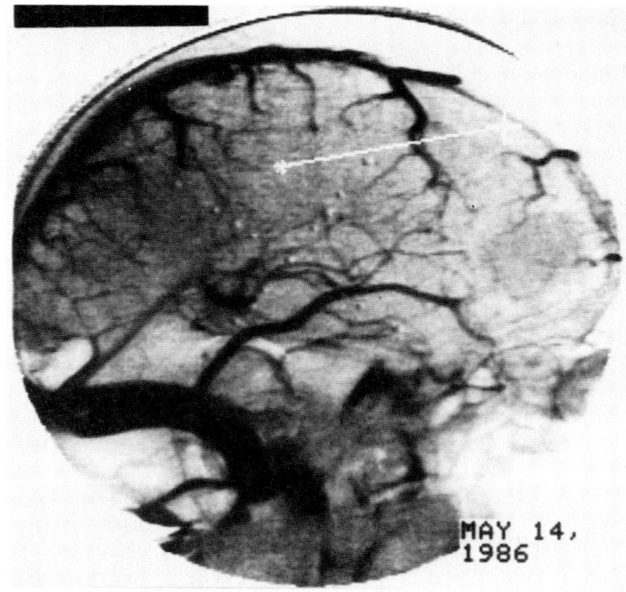


12a

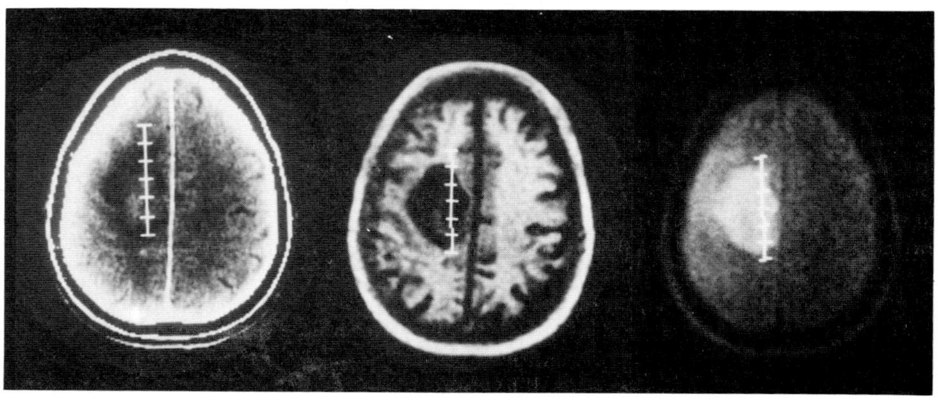

12b

## TRAJECTORY PLANNING

The biopsy probe is usually inserted through a twist drill or burr hole and directed by means of the stereotactic instrument through the lesion in question. An approach must be planned which avoids all vascular structures, provides the best sampling of the lesion, and avoids critical neuronal structures, e.g. cranial nerves, optic tract. In addition, it is best not to traverse major fissures of the brain (sylvian, Rolandic, interhemispheric), although in rare circumstances this can be considered. The planning of the optimal stereotactic trajectory for a biopsy procedure is best done preoperatively, and mechanical adjustments on the stereotactic frame, the approach angular settings and the number and location of each biopsy specimen obtained determined in advance. The following will describe our method for trajectory planning. Lesions in specific locations present special considerations and the plan for each of those locations will be described separately.

## SURGICAL APPROACHES

### Subcortical lesions

If a subcortical lesion is anterior to the Rolandic fissure, the approach is from an anterior to posterior direction. If the lesion is posterior to the central sulcus, it is approached from a posterior trajectory, usually performed with the patient rotated to the prone position. The location of the central sulcus can be determined by stereoscopic stereotactic arteriography or occasionally on stereotactic CT or MRI studies. Subinsular lesions may be approached from either in front or behind in the stereotactic frame, depending on whether the lesion lies more anteriorly or posteriorly. Basal ganglia lesions are best approached from a coronal entry point.

Thalamic lesions can be biopsied using many routes. An anterior thalamic lesion is best biopsied using a coronal approach, a pulvinar lesion can be sampled either from a coronal or posterior parietal entry point. Ventral thalamic lesions can be approached via the posterior temporal lobe. In this case, the patient is rotated in the stereotactic frame to a lateral decubitus position. Lesions of the pineal region and posterior third ventricle are biopsied with a probe directed from an anterior and lateral entry point. This trajectory should pass under the internal cerebral veins. Midbrain lesions are approached from a coronal entry point. Lesions in the pons are best accessed, in our experience, by passing the probe through a twist-drill opening in the lateral suboccipital squama, through the middle cerebellar peduncle. Here the stereotactic frame is placed in the inverted position and the surgery performed with the patient prone. Alternatively, central pontine lesions can also be approached from a coronal entry site. Cerebellar lesions are biopsied through the ipsilateral cerebellar hemisphere.

### Biopsy sampling

A stereotactic biopsy trajectory should be planned in order to traverse MRI-abnormal, CT-abnormal, and MRI- and CT-normal regions in order to obtain a representative sampling of a tumour. It is easier to plan a biopsy trajectory parallel to the CT slices and MR images. These trajectories can easily be displayed on stereotactic CT slices or MR images (*see Illustration 12b*). Occasionally this is not practical because of vascular structures that must be avoided.

Para-axial trajectories depend on surface vascular structures. The computer can calculate the distance along the trajectory to the target point and display a cursor on contiguous CT slices and MR images as the probe passes these.

## SURGICAL PROCEDURE

At our institution we routinely gather the stereotactic database on 1 day, and remove the stereotactic headholder. The treatment planning is done when convenient. The patient is returned to the operating room the next day and the stereotactic head frame is replaced.

Reapplication of the frame is simple: the surgeon taps the four fixation pins into the previously made drill holes, slides the sleeves over them and secures the sleeves with the colletts and caps after reproducing the micrometer measurements.

The calculated stereotactic frame adjustments are duplicated on the instrument. Stereotactic biopsy procedures can be done under local anaesthesia. However, we favour general anaesthesia for the following reasons. First, the trauma of passing a biopsy probe through a subcortical infiltrating tumour may precipitate a focal or generalized seizure, in spite of adequate anticonvulsant blood levels in a patient only under local anaesthesia. This is disconcerting for everyone concerned. Secondly, if arterial bleeding from a biopsy site should occur, an expedient stereotactically controlled craniotomy may be done to stop the bleeding if the patient is under general anaesthesia. Third, with his patient asleep, the surgeon is not under the emotional pressure of having an uncomfortable and complaining patient in the stereotactic frame. Rational decisions regarding further biopsy sampling or trajectories may be made.

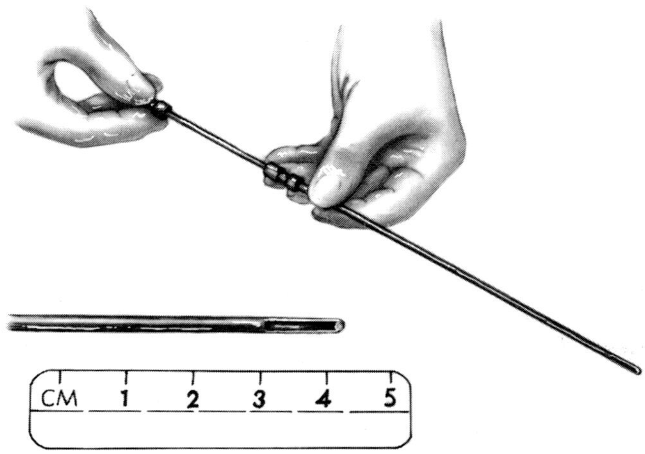


13

## 13

After preparing and draping the patient's head, a stereotactic guide tube penetrates a stab wound in the scalp, and anteroposterior and lateral teleradiographs are obtained in order to verify that the adjustments on the stereotactic frame are correct. The skull is penetrated using a ⅛-inch power-driven bit directed through the guide tube. The dura is opened with an insulated coagulation probe and unipolar cautery. The biopsy instrument is then directed to the position of the first biopsy specimen. We prefer a side-biting biopsy instrument that procures a 1-cm long, 1½-mm diameter cylinder of tissue. Multiple biopsies along a selected trajectory are obtained as the biopsy probe passes from normal tissue, through the tumour, and beyond, returning to normal tissue on the other side of the tumour. The position of each biopsy is confirmed by anteroposterior and lateral teleradiographs.

Bleeding is rarely encountered. It is manifested by the appearance of blood welling up through the biopsy cannula. If this occurs, the cannula should not be moved. As long as it remains in place, blood will go out of the cannula and not form an intracranial haematoma. Gentle saline irrigation through the cannula and occasional clearing of clotted blood from the cannula with an aspirator will be all that is required to manage the great majority of bleeding instances during stereotactic biopsy procedures.

## Results

Four hundred and twenty-two patients underwent computer-assisted stereotactic serial biopsies utilizing the method described above. The lesion locations and histology in this group of patients are summarized in *Tables 1* and *2*.

**Table 1 Lesion locations (422 patients)**

| | |
|---|---|
| Frontal | 94 |
| Parietal | 97 |
| Temporal | 47 |
| Occipital | 7 |
| Corpus callosum | 15 |
| Basal ganglia | 34 |
| Thalamus | 64 |
| Hypothalamus | 14 |
| Midbrain | 9 |
| Pineal | 12 |
| Pons | 19 |
| Cerebellum | 10 |
| Total | 422 |

**Table 2 Histologies (422 stereotactic biopsies)**

| | |
|---|---|
| Neoplastic (334):(79.1%) | |
| Astrocytomas | |
| Grade IV | 82 |
| Grade III | 52 |
| Grade II | 79 |
| Grade I (pilocytic) | 13 |
| Oligodendroglioma | 45 |
| Lymphoma | 21 |
| Metastatic | 25 |
| Meningioma | 6 |
| Germinoma | 11 |
| Non-neoplastic (83):(19.7%) | |
| Demyelinating | 21 |
| Infarct | 15 |
| Cryptic arteriovenous malformation | 8 |
| Radiation necrosis | 14 |
| Haematoma | 3 |
| Abscess | 9 |
| Miscellaneous | 13 |
| No tissue diagnosis (5):(1.2%) | |

The tissue sampling provided by the serial stereotactic biopsy technique resulted in a firm histological diagnosis in 417 of the 422 patients. In addition, all patients in this series had been referred for histological confirmation of their 'tumour' by stereotactic biopsy. However, 83 patients (19 per cent) had non-neoplastic lesions (*Table 2*).

Postoperative complications occurred in three patients. Two had clinical signs of local haemorrhage after the biopsy, and a third patient died from subarachnoid haemorrhage after stereotactic biopsy of a hypothalamic tumour.

## Discussion

Stereotactic biopsy procedures provide a low-risk method for establishing actual tissue diagnosis so that patients with non-neoplastic and benign lesions can be spared empirical radiation therapy, inappropriate chemotherapy, or unnecessary craniotomy. Serial stereotactic biopsies also provide information on the histological boundaries of a neoplasm, which is useful in treatment planning.

Radiation oncologists who must determine the size and location of radiation ports for external-beam radiation therapy, and neurosurgeons interested in stereotactic interstitial irradiation have usually depended on CT to define the tumour target-volume. However, intracranial glial neoplasms frequently extend beyond the limits defined by CT[20,37]. By CT it is impossible to differentiate simply between 'peritumoural oedema' and actual tumour infiltration[20,34,37]. Examination of the tissue samples obtained by stereotactic biopsy from hypodense and contrast-enhancing areas on CT is the only precise method by which the clinician may be sure of the presence or absence of tumour cells, and can better conceptualize the actual tumour volume to be treated[34].

Stereotactic interstitial irradiation[22,38] and computer-assisted stereotactic laser resection[17,18,36] are two means by which stereotactically defined tumour volumes may be treated. These procedures are described in detail elsewhere.

### FUTURE POSSIBILITIES

Traditionally, stereotactic surgery has been considered a subspeciality far removed from mainstream neurosurgery. However, conventional neurosurgical procedures previously based on the hand–eye coordination of the surgeon can be complemented by the three-dimensional precision provided by stereotactic methods. This has far reaching implications on the treatment of intra-axial tumours and vascular lesions, as well as some extra-axial lesions.

The addition of stereotactic technology to neurosurgical technical skills can only improve the accuracy with which intracranial procedures are done, improving the completeness of resection and reducing the morbidity. Stereotactic surgery is a vehicle by which the precision inherent in new imaging technologies can directly benefit the surgical patient. New developments in computer, laser, ultrasonic and electronic technologies will improve the precision and the efficiency with which these procedures are done, and in some cases reduce costs. Infiltrating tumours may be treated by the stereotactic implantation of interstitial fibreoptic bundle arrays for efficient activation of tumoricidal photodynamic chemicals. Interstitially placed chemodes may more efficiently deliver chemotherapeutic agents to infiltrating neoplasms. The future applications of stereotactic techniques are limited only by our imagination.

## *References*


1. Horsley, V., Clarke, R. H. (1908) The structure and functions of the cerebellum examined by a new method. Brain, 31, 45–124
2. Spiegel, E. A., Wycis, H. T., Marks, M., Lee, A. J. (1947) Stereotaxic apparatus for operations on the human brain. Science, 106, 349–350
3. Brown, R. A. (1979) A computerized tomography-computer graphics approach to stereotaxic localization. Journal of Neurosurgery, 50, 715–720
4. Apuzzo, M. L. J., Sabshin, J. K. (1983) Computed tomographic guidance stereotaxis in the management of intracranial mass lesions. Neurosurgery, 12, 277–285
5. Goerss, S., Kelly, P. J., Kall, B. A., Alker, G. J. Jr. (1982) A computed tomographic stereotactic adaptation system. Neurosurgery, 10, 375–379
6. Leksell, L., Jernberg, B. (1980) Stereotaxis and tomography: a technical note with 6 figures. Acta Neurochirurgica (Wien), 52, 1–7
7. Kelly, P. J., Gillingham, F. G. (1980) The long term results of stereotaxic surgery and L-dopa therapy in patients with Parkinson's disease: a ten year follow-up study. Journal of Neurosurgery, 53, 332–337
8. Horsley, V. (1909) The Linacre lecture. The function of the so-called motor area of the brain. British Medical Journal, ii, 125–132
9. Bucy, P. (1942) Cortical extirpation in the treatment of involuntary movements. Research Publication – Association for Research in Nervous and Mental Disease, 21, 551–595
10. Meyers, R. (1942) The modification of alternating tremors, rigidity and festination by surgery of the basal ganglia. Research Publication – Association for Research in Nervous and Mental Disease, 21, 602–665
11. Fenelon, F. (1950) Essais de traitment neurochirurgical du syndrome parkinsonnien par intervention directe sur les voies extrapyramidales immediatement sous-striopallidales (anse lenticulaire). Communication suivie de projection du film d'un des opérés pris avant at apres l'intervention. Revue Neurologique, 83, 437–440
12. Cooper, I. S., Poloukhine, N. (1955) Chemopallidectomy: a neurosurgical technique useful in geriatric parkinsonians. Journal of the American Geriatric Society, 3, 839–859
13. Guiot, G., Brion, S. (1953) Traitement des mouvements anormaux par la coagulation pallidale. Technique et resultats. Revue Neurologique (Paris), 89, 578–580
14. Cooper, I. S. (1976) Dystonia: surgical approaches to treatment and physiologic implications. In The Basal Ganglia, Yahr, M. D. (ed.), Research Publication – Association for Research in Nervous and Mental Disease, 55, pp. 369–384. New York: Raven Press
15. Hassler, R. (1955) The influence of stimulations and coagulations in the human thalamus on the tremor at rest and its physiopathologic mechanisms. In Proceedings of the Second International Congress on Neuropathology, London, pt. 2, pp. 637–642. Amsterdam: Excerpta Medica
16. Kelly, P. J. (1980) Microelectrode recording for the somatotopic placement of stereotactic thalamic lesions in the treatment of parkinsonian and cerebellar intention tremor. Applied Neurophysiology, 43, 262–266
17. Kelly, P. J. (1986) Computer-assisted stereotaxis: new approaches for the management of intracranial intra-axial tumors. Neurology, 36, 535–541
18. Kelly, P. J., Alker, G. J., Goerss, S. J. (1982) Computer-assisted stereotactic microsurgery for the treatment of intracranial neoplasms. Neurosurgery, 10, 324–331
19. Kelly, P. J., Alker, G. J. Jr., Kall, B. A., Goerss, S. J. (1984) A method of CT-based stereotactic biopsy with arteriographic control. Neurosurgery, 14, 172–177
20. Kelly, P. J., Daumas-Duport, C., Kispert, D. B., Kall, B. A., Scheithauer, B. W., Illig, J. J. (1987) Imaging-based stereotaxic serial biopsies in untreated intracranial glial neoplasms. Journal of Neurosurgery, 66, 685–874
21. Kelly, P. J., Earnest, F., Kall, B. A., Goerss, S. J., Scheithauer, B. (1985) Surgical options for patients with deep-seated brain tumors: computer-assisted stereotactic biopsy. Mayo Clinic Proceedings, 60, 223–229
22. Kelly, P. J., Kall, B. A., Goerss, S. J. (1984) Computer simulation for the stereotactic placement of interstitial radionuclide sources into CT-defined tumor volumes. Neurosurgery, 14, 442–448
23. Kelly, P. J., Kall, B. A., Goerss, S. (1983) Stereotactic CT scanning for the biopsy of intracranial lesions and functional neurosurgery. Applied Neurophysiology, 46, 193–199
24. Kall, B. A., Kelly, P. J., Goerss, S. J., Frieder, G. (1985) Methodology and clinical experience with computed tomograph and a computer-resident stereotactic atlas. Neurosurgery, 17, 400–407
25. Kelly, P. J., Derome, P., Guiot, G. (1978) Thalamic spatial variability and the surgical results of lesions placed with neurophysiologic control. Surgical Neurology, 9, 307–315
26. Guiot, G., Derome, P., Jedynak, P., Arfel, G., Walter, S. (1975) Permanence des indications de la chirurgie stéréotaxique dans le treblement parkinsonnien et certains mouvements anormaux rebelles. Annales de Medecine Interne, 126, 295–296
27. Krayenbuhl, H., Wyss, O. A. M., Yasargil, M. G. (1961) Bilateral thalamotomy and pallidotomy as treatment for bilateral parkinsonism. Journal of Neurosurgery, 18, 429–444
28. Krayenbuhl, H., Yasargil, M. G. (1962) Relief of intention tremor due to multiple sclerosis by stereotaxic thalamotomy. Confinia Neurologica, 22, 368–374
29. Bertrand, C., Molina-Negro, P., Martinez, S. N. (1979) Stereotactic targets for dystonias and dyskinesias: relationship to corticobulbar fibers and other adjoining structures. Advances in Neurology, 24, 395–399
30. Bertrand, C., Molina-Negro, P., Martinez, S. N. (1978) Combined stereotactic and peripheral surgical approach in spasmodic torticollis. Applied Neurophysiology, 41, 122–133
31. Edner, G. (1981) Stereotactic biopsy of intracranial space occupying lesions. Acta Neurochirurgica (Wien), 57, 213–234

32. Ostertag, C. B., Mennel, H. D., Kiessling, M. (1980) Stereotactic biopsy of brain tumors. Surgical Neurology, 14, 275–283

33. Lunsford, L. D., Martinez, A. J. (1984) Stereotactic exploration of the brain in the era of computed tomography. Surgical Neurology, 22, 222–230

34. Daumas-Duport, C., Monsaingeon, V., Szenthe, L., Szikla, G. (1982) Serial stereotactic biopsies: a double histological code of gliomas according to malignancy and 3–D configuration, as an aid to therapeutic decision and assessment of results. Applied Neurophysiology, 45, 431–437

35. Backlund, E. O. (1971) A new instrument for stereotaxic brain tumor biopsy. Acta Chirurgica Scandinavica, 137, 825–827

36. Kelly, P. J., Kall, B. A., Goerss, S. J., Earnest, F. (1986) Computer-assisted stereotaxic laser resection of intra-axial brain neoplasms. Journal of Neurosurgery, 64, 427–439

37. Scarabin, J. M., Pecker, J., Brucher, J. M., Vallée, B., Guégan, Y., Faivre, J. (1978) Stereotaxic exploration in 200 supratentorial brain tumors. Its value in addition to computerized tomography. Neuroradiology, 16, 591–593

38. Gutin, P. H., Phillips, T. L., Hosobuchi, Y., Wara, W. M., Mackay, A. R., Weaver, K. A. (1981) Permanent and removable implants for the brachytherapy of brain tumors. International Journal of Radiation Oncology, Biology, Physics, 7, 1371–1381

Illustrations by Robert Gordon

# Dorsal root entry zone coagulation

**Peter R. Bronec** MD
Division of Neurosurgery, Department of Surgery, Duke University Medical Center, Durham, North Carolina, USA

**Stephen C. Saris** MD
Surgical Neurology Branch, National Institute of Health, Bethesda, Maryland, USA

**Blaine S. Nashold Jr** MD
Division of Neurosurgery, Department of Surgery, Duke University Medical Center, Durham, North Carolina, USA

## Introduction

The dorsal root entry zone (DREZ) is the longest continuous region of grey matter in the spinal cord, extending from the caudal brainstem to the conus medullaris. It was first described as the substantia gelatinosa by the Italian neuroanatomist Rolando[1] in the 19th century. More recently, Rexed[2] identified ten cytologically distinct layers in the DREZ of the cat, and described an abundance of nociceptor neuron cell bodies in layers I–V (especially layer I) which contributed to the contralateral spinothalamic tract. Several bioactive peptides involved in the physiology of pain are found in the DREZ. For example, substance P, which is known to excite dorsal horn neurons responsive to noxious stimuli, is located in Rexed layers I, II, III and IV, while layers I, II, IV and VII contain either somatostatin, methionine or enkephalin, all of which inhibit nociceptive cell bodies[3].

Neuroanatomists have recognized the importance of the DREZ in the pathophysiology of pain. Recent neurophysiological experiments in animals have shown that root avulsion causes both marked neuronal hyperactivity in this zone[4] and an imbalance among the bioactive peptides. For example, in cats the concentration of substance P receptors increases after root avulsion and causes neuronal hyperexcitability[3]. These physiological and pharmacological changes in the DREZ after deafferentation are believed to be involved in the production of pain. DREZ lesioning was designed to destroy these regions of neuronal dysfunction, specifically Rexed layers I–V. The first human DREZ lesioning was performed in 1975 on a patient with chronic pain after a brachial plexus avulsion. Between 1975 and 1984, we have carried out 200 such operations with encouraging results.

### Indications

Thermocoagulation of the DREZ was designed to treat chronic pain syndromes resulting from deafferentation of second-order neurons. It is an operation which requires few specialized pieces of equipment and can be done with minimal risk to the patient. Its greatest success has been with a group of central pain syndromes which frequently do not respond to medical or surgical therapy: root avulsion, paraplegia-related pain, post-herpetic neuralgia and phantom limb pain (*see Table 1*). Less encouraging results have been obtained with post-thoracotomy pain and post-rhizotomy pain. A good result is generally defined as a sustained reduction in pain of at least 75 per cent requiring no further narcotic analgesics.

#### *Root avulsion*

Traumatic nerve root avulsions are most common from the cervical spinal cord (brachial plexus avulsion) but may also occur from the conus medullaris. They are most commonly seen with trauma sustained in motor vehicle accidents. Careful preoperative clinical evaluation and myelography are essential in order to determine the nerve roots which have been damaged and to identify pseudomeningoceles. The pain syndrome which results from root avulsion has been well described in the literature[5] and will not be discussed here. Approximately 75 per cent of these patients obtain a good result from DREZ thermocoagulation of the cervical cord or conus medullaris[6,7].

**Table 1 Results of dorsal root entry zone coagulation**

| *Indication* | *Number of patients* | *Good relief n (%)* | *Fair/poor relief n (%)* | *Range of follow-up* | *Median follow-up (years)* |
|---|---|---|---|---|---|
| Root avulsion | | | | | |
| brachial plexus | 26 | 18 (69) | 8 (31) | 5 months–6½ years | 2½ |
| lumbosacral plexus | 6 | 5 (83) | 1 (17) | 1–4 years | 2½ |
| Post-paraplegic pain | 56 | 28 (50) | 28 (50) | 6 months–6 years | 2 |
| Post-herpetic neuralgia | | | | | |
| spinal | 17* | 10 (59) | 7§ (41) | 6–25 months | 1 |
| trigeminal | 6 | 5 (83) | 1 (17) | 3–27 months | 1 |
| Phantom limb pain | 16 | 8† (50) | 8 (50) | 6 months–4 years | 2 |

* 15 thoracic, 1 cervical, 1 lumbar.
† Six of the nine patients with phantom limb pain and root avulsion had good results.
§ One patient had a residual band of pain adjacent to the region of DREZ lesioning but declined further surgery to extend the lesions.

### *Paraplegia*

Approximately 10 per cent of patients with traumatic paraplegia develop a central pain syndrome. Thorough clinical assessment preoperatively will reveal the level of injury and the presence of any trigger zones in the sensory transition region one to two dermatomes above the level of injury. Delayed computerized tomographic scanning of the cord after metrizamide injection is important to identify cysts in the spinal cord, which are present in up to 65 per cent of these patients. About 50 per cent of patients with paraplegia-related pain who have undergone DREZ coagulation at and two to three levels above the site of cord injury have had a good result[8]. Any spinal cord cyst is drained into the subarachnoid space at the time of DREZ lesioning.

### *Post-herpetic neuralgia*

A small percentage of patients with herpetic skin infections develop post-herpetic neuralgia. The majority of these infections occur in the thoracic dermatomes. However, herpes can also appear in the distribution of the cervical and lumbar roots, as well as the first division of the trigeminal nerve (herpes ophthalmicus). The pain typically remains confined to the dermatomes of previous cutaneous involvement. In the case of cervical, thoracic or lumbar root involvement, the correct level is identified by evoked potentials and is treated by coagulation of the DREZ. In our series, approximately three-quarters of such patients had a good outcome from surgery[9]. In the case of herpes ophthalmicus, the DREZ of the ipsilateral nucleus caudalis is coagulated. Initial results with this operation are very promising, although follow-up is as yet short. To date, five of six patients have had a good result.

### *Phantom limb pain*

Many patients who have had amputations develop pain in the stump and/or phantom limb. DREZ thermocoagulation improves patients with phantom pain, particularly if root avulsion is present. It is not indicated for stump pain, which is a peripheral rather than a deafferentation problem. In our small series, two-thirds of patients (six of nine) with phantom pain did well after a minimum follow-up of 6 months[10].

# Preoperative

## Preparation and position of patient

The night before surgery, the patient is started on dexamethasone 10 mg every 6 hours. After general anaesthesia has been induced, the patient is placed prone on an X-ray compatible operating table with bolsters at the shoulders and hips to reduce venous pressure. For cervical and upper thoracic procedures a cranial fixation device such as the Mayfield head holder is used. Before draping the patient, transcutaneous stimulating electrodes are applied for later intraoperative nerve root localization (*see Illustration 3*). In the case of thoracic procedures, a percutaneous flexible monopolar electrode is placed along the appropriate intercostal nerve under fluoroscopic guidance.

# The operations

## SPINAL DREZ COAGULATION

## 1

### The incision

The incision is planned to allow exposure of the involved spinal cord region plus one segment above and below. In the cervical region, the DREZ lies just rostral to its associated intervertebral foramen so that coagulation of the DREZ of C6 and C7, for example, would require a C5–C7 laminectomy. In the thoracic region, laminae are exposed two to three levels rostral to the affected dermatomes. Thus, T6 and T7 DREZ coagulation would require a T4–T6 laminectomy. A T10–L1 laminectomy is performed for coagulation of the DREZ of the conus medullaris.

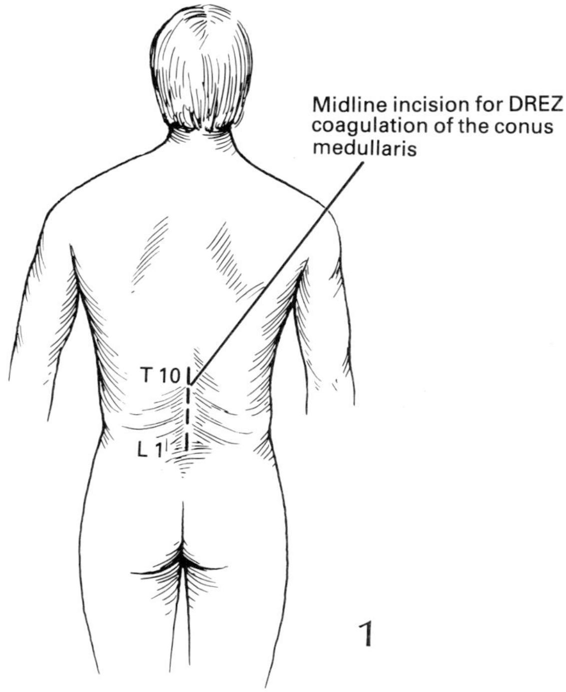


1

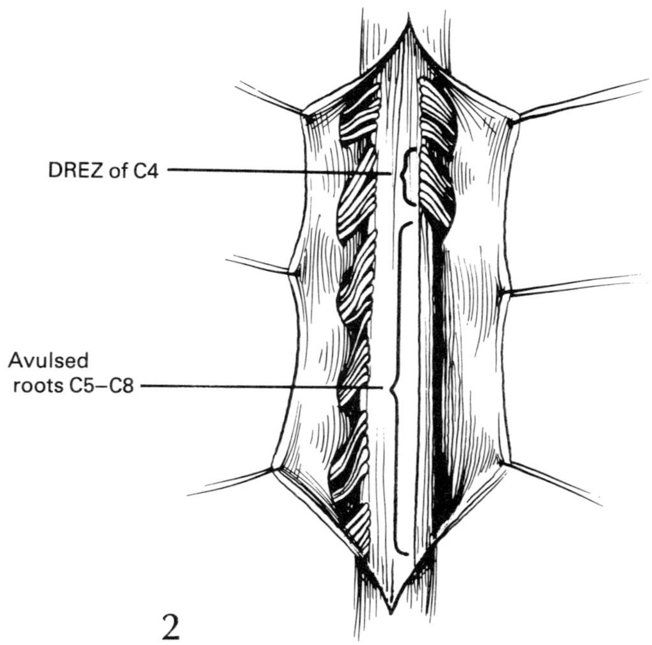


2

## 2

### Exposure

A standard laminectomy is performed. The dura is opened in the midline and retracted laterally with silk sutures. The arachnoid is opened directly over the DREZ (requiring two incisions for a bilateral procedure). For unilateral procedures, a hemilaminectomy and paramedian dural incision can be used, but this can be confining when attempting to record evoked potentials.

## Localization

3

In the cervical region, the level of the nerve root is identified by tracing it to its intervertebral foramen. In the case of root avulsions, the involved level is apparent. Before DREZ coagulation in the thoracic region or conus medullaris is started, a percutaneous monopolar electrode is placed near the intercostal, posterior tibial, sural or sciatic nerve. Intraoperatively, a multielectrode recording array is placed along the DREZ on the normal side. By evaluating the amplitude and latency characteristics of the evoked potentials at each electrode in the array, the site of maximal afferent activity is determined; this serves as an anatomical reference point.

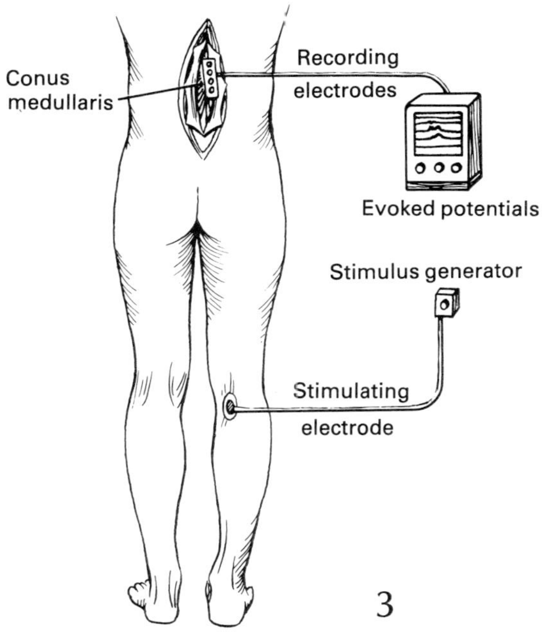


3

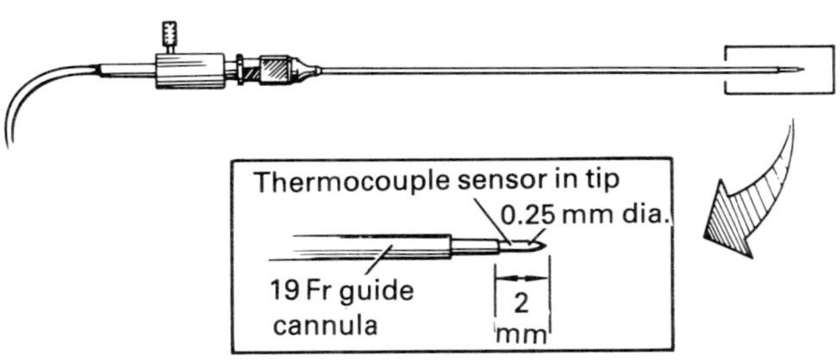


4

4

Radionics NCTD thermocouple temperature monitoring electrode (Burlington, Massachusetts, USA) with a tip diameter of 0.25 mm is used. It is insulated with a Teflon (El du Pont, UK) sheath which leaves only the distal 2 mm of the electrode exposed. A 19 Fr guide cannula is placed over the Teflon sheath for added stability.

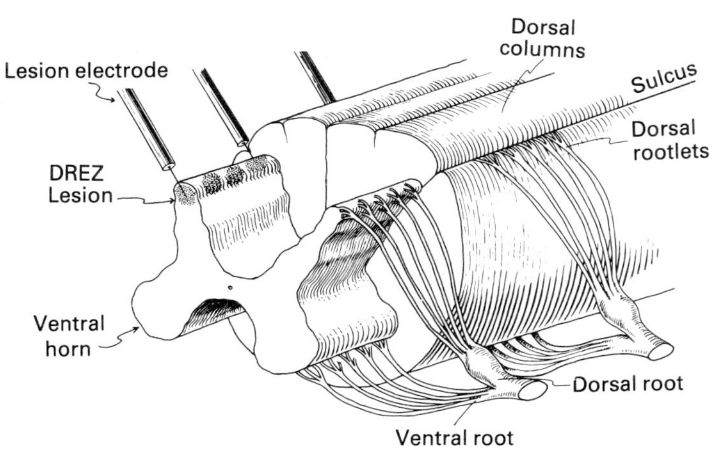


5

5

An operating microscope with a 300 mm lens and 12.5 power objective is used. The DREZ is identified as a small sulcus which runs lateral to the dorsal columns and through which the dorsal roots enter the cord. Arachnoid scars and blood vessels should be carefully mobilized from the DREZ. The lesions are made at 1 mm intervals through the affected levels and extended two segments rostral and one segment caudal to the region. Ten to fifteen lesions are required for each root level. The electrode is held perpendicular to the plane which is at a tangent to the cord at the DREZ. It is introduced to a depth of 2 mm, which is gauged by the Teflon sheath, and then heated to 75°C over a period of about 2 seconds. A 15-second lesion is then made. Although small blood vessels on the surface of the cord should be avoided if possible, incidental coagulation of a few minute vessels is inevitable. The electrode tip should be cleaned after each 15 lesions.

## Closure

After watertight dural closure, the muscle, fascia and subcutaneous tissue are closed in layers with interrupted sutures of slowly absorbable material. A monofilament, non-absorbable suture is used for the skin.

## NUCLEUS CAUDALIS THERMOCOAGULATION

# 6

### The incision

The patient is placed in the prone position with the head flexed and supported in a cranial fixation device. An incision is made from the inion to the area overlying the spinous tip of C4.

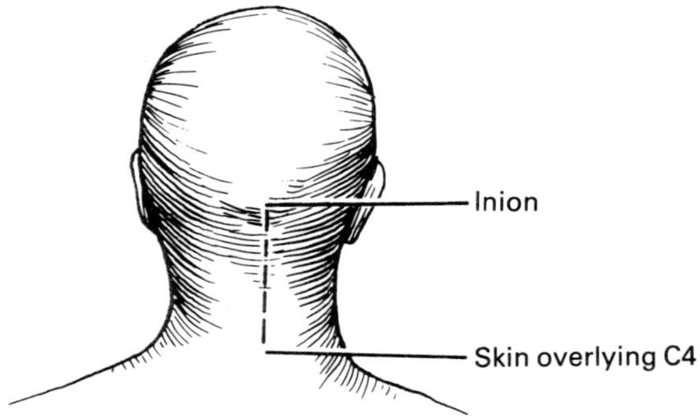


6

# 7

### Hindbrain exposure

A suboccipital craniectomy and C1-C3 laminectomy are performed. The dura is opened in a Y-shaped fashion to expose the caudal fourth ventricle, obex, dorsal medulla and dorsal roots of C2. The arachnoid is opened over the DREZ of C2 on the symptomatic side, and the opening extended rostrally over the cisterna magna.

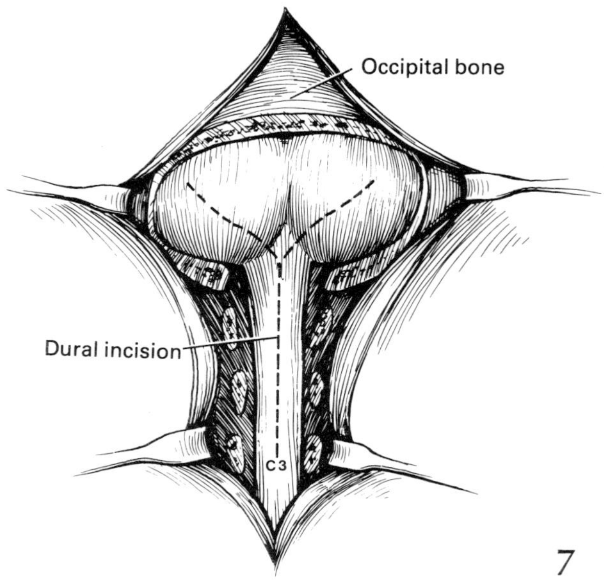


7

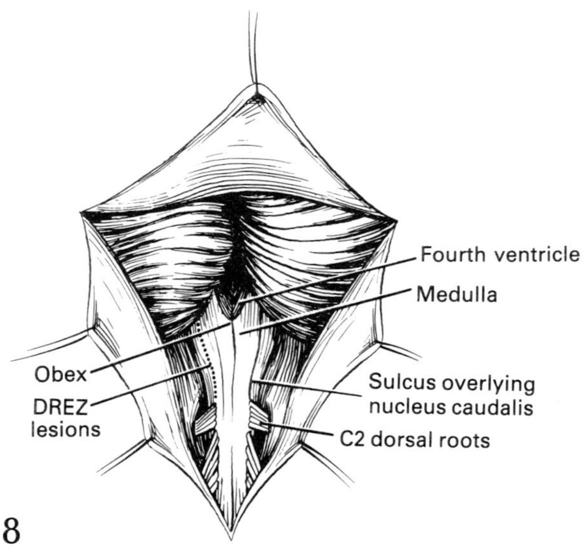


8

# 8

The C2 DREZ is then thermocoagulated as described above (*see Illustration 5*). The lesions are continued rostrally in the sulcus which overlies the nucleus caudalis. This sulcus starts at the rostral end of the spinal DREZ (at C2) and continues upward until 2–3 mm above the obex. As this sulcus ascends, it moves in a slightly lateral direction.

## Postoperative care and complications

All patients are kept in the intensive care unit overnight. Dexamethasone is continued for 5 days after surgery and then gradually reduced. After low thoracic and lumbar operations, patients are kept supine in bed for 5 days to avoid a cerebrospinal fluid leak. After high thoracic and cervical operations, the head of the bed is maintained at 30° for 5 days. Stitches are removed after 7–10 days.

The commonest minor complication is postoperative weakness of the ipsilateral leg. This loss of strength is minor and usually resolves after a few months. It is suspected to be secondary to oedema affecting the corticospinal tract; but the ascending spinocerebellar tracts or propriospinal tract may be involved. Less commonly, proprioception, pain and temperature sense are diminished distally as a result of surgery. Few major complications have occurred. One paraplegic patient lost residual hip function, while in another reflex bladder function was lost for several months even though the lesion did not involve sacral roots. These complications have been significantly reduced since the introduction of the smaller, temperature-controlled DREZ electrode. There has been no surgical mortality.

### *References*


1. Rolando, L. (1824) Ricerche Anatomiche sulla Struttura del Midollo Spinale. Torino: Dalla Stamperia Reale
2. Rexed, B. (1952) The cytoarchitectonic organisation of the spinal cord in the cat. Journal of Comparative Neurology, 96, 415–495
3. Blumenkopf, B. (1984) Neuropharmacology of the dorsal root entry zone. Neurosurgery, 15, 900–903
4. Ovelmen-Levitt, J., Johnson, B., Bedenbaugh, P., Nashold, B. S. Jr. (1984) Dorsal root rhizotomy and avulsion in the cat: a comparison of long term effects on dorsal horn neuronal activity. Neurosurgery, 15, 921–927
5. Parry, C. B. (1980) Pain in avulsion lesions of the brachial plexus. Pain, 9, 41–53
6. Nashold, B. S. Jr., Ostdahl, R. H. (1979) Dorsal root entry zone lesions for pain relief. Journal of Neurosurgery, 51, 59–69
7. Thomas, D. G. T., Sheehy, J. P. R. (1983) Dorsal root entry zone lesions (Nashold's procedure) for pain relief following brachial plexus avulsion. Journal of Neurology, Neurosurgery and Psychiatry, 46, 924–928
8. Nashold, B. S. Jr., Bullitt, E. (1981) Dorsal root entry zone lesions to control pain in paraplegics. Journal of Neurosurgery, 55, 414–419
9. Friedman, A. H., Nashold, B. S. Jr., Ovelmen-Levitt, J. (1984) Dorsal root entry zone lesions for the treatment of post-herpetic neuralgia. Journal of Neurosurgery, 60, 1258–1262
10. Stephen C. C., Saris, M. D., Robert, P., Jacono, M. D., Nashold, B. S. Jr. (1985) Dorsal root entry zone lesions for post-amputation pain. Journal of Neurosurgery, 62, 72–76

Illustrations by Robert N. Lane

# The craniosynostoses

**Richard Hayward** MB BS, FRCS
Consultant Neurosurgeon, The Hospital for Sick Children, London; National Hospitals for Nervous Diseases, London; St. Mary's Hospital, London, UK

## Introduction

This chapter will describe the management of those conditions in which an abnormality of head shape or size is produced by premature fusion of skull sutures. Occasionally such abnormalities may be associated with metabolic disorders[1], but these are rare and will not be discussed further.

In normal circumstances the size and shape of the skull vault is a passive reflection of the brain that it contains. For example, a child with hydrocephalus or subdural effusions will have a large skull, while one with microcephaly will have a skull that is small. In the presence of a normal brain, an abnormality of skull shape will usually only be produced if there is an abnormality of the sutures preventing the normal and even expansion of the vault. It was Virchow who first pointed out the simple rule governing the deformity that would be so produced. If a suture is fused prematurely there will be a restraint on growth perpendicular to it, while compensatory growth will occur along the axis of the suture. For example, premature fusion of the sagittal suture produces a head that is narrow from side to side, but elongated along the line of the suture, i.e. anteroposteriorly.

## Proposed classification

It has been customary in the past to classify the craniosynostoses according to the abnormalities of head shape that are produced. This certainly has some use for descriptive purposes, but as the relevant syndromes differ markedly in their aetiology, and their neurological and genetic implications, as well as in their surgical treatment, a different classification will be given here.

The classification according to skull shape is given in *Illustrations 1–6*. In this chapter the following basic classification will be used.

1. The simple craniosynostoses
2. The complex craniosynostoses
3. Total craniostenosis.

### The simple craniosynostoses

Here are included premature fusion of the sagittal suture, the metopic suture, one coronal suture or a lambdoid suture. These conditions usually occur in isolation, only rarely carry any genetic implications and are not usually associated with any impairment of brain function. Their aetiology remains unknown, but a good case has been made for the theory that they are caused by unusual pressures acting upon the fetal head within the last weeks of intrauterine life. For example, it has been suggested that premature descent of the fetal head into the pelvis can immobilize the skull at right angles to the sagittal suture and force it to fuse prematurely[2], or if the head is gripped more obliquely, cause a coronal suture to behave in a similar fashion[3]. In 1980 Graham and Smith[4] also describe two cases of metopic synostosis associated with abnormal constraints upon the fetal head.

A simple premature synostosis of a single skull suture will produce the following appearances.

## 1

*Sagittal synostosis.* This is usually more obvious posteriorly than anteriorly. The suture in front of the posterior fontanelle may be easily visible in the newborn as a prominent bony ridge. The head is typically narrow from side to side and lengthened from front to back. However, the usual asymmetry of the suture fusion results in the narrowing being most obvious posteriorly, while compensatory growth anteriorly results in what can be an unattractive bossing of the forehead.

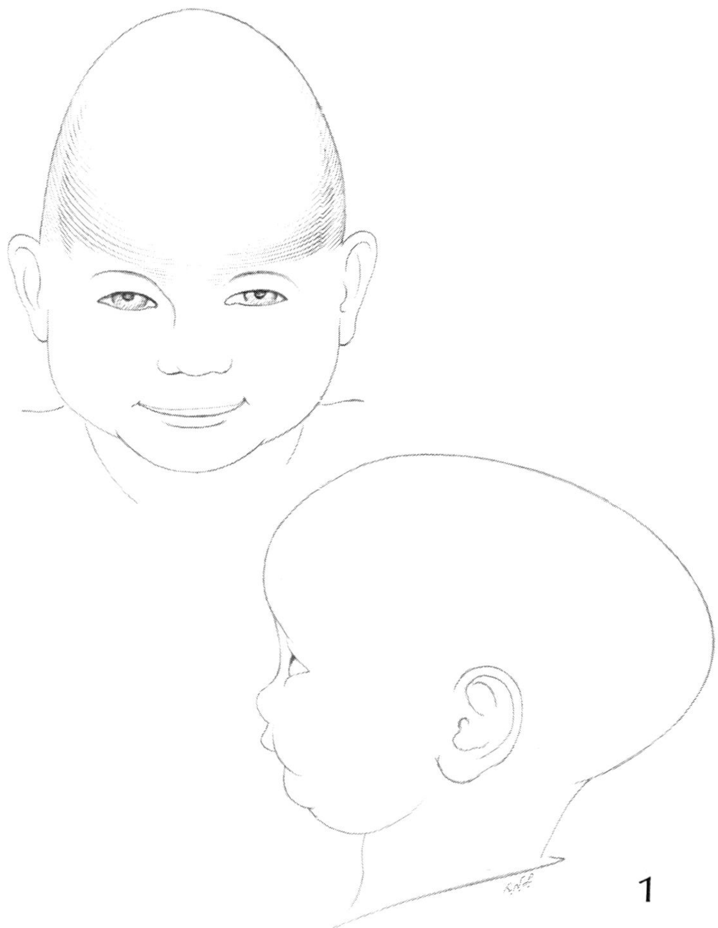

1

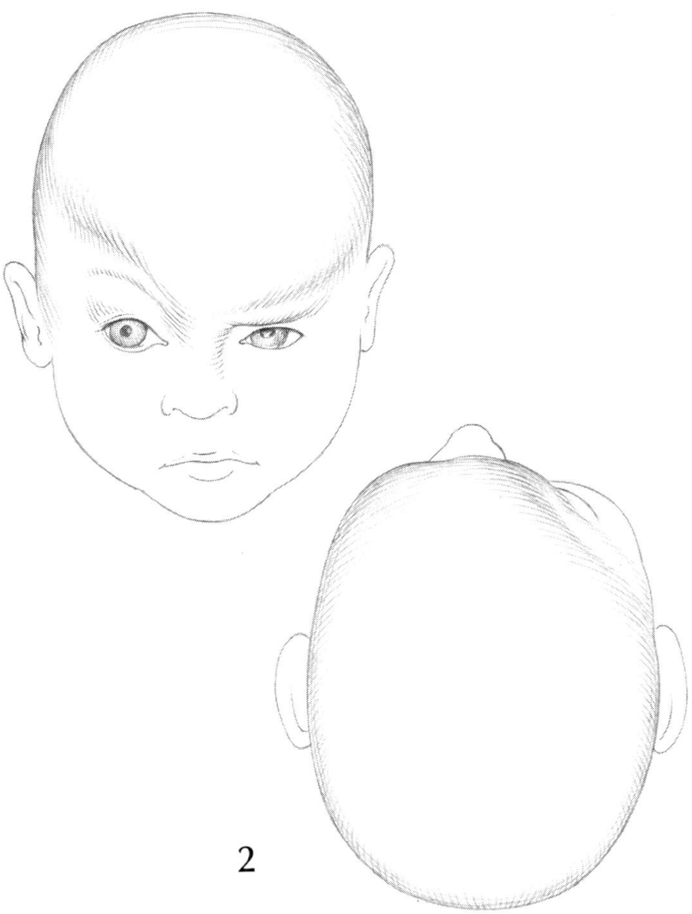

2

## 2

*Unicoronal synostosis.* There is a failure of the anterior fossa floor, and therefore of the superior orbital ridge on the affected side, to grow forwards. The bony contour behind the eyebrow is lost and the eyebrow itself is raised giving the child a permanently quizzical expression. Compensatory frontal expansion results in the frontal bone on the unaffected side becoming more prominent, while the eyebrow region appears drooped. It is often the appearance of this 'normal' side that prompts the parents to seek medical attention.

# 3

*Metopic synostosis.* This is a failure of the front of the anterior fossa, together with the frontal bones, to expand laterally. This results in hypotelorism, which may not necessarily produce any cosmetic disadvantage. However, the front of the head is triangular (trigonocephaly) and the suture itself is usually represented by an unattractive ridge down the centre of the forehead. When the child is viewed from above, the front of the head has the appearance of the bow of a ship.

*Lambdoid synostosis.* This is the least troublesome of the simple craniosynostoses. There is flattening of the occipital region on the affected side and often compensatory bulging on the other. The resulting deformity is often attributed to moulding of the head during parturition, but it fails to correct itself with time. A good head of hair is a most effective disguise and it is unusual for a unilateral lambdoid synostosis to require treatment.

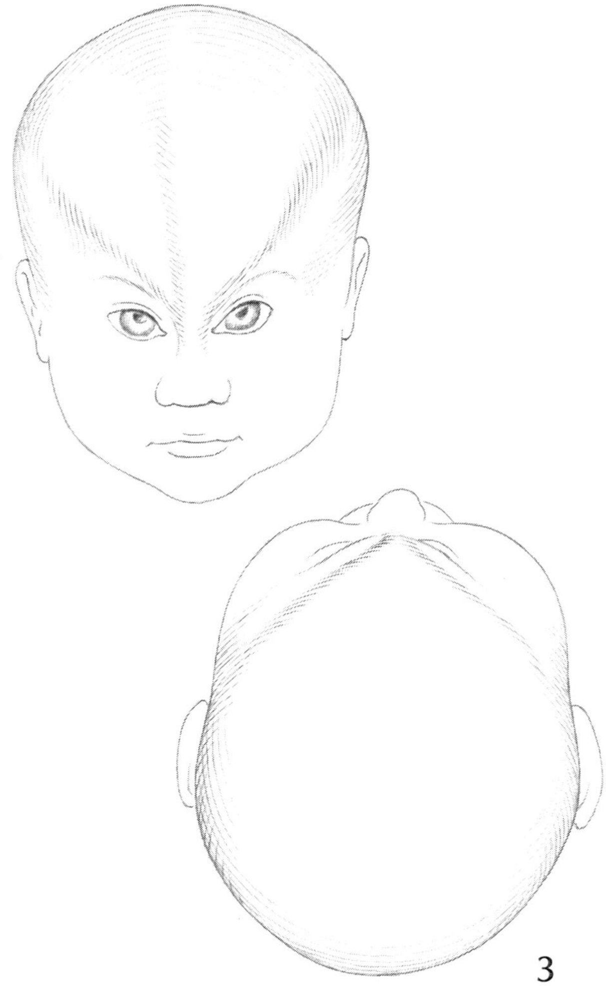

3

## The complex craniosynostoses

# 4 & 5

In this category occur the syndromes of Crouzon, Apert, Pfeiffer and Saethre-Chotzen, etc.[5,6]. All are autosomal dominant conditions, although most cases seen in neurosurgical departments represent new mutations. Not only are they often associated with other skeletal abnormalities, particularly of the digits, but they may be accompanied by varying degrees of mental retardation.

The common skull abnormality is a shortening of the skull base anteriorly associated with a bicoronal synostosis, although in some cases other sutures (particularly the sagittal) may also be fused prematurely. This produces a brachycephalic skull shape (*see Illustration 4*) (or occasionally turricephaly (*see Illustration 5*)) accompanied by recession of the middle third of the face. This in turn leads to deformities of the orbits and disturbs the dentition of the upper jaw.

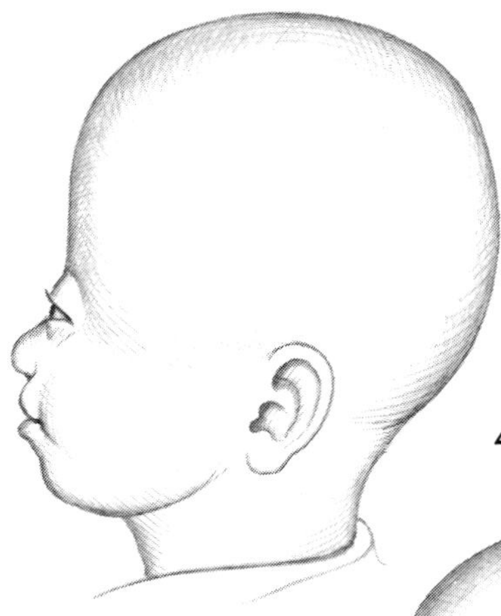

4

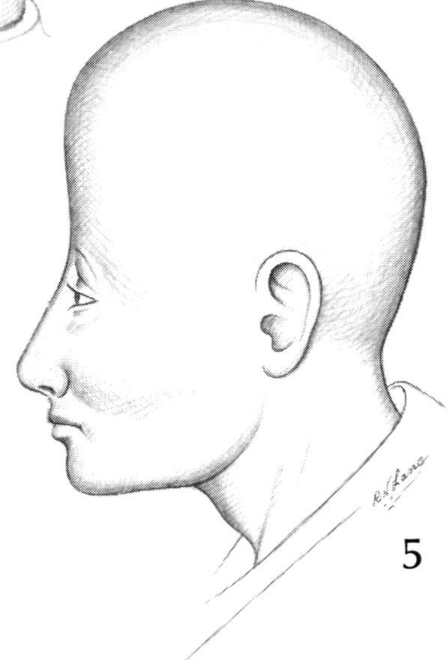

5

# 6

Differing degrees of synostosis compete with the pressure from expansion of the intracranial contents due to normal brain growth and, in severe cases, hydrocephalus, to produce abnormalities of appearance that can vary widely from case to case. At one end of the spectrum is the patient with a mild Crouzon's syndrome, who has a comparatively normal facial structure with some flattening of the supraorbital region and forehead, producing a mild turricephaly easily concealed by hair. At the other extreme is the child with the cloverleaf skull syndrome, where hydrocephalus, in the presence of a severe skull base stenosis and a bony constriction band around the equator of the skull (perhaps corresponding to the attachment of the tentorium posteriorly), forces the head to enlarge laterally through the still patent squamoparietal sutures and upwards through an enormous anterior fontanelle[7].

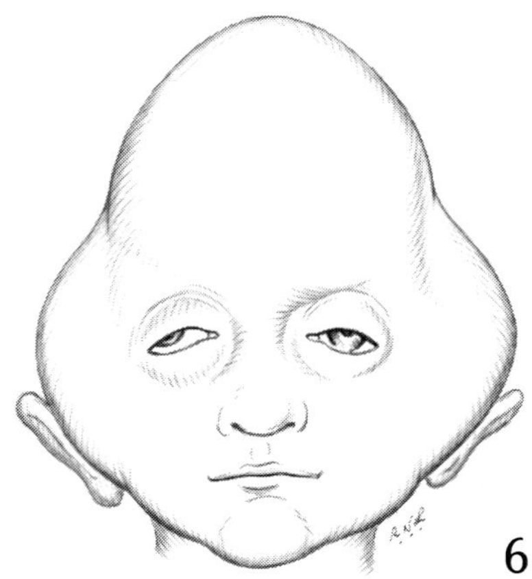

6

## Total craniostenosis

In this condition all the skull sutures are prematurely fused. In some cases it is merely an extension of one of the syndromes described under the complex synostoses, but in others it occurs independently, the condition being suspected when raised intracranial pressure is detected in a child whose facial and skull appearances may be normal, although measurement of the head circumference reveals that it is too small.

It should be emphasized that the above grouping of cases does not provide absolutely rigid lines of demarcation. Occasional cases of unicoronal synostosis may be seen as part of an inherited syndrome, and there are undoubted examples of bicoronal synostosis occurring sporadically without obvious genetic implications, which may represent a different aetiology to that associated with the syndromes listed under the complex craniosynostoses.

# Development of the skull

The bones of the skull vault develop in membrane, while those of the skull base develop from a cartilaginous precursor. The reason for this difference remains unknown. One theory is that bony vertebrate species have inherited a skull of insufficient size from their wholly cartilaginous forebears to accommodate their greatly increased brain volume. It is therefore 'necessary' for primitive, dermal bone to be incorporated in order to make up the skull vault. This dermal bone, which represents the scales of fishes, the dermal armour of reptiles and the bony scales of crocodiles, ossifies in membrane, a development that is still maintained in man[8]. However, whether this can be said to be the explanation for such other membrane-formed bones as those of the face, part of the clavicle and mandible, etc. is a subject beyond the purpose of this chapter. In any event, it may be relevant that in the complex craniostenoses (i.e. those which appear to be due most commonly to a genetic defect) the areas of maximum abnormality appear to be at junctional zones between bone developed in cartilage and bone developed in membrane (e.g. between skull base and skull vault, and between skull base and facial skeleton).

The development of the skull base remains poorly understood. The notochord, which is a potent embryonic inducer of bone, terminates at a point that is later represented by the junction on the clivus between occipital and sphenoid bones. It is the prechordal elements of the skull base which grow at the greatest rate during fetal life, and they are the very areas which are foreshortened in the complex craniosynostoses. However, in the most severe cases the restriction of skull base growth extends to involve the basiocciput as well.

The role of the sutures in the growth of the skull remains controversial. The sutures of the skull base are synchondroses, that is to say there is cartilage present between the bone ends (as befits their development). The bones of the skull vault, however, are fibrosynostoses and have fibrous tissue present between the bone ends. Do these skull vault sutures act as lines of active growth necessary for skull expansion, or are they merely passive lines of mesenchyme-derived fibrous tissue, lying between bony plates that are expanding insufficiently rapidly, compared to the expansion of the underlying brain, to be closed over until all brain growth has finally ceased? At the moment it appears that the latter is more likely to be the case. The experimental removal of a normal suture in an animal allows even more rapid expansion than normal across that area[9], while prevention of growth across a suture (e.g. by cementing struts across it) can lead to swift ossification of the intervening fibrous tissue and a subsequent solid fusion[10].

If the vault sutures have an entirely passive role, there are three possible processes that could lead to their premature fusion. Firstly, there could be a physical constraint placed upon them as has been suggested for the production of the simple craniosynostoses (*see above*). Secondly, failure of the skull base to expand could produce an immobility of the membrane bones of the vault, particularly close to the base, which would prevent the degree of expansion necessary to keep the vault sutures patent. In fact, in most of the complex craniosynostoses, vault sutures are obliterated and replaced by thickened bone where they approach the skull base. The rare but well documented cases of premature vault–suture fusion following excessive reduction of head size when hydrocephalus in a young infant has been overtreated may also be relevant in this instance[11]. Lastly, the sutures of the skull vault (and of the skull base) could be genetically directed towards premature fusion.

Of course, it may even be simplistic to assume that the basic pathology in the complex craniosynostoses lies in the sutures at all. A genetic defect similar to but more localized than that which affects patients with achondroplasia may turn out to be the primary fault. Such a concept has obvious relevance to our surgical treatments, which are all based on the theory that the sutures should be opened up in order to allow normal growth to take place.

Lastly, it should be noted that even in cases of total craniostenosis some growth of the head does occur. In other words, continuing expansion of the vault, although usually insufficient to prevent a rise in intracranial pressure, can occur in the absence of any patent vault sutures.

# The synostoses and mental retardation

There are several reasons why patients with craniosynostosis, particularly those with the complex syndromes, may be mentally retarded, and it is important to recognize them as some are clearly preventable by early surgery.

*Congenital abnormalities of the underlying brain* Although there are syndromes, especially those involving hypertelorism, in which developmental abnormalities of the underlying brain can be seen on the CT scan (e.g. agenesis of the corpus callosum, midline lipomas), such findings are rare in the synostoses. This CT evidence, of course, does not exclude the fact that the brain may be 'badly made', but it is uncommon to find the more familiar structural pointers towards such a conclusion.

*Hydrocephalus* There is no doubt that hydrocephalus has often been overlooked in these children in the past[12]. Older cases are still seen with a head both abnormal in shape and expanded due to arrested hydrocephalus, where mental retardation might have been avoided or lessened had CSF diversion been recommended at an earlier stage. The aetiology of the hydrocephalus is unknown, but may be related either to abnormalities of the skull base interfering with the normal passage of CSF through the basal cisterns, or to venous hypertension[13] (*see also* 'Chronic raised intracranial venous pressure', p. 497). It is usually only associated with the most severe cases amongst the complex craniostenoses, and it is essential for the production of the cloverleaf skull.

*Impairment of brain growth due to the craniostenosis* It is usually accepted that premature fusion of one skull suture is unlikely to produce any impairment of cerebral function (although it has been suggested that severe metopic synostosis can compress both frontal lobes). Indeed, it was once thought that *two* fused sutures were unlikely to affect brain function, but against this theory is the clinical evidence for raised intracranial pressure that exists, even in the absence of hydrocephalus, in some children with bicoronal synostosis[14], and also the evidence of the advance in development often seen after reconstructive surgery (*see below*). At the moment our policy is not to recommend surgery for the simple craniosynostoses on the basis that the condition is likely to interfere with brain development, but to concentrate instead on the cosmetic aspects. However, for the complex craniostenosis, 'freeing' the brain by providing it with more space is a most important part of both the recommendation and timing of surgery.

*Chronic raised intracranial venous pressure* The role of this is uncertain, but there can be no doubt that with the complex syndromes children often run a chronic raised intracranial venous pressure. This is partly due to the respiratory obstruction associated with their poor nasal airways, and some patients actually have choanal atresia. In others, there appear to be abnormalities of the venous sinuses, particularly the lateral sinuses, which are replaced by numerous irregular venous channels that nestle amongst tight dural folds, in thin convolutions of bone around the occipital region of the skull.

*Abnormal skull restraint occurring preterm* If the theory suggested earlier that prenatal constraints upon a child's head can lead to the development of one of the simple synostoses is correct, then it would not be unreasonable to assume that in severe cases there might also be some damage to the underlying brain. Therefore, when evidence of some degree of cerebral dysfunction is detected in a child with a single-suture synostosis and no other significant abnormalities, it should not necessarily be assumed that it is pressure owing to the failure of that suture to expand which is responsible.

## Indications for surgery

The indications for surgery are protection of brain function, protection of the eyes and cosmetic reasons.

### *Protection of brain function*

As explained above, brain function is unlikely to be compromised by a simple, single craniosynostosis. The indications for these operations, therefore, remain purely cosmetic. However, in the complex craniosynostoses, where two or more sutures are involved, protection of brain function is of extreme importance and the most important aim of early surgery is to provide an increased intracranial volume with, if possible, cosmetic improvements as well.

### *Protection of the eyes*

In several cases of complex (bicoronal) synostosis, the failure of the anterior skull base to advance may leave the patient with recession of both the supraorbital and infraorbital margins. The child may have difficulty in completely closing the eyelids, and therefore risk damage to the corneae. In extreme cases the eyeballs may dislocate themselves anterior to the lids, severely threatening vision unless immediate action to reduce them is taken.

Visual failure due to optic nerve compression in narrowed optic canals is well documented in the literature but, in my experience, remains an unusual complication.

### *Cosmetic*

In normal circumstances the growing brain pushes the surrounding skull ahead of it, but premature fusion of a suture produces an abnormal head shape due to restricted growth in one direction combined with compensatory growth in another. There are two possible ways in which a cosmetic improvement can be achieved by surgery. In the first, the bones may be removed and replaced in a new position; the patient will then look better immediately. In the other, fused sutures may be opened at a sufficiently early age so that advantage can be taken of the brain growth spurt, and the brain itself be allowed to push its bony surroundings into a better position. In these circumstances, the child may look unchanged at the end of the operation, but can be expected to improve over the weeks and months to come. On the whole, most operations combine both approaches.

## Timing of surgery

The sooner an operation is carried out after birth, the more chance there is of avoiding damage to the brain due to compression, and the more advantage can be taken of the brain growth that occurs during the first 6 months of life. However, against this desire for early operation must be set the hazards of carrying out major neurosurgical procedures in the newborn. After taking all the factors into consideration, it is best that none of the operations to be described in this section should be postponed much beyond the age of 3 months. A simple operation such as linear craniectomy for sagittal synostosis can, however, be performed much earlier.

An important question which remains unresolved is whether a frontal cranioplasty and supraorbital ridge advancement, performed early in the treatment of the complex craniosynostoses, will allow sufficient normal growth of the forehead, skull base and facial structures to occur over the following months to make further major craniofacial operations unnecessary. The operations in this category are those pioneered by Tessier[15], and include the dismantling of the middle third of the face along the classical Le Fort fracture lines[16], so as to advance the maxilla and correct hypertelorism.

At the moment the answer appears to be that the milder cases involving bicoronal synostosis are almost certainly saved from further surgery, and that in those more severe situations where subsequent operations have to be carried out, their performance is not too compromised by the earlier procedures[17]. However, it is exactly in the milder cases that normal facial growth is most likely to occur regardless of treatment.

## The team approach

Although the management of the simple craniosynostoses falls mainly within the province of the neurosurgeon alone, successful management of the complex problems requires a multidisciplinary approach. The interests of the patients are best served when they are managed in combined clinics, where both neurosurgeons and plastic surgeons with experience in the subject can meet together. Of equal importance is the assistance of ophthalmologists, ENT surgeons, psychologists, orthodontists, speech therapists, anaesthetists and geneticists. There is no excuse for these cases to be handled on an 'occasional' basis.

## Investigations

### *Skull X-rays*

All children should have conventional skull radiographs taken, together with tomography where indicated. These will show the following.

1. Which sutures are fused and which are patent. Typically there is thickening of bone along the fused suture which, particularly in sagittal synostosis, may be represented by a straight, radiolucent cleft between the adjacent bone ends.
2. The abnormal bone shape produced by the synostosis. In a unicoronal synostosis, for example, the affected orbital margin sweeps upwards and outwards into a 'Harlequin mask' position (*see Illustration 2*). There may also be duplication of the sphenoid ridge in these cases.
3. Evidence of raised intracranial pressure. Digital markings on the skull vault are always of significance in craniosynostosis. They tend to concentrate in those areas where brain growth is most restricted, e.g. frontally in cases of bicoronal synostosis. In a complete craniostenosis they may be present throughout the vault.

### *Computerized tomography (CT)*

A CT scan should always be performed for the following reasons.

1. The detection and assessment of hydrocephalus.
2. Detection of other intracranial congenital abnormalities which may have prognostic significance when it comes to predicting the patient's capacity for future intellectual development.
3. The detail of the bony abnormality imposed by the synostosis is often easier to detect by CT scanning. Reconstructions may also be useful, particularly in planning subsequent operations[18].

### *Intracranial pressure (ICP) monitoring*

In the simple synostoses there is unlikely to be any rise in ICP, and in the infant with a complex syndrome the anterior fontanelle, despite involvement of the coronal sutures, is usually sufficiently open to allow the ICP to be readily palpated. However, some children have abnormal fundal appearances in the absence of any other signs of raised ICP, and for them pressure monitoring may well help decide whether surgery is necessary for other than cosmetic reasons. A recent review of the subject is provided by Renier *et al.* [14].

## ANAESTHESIA

These operations should only be undertaken in units equipped to carry out major paediatric neurosurgical procedures. Patients are intubated, paralysed and receive intermittent positive-pressure ventilation. Scrupulous attention must be paid to the replacement of blood loss, as well as to recognition of the vagal stimulation that can occur (producing cardiac slowing or even arrest) during the orbital dissections. After lengthy operations it is best to ventilate smaller children electively for 24 hours.

# The operations

## SAGITTAL SYNOSTOSES[19]

## 7

This is the only operation for which a linear craniectomy along the line of the fused suture, if carried out early enough, is likely to be effective[19]. The fusion is usually more obvious posteriorly, where the suture is replaced by a bony ridge that can be easily palpated in the newborn. It is most important that the craniectomy runs all the way from the anterior to the posterior fontanelle. The operation is carried out with the child lying on its side or in the prone position.

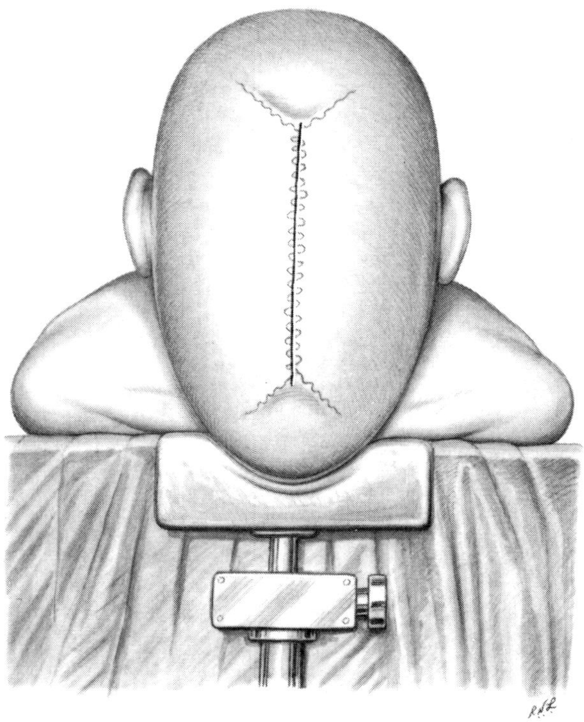

7

## 8 & 9

Either a linear incision is made in the midline joining anterior to posterior fontanelles or a vertex incision joining ear to ear. Self-retaining retractors are inserted to expose the line of the fused suture. The pericranium is stripped away from the midline for approximately 1.5 cm and excised. A burr hole is then made in the midline in order to expose the underlying dura. Bone nibblers are used to perform a linear craniectomy connecting anterior and posterior fontanelles. The width of the craniectomy should be 1 cm anteriorly but can widen to 2–2.5 cm posteriorly if the occipitoparietal region of the head is particularly narrow.

Bleeding from the bone is controlled using bone wax. A little Surgicel (Ethicon, UK) may be placed on the dura if there is venous oozing from the superior sagittal sinus. The wound is then closed in two layers using a subcutaneous absorbable suture and 4/0 nylon for the skin. A subgaleal Redivac drain is brought out through a stab incision adjacent to the wound. It may be removed after 48 hours. All that is required for a dressing is a strip of half-inch ribbon gauze held down to the wound with plastic spray. Sutures are removed after 7 days.

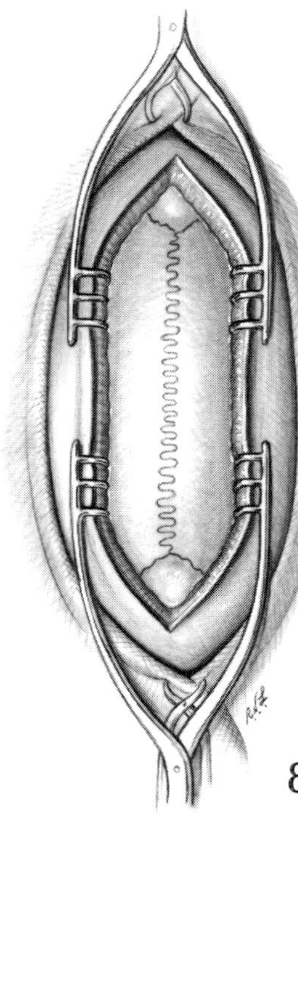

8

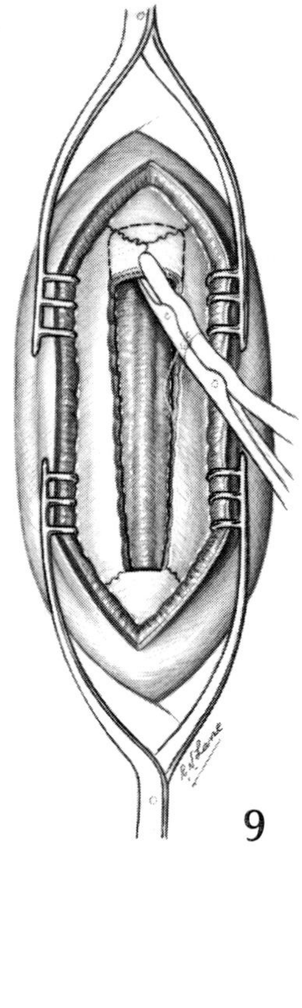

9

### A NOTE ON THE USE OF SILASTIC FILM

Many surgeons carrying out these operations line the bone edges with Silastic film (Dow Corning, UK) in order to delay their inevitable coming together and re-fusion. This means that foreign material is inserted (for life) in an infant, and there is an unavoidable increase in the risk of infection for what is, in the case of sagittal synostosis, an operation for purely cosmetic purposes. As the new bone formation occurs mainly from the dura, it seems unlikely that the Silastic lining will produce much in the way of delay, and my own policy now is to omit it in all reconstructions and craniectomies for craniosynostosis.

## METOPIC SYNOSTOSES

# 10 & 11

The child is placed in the supine position, with the head of the table raised in order to reduce venous bleeding. A coronal incision is made behind the hairline, coming down on each side to just in front of the ear. Bleeding from the skin edges is controlled using clips. The skin flap so formed is turned forwards, the subgaleal dissection ending at a point approximately one inch above the supraorbital ridge. (This is to preserve the supraorbital nerves.) A pericranial incision is now made in the coronal plane, on or just anterior to the coronal suture. This pericranial flap is now turned forwards, but the dissection is taken lower, to the supraorbital ridges themselves, so that the supraorbital vessels and nerves can be seen.

In the temporal region the dissection will run under the temporalis muscle, which should always be lifted up and carefully preserved without being cut as it can be replaced later over the junctions between the new bone positions.

A burr hole is made in the region of the pterion on each side. A bone incision is now made in the coronal plane joining the two burr holes up across the anterior fontanelle. Care is taken to preserve the dura when it is detached from the margins of the fontanelle. A second bone cut is now made joining the burr holes, but this time as low down on the supraorbital ridge as possible. The dura is freed from the bone, which it should now be possible to remove in one piece.

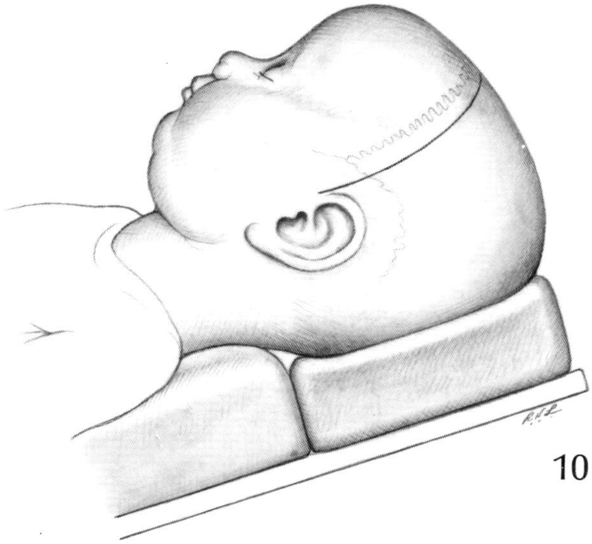

10

Unless the trigonocephaly produced by the metopic synostoses is very severe, it is usually possible to achieve an acceptable cosmetic result by remodelling of the frontal bones alone. However, in the more severe cases it may be necessary to cut out and reposition the supraorbital ridges, as described in the section on bicoronal synostosis.

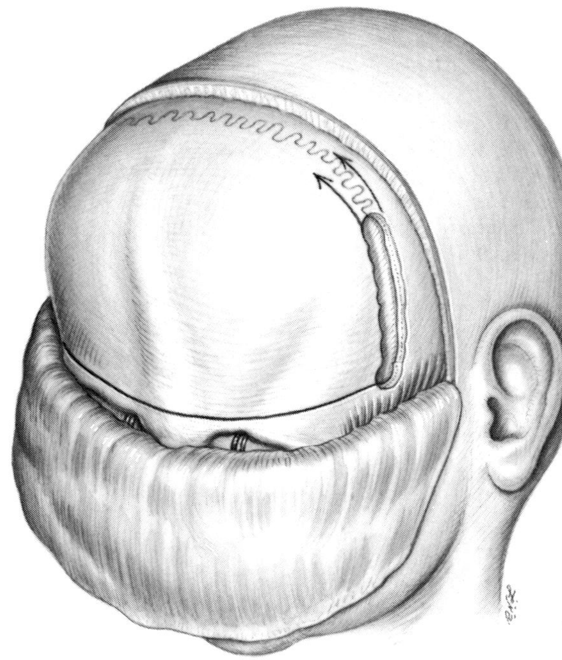

11

# 12, 13 & 14

The thickened ridge of the fused metopic suture is now cut out of the frontal bones using either bone forceps or an air drill. The upper part of the frontal bone plate close to the fontanelle usually has a more pleasing contour, and a 'V' is removed from it, the apex of which joins the metopic craniectomy. There are now three pieces of bone representing the frontal region, a small triangular piece and the two frontal halves. These latter are reversed and then joined as shown. The 'V' is used to fill the gap.

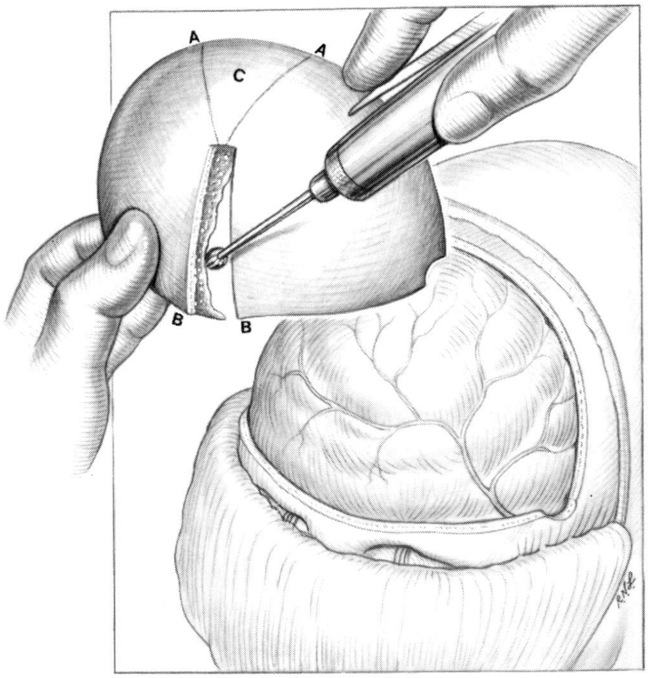


12

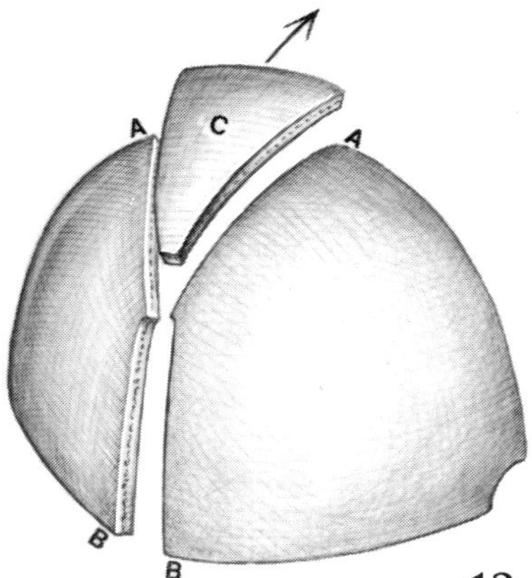


13

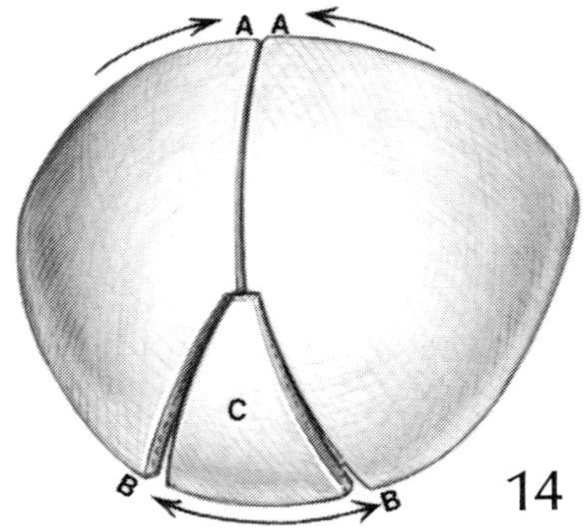


14

# 15

The new shell of frontal bone is replaced and the skin of the frontal flap pulled back so that the cosmetic effect can be evaluated. If this is satisfactory the bones can be attached to the supraorbital ridge in their new position. This is done using stainless steel wires passing through an appropriate number of small drill holes.

A subgaleal Redivac drain is used. The wound is closed with subcutaneous absorbable sutures and 4/0 nylon for the skin. A light ribbon gauze dressing is applied.

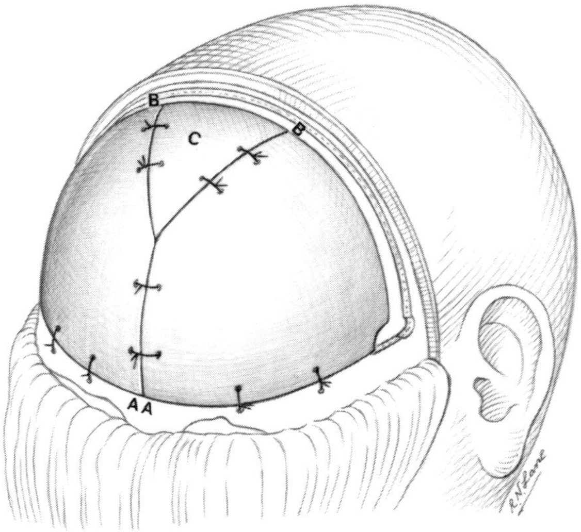


15

## A note on the use of vacuum drains after extensive craniectomies

Following this reconstruction and those to be described below, the patient is often left with a greatly expanded frontal extradural space. If this is exposed to a sudden severe drop in pressure, as can occur when the drain is opened, there may be immediate vasovagal effects, with a fall in blood pressure and pulse rate. Also, a violent 'sucking in' of the skin through the craniectomy may alter the new position of the bones if these have not been secured effectively enough. When in doubt, only minimal vacuum or just gravity drainage should be used.

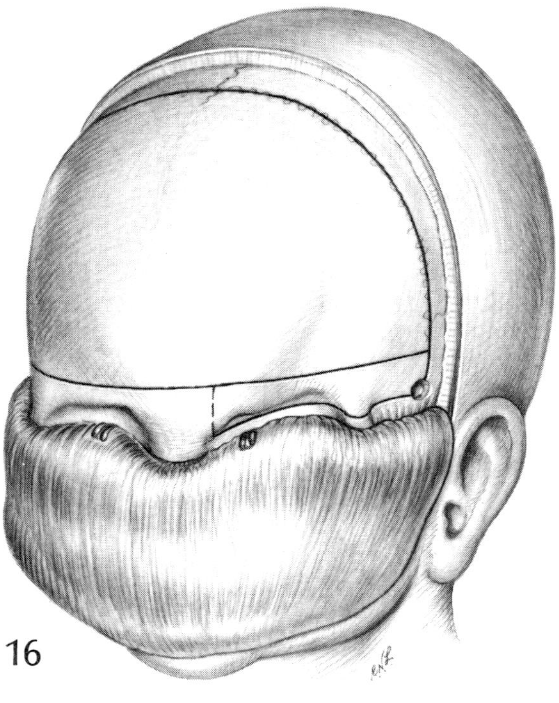

16

## UNICORONAL SYNOSTOSIS[20]

# 16

The child is positioned supine with the head of the table raised. Cleaning and draping is then carried out so that the face from the bridge of the nose upwards and the front half of the head are visible. This means that bilateral temporary tarsorrhaphy sutures must be inserted in order to protect the eyes. A coronal skin flap is turned as described in the previous section.

The pericranial flap is formed using the line of the fused and normal coronal sutures as a guide. However, on this occasion the flap is dissected further down and over the supraorbital ridge in order to enter the orbits. The supraorbital vessels and nerves can be identified in their grooves and dislocated from them in order to minimize damage. The pericranial section is now taken further downwards into the roof of the orbit on each side. At this stage it is usually not necessary to carry the dissection so far down on the normal side.

The two temporal burr holes and the supraorbital and coronal bone cuts are made as described for metopic synostosis. The complete frontal bone is removed and set aside.

# 17 & 18

The dura is now swept away from the lowest remaining part of the frontal bone and the orbital roof on the affected side. Bone cuts are then made along the lines shown until the supraorbital ridge is detached laterally from the frontal bone of the orbital roof. When this has been done, the supraorbital ridge should be attached only at the midline, where a little pressure provides a greenstick fracture to act as a hinge.

Unless excessive compensatory advancement of the 'normal' supraorbital ridge has occurred, it is usually unnecessary to isolate the ridge on that side.

The lateral part of the supraorbital ridge can now be advanced and held in its new position by the fingers of one hand, while the other hand pulls back the skin flap. This allows the cosmetic effect of the operation to be constantly evaluated. Having decided on the amount of advance necessary and on whether any raising or lowering or angulation of the ridge is required, the surgeon must now fix it securely in its new position. This is usually done using a strut of bone. Ideally this should connect the outer end of the supraorbital ridge to the frontal process of the zygomatic bone, but such a fixation can be both difficult and insecure, and it is sometimes necessary instead to run the strut posteriorly to the lateral part of the orbital plate of the frontal bone. The bone in the region of the pterion is often extremely thickened, and in this case it is advisable to carry out an extensive craniectomy of it.

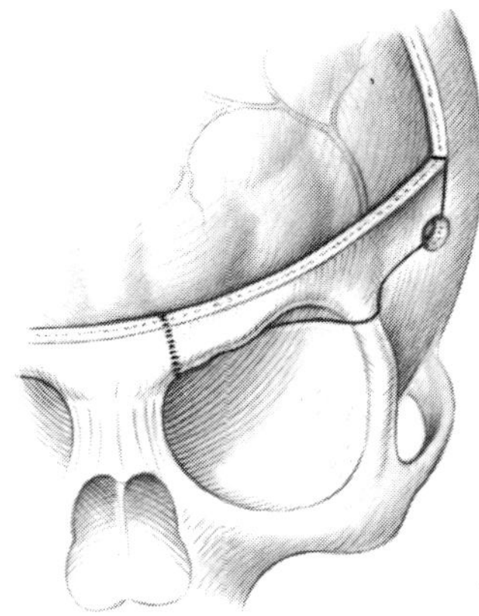

17

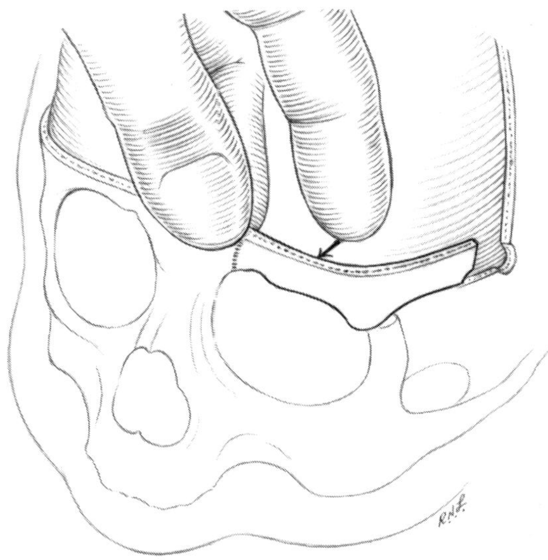

18

# 19

With the supraorbital ridge in a satisfactory position it is now necessary to reattach the frontal bone. On the affected side this has been too flat, while on the other, compensatory ballooning forward has usually occurred. A straight swap between the two sides (with the frontal bone being rotated through 180°) is the simplest solution where possible, but often it is necessary to trim the bone or even divide it into two again in order to gain a satisfactory appearance. It should not be fixed in position posteriorly across the line of the coronal sutures, as it is here that any further advance will take place as the brain grows during the months to come. If the frontal bone is attached only to the supraorbital ridges, then a 'floating forehead'[17] will be formed. A true floating forehead is produced when the supraorbital ridges themselves are secured only to facial structures, i.e. the root of the nose and the zygomatic bones.

The advance of the supraorbital ridges and the reconstruction of the forehead produce a bone gap of variable size in the plane of the coronal suture lines. This is an inevitable result of all these reconstructive procedures and is most obvious after surgery for a bicoronal synostosis (*see below*).

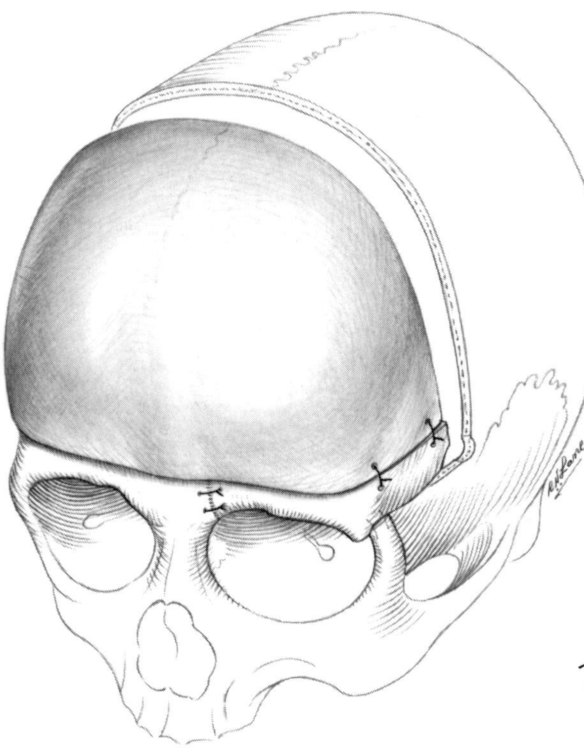

19

## BICORONAL SYNOSTOSES

### (The treatment of the complex craniostenoses)

The positioning of the patient, the cleaning, draping, tarsorrhaphies and incisions are as described in the previous section.

The pericranial flaps are brought down into the orbits and temporal fossae on both sides.

Temporal burr holes are made on each side. Before the frontal bone flap is cut out, the whole of the exposed skull should be carefully inspected to see which areas could be used at the end of the procedure to construct a satisfactory forehead. This is because in some cases the frontal bony contours are so abnormal that simple repositioning of existing parts is impossible and new bone will have to be taken from farther back. However, in most cases the coronal and supraorbital bone cuts can be carried out as described earlier. The latter is often made difficult by the presence of sharp septae of bone that run backwards from the supraorbital ridge and inwards from the region of the pterion. Their presence can be predicted from the axial CT scan. The dura in these areas is usually extremely thin, and it is not uncommon for small lacerations to be made in it. This produces a leakage of CSF which may be helpful in the subsequent separation of the dura from the supraorbital ridges, so no attempt at closure is made at this stage.

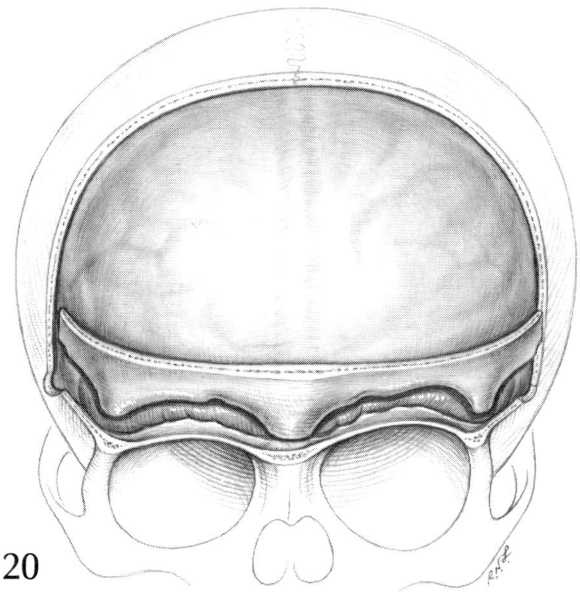

20

# 20

Both supraorbital ridges are cut out in the manner described for the treatment of unicoronal synostosis. If possible, the bone cut is continued posteriorly at each side to include a 'spar' of temporal bone. Not only may this help in subsequent fixations but it will also provide a more satisfactory contour to the final appearance of the forehead above and lateral to the orbits.

Sometimes it is possible to remove the bone in one block so that it resembles the upper part of a pair of spectacle frames. In other cases it is advisable to leave each ridge with a small greenstick fracture hinge anchoring it close to the midline. In a young child the supraorbital ridges are very prone to fracture in the region of the supraorbital grooves if they are handled roughly.

If any lacerations have been made in the dura they should be sutured with Vicryl (Ethicon, UK) after the mobilization of the supraorbital ridges has made access to the whole frontal dura much more convenient.

At this stage the supraorbital ridge should be inspected. Its shape is often unsatisfactory and it will need to be remodelled. This is done by thinning it at various points along its length using the air drill and then gently bending it to the desired contour. It can be fixed in its new shape by reinforcing it with a strut of bone taken from the posterior edge of the craniotomy and held in position with wire sutures.

## 21 & 22

Once again the surgeon's fingers are used to hold the supraorbital ridges forward while the skin is pulled back and a satisfactory appearance obtained. Even in a child of 3 months an advancement of no less than 2 cm (and if possible more) should be aimed for. It is always best to overcompensate for the amount of supraorbital ridge advance required. A child who looks perfect at the end of the operation will make the surgeon wish that he had done more when reviewed 6 months later. Overcorrection at this stage produces prominent bossing low down on both sides of the forehead, but this appearance, which may cause distress to parents who have not been warned about it, always improves over the next few months, and in any case can be lessened by leaving the spars of temporal bone attached to the supraorbital ridges. The ridges are now held forward in their new positions using struts of bone (which can easily be obtained from the parietal bones) in the manner described in the section on unicoronal synostosis.

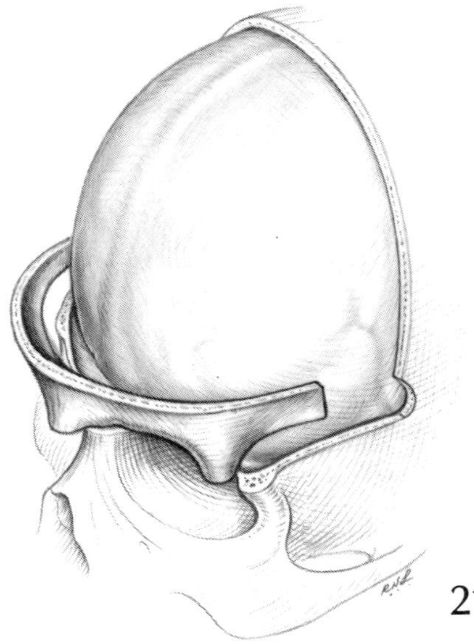

21

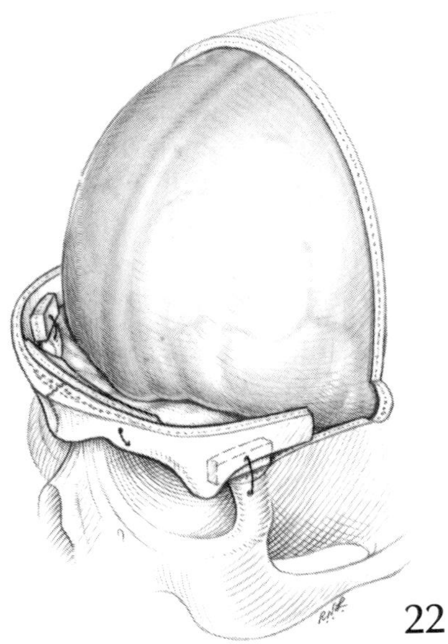

22

# 23

The frontal bone(s) are now inspected, shaped and tried in various different positions in order to achieve the best effect. There is a tendency to leave the patients with a broadening laterally, just above the supraorbital ridges, and particular care must be taken with this area. The frontal bones are then reattached to the supraorbital ridges to form a floating forehead.

The drainage, closure and dressing are as have been described already.

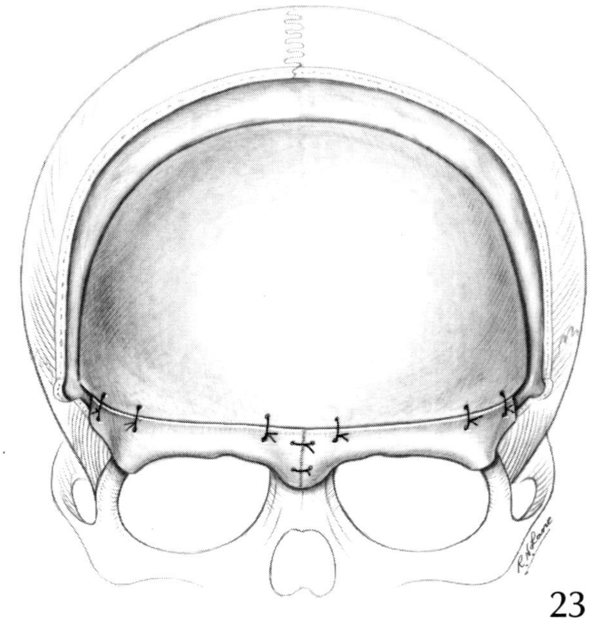

23

## TOTAL CRANIOSTENOSIS

When this occurs in the presence of one of the syndromes associated with the complex craniosynostoses (as is usually the case), the frontal cranioplasty and supraorbital ridge advancement described above may be enough to provide an increase in the intracranial volume sufficient to lower the intracranial pressure. The operation described in this section is to be used only when cosmetic indications for the operation are not present.

# 24

The child is positioned with the head of the table raised and the complete head shaved. The whole of the head is cleaned and draped, but it is not necessary to leave the orbits exposed, so tarsorrhaphies are not performed. An incision is made from ear to ear over the vertex of the head (the head in these cases is often conveniently spherical).

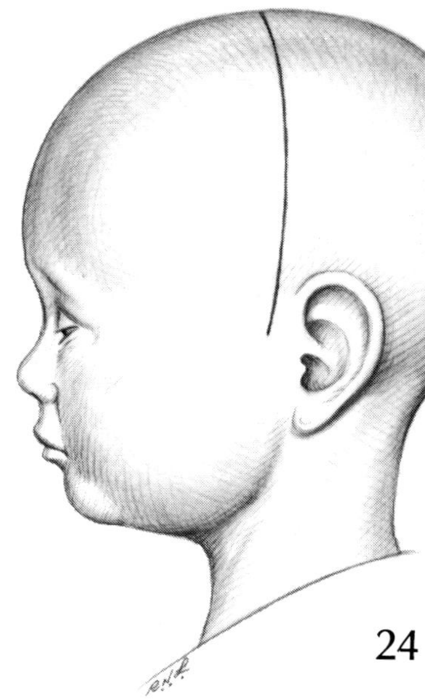

24

# 25 & 26

The skin flaps so formed are turned forwards and backwards as much as positioned with the head of the table raised and the complete head shaved. The whole of the head is cleaned and draped, but it is not necessary to leave the orbits exposed, so tarsorrhaphies are not performed. An incision is made from e formed still carry their attachments to the temporalis muscles on each side. The flaps are elevated and the bone cracked along the line of the fused squamoparietal sutures, where further bone removal can now be carried out. Effectively two flaps, each consisting of a parietal bone, have now been formed, each attached by a pedicle of temporalis muscle. The pericranium around their edges is trimmed back and the bone flaps replaced, and if necessary held loosely in position with a few pericranial sutures.

The drainage, closure and dressing of the wound are as described previously.

Although the dura has been left undisturbed by this operation, the raised pressure of the intradural contents, unhindered now by bone, will stretch it and force the freely floating flaps of bone further apart. Skull X-rays over the next few weeks will show an increase in size of the craniectomy defects as the realignment of the bones continues.

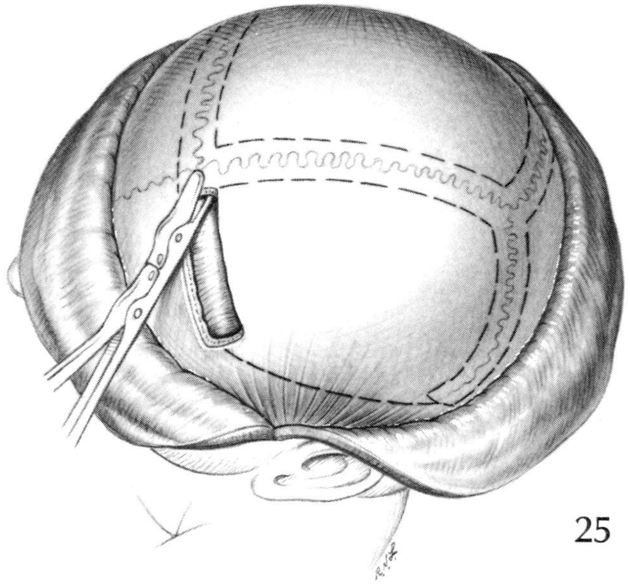

25

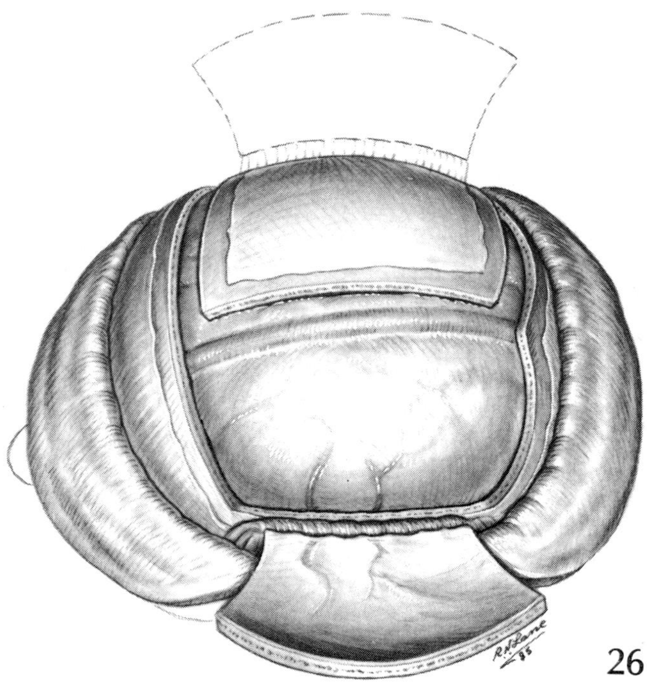

26

## Notes on the role of the neurosurgeon in combined craniofacial procedures

The operations described in this chapter for treatment of the complex craniostenoses reflect, not unnaturally, a neurosurgical bias. However, often the neurosurgeon is just one member of a team of surgeons operating, particularly on older patients, for complex craniofacial disorders, both congenital and acquired. Alteration of the facial skeleton may require an intracranial approach, especially when hypertelorism is to be corrected. An advance of the middle third of the face can be done extracranially, but if remodelling of the supraorbital region and forehead is also required, then clearly this can be carried out most conveniently at the same time.

At the very least then, the neurosurgeon's role (as in some combined operations for malignant disease of the head and neck) is a protective one. The frontal bone flap has to be elevated and then the dura stripped from the floor of the anterior fossa as far as, and sometimes beyond, the crista galli. The dural openings almost invariably produced by this dissection must be scrupulously repaired.

The details of the actual operative procedures for the correction of hypertelorism are beyond the scope of this chapter[21].

# Complications

### Sepsis

Operations for the treatment of craniosynostosis may be lengthy and the risk of infection is always present. Avoidance of foreign material reduces long-term complications, and some surgeons also advocate the use of a narrow spectrum antibiotic aimed at the organism most likely to cause problems (*Staphylococcus aureus*). If prophylactic antibiotics are employed they should be commenced at the time of premedication and then continued in a high dosage intravenously for 48 hours.

## Wound breakdown

Advancing the supraorbital ridges and frontal bones increases the size of the cranium and yet only the same amount of skin is available for the final closure. Fortunately, skin will stretch; but sometimes even after extensive undermining and incising the undersurface of the galea (which allows still more skin stretching), the effectiveness of the operation is marred by fears of failing to achieve closure. Care should always be taken to avoid a situation where, at the end of the procedure, areas of tight, white skin can be seen pulled taut over the bone prominences produced by the advance.

If a breakdown does occur it may be necessary to reduce the amount of the advance before resuturing, or to swing a large flap from the posterior part of the scalp in order to take tension off the suture line. Hopefully, the implantable skin expanders which are now becoming available will lessen the problems of closure by allowing extra tissue to be produced before the definitive operation.

## Cerebrospinal fluid leakage

A subgaleal collection of CSF can often be controlled by serial aspirations combined with as firm a bandage as the surgeon's confidence in the strength of his reconstruction will allow. External leakage requires the insertion of a lumbar drain. This is usually sufficient to achieve control, but occasionally it is necessary to re-explore the wound or, where this is not desirable, to insert a lumboperitoneal shunt.

## Epilepsy

Epilepsy is a rare complication of these procedures. For the more extensive reconstructions we use prophylactic anticonvulsants for 3 months in an infant, and for 1 year in an older child.

# Results of surgery for the craniosynostoses

There is no doubt that the milder the abnormality, the better the cosmetic result of surgery. For example, a child with a simple sagittal synostosis which was operated on early should present a head shape that is essentially normal within 2 or 3 months of operation. A good result can also be expected following treatment of the other simple craniosynostoses. However, with the bicoronal synostoses there is a wide spectrum of results. Once again, milder cases are very effectively treated, and so are those children with Crouzon's syndrome who have the straight or concave forehead of turricephaly. However, although improvements can undoubtedly be obtained in the appearance of children severely affected by Apert's syndrome or possessing a cloverleaf skull, the rewards in terms of restoring normality are much smaller, and the parents should always be warned of these surgical limitations.

Once again, it should be emphasized that an improvement in appearance requires not only (in most cases) a surgical reshaping, but also the push provided by the growing brain to encourage and maintain a more normal head shape. Therefore, these operations should always be carried out as early as is thought to be compatible with the child's capacity to cope with the rigours of the procedure.

Whether or not the degree of maxillary hypoplasia in the complex craniostenoses is altered by early operation remains unproven. After all, the operations open up the sutures of the cranial vault but come down to the skull base at only the extreme anterior end of the foreshortened anterior fossa. If the primary abnormality lies in the frontoethmoid and frontosphenoid sutures, which such surgery is unlikely to open up (despite some reports[22]), and if the maxilla is dependent upon its attachments to these areas for its subsequent growth, or is primarily involved in the disease process as well, then it would hardly be surprising if the operations already described have little or no effect upon subsequent maxillary growth.

Such patients may therefore require advancement of the maxilla at a later date, and it is essential that they have access to combined clinics where their problems can be discussed with faciomaxillary surgeons.

However, there is one cosmetic effect which is seen very soon after the operations performed on all infants with the complex craniostenoses, and this is an apparent resetting of the face so that the angle at which it lies in relation to the forehead appears greatly improved.

Surgery to correct hypertelorism can produce an excellent result if judgement is confined to a radiological assessment of the new positions of the bony orbits. However, the patient's appearance may not have benefited to the same degree. This is because unless it is possible to remove much of the tissue that lies between the middle and posterior parts of the orbits (usually expanded ethmoid sinuses and sometimes a downward prolongation of the anterior cranial fossa), the orbital contents cannot move medially to the same extent as the anterior orbital rims. Therefore, the globes of the eyes take up a relatively more lateral position within the orbits, and an approximation of 40 mm for the orbital margins may reduce the interpupillary distance by only 15–20 mm.

## References


1. Lemire, R. J., Loeser, J. D., Leech, R. W., Alvord, E. C. (1975) Normal and Abnormal Development of the Human Nervous System. New York: Harper and Row

2. Graham, J. M., deSaxe, M., Smith, D. W. (1979) Sagittal craniostenosis: fetal head constraint as one possible cause. Journal of Pediatrics, 95, 747–750

3. Graham, J. M., Badura, R. J., Smith, D. W. (1980) Coronal craniostenosis: fetal head constraint as one possible cause. Pediatrics, 65, 995–999

4. Graham, J. M., Smith, D. W. (1980) Metopic craniostenosis as a consequence of fetal head constraint: Two interesting experiments of nature. Pediatrics, 65, 1000–1002

5. Carter, C. O., Till, K., Fraser, V., Coffey, R. (1982) A family study of craniosynostosis, with probable recognition of a distinct syndrome. Journal of Medical Genetics, 19, 280–285

6. Cohen, M. M. (1977) Genetic perspectives on craniosynostosis and syndromes with craniosynostosis. Journal of Neurosurgery, 47, 886–898

7. Zuleta, A., Basauri, L. (1984) Cloverleaf skull syndrome. Child's Brain, 11, 418–427

8. Keith, A. (1948) Human embryology and morphology. 6th Edition Edward Arnold: London

9. Persson, K. M., Roy, W. A., Persing, J. A., Rodeheaver, G. T., Winn, H. R. (1979) Craniofacial growth following experimental craniosynostosis and craniectomy in rabbits. Journal of Neurosurgery, 50, 187–197

10. Nappen, D. L., Kokich, V. G. (1983) Experimental craniosynostosis in growing rabbits – the role of the periosteum. Journal of Neurosurgery, 58, 101–108

11. Andersson, H. (1966) Craniosynostosis as a complication after operation for hydrocephalus. Acta Paediatrica Scandinavica, 55, 192–196

12. Fishman, M. A., Hogan, G. R., Dodge, P. R. (1971) The concurrence of hydrocephalus and craniosynostosis. Journal of Neurosurgery, 34, 621–629

13. Sainte-Rose, C., LaCombe, J., Pierre-Kahn, A., Renier, D., Hirsch, J. F. (1984) Intracranial venous hypertension: cause or consequence of hydrocephalus in infants. Journal of Neurosurgery, 60, 727–736

14. Renier, D., Sainte-Rose, C., Marchac, D., Hirsch, J. F. (1982) Intracranial pressure in craniostenosis. Journal of Neurosurgery, 57, 370–377

15. Tessier, P. (1967) Ostéotomies totales de la face syndrome de crouzon syndrome d'apert oxycéphalies. Scaphacéphalies. Turricéphalies. Annales de Chirurgie Plastique, 12, 273–286

16. Liversedge, R. (1979) Crush injuries of the face. British Journal of Hospital Medicine, 21, 120–136

17. Marchac, D., Renier, D. (1983) Craniofacial surgery for craniosynostosis. Little, Brown

18. Furuya, Y., Edwards, M. S., Alpers, C. E., Tress, B., Norman, D., Ousterhout, D. (1984) Computerized tomography of cranial sutures. Part 2: Abnormalities of sutures and skull deformity in craniosynostosis. Journal of Neurosurgery, 61, 59–70

19. Vollmer, D. G., Jane, J. A., Park, T. S., Persing, J. A. (1984) Variants of sagittal synostosis: strategies for surgical correction. Journal of Neurosurgery, 61, 557–562

20. Jane, J. A., Park, T. S., Zide, B. M., Lambruschi, P., Persing, J. A., Edgerton, M. J. (1984) Alternative techniques in the treatment of unilateral coronal synostosis. Journal of Neurosurgery, 61, 550–556

21. David, D. J. (1984) New perspectives in the management of severe cranio-facial deformity. Annals of the Royal College of Surgeons of England, 66, 270–279

22. Hoffman, H. J., Hendrick, E. B. (1979) Early neurosurgical repair in craniofacial dysmorphism. Journal of Neurosurgery, 51, 796–803

# Index